# Thyroid: A Growing Concern

# Thyroid: A Growing Concern

Edited by Dakota Marshall

hayle
medical

New York

Hayle Medical,
750 Third Avenue, 9th Floor,
New York, NY 10017, USA

Visit us on the World Wide Web at:
www.haylemedical.com



ISBN: 978-1-63241-599-8

The publisher's policy is to use permanent paper from mills that operate a sustainable forestry policy. Furthermore, the publisher ensures that the text paper and cover boards used have met acceptable environmental accreditation standards.



Printed in China.

**Cataloging-in-Publication Data**

Thyroid : a growing concern / edited by Dakota Marshall.
p. cm.
Includes bibliographical references and index.
ISBN 978-1-63241-599-8
1. Thyroid gland. 2. Thyroid gland--Diseases. I. Marshall, Dakota.
RC655 .T49 2019
612.44--dc23

# Table of Contents

# Preface

The thyroid gland is an endocrine gland in the neck, which secretes thyroid hormones. These are responsible for protein synthesis and maintenance of the metabolic rate of the body. The thyroid is susceptible to a number of diseases. The conditions of the thyroid gland can be classified into five types- hypothyroidism, hyperthyroidism, structural abnormalities, benign or cancerous tumors and abnormal thyroid function without clinical symptoms. The gland can develop several nodules. Thyroid nodules may either be hyperplasia or a thyroid neoplasm. Goitres can be uninodular or multinodular or can be diffuse. For the diagnosis of thyroid diseases, the examination of the thyroid gland is crucial. This includes the search for abnormal masses and assessment of thyroid size. Systemic signs such as hair loss, weight gain or loss, swelling of the calves and protrusion of the eyes are some symptomatic signs of an underlying thyroid condition. Hypothyroidism affects around 3-10% adults, with women and the elderly being the most affected. It is estimated that one-third of the world's population has low iodine levels in diet, resulting in high prevalence of goiter. Depending on the diagnosis, medication, surgery and radioiodine therapy may be used for the treatment of thyroid disease. This book explores all the important aspects of thyroid disease in the present day scenario. The various studies that are constantly contributing towards advancing the understanding of thyroid function and pathology are examined in detail. It is an essential guide for both academicians and those who wish to pursue the study of endocrine and metabolic disorders.

This book unites the global concepts and researches in an organized manner for a comprehensive understanding of the subject. It is a ripe text for all researchers, students, scientists or anyone else who is interested in acquiring a better knowledge of this dynamic field.

I extend my sincere thanks to the contributors for such eloquent research chapters. Finally, I thank my family for being a source of support and help.

**Editor**

# 1

# Advantages and disadvantages of 3D ultrasound of thyroid nodules including thin slice volume rendering

Rafal Zenon Slapa[1*], Wieslaw Stanislaw Jakubowski[1], Jadwiga Slowinska-Srzednicka[2], Kazimierz Tomasz Szopinski[1,3]

**Abstract**

**Background:** The purpose of this study was to assess the advantages and disadvantages of 3D gray-scale and power Doppler ultrasound, including thin slice volume rendering (TSVR), applied for evaluation of thyroid nodules.

**Methods:** The retrospective evaluation by two observers of volumes of 71 thyroid nodules (55 benign, 16 cancers) was performed using a new TSVR technique. Dedicated 4D ultrasound scanner with an automatic 6-12 MHz 4D probe was used. Statistical analysis was performed with Stata v. 8.2.

**Results:** Multiple logistic regression analysis demonstrated that independent risk factors of thyroid cancers identified by 3D ultrasound include: (a) ill-defined borders of the nodule on MPR presentation, (b) a lobulated shape of the nodule in the c-plane and (c) a density of central vessels in the nodule within the minimal or maximal ranges. Combination of features provided sensitivity 100% and specificity 60-69% for thyroid cancer. Calcification/microcalcification-like echogenic foci on 3D ultrasound proved not to be a risk factor of thyroid cancer.

Storage of the 3D data of the whole nodules enabled subsequent evaluation of new parameters and with new rendering algorithms.

**Conclusions:** Our results indicate that 3D ultrasound is a practical and reproducible method for the evaluation of thyroid nodules. 3D ultrasound stores volumes comprising the whole lesion or organ. Future detailed evaluations of the data are possible, looking for features that were not fully appreciated at the time of collection or applying new algorithms for volume rendering in order to gain important information. Three-dimensional ultrasound data could be included in thyroid cancer databases. Further multicenter large scale studies are warranted.

## Background

Thyroid incidentalomas are frequent and their prevalence when identified by high-resolution ultrasound is up to 67%, although most of these lesions are benign [1]. Despite the great deal of accumulated knowledge on the diagnosis and treatment of thyroid nodules, the management of thyroid carcinoma has yet to be optimized [2-6]. The recent development of three-dimensional (3D) imaging has greatly enhanced radiologic data acquisition, evaluation and storage. Ultrasound is the most useful modality for imaging thyroid nodules and it appears that 3D ultrasound could add a new dimension to thyroid cancer studies.

Three-dimensional ultrasound has been investigated for more than 20 years [7]. Due to recent developments in computer techniques and scanner technology, the acquisition of volumes with automatic three-dimensional (3D) probes has become less complicated and the quality of the images acquired by 3D ultrasound has improved to become comparable to conventional sonographic images.

There have been few reports on the examination of thyroid gland and thyroid nodule volumes by 3D ultrasound [8,9]. The presentation, size and vasculature of fetal thyroid goiter has also been evaluated with 3D ultrasound [10]. We have previously investigated the possibilities of evaluating thyroid nodules with

* Correspondence: r.slapa@acn.waw.pl
[1]Department of Diagnostic Imaging, Second Faculty of Medicine with the English Division and the Physiotherapy Division, Medical University of Warsaw, ul. Kondratowicza 8, 03-242 Warsaw, Poland
Full list of author information is available at the end of the article

gray-scale 3D ultrasound [11]. However, to the best of our knowledge, no previous report has described the characterization of thyroid nodules by combined gray-scale and power Doppler 3D ultrasound with evaluation of independent risk factors of thyroid cancer.

The aims of the present study were: (1) Evaluation of the feasibility and effectiveness of 3D ultrasound in differential diagnosis of thyroid nodules; (2) Description of classic and new features of thyroid nodules; (3) Identification of independent risk factors of thyroid cancer in 3D ultrasound data by multiple logistic regression analysis; (4) Analysis of feasibility of 3D ultrasound for application in thyroid cancer databases.

## Methods

The study was carried out in compliance with Helsinki Declaration. From years 2003-2005, 92 thyroid nodules in 82 patients referred for fine needle biopsy (FNB) were examined with 3D gray-scale and power Doppler sonography. Seventy-one thyroid nodules larger than 7 mm in 65 patients with established diagnosis (benign nodule or cancer) by FNB and/or pathology after surgery were evaluated retrospectively in 3D sonography volumes [Table 1]. The purpose and procedure was explained to the patients and their informed consent was obtained. Initially patients were prospectively evaluated using conventional sonography of the whole thyroid gland and the neck lymph nodes. In multinodular goiter, suspicious nodules were identified by the presence of any combination of the following criteria: dominant (the largest or enlarging) nodule, hypoechoic nodule, nodule with poorly defined borders, calcification/microcalcification-like echogenic foci (CAL), and increased central vasculature [12-15]. Thyroid nodules in patients with carcinoma established by FNB diagnosis before 3D sonography were also included in the study.

Final diagnoses were established by FNB and pathology after surgery for all 16 carcinomas (15 papillary cancers, 1 medullary cancer) and 12 benign nodules, and by multiple FNB and at least 2 years follow up for 43 benign nodules. FNB was guided by ultrasound imaging. The FNB diagnoses were organized into 4 categories - (1) inadequate material (unsatisfactory or nondiagnostic): smears with few or no follicular cells; (2) benign or negative: group including colloid nodule, Hashimoto's thyroiditis, cyst, thyroiditis; (3) suspicious or indeterminate: cytologic results that suggest a malignant lesion but do not completely fulfill the criteria for definitive diagnosis, including follicular neoplasms, Hürthle cell tumors and atypical papillary tumors; (4) malignant or positive: group consisting of primary thyroid cancers [16]. Nodules diagnosed with FNB a follicular neoplasm that were not subjected to surgery were excluded from the retrospective analysis.

**Table 1 General findings of 71 retrospectively analyzed thyroid nodules**

| | Benign nodule | Cancer |
|---|---|---|
| Number of nodules | 55 | 16 |
| Nodules in multinodular goiter | 45 | 14 |
| Solitary nodules | 10 | 2 |
| Women | 46 | 9 |
| Men | 4 | 6 |
| Age of patients (years) | 22-76 | 26-70 |

Three-dimensional ultrasound studies were performed using a dedicated 4D sonographic scanner (Voluson 730; GE Medical Systems, Kretz Ultrasound, Zipf, Austria) equipped with an automatic linear 6-12 MHz 4D probe. All volumes were registered on a magneto-optical disk. The images were transferred to a personal computer and evaluated with 3D VIEW 2000 software (GE Medical Systems, Kretz Ultrasound, Zipf, Austria), which provides the same viewing interface as the scanner.

Gray-scale and power Doppler volumes were acquired. Power Doppler studies were performed with pulse repetition frequency (PRF) and color gain set just above the noise level (PRF = 0.9 kHz) and with the wall motion filter set to "low" to optimize for slow flow detection. Two radiologists blinded to the results of the FNB and pathology examinations independently reviewed the images.

Contiguous slices, from one border to the opposite border of the nodule were evaluated interactively from gray-scale volumes. The nodule shape in the plane parallel to the ultrasound probe surface (c-plane), echogenicity, margins of the nodule and presence of calcification/microcalcification-like echogenic foci (CAL) in the plane of the array of probe crystals (a-plane), were evaluated in multiplanar reformation (MPR) mode and with our original method of thin-slice volume rendering using a smooth surface algorithm [11].

In the evaluation of vessels on rendered 3D power Doppler volumes of whole nodules, the peripheral and central vessels overlapped and classification of the vascularization was difficult, especially in cases where it was abundant [Figure 1, Additional file 1]. Thus, we applied original thin-slice volume rendering of color data alone, employing the 100% color max algorithm [Figure 2, 3, Additional file 2]. The thickness of the slice was approximately 15-25% of the maximal nodule diameter. To define the location of nodule borders on a volume-rendered image, it was displayed on the same screen as the MPR presentation of gray-scale with color. The vessels were evaluated interactively with 360° rotation of the volume around the central axis of the nodule

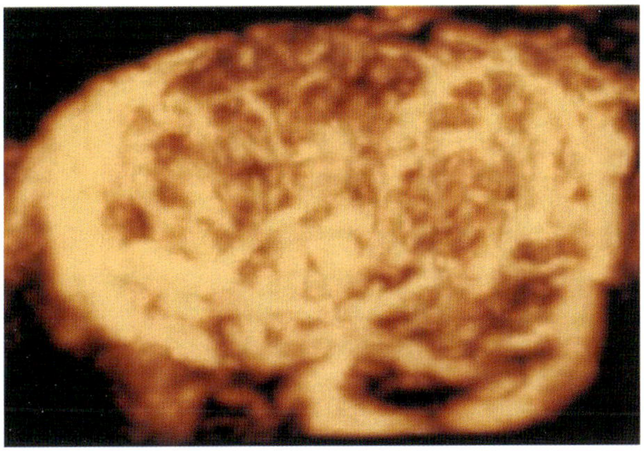

**Figure 1 Three-dimensional power Doppler ultrasound of Hürthle cell adenoma: presentation of the whole nodule**. On the 3D rendered image of the whole nodule the peripheral and central vessels overlap making the evaluation of the abundant vascularization difficult. (See also: Additional file 1).

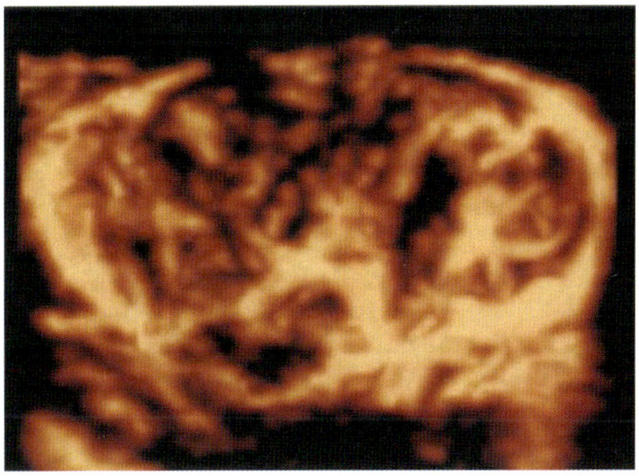

**Figure 3 Three-dimensional power Doppler ultrasound of Hürthle cell adenoma: presentation with thin-slice rendering method (the nodule from figure 1)**. Thin-slice rendering permits evaluation of the central and peripheral vessels (See also: Additional file 2).

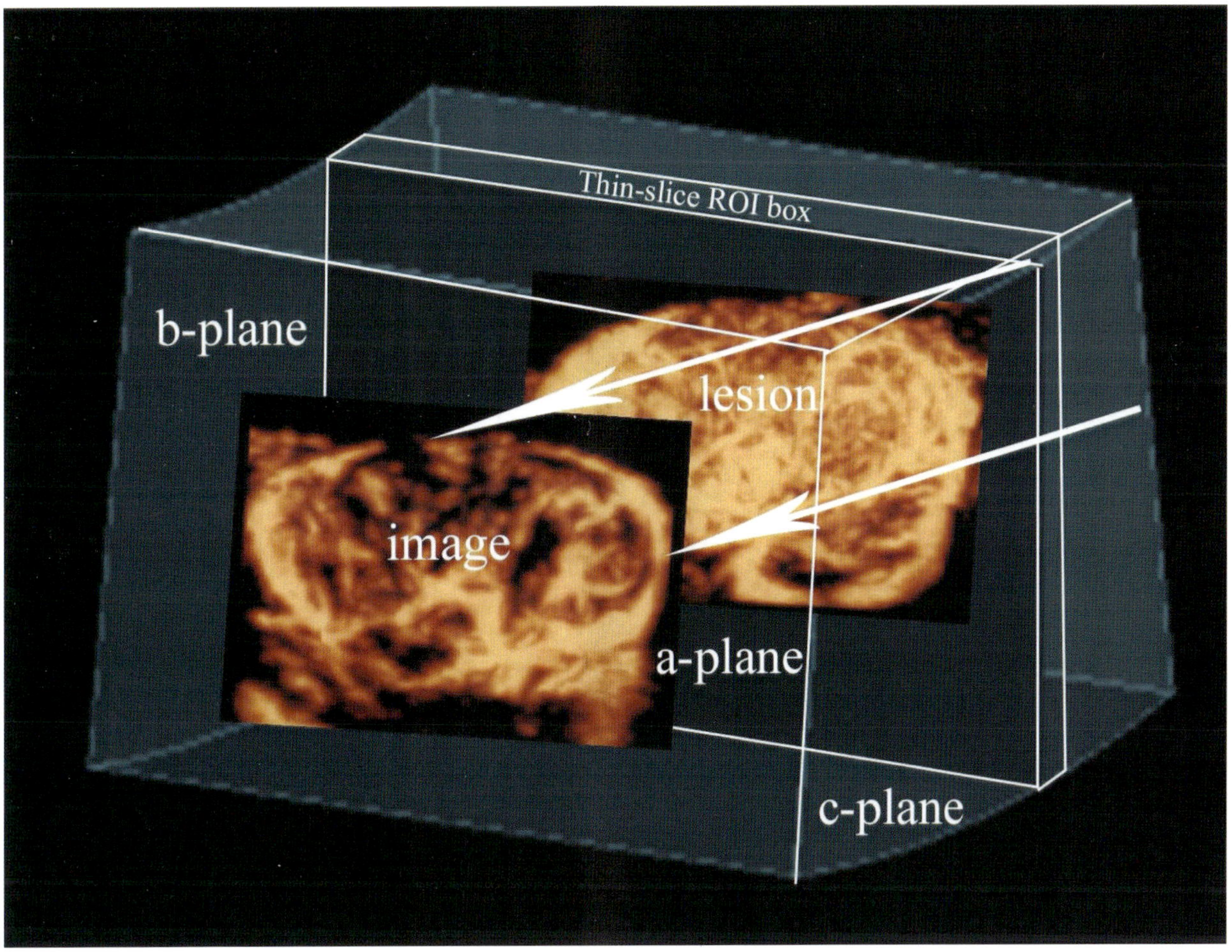


**Figure 2 Schematic presentation of the 3D sonographic method: thin-slice volume rendering of vessels visualized with power Doppler**. The Color max algorithm is applied to the thin-slice region of interest (ROI) box, with the resultant 2D image of the vessels in the a-plane.

joining the anterior and posterior surfaces of the thyroid gland. The pattern of nodule vascularization, central vessel alignment, maximal extent of the peripheral vessel component and maximal area of the central vessel component were evaluated.

Statistical analysis was performed with Stata v. 8.2 (Stata Statistical Software: Release 8.2, Stata Corporation, College Station, TX, USA). The agreement between the observers and the gray-scale techniques (MPR and thin-slice rendering) was evaluated with $\kappa$ statistics using the scale of Landis and Koch: $\kappa < 0$ denotes poor reproducibility, 0-0.20 slight, 0.21-0.40 fair, 0.41-0.60 moderate, 0.61-0.80 substantial, and 0.81-1.00 almost perfect reproducibility [17]. For evaluation of the independent risk factors of thyroid cancer identified by 3D ultrasound, multiple logistic regression analysis was applied. To assess the echogenicity of thyroid nodules, the Fisher exact test was applied. The significance threshold was set at 0.05.

## Results

### Gray-scale 3D ultrasound

A summary of features of nodules examined with 3D gray-scale ultrasound is presented in Table 2. The Fisher exact test indicated that the percentage of cancers is significantly higher in the group of hypoechoic and mixed echogenicity nodules ($p = 0.015$). The feature of ill-defined nodule borders was 63-69% sensitive and 82-85% specific in the case of thyroid cancer. The sensitivity and specificity of CAL in MPR presentation were respectively, 81-88% and 38-44%, and with thin-slice rendering, 88-94% and 22-25%. In the case of one cancer, thin-slice rendering revealed CAL that was not observed in MPR presentation. Analysis of the shape of the nodule in the c-plane was possible in 44-54% of cases in MPR presentation and in 100% of cases with thin-slice rendering. The analysis in the c-plane was therefore performed using thin-slice rendered images. A lobulated shape was 94-100% sensitive and 47-58% specific for thyroid cancer. The level of agreement between observers and between techniques is presented in Tables 3 and 4.

### Analysis of vascularization of thyroid nodules in 3D power Doppler ultrasound

Analysis of vascularization of benign thyroid nodules and thyroid cancers by thin-slice rendering of 3D power Doppler ultrasound is presented in Table 5. Agreement

**Table 2 Features of benign thyroid nodules and thyroid cancer in 3D gray-scale ultrasound [echogenicity, borders, calcification/microcalcification-like echogenic foci (CAL), shape in c-plane (parallel to ultrasound probe)] in multiplanar reformation mode (MPR) and by thin-slice rendering with surface algorithm (Surf)**

| | | BENIGN *Observer 1* | BENIGN *Observer 2* | CANCER *Observer 1* | CANCER *Observer 2* |
|---|---|---|---|---|---|
| *ECHOGENICITY:* | | | | | |
| **Hypoechoic** | **MPR** | 20 | 22 | 12 | 11 |
| | **Surf** | 20 | 21 | 11 | 12 |
| **Mixed** | **MPR** | 17 | 17 | 4 | 5 |
| | **Surf** | 22 | 20 | 5 | 4 |
| **Isoechoic** | **MPR** | 17 | 15 | | |
| | **Surf** | 12 | 13 | | |
| **Hyperechoic** | **MPR** | 1 | 1 | | |
| | **Surf** | 1 | 1 | | |
| *BORDERS:* | | | | | |
| **Ill-defined** | **MPR** | 8 | 10 | 10 | 11 |
| | **Surf** | 5 | 10 | 8 | 9 |
| **Well-defined** | **MPR** | 47 | 45 | 6 | 5 |
| | **Surf** | 50 | 45 | 8 | 7 |
| *CALCIFICATION/MICROCALCIFICATION-LIKE ECHOGENIC FOCI* | | | | | |
| **Present** | **MPR** | 31 | 34 | 14 | 13 |
| | **Surf** | 43 | 41 | 15 | 14 |
| **Absent** | **MPR** | 24 | 21 | 2 | 3 |
| | **Surf** | 12 | 14 | 1 | 2 |
| *SHAPE IN C-PLANE* | | | | | |
| **Lobulated** | **Surf** | 23 | 29 | 16 | 15 |
| **Oval** | **Surf** | 32 | 26 | 0 | 1 |

(mixed) echogenicity - hypo- and isoechogenic.

**Table 3 Observer agreement ($\kappa$ statistics) over the evaluation of features of thyroid nodules in multiplanar reformation mode (MPR) and by thin-slice rendering with surface algorithm (Surf)**

| | | $\kappa$ | p |
|---|---|---|---|
| Echogenicity | MPR | 0.70 | < 0.0001 |
| Echogenicity | Surf | 0.71 | < 0.0001 |
| Borders | MPR | 0.82 | < 0.0001 |
| Borders | Surf | 0.60 | < 0.0001 |
| CAL | MPR | 0.57 | < 0.0001 |
| CAL | Surf | 0.44 | = 0.0002 |
| Shape in c-plane | Surf | 0.57 | < 0.0001 |

calcification/microcalcification-like echogenic foci (CAL); c-plane - plane parallel to ultrasound probe.

between observers in the evaluation of vascularization of thyroid nodules is presented in Table 6.

The pattern of vascularization of benign nodules was predominantly peripheral/central (seen in 85% of nodules), followed by a peripheral pattern (seen in 7-15% of nodules). No vessels were visible in 4-7% of nodules. Cancers presented predominantly peripheral/central vascularization (seen in 75% of cancers), followed by a central pattern (seen in 12.5% of cancers). No vessels were visible in 12.5% of cancers.

The regularity of central vessel alignment could not be evaluated in 50-56% of cancers.

A density of central vessels in ranges 1 and 4 [Figure 4, 5], correlated with an increased probability of cancer, described in logistic regression analysis (discussed below); this feature was 75-81% sensitive and 49-56% specific for a diagnosis of thyroid cancer.

### Multiple logistic regression analysis of 3D ultrasound of thyroid nodules

Multiple logistic regression analysis was applied for differential diagnosis of thyroid nodules [Table 7].

The analysis revealed 3 statistically significant independent risk factors of thyroid cancer in 3D ultrasound data: ill-defined nodule borders on the a-plane in MPR mode; lobulated shape of the nodule in the c-plane on thin-slice rendering; and maximal area of the central vessel component within ranges 1 (1-25%) or 4 (76-100%). Our model of multiple logistic regression analysis proved to be highly predictive (area under ROC curve = 0.87) [Figure 6].

**Table 4 The agreement ($\kappa$ statistics) between features of thyroid nodules evaluated in multiplanar reformation mode and by thin-slice rendering with surface algorithm**

| | OBSERVER 1 | | OBSERVER 2 | |
|---|---|---|---|---|
| | $\kappa$ | p | $\kappa$ | p |
| Echogenicity | 0.85 | < 0.0001 | 0.91 | < 0.0001 |
| Borders | 0.80 | < 0.0001 | 0.93 | < 0.0001 |
| CAL | 0.56 | < 0.0001 | 0.73 | < 0.0001 |

calcification/microcalcification-like echogenic foci (CAL).

To optimize the detection of thyroid cancers, the sensitivity and specificity for combinations of parameters for hypoechoic or mixed echogenicity nodules displaying at least one risk factor were calculated. The best combination was for ill-defined borders in MPR mode or lobulated shape in the c-plane - sensitivity 100% and specificity 60-69%; the application of these criteria for referral to FNB would had decreased the number of biopsies from 71 to 38 without missing a malignant nodule.

## Discussion

The designation of thyroid nodules for FNB is especially important in multinodular goiter. This condition is often diagnosed by ultrasound examination, especially in the elderly and in people living in iodine-deficient areas. However, multinodular goiter can no longer be regarded as an indicator of benignity of thyroid nodules. Multiple studies have found a similar incidence of cancer in patients with a multinodular goiter and in those with a solitary nodule. In Poland over 50% of differentiated thyroid cancers are diagnosed in patients with multinodular goiter. In our study subjects, 14 of 16 cancers were localized in multinodular goiters. It is often impossible to subject all nodules in a multinodular goiter to FNB and this is why it is so important to use ultrasound examination to identify the nodules with suspicious features that require FNB [2,3,18-20].

So far, a few risk factors of thyroid cancer have been identified in studies using ultrasound. However, no single ultrasound feature has been identified that is 100% sensitive and specific for thyroid cancer. To increase the sensitivity and specificity, the use of combinations of different features has been proposed [21].

Gray-scale 3D ultrasound has recently been applied to the investigation of thyroid nodules [11]. The general advantages of three-dimensional ultrasound include following ones:

- Separation in time of image aquisition and analysis,
- Saving of examination room time,
- Less time on scanning - less injury problems,
- Diversyfication of sonographers work (scanning, reconstruction),
- Less operator dependent,
- Increase of confidence in diagnosis,
- Possibility of remote consultation,
- Precise evaluation of lesion diameters and volumes,
- Additional, unlimited planes of visualization,

**Table 5 Analysis of vascularization of benign thyroid nodules and thyroid cancers in 3D power Doppler ultrasound evaluated with thin-slice rendering**

| | | BENIGN *Observer 1* | BENIGN *Observer 2* | CANCER *Observer 1* | CANCER *Observer 2* |
|---|---|---|---|---|---|
| | *PERIPHERAL VESSELS % of the circumference of the nodule* | | | | |
| **0** | **0 - 10** | 4 | 2 | 4 | 4 |
| **1** | **11-25** | 4 | 5 | 1 | 1 |
| **2** | **26-50** | 10 | 10 | 4 | 4 |
| **3** | **51-75** | 7 | 10 | 4 | 3 |
| **4** | **76-100** | 30 | 28 | 3 | 4 |
| | *CENTRAL VESSELS % of the area of the nodule* | | | | |
| **0** | **0** | 8 | 10 | 2 | 2 |
| **1** | **1-25** | 13 | 12 | 8 | 9 |
| **2** | **26-50** | 8 | 7 | 1 | 0 |
| **3** | **51-75** | 13 | 10 | 2 | 1 |
| **4** | **76-100** | 13 | 16 | 3 | 4 |
| | *ALIGNMENT OF CENTRAL VESSELS:* | | | | |
| **Regular** | | 38 | 35 | 5 | 6 |
| **Chaotic** | | 5 | 5 | 3 | 1 |
| **Not possible to define** | | 12 | 15 | 8 | 9 |

- ≫ Unlimited combinations of rendering algorithms - new information,
- ≫ Presentation of data similar to CT or MR (TUI),
- ≫ Convenient presentation for clinician and for teaching,
- ≫ Possibility of inclusion in patients data bases with future evaluation of new features or even with new rendering algorithms.

The present study describes thyroid cancer risk factors based on gray-scale and power Doppler 3D ultrasound. Three-dimensional ultrasound permits the evaluation of tissues by the application of different rendering algorithms in countless combinations. For the evaluation of volume data, we applied the original thin-slice method. Each gray-scale ultrasound volume was evaluated with a surface algorithm that enabled reduction of noise and speckles, and improved contrast. These features improved visualization of the lesions on images parallel to the ultrasound probe and were also more sensitive for high echoes of the calcification/microcalcification type. Due to characteristics of the software applied, the thickness of the evaluated slices was approximately 15-25% of the maximal diameter of the lesion. A new software tool called static Volume Contrast Imaging (VCI) (applied to some archived volumes in our study) enables the evaluation of the lesion with different combinations of rendering algorithms (including surface) with a fixed thin-slice thickness of as little as 2 mm [Figure 7]. In addition, a new option called Tomographic Ultrasound Imaging (TUI) allows the presentation of a series of slices (e.g. covering the whole lesion) in a similar way to magnetic resonance or computed tomography data [Figure 8]. Both VCI and TUI should greatly enhance and accelerate the evaluation of features of thyroid nodules with the thin-slice method.

**Table 6 Observer agreement ($\kappa$ statistics) over the evaluation of vascularization of thyroid nodules by 3D power Doppler ultrasound with thin-slice rendering**

| | $\kappa$ | P |
|---|---|---|
| Extent of peripheral vessels | 0.93 | < 0.0001 |
| Area of central vessels | 0.95 | < 0.0001 |
| Alignment of central vessels | 0.72 | < 0.0001 |

In published 2D color or power Doppler studies of thyroid cancers, increased central vascularization with irregular alignment was found. However, the criteria used to evaluate central vascularization were not uniform, so it is difficult to compare the data [4,12,13,15].

The vascular net of the nodule may be visualized with 3D power Doppler ultrasound. However, due to the overlaying of peripheral and central vessels when the whole lesion was included in rendering (particularly confusing in highly vascularized nodules), we applied the original thin-slice method for the evaluation of vascularization. This permits the visualization of longer fragments of vessels rather than the cross-sections that may be seen with conventional power Doppler ultrasound. However, in at least half of thyroid cancers, the

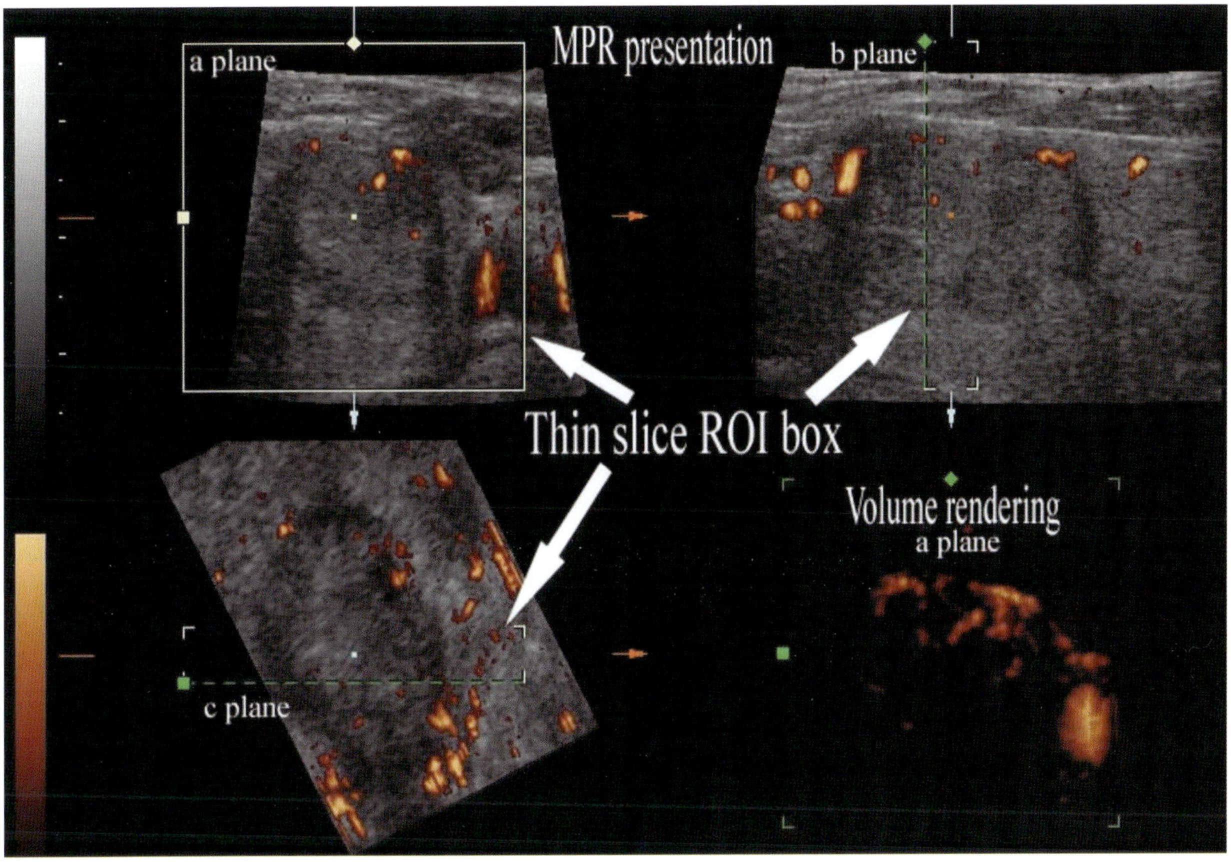


**Figure 4 Three-dimensional power Doppler ultrasound of papillary cancer with low density of vessels**. Multiplanar reformation (MPR) mode presentation and thin-slice volume rendering (lower right corner). The maximal density of the vessels was evaluated on the volume-rendered image (in the a-plane). The borders of the cancer on the a-plane image in MPR were correlated with the distribution of vessels on the volume-rendered image. The density of the vessels is in the lowest range: 1 = (1-25%) of area of the nodule; ROI - region of interest.

thin-slice method did not allow evaluation of the regularity of the central vessels; in most of these nodules, this could be related to the lowest density of central vessels and in some cases, to the highest density of central vessels.

In many nodules, central vascularization is not homogenous and the choice of the plane for evaluation and documentation in 2D ultrasound examination depends on the operator. In evaluations based on archived images from earlier 2D examination, alternative sections are not always available for inspection. In our study using 3D power Doppler ultrasound, the vessels of the whole nodule were evaluated during a 360° rotation of the volume around the antero-posterior axis and the section used to describe the vascularization was chosen by the radiologist. To increase the objectivity of the evaluation, a five point score describing the visually estimated percentage of the area of the nodule covered by central vessels was applied. To correlate the present study with previously published 2D studies that identified increased central vascularization in cancers, the image with maximal density of vessels was chosen for the rating. Central vessel densities in the lowest range (1-25% of nodule area) were found in over half of the cancers, despite optimization of power Doppler acquisition for slow flow and evaluation of vessels in slices with a thickness of 15-25% of the maximal diameter of the nodule. Thus, in contrast to many previous reports, poor central vascularization was frequently observed in thyroid cancers in this study. It is noteworthy that our material included many small cancers that may be hypovascular because of their high fibrous component [4,22].

There is usually some degree of observer variation in both the clinical evaluation and interpretation of imaging studies of thyroid disorders, and this must always be taken into account in decision-making. In previous 2D ultrasound examinations of thyroid nodules, poor reproducibility was reported in the evaluation of echogenicity, borders and volume; while good reproducibility was found in the evaluation of presence of calcifications, central vessels or cystic components [23-26]. However 3D ultrasound in the present study proved to deliver

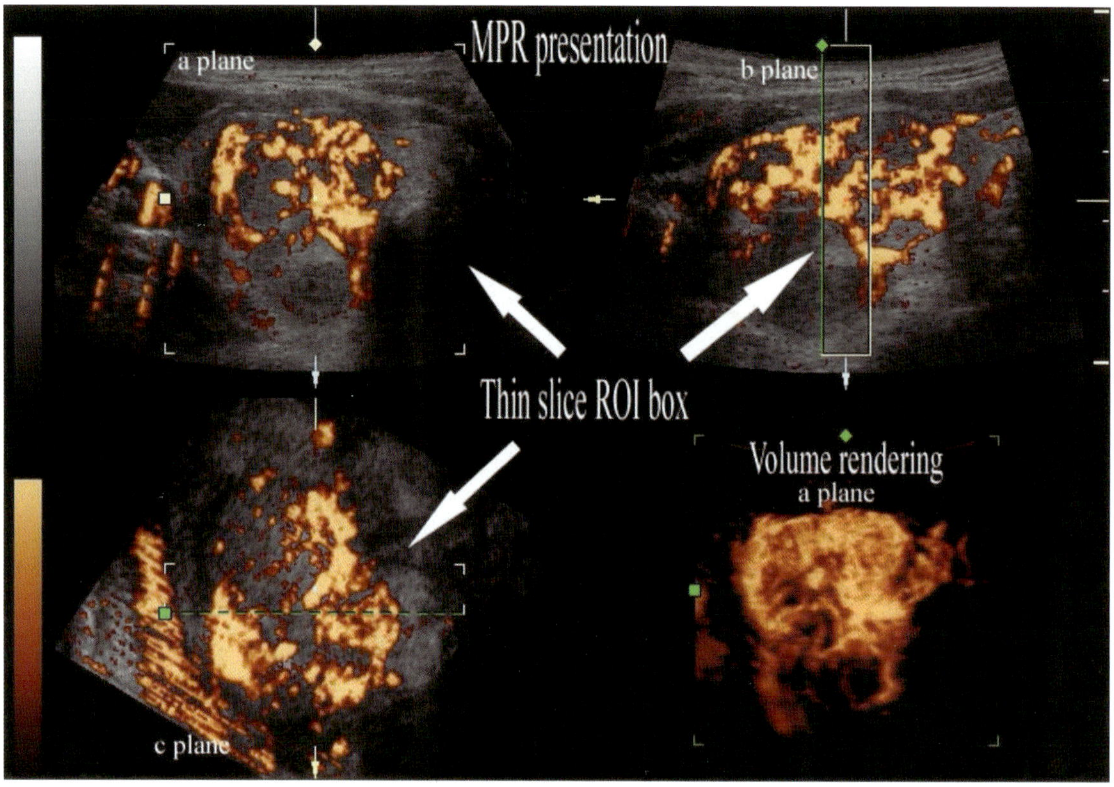


**Figure 5 Three-dimensional power Doppler ultrasound of papillary cancer with high density of vessels.** Multiplanar reformation (MPR) mode presentation and thin-slice volume rendering (lower right corner). The density of the vessels is in the highest range: 4 = (76-100%) of area of the nodule; ROI - region of interest.

overall good interobserver reproducibility in evaluation of thyroid nodule features. The poorest agreement on evaluation of gray-scale features on 3D ultrasound was at least moderate ($\kappa \geq 0.41$). Least agreement between observers and between techniques occurred in the evaluation of CAL.

The evaluation of 3D power Doppler ultrasound proved to deliver even better interobserver reproducibility. The $\kappa$ statistics for evaluation of vascularization revealed at least substantial agreement between observers ($\kappa \geq 0.61$).

The differences in reproducibility of certain features of nodules between previous 2D studies [25] and 3D ultrasound may be partly due to peculiarities of evaluation

**Table 7 Evaluation of 3D ultrasound features of thyroid cancer with multiple logistic regression analysis.**

| | OR | P |
|---|---|---|
| Ill-defined borders (a-plane, MPR mode) | 8.3 | 0.005 |
| Ill-defined borders (a-plane, thin-slice rendering) | | > 0.1 |
| Presence of calcification/microcalcification-like echogenic foci | | > 0.1 |
| Lobulated shape (c-plane, thin-slice rendering) | 10 | 0.044 |
| Extent of peripheral vessels | | > 0.1 |
| Central vessels: (1-25%) or (76-100%) of the area of the nodule | 7.3 | 0.016 |
| Alignment of central vessels | | > 0.1 |

odds ratio (OR); a-plane - plane of the array of probe crystals; c-plane - plane parallel to ultrasound probe surface; multiplanar reformation mode (MPR); thin-slice rendering with surface algorithm.

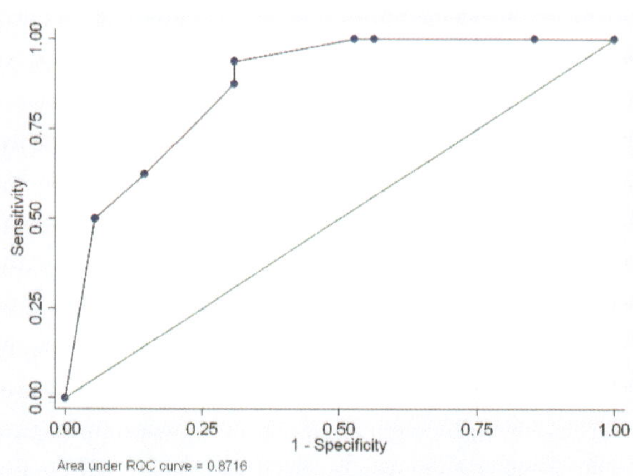


**Figure 6 The receiver operating characteristic (ROC) curve for multiple logistic regression analysis of 3D ultrasound features of thyroid cancers.** The model is highly predictive (area under ROC curve = 0.87).

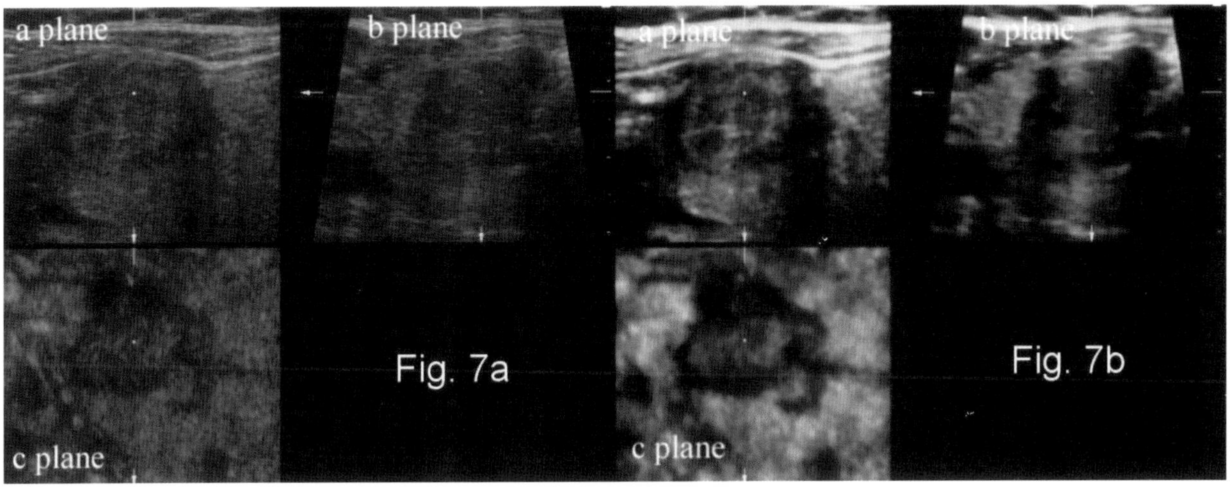


**Figure 7 Multiplanar reformation (MPR) presentation of three-dimensional gray-scale ultrasound of papillary thyroid cancer without and with static volume imaging mode**. (a) classic MPR presentation; (b) MPR presentation of the lesion with a new 3D postprocessing technique - static volume contrast imaging (VCI). Thin-slice volumes of 2 mm thickness with the surface rendering algorithm increases the contrast and reduces the noise on the resultant images.

using the two techniques. With conventional ultrasound, often selected images of the nodule are evaluated retrospectively, whereas with 3D ultrasound, continuous images through the whole nodule are evaluated interactively.

We applied multiple logistic regression analysis to assess the risk factors of thyroid carcinoma identified by 3D ultrasound. Numerous features of thyroid nodules were investigated by gray-scale and power Doppler ultrasound. Our study revealed 3 independent risk factors of thyroid cancer:

✓ ill-defined nodule borders on MPR (sensitivity 63-69% and specificity 82-85%) - a feature known from 2D ultrasound studies,
✓ lobulated shape of the nodule in the plane parallel to the ultrasound probe (sensitivity 94-100% and specificity 47-58%) - a new feature specific to 3D ultrasound,

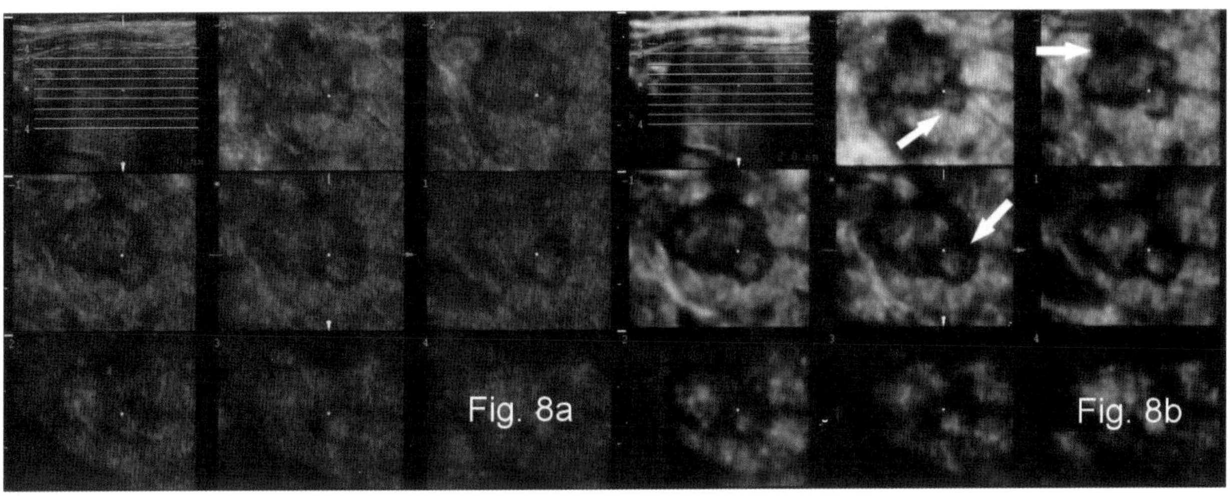


**Figure 8 Presentation of three-dimensional gray-scale ultrasound of papillary thyroid cancer with a new 3D postprocessing technique - tomographic ultrasound imaging (TUI)**. (a) a set of sequential slices 2 mm apart in the c-plane (plane parallel to the surface of the ultrasound probe) covering the whole nodule and localizer in the axial plane (upper left corner); (b) TUI of the whole nodule with static volume contrast imaging (VCI) - a set of c-plane images as a result of rendering of sequential thin slice volumes (2 mm thickness) with the surface algorithm and axial localizer (upper left corner). On coronal images the lobulations of the carcinoma (arrows) are more readily distinguished than in Fig. 8(a) due to improved contrast and reduced noise.

✓ density of central vascularization within the lowest or highest ranges (sensitivity 75-81% and specificity 49-56%) - the high percentage of cancers with a vessel density within the lowest range is a novel finding.

Ill-defined borders are an established risk factor of thyroid cancer. Moreover, ill-defined borders are a feature of aggressive behavior in papillary microcancer of the thyroid [12,27-29], which highlights the importance of investigating nodules presenting with an ill-defined border.

We analyzed the shape of thyroid nodules in the plane parallel to the ultrasound probe. A lobulated shape proved to be an independent predictor of thyroid cancer. In previous studies using conventional ultrasound, a lobulated shape was described as a feature of nodule borders. However, due to our combined observation of micro- and macrolobulated appearance, we established that this feature describes nodule shape. The disorganized tumor growth that produces the lobulated shape may be related to optimization of the supply of nutrients in an environment containing a heterogenous net of thyroid vessels [30]. The more frequent appearance of lobulated cancers in the plane parallel to the ultrasound probe (c-plane), in contrast to findings in 2D ultrasound studies [27,29], may be attributed to the arrangement of vessels in the thyroid gland and differences in the analysis of conventional ultrasound images compared to the analysis of 3D ultrasound volumes. Moreover, the plane parallel to ultrasound probe - the coronal plane in the case of thyroid examination - is characterized by the largest surface and provides the most space in the gland for the propagation of side lobes resulting in a lobulated shape.

There have been attempts to join individual volumes to obtain a volume encompassing the whole thyroid. Such an approach would enable physicians to fully archive the anatomy and pathology and to compare them during a follow-up [31].

Maybe in the future construction of three-dimensional probes with wider field of view (automatic 3D probes with wider footprint together with application of trapezoid field of view) would facilitate the acquisition of the volume covering the whole lobe or even the whole thyroid.

Even the new generation of elastography, called supersonic shear wave elastography [32,33] has already been equipped with three dimensional imaging capabilities at the end of year 2010. As in the real world, biological objects are three-dimensional, their three-dimensional analysis seems to be the most precise and desirable one.

According to Mitchell et al. an optimal management strategy for thyroid incidentalomas could be developed using an evidence-based approach in which systematic evaluation of obtained data is used. All physicians involved in the care of those with thyroid disease (radiologists, along with endocrinologists and surgeons) should be encouraged to submit data to national databases and participate in properly randomized studies to address the optimal management strategy in the treatment of incidentally detected thyroid nodules [34]. As high-resolution ultrasound is the most useful modality for imaging thyroid nodules, the databases should contain the most complete ultrasound documentation. Our study indicates that, the most appropriate technique for this purpose appears to be 3D ultrasound as it stores volumes describing the whole lesion or organ. Future detailed evaluations of the data are possible, looking for features that were not fully appreciated at the time of collection or applying new algorithms for volume rendering in order to glean important information.

## Conclusions

(1) Three-dimensional ultrasound is a practical and reproducible method for the evaluation of thyroid nodules. It enables precise, sonographic, volumetric evaluation of morphology of thyroid lesions as: echogenicity and shape of the lesion, its borders, calcification/microcalcification-like echogenic foci and vascularization;

(2) Three-dimensional ultrasound stores volumes comprising the whole lesion or organ. Future detailed evaluations of the data are possible, looking for features that were not fully appreciated at the time of collection or applying new algorithms for volume rendering in order to gain important information.

(3) Three-dimensional ultrasound data could be included in thyroid cancer databases.

(4) Further multicenter large scale studies are warranted.

**Acknowledgements**

This study was supported by the KBN (Research Council of Polish Government) grant 3 P05B 100 23 over the period 2002-2005.
This publication was financially supported by the Ministry of Science and Higher Education of Poland - the grant of the Polish Thyroid Association.
Parts of this publication are excerpts from R.Z. Slapa theses for associate professor degree in Medical University of Warsaw (2009), entitled: "Application of three-dimensional ultrasound in diagnostics of focal thyroid lesions" and published in Polish language, Medical University of Warsaw, Warsaw 2007.
We thank John Gittins PhD (Great Britain) for editing and proofreading the manuscript.

**Author details**

[1]Department of Diagnostic Imaging, Second Faculty of Medicine with the English Division and the Physiotherapy Division, Medical University of Warsaw, ul. Kondratowicza 8, 03-242 Warsaw, Poland. [2]Department of Endocrinology, Centre for Postgraduate Medical Education, Warsaw, Poland. [3]Interdisciplinary Centre for Mathematical and Computational Modelling, Warsaw University, Warsaw, Poland.

**Authors' contributions**

RZS conceived, designed, coordinated and evaluated the study, carried out the ultrasound examinations and wrote the manuscript, WSJ participated in design, coordination and evaluation of the study, JSS governed clinical part of the study: patient selection, evaluation, consultations and establishment of final diagnosis, KTS participated in the design and evaluation of the study. All authors have read and approved the final manuscript.

**Competing interests**

The authors declare that they have no competing interests.

**References**


1. Tan GH, Gharib H: Thyroid incidentalomas: management approaches to nonpalpable nodules discovered incidentally on thyroid imaging. *Ann Intern Med* 1997, **126**:226-231.
2. Hegedus L, Bonnema SJ, Bennedbaek FN: Management of simple nodular goiter: current status and future perspectives. *Endocr Rev* 2003, **24**:102-132.
3. Cooper DS, Doherty GM, Haugen BR, Kloos RT, Lee SL, Mandel SJ, Mazzaferri EL, McIver B, Sherman SI, Tuttle RM: American Thyroid Association Guidelines Taskforce. Management guidelines for patients with thyroid nodules and differentiated thyroid cancer. *Thyroid* 2006, **16**:109-142.
4. AACE/AME task force on thyroid nodules: American association of clinical endocrinologists and associacione medici endocrinologi medical guidelines for clinical practice for the diagnosis and management of thyroid nodules. *Endocr Pract* 2006, **12(1)**:63-102.
5. Pacini F, Schlumberger M, Dralle H, Elisei R, Smit JW, Wiersinga W, European Thyroid Cancer Taskforce: European consensus for the management of patients with differentiated thyroid carcinoma of the follicular epithelium. *Eur J Endocrinol* 2006, **154**:787-803.
6. Rosen JE, Stone MD: Contemporary diagnostic approach to the thyroid nodule. *J Surg Oncol* 2006, **94**:649-661.
7. Rankin RN, Fenster A, Downey DB, Munk PL, Levin MF, Vellet AD: Three-dimensional sonographic reconstruction: techniques and diagnostic applications. *Am J Roentgenol* 1993, **161(4)**:695-702.
8. Schlogl S, Werner E, Lassmann M, Terekhova J, Muffert S, Seybold S, Reiners C: The use of three-dimensional ultrasound for thyroid volumetry. *Thyroid* 2001, **11**:569-574.
9. Lyshchik A, Drozd V, Schloegl S, Reiners C: Three-Dimensional ultrasonography for volume measurement of thyroid nodules in children. *J Ultrasound Med* 2004, **23**:247-254.
10. Nath CA, Oyelese Y, Yeo L, Chavez M, Kontopoulos EV, Giannina G, Smulian JC, Vintzileos AM: Three-dimensional sonography in the evaluation and management of fetal goiter. *Ultrasound Obstet Gynecol* 2005, **25**:312-314.
11. Slapa RZ, Slowinska-Srzednicka J, Szopinski K, Jakubowski W: Gray-scale three-dimensional sonography of thyroid nodules: feasibility of the method and preliminary studies. *Eur Radiol* 2006, **16**:428-436.
12. Papini E, Guglielmi R, Bianchini A, Crescenzi A, Taccogna S, Nardi F, Panunzi C, Rinaldi R, Toscano V, Pacella CM: Risk of malignancy in nonpalpable thyroid nodules: predictive value of ultrasound and color-Doppler features. *J Clin Endocrinol Metab* 2002, **87**:1941-1946.
13. Chan BK, Desser TS, McDougall IR, Weigel RJ, Jeffrey RB Jr: Common and uncommon sonographic features of papillary thyroid carcinoma. *J Ultrasound Med* 2003, **22**:1083-1090.
14. Kim E-K, Park CS, Chung WY, Oh KK, Kim DI, Lee JT, Yoo HS: New sonographic criteria for recommending fine-needle aspiration biopsy of nonpalpable solid nodules of the thyroid. *AJR* 2002, **178**:687-691.
15. Frates MC, Benson CB, Doubilet PM, Cibas ES, Marqusee E: Can color Doppler sonography aid in the prediction of malignancy of thyroid nodules. *J Ultrasound Med* 2003, **22**:127-131.
16. Gharib H, Papini E, Valcavi R, Baskin HJ, Crescenzi A, Dottorini ME, Duick DS, Guglielmi R, Hamilton CR Jr, Zeiger MA, Zini M, AACE/AME Task Force on Thyroid Nodules: American Association of Clinical Endocrinologists and Associazione Medici Endocrinologi medical guidelines for clinical practice for diagnosis and management of thyroid nodules. *Endocr Pract* 2006, **12**:63-102.
17. Landis JR, Koch GG: An application of hierarchical kappa-type statistics in the assessment of majority agreement among multiple observers. *Biometrics* 1977, **33**:363-374.
18. Gandolfi PP, Frisina A, Raffa M, Renda F, Rocchetti O, Ruggeri C, Tombolini A: The incidence of thyroid carcinoma in multinodular goiter: retrospective analysis. *Acta Biomed* 2004, **75**:114-117.
19. Frates MC, Benson CB, Doubilet PM, Kunreuther E, Contreras M, Cibas ES, Orcutt J, Moore FD Jr, Larsen PR, Marqusee E, Alexander EK: Prevalence and distribution of carcinoma in patients with solitary and multiple thyroid nodules on sonography. *J Clin Endocrinol Metab* 2006, **91**:3411-3417.
20. Nauman J: Preface to Polish edition. Schilddrüsen-Sonographie.Edited by: Klima G. Urban 1997:.
21. Butros R, Boyvat F, Ozyer U, Bilezikci B, Arat Z, Aytekin C, Guvener N, Demirhan B: Management of infracentimetric thyroid nodules with respect to ultrasonographic features. *Eur Radiol* 2007, **17**:1358-1364.
22. Pacella CM, Guglielmi R, Fabbrini R, Bianchini A, Rinaldi R, Panunzi C, Pacella S, Crescenzi A, Papini E: Papillary carcinoma in small hypoechoic thyroid nodules: predictive value of echo color Doppler evaluation. *Preliminary results J Exp Clin Cancer Res* 1998, **17(1)**:127-128.
23. Jarlov AE: Observer variation in the diagnosis of thyroid disorders. Criteria for and impact on diagnostic decision-making. *Dan Med Bull* 2000, **47(5)**:328-339.
24. Gallo M, Pesenti M, Valcavi R: Ultrasound thyroid nodule measurements: the "gold standard" and its limitations in clinical decision making. *Endocrine Practice* 2003, **9**:194-199.
25. Wienke JR, Chong WK, Fielding JR, Zou KH, Mittelstaedt CA: Sonographic features of benign thyroid nodules: interobserver reliability and overlap with malignancy. *J Ultrasound Med* 2003, **22**:1027-1031.
26. Brauer VFH, Eder P, Miehle K, Wiesner TD, Hasenclever H, Paschke R: Interobserver variation for ultrasound determination of thyroid nodule volumes. *Thyroid* 2005, **15**:1169-1175.
27. Yuan WH, Chiou HJ, Chou YH, Hsu HC, Tiu CM, Cheng CY, Lee CH: Gray-scale and color Doppler ultrasonographic manifestations of papillary thyroid carcinoma: analysis of 51 cases. *Clin Imaging* 2006, **30**:394-401.
28. Ito Y, Kobayashi K, Tomoda C, Uruno T, Takamura Y, Miya A, Matsuzuka F, Kuma K, Miyauchi A: Ill-defined edge on ultrasonographic examination can be a marker of aggressive characteristic of papillary thyroid microcarcinoma. *World J Surg* 2005, **29**:1007-1011.
29. Shimura H, Haraguchi K, Hiejima Y, Fukunari N, Fujimoto Y, Katagiri M, Koyanagi N, Kurita T, Miyakawa M, Miyamoto Y, Suzuki N, Suzuki S, Kanbe M, Kato Y, Murakami T, Tohno E, Tsunoda-Shimizu H, Yamada K, Ueno E, Kobayashi K, Kobayashi T, Yokozawa T, Kitaoka M: Distinct diagnostic criteria for ultrasonographic examination of papillary thyroid carcinoma: a multicenter study. *Thyroid* 2005, **15**:251-258.
30. Vaupel P, Kallinowski F, Okunieff P: Blood flow, oxygen consumption and tissue oxygenation of human tumors. *Adv Exp Med Biol* 1990, **277**:895-905.
31. Szopinski KT, Mroz C, Przelaskowski A, Mlosek RK, Sieluzycka J, Slapa RZ: A new method of merging and reviewing of 3D ultrasound data sets - application in breast and thyroid sonography. *Eur Radiol* 2007, **17(supp 1)**:178.
32. Tanter M, Bercoff J, Athanasiou A, Deffieux T, Gennisson J-L, Montaldo G, Muller M, Tardivon A, Fink M: Quantitative assessment of breast lesion viscoelasticity: Initial clinical results using supersonic shear imaging. *Ultrasound Med Biol* 2008, **34(9)**:1373-1386.
33. Sebag F, Vaillant-Lombard J, Berbis J, Griset V, Henry JF, Petit P, Olivier C: Shear wave elastography: a new ultrasound imaging mode for the differential diagnosis of benign and malignant thyroid nodules. *J Clin Endocrinol Metab* 2010, **95**:5281-8.
34. Mitchell J, Parangi S: The thyroid incidentaloma: an increasingly frequent consequence of radiologic imaging. *Semin Ultrasound CT MR* 2005, **26**:37-46.

# 2

# Cytometric evaluation of intracellular IFN-γ and IL-4 levels in thyroid follicular cells from patients with autoimmune thyroid diseases

Artur Bossowski[1*], Jerzy Harasymczuk[2], Anna Moniuszko[3], Anna Bossowska[4], Maciej Hilczer[5] and Karol Ratomski[6]

**Abstract**

**Background:** In recent few years is underlined that altered balance of pro- and anti-inflammatory cytokines play an important role in the pathogenesis of AITD.

The aim of this study was to estimate intracellular INF-γ and IL-4 levels in thyroid-infiltrating lymphocytes and thyrocytes isolated from thyroid tissues in 54 adolescent patients aged 8-21 years, with Graves' disease (GD; n = 18), Hashimoto's thyroiditis (HT; n = 18) and non-toxic multinodular goiter (NTMG; n = 18).

**Methods:** Fresh thyroid tissues were taken on culture medium RPMI -1640, it was mechanically prepared. In next step were added cell activators -12- myristate 13- the acetate (PMA) and Ionomycin as well as the inhibitor of transportation of proteins - Breferdin A. They were cultured 24 hours in 50 ml flasks at 37°C in a 5-95% CO2-air water-saturated atmosphere. After that, thyrocytes were identified by mouse mAb directed against human TPO epitope 64 conjugated with rabbit anti-mouse antibodies IgG (Fab')$_2$ labeled by FITC. After incubation at room temperature to each of samples added reagent A fixative the cellular membrane. In next step into the cell suspensions were added reagent B to permeabilization of cellular membrane and specific anti-IL-4-PE or anti-IFN-γ-PE mAbs. Identification of intracellular cytokines in T lymphocytes was performed in the same procedure with application of anti-CD4-PerCP and anti-CD8-PerCP mAbs specific for T lymphocytes. The cells were analyzed in a flow cytometry (Coulter EPICS XL).

**Results:** In examined group of patients with GD we observed statistically significant higher mean percentage of cells with phenotype CD4+IL-4 ($p < 0.05$; $p < 0.025$), CD8+IL-4 ($p < 0.033$; $p < 0.01$) and TFCs-IL-4+ ($p < 0.05$; $p < 0.01$) in comparison to patients with HT and NTMG. The analysis of mean percentages of positive TILs and TFCs with intracellular INF-g levels in patients with HT revealed statistically significant increase percentage of CD4+INF-γ ($p < 0.04$; $p < 0.001$), CD8+ INF-γ (NS; $p < 0.025$), TFCs+INF-γ ($p < 0.03$; $p < 0.001$) cells in comparison to the percentage of positive cells from patients with GD and NTMG.

**Conclusions:** We conclude that human thyrocytes in autoimmune thyroid disorders could be a source of cytokine production and that their activation influences local interaction with T lymphocytes inflowing to the thyroid gland.

**Keywords:** thyrocytes, cytokines, Graves, disease, Hashimoto?'?s thyroiditis

## Background

Graves' disease (GD) and Hashimoto's thyroiditis (HT) are a common autoimmune disorders. It was proven, that subpopulation of Th1 plays an important role in induction of classical mechanisms of late type reaction and that produced by CD4+ IFN-γ is an activator of macrophages and stimulates production of IgG2a. Th1 cells through the influencing on differentiation of cytotoxic lymphocytes CD8+, modulate also inflammatory reaction in response to the antigen stimulation [1]. CD4+ cells, which belong to subpopulation Th2 stimulate immunological response of B lymphocytes. There are some studies evaluating cytokines in these diseases, demonstrating the production of IL-4 and TNF- by infiltrating T cells and macrophages. However, the specific role of these molecules in the pathogenesis of autoimmune thyroid

* Correspondence: abossowski@hotmail.com
[1]Department of Pediatrics, Endocrinology, Diabetology with the Cardiology Division, Medical University. Bialystok 15-089. Poland
Full list of author information is available at the end of the article

diseases (AITD) is still debated [2-4]. We presume that an altered balance of pro- and anti-inflammatory cytokines may play an important role in the pathogenesis of autoimmune thyroiditis.

T-helper 1 (Th1) cell-mediated inflammatory responses predominate in the early pathogenesis of GD, whereas Th2 cell-mediated immunity may play a role in later stages. Th1 cells produce IFN-gamma and Th2 cells produce IL-4. Nanba T et al. reported that IFN-gamma and IL-4 gene polymorphisms, which are related to higher IFN-gamma and lower IL-4 production, respectively, are more frequent in patients with severe HT than in those mild HT. They investigated the proportion of peripheral Th1 and Th2 cells in patients with AITD and concluded that the peripheral Th1/Th2 cell ratio is related to the severity of HT and is related to the intractability of GD. They hypothesize that these patterns of peripheral Th cell subsets may be expressed within the thyroid [5].

The aim of this study was to estimate intracellular INF-γ and IL-4 levels in thyroid-infiltrating lymphocytes (TILs), and in thyroid follicular cells with application of mouse monoclonal antibodies type #64 which recognize B antigen regions of TPO (thyroid peroxidase) in patients with AITD and NTMG.

## Patients and methods

The study was performed in a group of 54 adolescent patients (14 boys and 42 girls), aged 8-21 years, with Graves' disease (GD; n = 18, mean age 16.4 ± 3.3 years), Hashimoto's thyroiditis (HT; n = 18, mean age 16.8 ± 2.8 years) and non-toxic multinodular goiter (n = 18, mean age 16 ± 3 years), hospitalized in the Department Pediatrics, Endocrinology, Diabetology with the Cardiology Division, Medical University of Białystok. The patients underwent total or subtotal thyroidectomy in the 1st Department of General Surgery, Medical University of Białystok or in the Department of Pediatric Surgery, Traumatology and Urology, Poznań University of Medical Sciences. The diagnosis was established based on clinical examinations confirmed by laboratory, ultrasonographic and scintigraphic investigations with the use of $^{131}I$ (in case of nodular goiter with symptoms of hyperthyroidism). Additionally, fine-needle aspiration biopsies in HT and nodular goiter were performed in the Department of Patomorphology, Medical University of Białystok. The qualifying criteria for patients with GD were as follows: large goiter, presence of ophthalmopathy, antibodies against receptor for thyroid stimulating hormone (TRAb) > 5, positive titers of antithyroid peroxidase (anti-TPO) or anti-thyroglobulin (anti-TG) antibodies, and persisting over 2-3 months since the diagnosis of thyroid- stimulating hormone (TSH) < 0.45. Methimazole therapy, at the initial dose of 0.5-1.0 mg/kg/day, was used in combination with propranolol 0.5-1.0 mg/kg/day to treat hyperthyroidism in the course of GD. A further reduction in methimazole dose and obtaining euthyrosis prior to surgery depended on clinical-biochemical parameters. Average daily doses of this antithyroid drug were 10-15 mg. Patients with HT received treatment exclusively with L-thyroxine (mean 75 ± 25 mg/24 h) for the period of 6-12 months (mean 8 months) since the diagnosis.

The function of the thyroid gland in patients with GD was assessed at the time of diagnosis and prior to surgery. Thyroid function was evaluated based on thyroid hormones and TSH tests performed jointly with the measurement of titers of antithyroid antibodies (ATPO, ATG, TRAK).

Our study was approved by the Committee for Ethics and Supervision on Human and Animal Research of the Medical University in Białystok. An informed consent was given by the participating children and their parents.

### Determination of the Antithyroid Antibody Titers and Thyroid Hormone Concentration

Blood for analysis was collected on empty stomach in the morning hours from the basilic vein and centrifuged for 10 min at 2,000 rotations/min. Sera were stored at -20° until the required number was collected. Thyroid stimulating hormone receptor antibodies (TRAbs) were routinely determined by a radioreceptor assay (TRAK-human kits, Brahms Diagnostica GmbH, Berlin, Germany), in which the value < 1 U/l was treated as negative, 1.0-1.5 U/l as a grey zone and the values > 1.5 U/l were considered positive. Antithyroperoxidase antibodies (TPO-Abs) and antithyroglobulin antibodies (TG-Abs) were determined using immunodiagnostic test Varelisa (Variable Enzyme Linked Immno Sorbent Assay, Pharmacia

Upjohn Diagnostics GmbH Co.KG. Freiburg, Germany). Normal range for TG-Abs was < 500 IU/ml and for TPO-Abs was < 50 IU/ml. The levels of fT4, fT3 and hTSH in blood serum were determined on a mini-analyzer (Bio Merieux, France), based on test VIDAS (Bio Merieux, France), combining the immunoenzymatic method with the final fluorescence measurement (ELFA). Normal range of fT4 was 0.71-1.55 ng/dl, fT3–2.6-5.4 ng/dl and hTSH–0.32-5.0 μIU/ml.

### Thyrocyte preparations

The thyroid tissue samples were analyzed following the previously described techniques [6,7]. Briefly, postoperative 1.0 cm/1.0 cm thyroid sections were collected to test-tubes with RPMI-1640 medium. Initially, the material was minced mechanically and digested with a mixture of collagenase type IV-S (Sigma) in Hanks balanced saline solution (HESS). To eliminate non-adherent cells from thyrocyte preparations, the dispersed cells were cultured for

24 h with minimum essential medium (MEM), containing 10% fetal bovine serum and Ham F12 medium, supplemented with 20 mm HEPES buffer, 2 mm L-glutamine, 100 U/ml penicillin, and 100 µg/ml streptomycin (Sigma). They were cultured in 50 ml flasks (Falcon Plastics, Becton-Dickinson, USA) at 37°C in a 5-95% CO2-air water-saturated atmosphere. The following day, the non-adherent cells (predominantly lymphoid cells and erythrocytes) were removed from culture supernatants for lymphocyte isolation. Trypsinization was performed at confluence (Figure 1).

#### Identification of thyrocyte populations

Purity of thyroid cells was tested by flow cytometry as previously described [7]. Briefly, the isolated cells diluted in RPMI 1640 medium were rinsed twice with a buffer containing PBS, 0.5% bovine albumin and 2 mM EDTA, and suspended in 1 ml PBS. After that, 50 µl portions of cell suspension were placed in a test-tube, adding 10 µl of mouse monoclonal antibody (mAb) at 400 µg/ml concentration directed against human TPO epitope 64

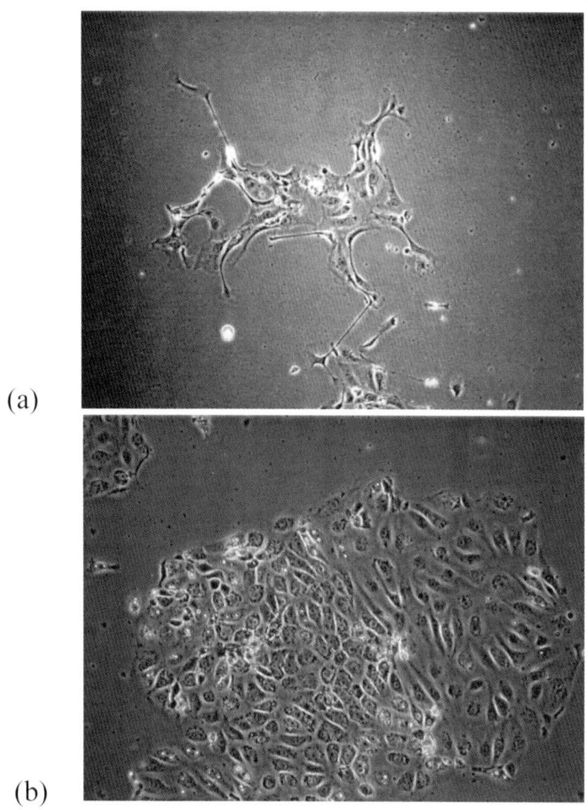

Figure 1 Thyrocytes in suspension in culture medium (a) formed monolayers on plastic plates after 24 h in culture (b).

reacting with domain B. Following 30 min incubation at 4°C, the cells were rinsed three times with a buffer of PBS + 0.5% bovine albumin + 2 mM EDTA. Then, 20 µl of rabbit antibody $F(ab')_2$ conjugated with FITC (FITC-coupled $F(ab')_2$ antimouse IgG, DAKO) was added. After 30 min incubation at 4°C, cell suspensions were rinsed three times again in the buffer described above. Then, the samples were submitted to analysis in a flow cytometer (Coulter EPICS XL).

The unspecific binding of monoclonal antibodies to the thyrocytes was evaluated by the use of irrelevant IgG of the same isotype as the used antibodies. The specificity of the reaction was checked by immunoprecipitation of mAbs by highly purified human TPO.

#### Identification of intracellular IL-4 and IFN-γ levels in thyrocytes by flow cytometry

Fresh thyroid tissues were taken on culture medium RPMI -1640, it was mechanically prepared (described as above). Briefly, the cell suspensions were rinsed three times with PBS, and later were added cell activators - 12 - myristate 13 - the acetate (the PMA - 50 ng/ml) and Ionomycin (1 mM) as well as the inhibitor of transportation of proteins - Breferdin A (3 mmol/ml). They were cultured 24 hours in 50 ml flasks at 37°C in a 5-95% CO2-air water-saturated atmosphere. After that, 10 µl of mouse monoclonal antibody (mAb) directed against human TPO epitope 64 was added into the suspension. After 15 minutes of incubation at room temperature to each of samples added 100 µl of reagent A fixative the cellular membrane (IntraStain-Dako, Denmark). In next step we conjugated this complex with rabbit anti-mouse antibodies IgG $(Fab')_2$ labeled by FITC and than incubated by next 15 minutes (identified as above). Then, the cell suspensions were rinsed three times with PBS and were added 100 µl of reagent B to permeabilization the cellular membrane (IntraStain-Dako, Denmark) and 20 µl specific anti-IL-4-PE ($IgG_1$, BD) or anti-IFN-γ-PE ($IgG_1$, BD) monoclonal antibody, and murine $IgG_1$ as negative control, then incubated for 30 min at 4°C. After two washes with PBS supplemented with 5% BSA, the cells were immediately analyzed in a flow cytometry (Coulter EPICS XL) (Figure 2, Figure 3).

#### Identification of intracellular IL-4 and IFN-γ levels in lymphocyte populations by flow cytometry

The percentage of lymphocytes was determined as previously described [8]. Briefly, after 24 h of incubation with cell activators and inhibitor of transportation of proteins (described above), the non-adherent cells (predominantly lymphoid cells and erythrocytes) were removed from culture supernatants for lymphocyte isolation. In the next step, 10 µl anti-CD4-PerCP and anti-CD8-PerCP (IgG1, BD) monoclonal Abs were used for

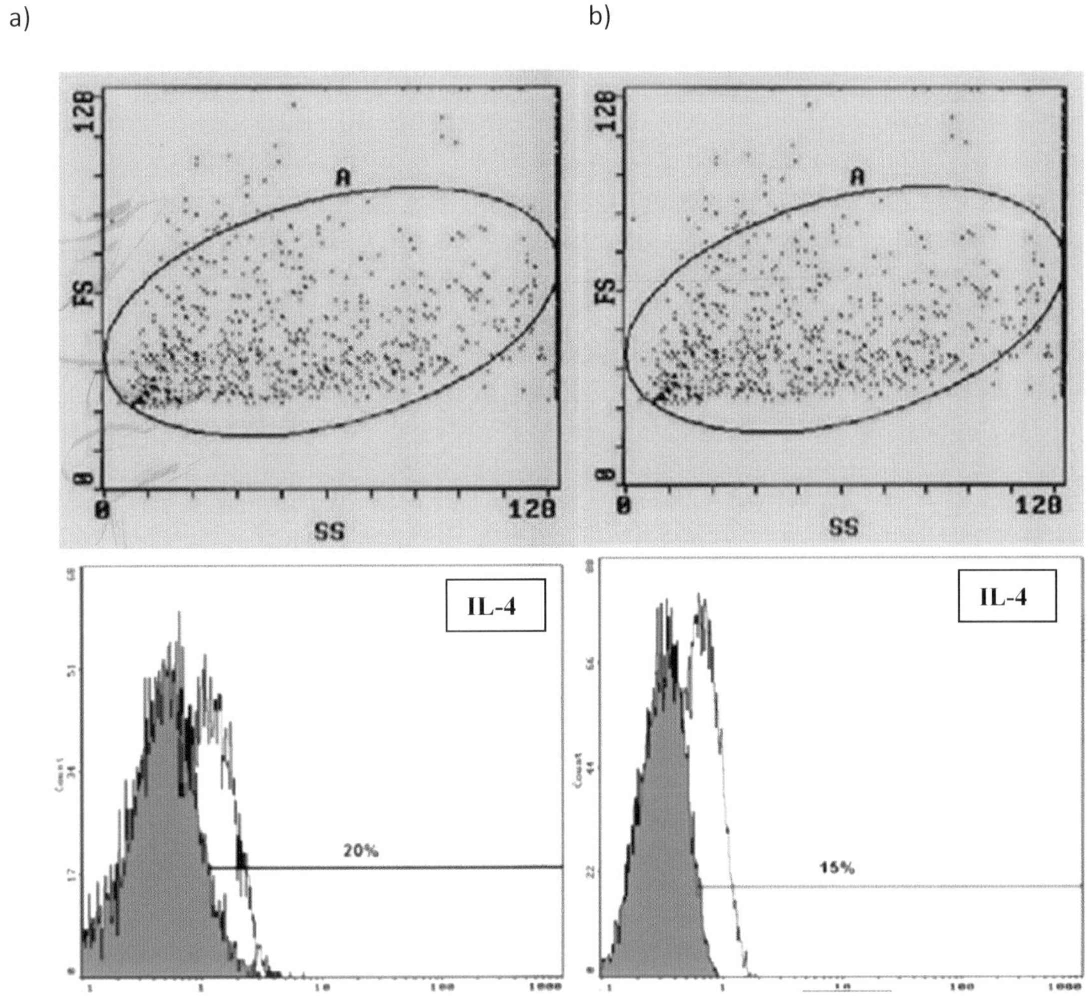


**Figure 2 Identification of IL-4 in thyroid follicular cells in patients with GD and HT using flow cytometry**. (a) Flow cytometric dot plots of dispersed TFCs from a representative patient with GD. Scatter plot of gating thyrocytes (left upper panel). Flow cytometric detection of IL-4 in thyrocytes from patients with GD (left down panel). Cells were labeled with control IgG1 (grey) or anti-IL-4 mAb (white). (b) Flow cytometric dot plots of dispersed TFCs from a representative patient with HT. Scatter plot of gating thyrocytes (right upper panel). Flow cytometric detection of IL-4 in thyrocytes from patients with HT (right down panel). Cells were labeled with control IgG1 (grey) or anti-IL-4 mAb (white).

direct staining of membrane molecules specific for T lymphocytes. After 15 minutes of incubation at room temperature to each of samples added 100 μl of reagent A fixative the cellular membrane (IntraStain-Dako, Denmark) and incubated by next 15 minutes. Then, the cell suspensions were rinsed three times with PBS and were added 100 μl of reagent B to permeabilization the cellular membrane (IntraStain-Dako, Denmark) and 20 μl specific anti-IL-4-PE ($IgG_1$, BD) or anti-IFN-γ-PE ($IgG_1$, BD) monoclonal antibody, with murine $IgG_1$ as negative control. The cells were analyzed in a flow cytometry (Coulter EPICS XL).

### Statistical analysis

The results were analyzed using Statistica 9.0 software. The mean values of immune parameters between groups were evaluated using Student's t test, U Mann-Whitney's test or Fisher's exact probability test. Correlation was assessed by Spearman's signed ranks test. $P < 0.05$ was considered significant.

## Results

Table 1 presents the characteristics and laboratory findings in patients with GD (prior to methimazole treatment and then in the state of clinico-biological euthyrosis before surgery), with HT and with nontoxic nodular goiter (NTMG; prior to treatment). Patients with > 1 cm nodular lesions in ultrasonography underwent fine-needle aspiration biopsy (BAC), which showed benign colloid nodular goiter. Scintigraphy additionally performed in 3 patients with nodular goiter and clinical symptoms of hyperthyroidism showed a selective

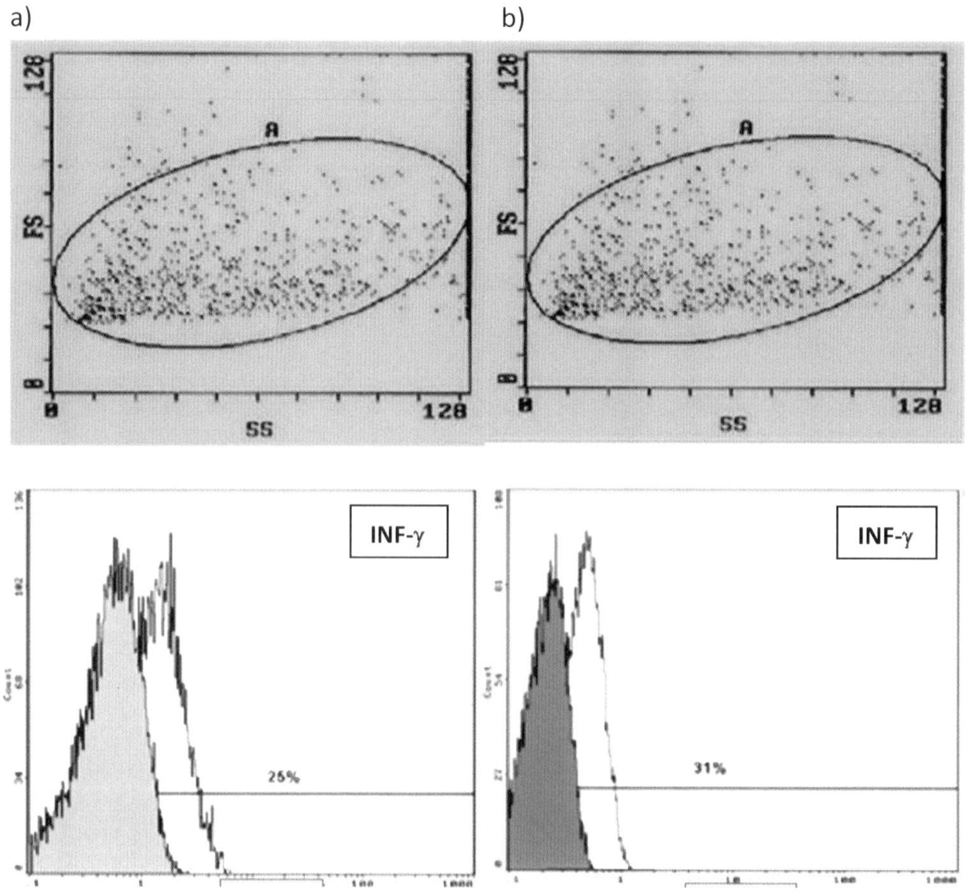


**Figure 3 Identification of INF-γ in thyroid follicular cells in patients with GD and HT using flow cytometry**. (a) Flow cytometric dot plots of dispersed TFCs from a representative patient with GD. Scatter plot of gating thyrocytes (left upper panel). Flow cytometric detection of INF-γ in thyrocytes from patients with GD (left down panel). Cells were labeled with control IgG1 (grey) or anti-INF-γ mAb (white). (b) Flow cytometric dot plots of dispersed TFCs from a representative patient with HT. Scatter plot of gating thyrocytes (right upper panel). Flow cytometric detection of INF-γ in thyrocytes from patients with HT (right down panel). Cells were labeled with control IgG1 (grey) or anti-INF-γ mAb (white).

increase in the accumulation of radioactive iodine within the area of single nodular lesions.

In the analysis of the thyroid peroxidase antigen by flow cytometry method, anti-human native TPO mouse monoclonal antibodies were used. The assessment of the percentage of thyroid cells with mAb #64TPO epitope expression showed no significant differences between GD and HT patients (73 vs.65%, NS) at a concentration of 400 mg/ml of anti-TPO antibodies. When the concentration of anti-TPO antibodies decreased, the mean percentage of thyroid cells with antigen region #64 expression was reduced.

Patients with GD showed a higher percentage of CD4+IL-4, CD8+IL-4 and TFC-IL-4+ cells, compared to patients with HT ($p < 0.05$, $p < 0.033$, $p < 0.05$, respectively) and NTMG (controls) ($p < 0.025$, $p < 0.01$, $p < 0.01$, respectively) (Figure 4). There was no difference between the proportions of these CD4+IL-4, CD8+IL-4 and TFC-IL-4+ cell populations in cases with HT and NTMG.

The analysis of mean percentages of positive TILs and TFCs with intracellular INF-g levels in patients with HT revealed statistically significant increase percentage of CD4+INF-γ, CD8+ INF-γ, TFC+INF-γ cells, compared to the percentage of positive cells from patients with GD ($p < 0.04$, NS, $p < 0.03$, respectively) and NTMG ($p < 0.001$, $p < 0.025$, $p < 0.001$, respectively) (Figure 5).

In the present study, the relationship between antithyroid antibodies and the percentage of TFCs and T cells with the expression of cytokines was evaluated. In patients with untreated GD there was a statistically significant positive correlation between the percentage of TFCs-IL4+ and CD4+IL-4 T cells and the concentration of TRAK antibodies ($R = 0.62$, $p < 0.02$; $R = 0.34$, $p < 0.04$, respectively). However, no such correlations were

**Table 1 Data of patients with GD before methimazole therapy, after six months of therapy (prior to surgery) in non-toxic multinodular goiter and HT**

| | Untreated GD group Group A | Group after six months of methimazole therapy Group A' | Group with HT Group B | Group with non-toxic multinodular goiter Group C | P |
|---|---|---|---|---|---|
| Age (years) | 15.4 ± 2.1 | 16.4 ± 3.3 | 16.8 ± 2.8 | 15.8 ± 1.8 | NS, NS*, NS** |
| n | 18 | 18 | 18 | 18 | |
| Weight (kg) | 57 ± 11.0 | 59 ± 7 | 63 ± 8 | 62 ± 7 | NS, NS*, NS** |
| Height (cm) | 166 ± 3 | 169 ± 1 | 170 ± 5 | 169 ± 7 | NS, NS*, NS** |
| BSA ($m^2$) | 1.66 | 1.68 | 1.7 | 1.67 | NS, NS*, NS** |
| anti-TPO (IU/ml) | 1250 ± 350 | 650 ± 250 \ | 1550 ± 500 | 41.3 ± 38 | p < 0.0001, p* < 0.01, p** < 0.001 |
| anti-TG (IU/ml) | 630 ± 262 | 360 ± 40 | 820 ± 150 | 180 ± 86 | p < 0.001, p* < 0.01, p** < 0.001 |
| TRAb (U/l) | > 5 positive | > 3 positive | (-) | (-) | |
| fT4 (ng/dl) | 5.9 ± 2.0 | 2.04 ± 0.3 | 1.29 ± 0.2 | 1.1 ± 0.2 | p < 0.001, NS*, NS** |
| fT3 (ng/dl) | 8.85 ± 2.1 | 3.8 ± 0.5 | 3.64 ± 0.21 | 2.94 ± 0.21 | p < 0.002, NS*, NS** |
| TSH (μIU/ml) | 0.03 ± 0.01 | 1.3 ± 0.2 | 3.1 ± 0.5 | 2.9 ± 0.3 | p < 0.001 p* < 0.01, NS** |

GD- Graves' disease HT- Hashimoto's thyroiditis NTMG-non-toxic multinodular goiter

p, Statistical significance between group A and C; p*, statistical significance between group A' and C; p**, statistical significance between group B and C; X, standard deviation; NS, no statistical significance.

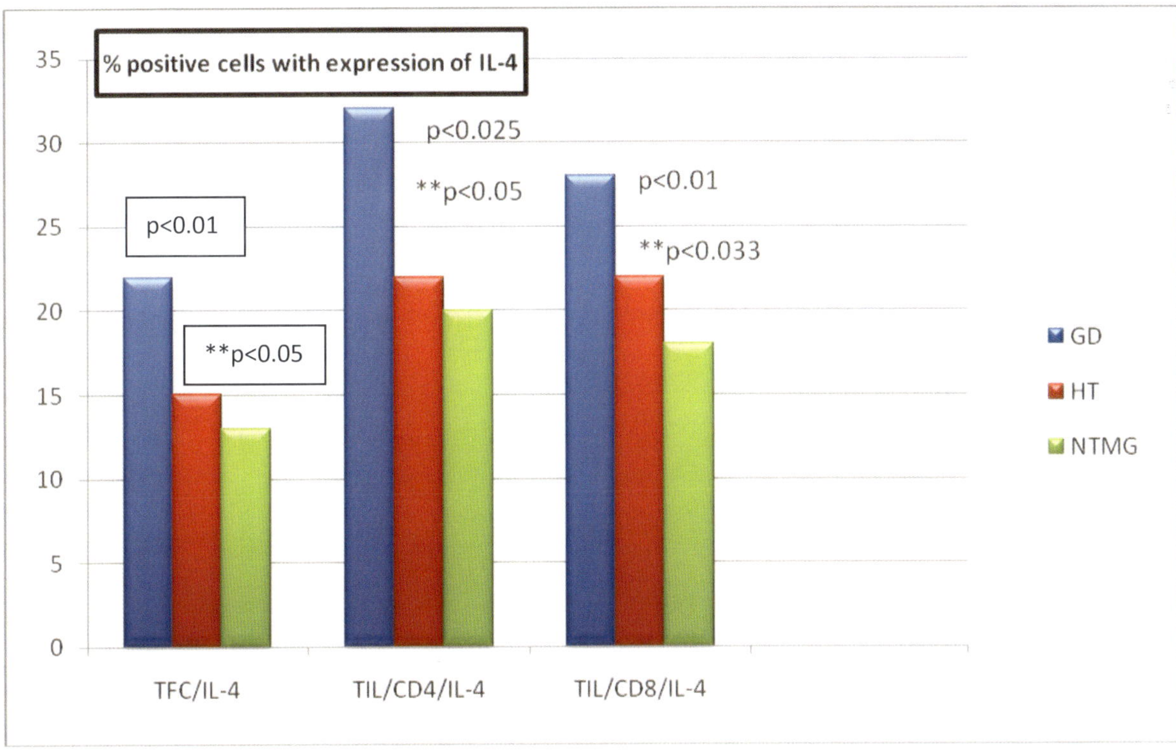


**Figure 4** Mean percentages of positive TFCs and TILs with intracellular expression of IL-4 in examined patients.

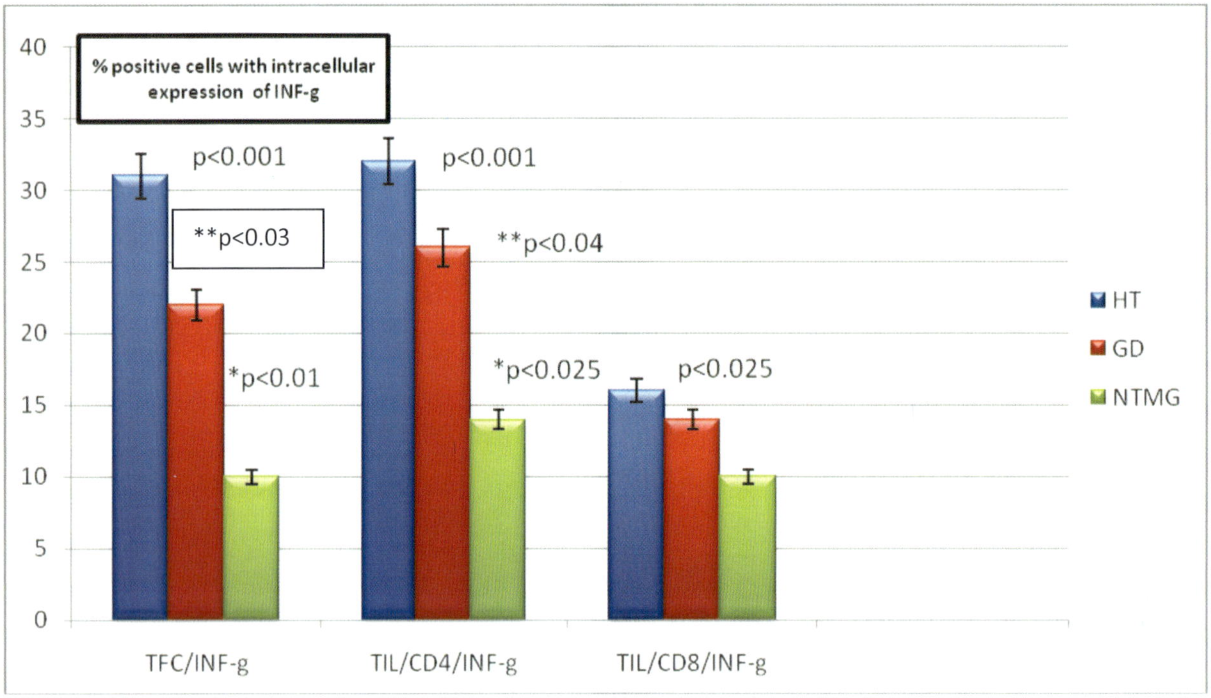


**Figure 5** Mean percentages of positive TFCs and TILs with intracellular expression of INF-g in examined patients.

noted in regard to patients with HT and non-toxic multinodular goiter. There were no significant correlations between thyroid hormones and the percentage of intrathyroid lymphocytes and TFCs with IL-4 and INF-γ expression.

## Discussion

An altered balance of pro- and anti-inflammatory cytokines is thought to play an important role in the pathogenesis of autoimmune thyroid diseases. Disruption of thyroid self tolerance, usually after an infection, generates abnormal thyroid-immune interactions, implicating an array of cytokines and their receptors. Thyrocytes achieve antigen presenting cell properties, which stimulate effectors immune cells: Th1 and Th2, in the context of defective immunomodulatory T regulatory cells, resulting in thyroid lymphocytic infiltration and activation of B cells, with production of antibodies against thyroid antigens, thyroid destruction or stimulation, depending on the Th1-Th2 balance [9].

Over the last decade many researchers have proven, that T cell recognition of autoantigens had shown considerable intra- and interindividual heterogeneity, and a mixed pattern of cytokine production indicates that both the Th1 and Th2 limbs of the helper T cell response are involved in all types of autoimmune thyroiditis. HT glands activate T cells that display a predominantly Th1 phenotype. The Th1 pattern produces IL-2, IFN-γ, and TNF-α, with a relative absence of IL-4 or -10, suggesting that these cells support a predominantly T cell-mediated induction of apoptosis [10]. In contrast, GD thyrocytes do not undergo apoptosis and are characterized by a predominantly Th2 infiltrate [11]. The Th2 pattern produces relatively less IL-2, TNF- α, and IFN- γ, and more IL-4, -5, and -10, indicating a tendency toward B-cell maturation and an antibody-mediated immune response [10].

Secretion of cytokines within the thyroid accounts for the accumulation and expansion of the intrathyroidal lymphocyte pool. Also, the thyroid cells themselves contribute to this secretion. The thyroid cells also produce a number of proinflammatory molecules which will tend to exacerbate the autoimmune process, eg. IFN- γ and IL-4 [12].

IFN- γ, a prototypic proinflammatory cytokine produced by several different cell types, including the Th1 subset of CD4(+) T cells, plays an important role in inflammation and autoimmune diseases [13]. Carella C et al. observed that INF- γ is the cytokine most clearly associated with AITD, especially hypothyroidism, despite being neither Th1- nor Th2-dependent [14]. Phenekos C et al. found that patients with HT had higher INF- γ levels compared to patients with TNG, GD and controls. In contrast, patients with GD had higher serum levels of IL-4 in comparison with patients with HT. These results were similar to the results of our study. Therefore, we can also conclude, that a Th1 pattern of immune response characteristic of cellular immunity is dominant in HT, whereas the predominance of Th2 cytokines in GD indicates a humoral pattern of immune reaction [15].

IL-4 is produced by Th2, mastocytes and basophiles. The IL-4 is involved in both humoral and cellular immunity. Chen RH et al. tested whether the IL-4 gene could be used as a genetic marker to predict the development of AITD among the Chinese population of Taiwan. They found no significant difference in the frequencies of presence of genotype and allelic variants for the IL-4 gene at both the intron 3 and the promoter regions between the normal control group and each of the two patient groups. These findings suggest that the IL-4 gene polymorphisms that arise at either intron 3 or promoter -590 positions are not suitable genetic markers for AITD among Taiwanese Chinese [16].

Because GD and HT are a common autoimmune disorders with genetic predisposition, the expression of genes coding cytokines was measured. Zhu W et al. observed strong evidence that the Chr.5q31-33 region, which contains the immune response various cytokine genes eg. IL-4, is linked to autoimmune thyroid disorders in Chinese and Japanese populations [17]. Also Khalilzadeh O et al. observed the association between GD and the polymorphisms in anti-inflammatory cytokine IL-4 [18].

Alnaqdy A et al. noticed that patients with GD showed significantly higher levels of IL-4 and IFN- γ compared with the normal controls. There was also a significant increase in serum levels of IL-4 in the treated group, compared to the untreated group. IL-4, and IFN-γ, showed a high prevalence in Omani patients with GD. Thus, cytokines and autoantibodies may prove useful in the diagnosis of GD and in assessing prognosis [19].

Worth emphasizing is fact, that IL- 4 in GD prevents adhesion molecules expression in order not to damage thyrocytes. In our study production of IL-4 in thyrocytes of patients with GD was elevated, what may be responsible for protection of these cells against immune damage or reduction of their apoptosis. Stassi G et al. suggested that, infiltration of Th2 lymphocytes and production of IL-4 and IL-10 by thyrocytes in patients with GD can induce the expression of antiapoptotic molecules and leading thyrocyte resistance to CD95-mediated apoptosis [20]. On the other hand, in patients with HT we detected in thyrocytes elevated level of IFN- γ, what may be responsible for prolongation of inflammatory process within thyroid gland.

In conclusion, our findings suggest that the human thyrocytes in autoimmune thyroid disorders could be a source of cytokine production and that their activation influences local interaction with T lymphocytes inflowing. The alteration of intracellular cytokine levels in T cells within thyroid gland suggest predominance role of Th1 immune response in HT, and development of Th2 immune response in GD.

### Abbreviations

**PerCP**: peridinin chlorophyll protein; **FITC**: fluorescein isothiocyanate; **PE**: phycoerythrin; **fT3**: free triiodothyronine; **fT4**: free thyroxine; **TSH**: thyroid stimulating hormone; **TRAbs**: antibodies against receptor for thyroid stimulating hormone; **TPO-Abs**: antithyroid peroxidase antibodies; **hTPO**: human thyroid peroxidase; **TG-Abs**: antithyroglobulin antibodies; **AITD**: autoimmune thyroid disease; **GD**: Graves' disease; **NTMG**: non-toxic multinodular goiter; **HT**: Hashimoto's thyroiditis; **mAb**: monoclonal antibodies; **TFC**: thyroid follicular cell; **ITLs**: intrathyroidal T lymphocytes.

### Acknowledgements and Funding

This study was supported byMinistry of Science and Higher Education Grantnumber N N407 21 6640. The publishing costs are covered by grant number N N407 21 6640.

### Author details

[1]Department of Pediatrics, Endocrinology, Diabetology with the Cardiology Division, Medical University. Bialystok 15-089. Poland. [2]Department of Pediatric Surgery, Traumatology and Urology. University of Medical Sciences, Poznań 60-967. Poland. [3]Department of Infectious Diseases and Neuroinfections. Medical University. Białystok 15-089. Poland. [4]Division of Cardiology. Internal Affair and Administration Ministry Hospital. Białystok 15-089. Poland. [5]Department of Endocrinology and Metabolic Diseases. Medical University. Łódź 93-338. Poland. [6]Dep. of Pediatric Laboratory Diagnostic. Medical University. Bialystok 15-089. Poland.

### Authors' contributions

AB(1) participated in the designing of the study, collecting of clinical data and drafting the manuscript. MH and AB(4) performed the statistical analysis and helped to draft the manuscript. JH performed thyroid surgery and collected the clinical material. KR participated in the cytometric analysis. AM participated in the design of the study and drafted the manuscript. All authors read and approved the final manuscript.

### Competing interests

The authors declare that they have no competing interests.

### References

1. Mosmann TR, Coffman RL: **TH1 and TH2 cells: different patterns of lymphokine secretion lead to different functional properties.** *Annu Rev Immunol* 1989, **7**:145-173.
2. Paschke R, Schuppert F, Taton M, Velu T: **Intrathyroidal cytokine expression profiles in autoimmune thyroiditis.** *J Immunol* 1994, **141**:309-315.
3. Watson PF, Pickerill AP, Davies R, Weetman AP: **Analysis of cytokine gene expression in Graves' disease and multinodular goitre.** *Clin Endocrinol Metab* 1994, **79**:355-360.
4. Ajjan RA, Watson PF, McIntosh RS, Weetman AP: **Intra-thyroidal cytokine gene expression in Hashimoto's thyroiditis.** *Clin Exp Immunol* 1996, **105**:523-528.
5. Nanba T, Watanabe M, Inoue N, Iwatani Y: **Increases of the Th1/Th2 cell ratio in severe Hashimoto's disease and in the proportion of Th17 cells in intractable Graves' disease.** *Thyroid* 2009, **5**:495-501.
6. Rasmussen AK, Feldt-Rasmussn U, Brandt M, Hartoft-Nielsen ML, Carayon P, Buschard K: **Thyrotropin stimulates specifically the expression of the autoantibody binding domains of the thyroperoxidase molecule.** *Autoimmunity* 1999, **29**:323-331.
7. Bossowski A, Stasiak-Barmuta A, Czarnocka B, Urban M, Dadan J: **Application of mAbs for identification of antigen regions of human thyroid peroxidase in adolescents with Graves' disease and non-toxic multinodular goiter by flow cytometry.** *Autoimmunity* 2005, **38**:605-11.

8. Stassi G, Todaro M, Bucchieri F, Stoppacciaro A, Farina F, Zummo G, Testi R, De Maria R: **Fas/Fas ligand-driven T cell apoptosis as a conseqence of ineffective thyroid immunoprivilege in Hashimoto's thyroiditis.** *J Immunol* 1999, **162**:263-267.
9. Lichiardopol C, Moţa M: **The thyroid and autoimmunity.** *Rom J Intern Med* 2009, **47**:207-15.
10. McIver B, Morris JC: **The pathogenesis of Graves' disease.** *Endocrinol Metab Clin North Am* 1998, **27**:73-89.
11. Stassi G, Zeuner A, Di Liberto D, Todaro M, Ricci-Vitiani L, De Maria R: **Fas-FasL in Hashimoto's thyroiditis.** *J Clin Immunol* 2001, **21**:19-23.
12. Weetman AP: **Cellular immune responses in autoimmune thyroid disease.** *Clinical Endocrinology* 2004, **61**:405-413.
13. Fang Y, Yu S, Braley-Mullen H: **Contrasting roles of IFN-gamma in murine models of autoimmune thyroid diseases.** *Thyroid* 2007, **17**:989-94.
14. Carella C, Mazziotti G, Morisco F, Manganella G, Rotondi M, Tuccillo C, Sorvillo F, Caporaso N, Amato G: **Long-term outcome of interferon-γ-induced thyroid autoimmunity and prognostic influence of thyroid autoantibody pattern at the end of treatment.** *Journal of Clinical Endocrinology and Metabolism* 2001, **86**:1925-1929.
15. Phenekos C, Vryonidou A, Gritzapis AD, Baxevanis CN, Goula M, Papamichail M: **Th1 and Th2 serum cytokine profiles characterize patients with Hashimoto's thyroiditis (Th1) and Graves' disease (Th2).** *Euroimmunomodulation* 2004, **11**:209-13.
16. Chen RH, Chang CT, Wang TY, Chen CC, Tsai CH, Tsai FJ: **Lack of association between interleukin-4 gene polymorphisms and autoimmune thyroid diseases amongst Taiwanese Chinese.** *Endocrine* 2007, , **32**: 170-4.
17. Zhu W, Liu N, Zhao Y, Jia H, Cui B, Ning G: **Association analysis of polymorphisms in IL-3, IL-4, IL-5, IL-9 and IL-13 with Graves' disease.** *J Endocrinol Invest* 2010, **03**:22.
18. Khalilzadeh O, Anvari M, Momen-Heravi F, Esteghamati A, Rashidi A, Mahmoudi M, Nikbin B, Amirzargar A: **Gene polymorphisms of interleukin-4, interleukin-10 and transforming growth factor-beta in Graves' disease.** *Clin Exp Med* 2010, **10**:123-8.
19. Alnaqdy A, Al-Maskari M: **Levels of cytokines and thyroid autoantibodies in Omani patients with Graves' disease.** *Br J Biomed Sci* 2007, **64**:164-7.
20. Stassi G, De Maria R: **Autoimmune thyroid disease: Newmodels of cell death in autoimmunity.** *Nat Rev Immunol* 2002, **2**:195-204.

# 3

# Do IGF-I concentrations better reflect growth hormone (GH) action in children with short stature than the results of GH stimulating tests? Evidence from the simultaneous assessment of thyroid function

Joanna Smyczyńska[1,3], Renata Stawerska[1,3], Andrzej Lewiński[2,3*], Maciej Hilczer[1,3]

**Abstract**

**Background:** The diagnosis of growth hormone (GH) deficiency (GHD) in short children seems unquestionable when both GH peak in stimulating tests (GHST) and IGF-I concentration are decreased. However, the discrepancies between the results of GHST and IGF-I secretion are observed. It seems purposeful to determine the significance of GHST and IGF-I assessment in diagnosing GHD. The relationship between GH secretion and thyroid function, as well as GH influence on the peripheral thyroxine ($T_4$) to triiodothyronine ($T_3$) deiodination, mediated by IGF-I, were identified. Thus, clear differences in thyroid function between GH-deficient and non-GH-deficient subjects should exist.

**Methods:** Analysis comprised 800 children (541 boys), age 11.6 ± 3.1 years (mean ± SD), with short stature, in whom two (2) standard GHST (with clonidine and with glucagon) were performed and IGF-I, free $T_4$ ($FT_4$), free $T_3$ ($FT_3$) and TSH serum concentrations were assessed. The patients were qualified to the following groups: GHD - decreased GH peak in GHST and IGF-I SDS (n = 81), ISS - normal GH peak and IGF-I SDS (n = 347), low GH - normal IGF-I SDS, and decreased GH peak (n = 212), low IGF - decreased IGF-I SDS, and normal GH peak (n = 160). The relationships among the results of particular tests were evaluated.

**Results:** In the groups with decreased IGF-I concentrations (GHD Group and low IGF Group), the more severe deficit of height was observed, together with higher TSH and $FT_4$ but lower $FT_3$ levels than in groups with normal IGF-I concentrations (ISS Group and low GH Group), independently of the results of GHST. TSH, $FT_4$ and $FT_3$ concentrations were - respectively - similar in two groups with decreased IGF-I secretion, as well as in two groups with normal IGF-I levels. Significant correlations were found between patients' height SDS and IGF-I SDS, between $FT_3$ and IGF-I SDS (positive), and between $FT_4$ and IGF-I SDS (negative), with no correlation between GH peak and any of the parameters analyzed.

**Conclusion:** The assessment of thyroid function in children with short stature provides the evidence that measurement of IGF-I concentration may be a procedure reliable at least to the some degree in diagnosing GHD as the results of GHST.

* Correspondence: alewin@csk.umed.lodz.pl
[2]Department of Endocrinology and Metabolic Diseases, Medical University of Lodz, Lodz, Poland
Full list of author information is available at the end of the article

## Background

The growth hormone (GH) secretion is routinely evaluated in children with short stature, on the ground of the results of GH stimulating tests (GHST) with different pharmacological stimuli [1,2]. Insulin-like growth factor-I (IGF-I) is the main peripheral mediator of GH activity. The assessment of IGF-I secretion is an important diagnostic tool, as its synthesis is GH-dependent, whereas serum concentration - on the contrary to GH levels - relatively stable [3]. The diagnosis of GH deficiency (GHD) seems unquestionable when both GH peak in GHST and IGF-I concentration are decreased. Consistently, GHD may be excluded in the patients, in whom both GH and IGF-I secretion are normal. In such cases, the diagnosis of idiopathic short stature (ISS) seems to be the most adequate after careful exclusion of other possible causes of short stature (including genetically-determined syndromes, chronic diseases, malnutrition, *etc.*). However, in clinical practice, the discrepancies either between the results of GHST and IGF-I secretion or between the results of particular GHST are - quite frequently - observed. According to current recommendations, two (2) different GHST are required in every case and their results should be interpreted together [1,2]. The problem of the poor reproducibility of GHST was raised - among others - by Rosenfeld et al. [4] and Price et al. [5]. Next, the possibility of obtaining normal results of GHST in children, previously diagnosed as GH-deficient (*i.e.* in children with subnormal GH response to pharmacological stimulation in past) was documented in several studies [5-8]. The relationships between GH secretion, more presently - between the results of GHST and IGF-I levels were assessed in numerous studies. Unfortunately, their results are incoherent, either confirming [9-12] or denying [13-16] the correlation between GH peak in GHST and IGF-I secretion. In 2005, Cianfarani et al. [3] stated that IGF-I concentrations were reliable indicators of daily GH secretion, due to their GH dependency and relative stability in circulation. Similar were the results of much earlier observations of Rosenfeld et al. [17] and Shalet et al. [18]. In one of our previous studies [19], the stability of IGF-I concentration was also proved, despite divergent results of the repeated GHST.

Taking into account all the doubts concerning diagnosing GHD in children, it seems purposeful to search for other indices that could be helpful in the evaluation of GH secretory status. Particularly, further studies on determining the significance of both GHST and IGF-I assessment among the diagnostic procedures seem promising.

The relationships between GH secretion and thyroid function, as well as GH influence on the peripheral thyroxine ($T_4$) to triiodothyronine ($T_3$) deiodination were identified during the observations of patients with GHD, either untreated or subjected to GH therapy. The first studies, carried out about 30 years ago, revealed an increase of $T_4$ to $T_3$ conversion, leading to an increase of extrathyroidal $T_3$ concentration, together with a decrease of $T_4$ concentration during GH administration [20,21]. These observations were also confirmed by the results of subsequent studies. In 1989, Jørgensen et al. [22] confirmed the observation that GH replacement induced an enhancement of $T_4$ to $T_3$ deiodination. In 1994, the same research group [23] demonstrated that in the adult patients with GHD the levels of $T_3$ remained decreased, even in the course of $T_4$ substitution, while normalizing during GH replacement therapy (parallel to the decrease of TSH levels). The key role of IGF-I in stimulating the process of $T_4$ to $T_3$ deiodination was also suggested by Jørgensen et al. [24].

On the other hand, the influence of thyroid function disorders on GH secretion, as well as on IGF system, was also described. Thus, it was shown that hypothyroidism (HypoT) - even in its subclinical form - might affect IGF-I secretion [25]. Moreover, it was previously supposed that the effects of thyroid hormone on IGF-I secretion could be independent from GH mediation [26,27]. In particular, a significant decrease of IGF-I and IGF binding protein-3 (IGFBP-3) concentrations was documented in the patients with HypoT, both in adults [28] and in children [29]. Furthermore, it was shown that $T_4$ replacement therapy improved the previously decreased GH and IGF-I secretion, however, with no complete recovery [30].

As it was mentioned before, a decrease of $T_4$ to $T_3$ deiodination, leading to the decrease of $T_3$ concentration with reference to $T_4$ level, should be observed in GH-deficient patients. Ceratinly, the individual variances of the thyroid function or/and in the activity of peripheral deiodinases must also be taken into account. Nevertheless, it seems that in the study including large groups of patients, the clear differences between GH-deficient and non-GH-deficient subjects should be identified.

The aim of current study was to compare the selected indices of thyroid function in children with short stature, diagnosed towards GHD, with reference to both the results of GHST and IGF-I secretion. In fact, we expected to reveal the differences between the groups with either normal or subnormal results of GHST and/or between those with either normal or decreased IGF-I levels, as since such observations could contribute to optimizing the assessment of GH secretory status in children with short stature.

## Methods

The retrospective analysis comprised 800 children (541 boys, 259 girls), age 11.6 ± 3.1 years (mean ± SD), with short stature (*i.e.*, patient's height below 3rd centile for age and sex), diagnosed at our Department (2001-2010). All the children underwent the following diagnostic procedures:

- patients' height was measured on admission to the hospital and was expressed as height SDS (hSDS) for age and sex for Polish children [31]; taking into account the normal distribution of heights in the population of children, an exact value -1.88 was assumed as hSDS for 3rd centile;
- two (2) GHST were performed in children admitted to the hospital, remaining fasting, in the morning hours. For stimulation, clonidine in a dose of 0.15 mg/m$^2$ *p.o.* (1st test), and glucagon in a dose of 30 µg/kg *i.m.*, not exceeding 1 mg (2nd test) were used. Blood samples for GH estimation were collected every 30 min from 0 to 120 min in the tests with clonidine and at 0, 90, 120, 150 and 180 min in the test with glucagon;
- serum IGF-I, free $T_4$ ($FT_4$), free $T_3$ ($FT_3$) and TSH concentrations were measured in single blood samples, obtained in 0 min of 1st stimulating test, just before clonidine administration.

The main assumption of the study was to include the patients either with ISS or with isolated non-acquired GHD only. In order to avoid the possible influence of disorders of thyroid function on GH and/or IGF-I secretion and action, only the children with values of TSH, $FT_4$, and $FT_3$ concentrations within the reference range were included into the analysis. The exclusion criteria encompassed any chronic diseases, other hormonal deficiencies, acquired GHD, Turner syndrome in girls, other genetically determined syndromes, malnutrition and obesity (assessed as body mass index either below or over the reference range respectively for age and sex [31]).

The concentrations of GH were measured by the two-site chemiluminescent enzyme immunometric assay (hGH IMMULITE, DPC) for the quantitative measurement of human GH, calibrated to WHO IRP 80/505 standard. The analytical sensitivity of the assay was up to 0.01 ng/ml, the calibration range up to 40 ng/ml, the sensitivity of 0.01 ng/ml, the intra-assay coefficient of variation (CV) of 5.3-6.5% and the inter-assay CV of 5.5-6.2%. The cut-off value for normal and subnormal GH peak in response to stimulation was 10.0 ng/ml according to current recommendations [1,2].

Serum IGF-I concentrations were assessed by Immulite, DPC assays; WHO NIBSC 1st IRR 87/518 standard was applied, with analytical sensitivity 20 ng/ml, calibration range up to 1600 ng/ml, intra-assay CV - 3.1-4.3% and inter-assay CV - 5.8-8.4%. For comparison among children of different age and sex, IGF-I concentrations were expressed as IGF-I SDS, according to DPC reference data. As it was stated before, IGF-I values higher than -1.0 SD reflected a normal GH secretion [3]. Thus, we decided to select just that threshold value as the cut-off level for normal and decreased IGF-I secretion in our study.

Serum TSH, $FT_4$ and $FT_3$ concentrations were measured by the electroimmunochemiluminescent method (ECLIA), Roche, Elecsys®Systems 1010/2010/modular analytics E170. For TSH, the analytical sensitivity was 0.005 µIU/ml, range - up to 100 µIU/ml, intra-assay coefficient of variance (CV) - 1.5-8.6%, accuracy - 1.1-3.0%. The analytical range for $FT_4$ was 0.023-7.77 ng/ml, intra-assay CV - 1.4-2.9%, accuracy - 2.7-6.6%. For $FT_3$, the analytical range was 0.26-32.55 pg/ml, intra-assay CV - 3.7-9.5%, accuracy - 3.8-11.2%. For the assessment of $FT_3/FT_4$ molar ratio, the concentrations of $FT_4$ and $FT_3$ were expressed as molar ones.

According to the results of GHST (normal or subnormal) and to IGF-I secretion (normal or decreased), the patients were qualified to the following groups:

- **GHD** - the patients with decreased both GH peak in GHST and IGF-I SDS (n = 81);
- **ISS** - the patients with normal both the results of GHST and IGF-I SDS (n = 347);
- **low GH** - the patients with normal IGF-I SDS, despite decreased GH peak in GHST (n = 212);
- **low IGF** - the patients with decreased IGF-I SDS, despite normal GH peak in GHST (n = 160).

The analysis of the relationships between the components of somatotrophic axis (the results of GHST, IGF-I concentration) and the components of the pituitary - thyroid axis (TSH, $FT_4$ and $FT_3$ concentrations) were assessed. Statistical analysis included Kruskal-Wallis' nonparametric test for independent samples, as well as the assessment of correlations between patient's height and the results of particular hormonal tests.

## Results

The deficit of height (expressed as hSDS for age and sex) proved to be the most expressed in **low IGF Group** (*i.e.* in the patients with low IGF-I and normal GH peak in GHST), being significantly lower than that in both **ISS Group** ($p < 0.001$) and **low GH Group** ($p < 0.001$), as well as than that in **GHD Group** ($p = 0.031$). Interestingly, both the mean value and the distribution of hSDS values in **ISS Group** and in **low GH Group** (*i.e.* in the groups of patients with normal IGF-I secretion) were similar, despite completely different results of GHST in them. Moreover, hSDS values in these groups were also higher than those in the groups with decreased IGF-I, *i.e.* **GHD Group** and **low IGF Group** (also independently of the results of GHST).

The levels of TSH were also very similar in **ISS Group** and in **low GH Group**, being - at the same time - lower than both in **GHD Group** (the differences insignificant - NS) and than in **low IGF Group** (NS and p = 0.032, respectively), while the difference between **GHD Group** and **low IGF Group** was insignificant.

Moreover, $FT_4$ concentrations turned out to be very similar in **ISS Group** and in **low GH Group**, being also significantly lower than both in **GHD Group** ($p < 0.001$ and $p = 0.002$, respectively) and in **low IGF Group** ($p < 0.001$ for both pairs compared).

Interestingly, there was no significant difference in $FT_3$ concentrations between **ISS Group** and **low GH Group**, while in these two groups, $FT_3$ concentrations were significantly higher than those in both **GHD Group** ($p = 0.012$ and $p = 0.010$, respectively) and **low IGF Group** ($p = 0.001$ for both pairs compared). The difference between **GHD Group** and **low IGF Group** did not reach the border of significance.

Finally, $FT_3/FT_4$ molar ratio was similar in **ISS Group** and **low GH Group**, being - in these two groups - significantly higher ($p < 0.0001$) than those in **GHD Group** and in **low IGF Group**, while the difference between the latter two groups was also insignificant. More detailed data, are presented Table 1 and Figures 1, 2, 3, 4 and 5.

Summing up, in groups of patients with decreased IGF-I concentrations (*i.e.* in **GHD Group** and in **low IGF Group**), the more severe deficit of height was observed, together with higher TSH and $FT_4$ levels but lower $FT_3$ concentrations than those in groups with normal IGF-I concentrations (*i.e.* in **ISS Group** and in **low GH Group**). All the assessed parameters of thyroid function presented similar in the two groups with decreased IGF-I secretion (*i.e.* **GHD Group** and **low IGF Group**). There were no important differences between groups with normal IGF-I levels (*i.e.* **ISS Group** and **low GH Group**).

As a matter of fact, there were no strong correlations between the assessed indices of thyroid function (TSH, free thyroid hormones) and the parameters of somatotrophic axis (GH peak in GHST, IGF-I). However, a significant, positive correlation was found between patients' hSDS and IGF-I SDS ($r = 0.25$, $p < 0.05$), while there was no correlation between hSDS and GH peak in GHST ($r = 0.03$, NS). A positive correlation was also observed between IGF-I SDS and $FT_3$ concentration ($r = 0.24$, $p < 0.05$), together with a negative one between IGF-I SDS and $FT_4$ ($r = -0.20$, $p < 0.05$) and with no correlation between IGF-I SDS and TSH level ($r = -0.06$, NS). Thus, the observed correlations seem to be independent from TSH level, while an increase of IGF-I concentration may be related to the increase of $FT_3$ and decrease of $FT_4$. Moreover, there was no correlation between GH peak and any of the parameters analyzed. Detailed data are shown in Table 2.

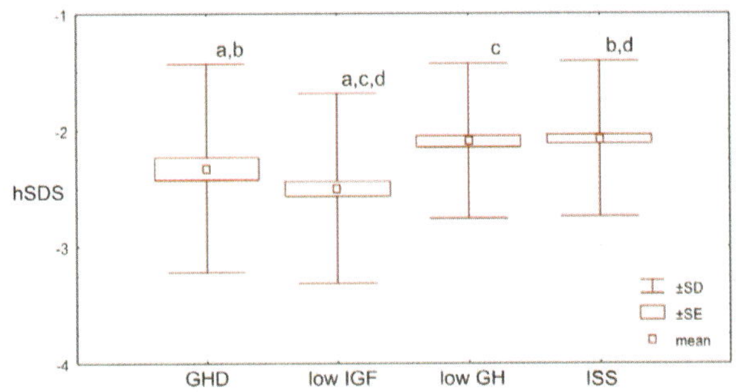


**Figure 1 Patients' height (expressed as hSDS) in particular groups of children**. Significant differences: a,b - $p < 0.05$; c,d - $p < 0.001$.

## Discussion

In our study, groups with decreased IGF-I levels (*i.e.*, GHD Group and low IGF-I Group) presented with the relatively higher TSH and $FT_4$ but lower $FT_3$ concentrations than those with normal IGF-I secretion, independently from either subnormal or normal GH peak in GHST. It should be recalled that GHD leads to the decrease of peripheral $T_4$ to $T_3$ deiodination [20-23]. Thus, the observed lower $FT_3$ concentrations in both

**Table 1 Patients' height and thyroid function in particular groups of children**

| Group | GHD | low IGF-I | low GH | ISS |
|---|---|---|---|---|
| **max GH** [ng/ml] | < 10 ng/ml | ≥10 ng/ml | < 10 ng/ml | ≥10 ng/ml |
| **IGF-I SDS** | < -1.0 | < -1.0 | ≥-1.0 | ≥-1.0 |
| **hSDS** for age and sex | -2.31 ± 0.88 [a,b] | -2.50 ± 0.81 [a,c,d] | -2.10 ± 0.66 [c] | -2.08 ± 0.67 [b,d] |
| **TSH** [mIU/l] | 2.33 ± 1.27 | 2.40 ± 1.01 [e] | 2.17 ± 0.75 [e] | 2.17 ± 1.08 |
| **$FT_4$** [ng/dl] | 1.25 ± 0.23 [f,g] | 1.28 ± 0.23 [h,i] | 1.16 ± 0.20 [f,h] | 1.17 ± 0.24 [g,i] |
| **$FT_3$** [pg/ml] | 4.03 ± 0.83 [j,k] | 4.09 ± 0.80 [l,m] | 4.44 ± 0.80 [j,l] | 4.35 ± 0.74 [k,m] |
| **$FT_3/FT_4$** [molar ratio] | 0.40 ± 0.11 [n,o] | 0.39 ± 0.10 [p,r] | 0.48 ± 0.14 [n,p] | 0.46 ± 0.12 [o,r] |

Significant differences: a,b - $p < 0.05$; c,d - $p < 0.001$; e-$p < 0.05$; f-$p < 0.005$; g,h,i,j - $p < 0.01$; k,l,m - $p < 0.001$; n,o,p,r - $p < 0.0001$.

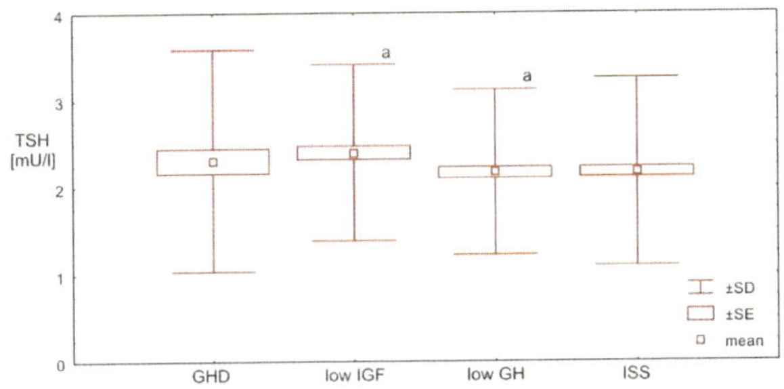


**Figure 2** TSH secretion in particular groups of patients. Significant difference: a - $p < 0.05$.

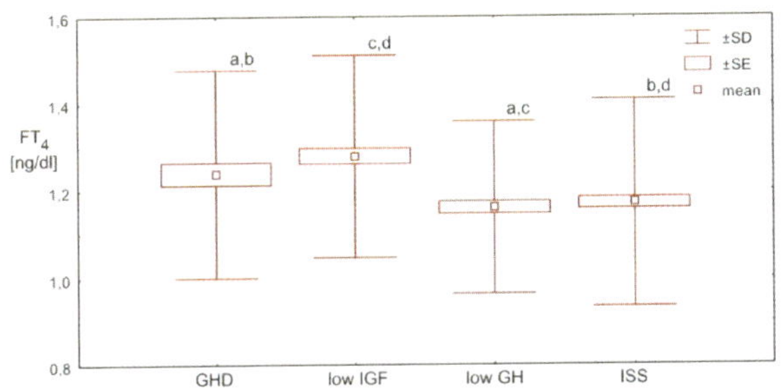


**Figure 3** $FT_4$ secretion in particular groups of patients. Significant differences: a - $p < 0.005$; b,c,d - $p < 0.01$.

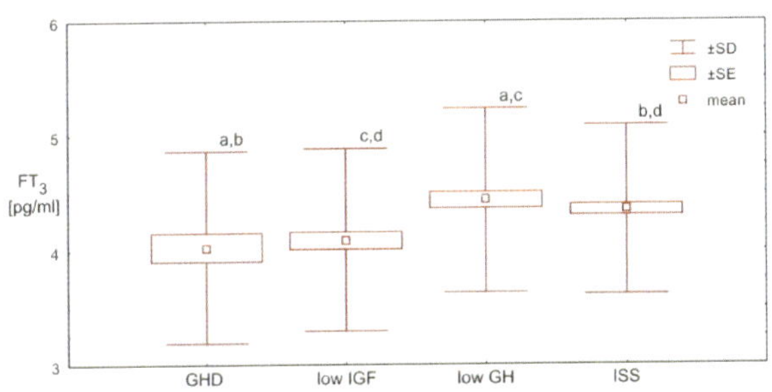


**Figure 4** $FT_3$ concentrations in particular groups of patients. Significant differences: a - $p < 0.01$; b,c,d - $p < 0.001$.

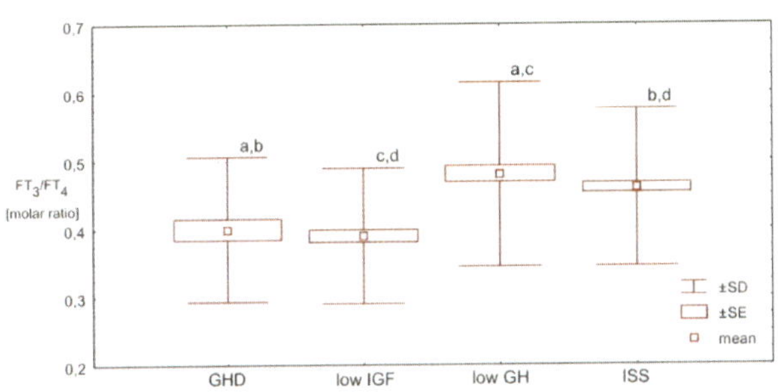


**Figure 5** Molar ratio $FT_3/FT_4$ in particular groups of patients. Significant differences: a,b,c,d - $p < 0.0001$.

**Table 2 Correlations between the indices of thyroid function and the components of somatotrophic axis**

| | hSDS | GH peak [ng/ml] | IGF-I SDS | TSH [mIU/l] | $FT_4$ [ng/dl] | $FT_3$ [pg/ml] |
|---|---|---|---|---|---|---|
| **hSDS** | | 0.03 | **0.25*** | -0.05 | 0.05 | 0.13* |
| **GH peak** [ng/ml] | 0.03 | | 0.12* | 0.01 | 0.12* | 0.00 |
| **IGF-ISDS** | **0.25*** | 0.12* | | -0.06 | **-0.20*** | **0.24*** |
| **TSH** [mIU/l] | -0.05 | 0.01 | -0.06 | | 0.12* | 0.10* |
| **$FT_4$** [ng/dl] | 0.05 | 0.12* | **-0.20*** | 0.12* | | 0.03 |
| **$FT_3$** [pg/ml] | 0.13* | 0.00 | **0.24*** | 0.10* | 0.03 | |

Correlations marked * are significant ($p < 0.05$).

groups with decreased IGF-I, despite even higher $FT_4$ levels in them seem to correspond with GHD in these patients. Moreover, the very similar $FT_4$, $FT_3$ and TSH concentrations in both groups with normal IGF-I levels (*i.e.*, in ISS Group and low GH Group), independently from either normal or subnormal results of GHST, should be stressed. We are convinced that these observations speak against the disorders of thyroid function related to GHD in both groups with normal IGF-I secretion, especially since we certainly do not expect such disorders in patients with ISS.

According to previous suggestions that IGF-I may be a mediator of GH action on stimulating peripheral $T_4$ deiodination [24], the results of current study seem quite reliable. The quoted observation allows to explain the results obtained in GHD Group, ISS Group, and - to some extent - in low IGF Group. In fact, in the latter group, either decreased GH sensitivity or other completely overlooked diseases, present in most of children, should be assumed as the only possible cause of decreased IGF-I secretion. Taking into account both the relatively low incidence of GH insensitivity and the exclusion criteria, such possibility seems, however, poorly justified. Next, the results, obtained in low GH Group do not seem to be explained by anything - except for the falsely positive (*i.e.*, falsely decreased) GH peaks in both performed GHST. In these patients, not only IGF-I concentrations are normal but also they correspond to the similar thyroid status as we observed in ISS Group.

As it was mentioned before, the discrepancies between the results of GHST and IGF-I secretion were reported in numerous studies [9-12], being explained either by the individual differences in GH sensitivity [32] or by the lack of concordance between GH secretion under physiological conditions and the results of GHST [33-35]. The conclusions, derived from these observations were also non-consistent. For instance, Rasat et al. [36] proposed IGF-I assessment as a screening procedure in diagnosing GHD. Similar was the statement of

Rosenfeld [37-39]. However, there is also a strong evidence that it may be impossible to predict the results of GHST on the ground of IGF-I concentration [9,12-14,16,40-42]. It seems very important to adequately answer the question, which (if any) of these procedures is the most reliable one in GHD diagnosing. According to current recommendations [1,2], GHST are the main tools for the assessment of GH secretion. However, some other options were also proposed. Thus, Badaru and Wilson [43] stated that IGF-I assessment had of no less importance than the results of GHST. Similarly, Loche at al. [7] suggested that the diagnosis of GHD should not exclusively be based on the results of GHST. In 2009, Lemaire et al. [44] proposed the assessment of growth rate and IGF-I concentration as the screening procedures in children suspected for GHD, in order to reduce the necessity of subjecting the patients to GHST. The results of our previous studies [19,45] also speak for the significance of IGF-I assessment in GHD diagnosing, thus bringing into question the credibility of GHST.

Another issue, however not analyzed in the current study, is an assessment of spontaneous GH secretion. Although - up to now - this procedure has not been recommended for clinical practice according to international guidelines [2], the data exist that GH administration to short children with decreased stimulated but normal spontaneous GH secretion is not associated with an increase of final height [46]. It seems that not only decreased spontaneous GH secretion should be taken into account in short children with low IGF-I concentrations (leading to the diagnosis of neurosecretory dysfunction) but also normal spontaneous GH secretion must be considered in the patients with normal IGF-I levels, despite decreased GH peak in GHST. It should also be taken into account that the relatively high incidence of falsely positive results of the two (2) GHST, performed in an individual patient was revealed in one of our previous studies [47]. As in Poland the assessment of spontaneous GH secretion after falling asleep was introduced as an obligatory procedure (screening) in diagnosing GHD in children, our research team intends to assess prospectively both IGF-I secretion and thyroid function with respect to nocturnal GH secretion.

## Conclusion

It seems that the assessment of thyroid function, while diagnosing GHD in children with short stature, provides the evidence that IGF-I concentration may be no less reliable indicator of GH action than the results of GHST, at least in children suspected for idiopathic, isolated GHD and after exclusion of other causes of impaired IGF-I secretion.

### Abbreviations

CV: coefficient of variation; $FT_4$: free thyroxine; $FT_3$: free triiodothyronine; GH: growth hormone; GHD: growth hormone deficiency; GHST: growth hormone stimulating tests; hSDS: height standard deviation score; Hypo-T: hypothyroidism; IGF-I: insulin-like growth factor-I; IGFBP-3: insulin-like growth factors binding protein-3; ISS: idiopathic short stature; SD: standard deviation; SDS: standard deviation score; $T_4$: thyroxine; $T_3$: triiodotyronine; TSH: thyroid stimulating hormone (thyrotropin)

### Author details

[1]Department of Pediatric Endocrinology, Medical University of Lodz, Lodz, Poland. [2]Department of Endocrinology and Metabolic Diseases, Medical University of Lodz, Lodz, Poland. [3]Department of Endocrinology and Metabolic Diseases, Polish Mother's Memorial Hospital - Research Institute in Lodz, Poland.

### Authors' contributions

JS designed the study, qualified the patients and performed statistical analysis. RS participated in performing hormonal studies and in statistical analysis. AL participated in drawing up the study protocol and coordinated the study. MH, the senior author, wrote the manuscript. All authors read and approved the final manuscript

### Competing interests

The authors declare that they have no competing interests.

### References

1. Saggese G, Ranke MB, Saenger P, Rosenfeld RG, Tanaka T, Chaussain JL, Savage MO: **Diagnosis and treatment of growth hormone deficiency in children and adolescents: towards a consensus.** *Horm Res* 1998, **50**:320-340.
2. GH Research Society: **Consensus guidelines for the diagnosis and treatment of growth hormone deficiency in childhood and adolescence: summary statement of the GH Research Society.** *J Clin Endocrinol Metab* 2000, **85**:3990-3993.
3. Cianfarani S, Liguori A, Germani D: **IGF-I and IGFBP-3 assessment in the management of childhood onset growth hormone deficiency.** *Endocr Dev* 2005, **9**:66-75.
4. Rosenfeld RG, Albertsson-Wikland K, Cassorla F, Frasier SD, Hasegawa Y, Hintz RL, Lafranch S, Lippe B, Loriaux L, Melmed S, Preece MA, Ranke MB, Reiter EO, Rogol AD, Underwood LE, Werther GA: **Diagnostic controversy: the diagnosis of childhood growth hormone deficiency revisited.** *J Clin Endocrinol Metab* 1995, **80**:1532-1540.
5. Price DA: **GH testing in KIGS: the clinical reality.** In *Growth Hormone Therapy in KIGS - 10 Years' Experience.* Edited by: Ranke MB, Wilton P. Johann Ambrosius Barth Verlag, Leipzig, Hiedelberg; 1999:73-80.
6. Zadik Z, Chalew SA, Gilula Z, Kowarski AA: **Reproducibility of growth hormone testing procedures: a comparison between 24-hour integrated concentration and pharmacological stimulation.** *J Clin Endocrinol Metab* 1990, **71**:1127-1130.
7. Loche S, Bizzarri C, Maghine M, Faedda A, Tziala C, Autelli M, Casini MR, Cappa M: **Results of early reevaluation of growth hormone secretion in children with apparent growth hormone deficiency.** *J Pediatr* 2002, **140**:445-449.
8. Thomas M, Massa G, Maes M, Beckers D, Craen M, Francois I, Heinrichs C, Bourguignon JP, Belgian Study Group for Paediatric Endocrinology (BSGPE): **Growth hormone (GH) secretion in patients with childhood-onset GH deficiency: retesting after one year of therapy and at final height.** *Horm Res* 2003, **59**:7-15.
9. Rosenfeld RG, Wilson DM, Lee PD, Hintz RL: **Insulin-like growth factors I and II in evaluation of growth retardation.** *J Pediatr* 1986, **109**:428-433.
10. Nunez SB, Municchi G, Barnes KM, Rose SR: **Insulin-like growth factor I (IGF-I) and IGF-binding protein-3 concentrations compared to stimulated and night growth hormone in the evaluation of short children - a clinical research center study.** *J Clin Endocrinol Metab* 1996, **81**:1927-1932.
11. Koch A, Dorr HG: **Insulin-like growth factor-I and its binding protein-3 in serum: are they good screening properties for the diagnosis of growth hormone deficiency?** *Eur J Clin Chem Clin Biochem* 1997, **35**:379-385.

12. Tillmann V, Buckler JM, Kibirige MS, Price DA, Shalet SM, Wales JK, Addison MG, Gill MS, Whatmore AJ, Clayton PE: Biochemical tests in the diagnosis of childhood growth hormone deficiency. *J Clin Endocrinol Metab* 1997, **82**:531-535.
13. Hindmarsh PC, Swift PGF: An assessment of growth hormone provocation tests. *Arch Dis Child* 1995, **72**:362-368.
14. Mitchell H, Dattani V, Nanduri P, Hindmarsh PC, Preece MA, Brook CDG: Failure of IGF-I and IGFBP-3 to diagnose growth hormone insufficiency. *Arch Dis Child* 1999, **80**:443-447.
15. Bouquete HR, Sobrado PG, Fideleff HL, Sequera AM, Giaccio AV, Suarez MG, Rubial GF, Miras M: Evaluation of diagnostic accuracy of insulin-like growth factor (IGF)-I and IGF-binding protein-3 in growth hormone-deficient children and adults using ROC plot analysis. *J Clin Endocrinol Metab* 2003, **88**:4702-4708.
16. Haghshenas Z, Sotoudeh K, Karamifar H, Karamizadeh Z, Amirhakimi G: The role of insulin like growth factor (IGF)-1 and IGF-binding protein-3 in diagnosis of Growth Hormone Deficiency in short stature children. *Indian J Pediatr* 2009, **76**:699-703.
17. Rosenfeld RG, Lamson G, Pham H, Oh Y, Conover C, De-Leon DD, Donovan SM, Ocrant I, Guidice L: Insulin-like growth factor binding proteins. *Recent Prog Horm Res* 1990, **46**:99-164.
18. Shalet SM, Toogood A, Rahim A, Brennan BMD: The diagnosis of growth hormone deficiency in children and adults. *Endocrine Rev* 1998, **19**:203-223.
19. Hilczer M, Smyczynska J, Stawerska R, Lewinski A: Stability of IGF-I concentration despite divergent results of repeated GH stimulating tests indicates poor reproducibility of test results. *Endocr Regul* 2006, **40**:37-45.
20. Gács G, Bános C: The effect of growth hormone on the plasma levels of T4, free-T4, T3, reverse T3 an TBG in hypopituitary patients. *Acta Endocrinol (Copenh)* 1981, **96**:475-479.
21. Rezvani I, DiGeorge AM, Dowshen SA, Bourdony CJ: Action of human growth hormone (hGH) on extrathyroidal conversion of thyroxine (T4) to triiodothyronine (T3) in children with hypopituitarism. *Pediatr Res* 1981, **15**:6-9.
22. Jørgensen JO, Pedersen SA, Laurberg P, Weeke J, Skakkebaek NE, Christiansen JS: Effects of growth hormone therapy on thyroid function of growth hormone-deficient adults with and without concomitant thyroxine-substituted central hypothyroidism. *J Clin Endocrinol Metab* 1989, **69**:1127-1132.
23. Jørgensen JO, Møller J, Laursen T, Orskov H, Christiansen JS, Weeke J: Growth hormone administration stimulates energy expenditure and extrathyroidal conversion of thyroxine to triiodothyronine in a dose-dependent manner and suppresses circadian thyrotrophin levels: studies in GH-deficient adults. *Clin Endocrinol (Oxf)* 1994, **41**:609-614.
24. Jørgensen JO, Møller J, Skakkebaek NE, Weeke J, Christiansen JS: Thyroid function during growth hormone therapy. *Horm Res* 1992, **38(Suppl 1)**:63-67.
25. Akin F, Yaylali GF, Turgut S, Kaptanoglu B: Growth hormone/insulin-like growth factor axis in patients with subclinical thyroid dysfunction. *Growth Horm IGF Res* 2009, **19**:252-255.
26. Näntö-Salonen K, Muller HL, Hoffman AR, Vu TH, Rosenfeld RG: Mechanisms of thyroid hormone action on the insulin-like growth factor system: all thyroid hormone effects are not growth hormone mediated. *Endocrinology* 1993, **132**:781-788.
27. Inukai T, Takanashi K, Takebayashi K, Fujiwara Y, Tayama K, Takemura Y: Thyroid hormone modulates insulin-like growth factor-I(IGF-I) and IGF-binding protein-3, without mediation by growth hormone, in patients with autoimmune thyroid diseases. *Horm Metab Res* 1999, **31**:576-579.
28. Iglesias P, Bayón C, Méndez J, Gancedo PG, Grande C, Diez JJ: Serum insulin-like growth factor type 1, insulin-like growth factor-binding protein-1, and insulin-like growth factor-binding protein-3 concentrations in patients with thyroid dysfunction. *Thyroid* 2001, **11**:1043-1048.
29. Purandare A, Co Ng L, Godil M, Ahnn SH, Wilson TA: Effect of hypothyroidism and its treatment on the IGF system in infants and children. *J Pediatr Endocrinol Metab* 2003, **16**:35-42.
30. Soliman AT, Omar M, El Awwa A, Rizk MM, El Alaily RK, Bedair EM: Linear growth, growth-hormone secretion and IGF-I generation in children with neglected hypothyroidism before and after thyroxine replacement. *J Trop Pediatr* 2008, **54**:347-349.
31. Palczewska I, Niedźwiecka Z: Indices of somatic development of Warsaw children and adolescents. *Medycyna Wieku Rozwojowego* 2001, **5(suppl. I/2)**:17-118, (in Polish).
32. Clayton PE: The Role of Insulin-Like Growth Factors in the Diagnosis of Growth Hormone Deficiency. In *Growth Hormone Therapy in KIGS - 10 Years' Experience.* Edited by: Ranke MB, Wilton P. Johann Ambrosius Barth Verlag, Leipzig, Hiedelberg; 1999:53-64.
33. Bercu BB, Schulman D, Root AW, Spiliotis BE: Growth hormone provocative testing frequently does not reflect endogenous GH secretion. *J Clin Endocrinol Metab* 1986, **63**:709-716.
34. Donaldson DL, Pan F, Hollowell JG, Stevenson JL, Gifford RA, Moore WV: Reliability of stimulated and spontaneous growth hormone levels in identifying the child with low GH secretion. *J Clin Endocrinol Metab* 1991, **72**:647-652.
35. Ropelato MG, Martinez A, Heinrich JJ, Bergada C: Reproducibility of growth hormone secretion tests. *J Pediatr Endocrinol Metab* 1996, **9**:41-50.
36. Rasat R, Livesey JL, Espiner EA, Abbott D, Donald RA: IGF-1 and IGFBP-3 screening for disorders of growth hormone secretion. *N Z Med J* 1996, **109**:156-159.
37. Rosenfeld RG: Biochemical diagnostic strategies in the evaluation of short stature: the diagnosis of insulin-like growth factor deficiency. *Horm Res* 1996, **46**:170-173.
38. Rosenfeld RG: An endocrinologist's approach to the growth hormone - insulin-like growth factor axis. *Acta Paediatr Suppl* 1997, **423**:17-19.
39. Rosenfeld RG: Editorial: Is growth hormone deficiency a viable diagnosis? *J Clin Endocrinol Metab* 1997, **82**:349-351.
40. Juul A, Dalgaard P, Blum WF, Bang P, Hall K, Michaelsen KF, Müller J, Skakkebaek N: Serum levels of insulin-like growth factor (IGF) binding protein 3 (IGFBP-3) in healthy infants, children and adolescents: the relation to IGF-I, IGF-II, IGFBP-1, IGFBP-2, age, sex, body mass index, and pubertal maturation. *J Clin Endocrinol Metab* 1995, **80**:2534-2542.
41. Ranke MB, Schweitzer R, Elmlinger MW, Weber K, Binder G, Schwarze CP, Wollmann HA: Significance of basal IGF-I, IGFBP-3 and IGFBP-2 measurements in the diagnostics of short stature in children. *Horm Res* 2000, **54**:60-68.
42. Bouquete HR, Sobrado PG, Fideleff HL, Sequera AM, Giaccio AV, Suarez MG, Rubial GF, Miras M: Evaluation of diagnostic accuracy of insulin-like growth factor (IGF)-I and IGF-binding protein-3 in growth hormone-deficient children and adults using ROC plot analysis. *J Clin Endocrinol Metab* 2003, **88**:4702-4708.
43. Badaru A, Wilson DM: Alternatives to growth hormone stimulation testing in children. *Trends Endocrinol Metab* 2004, **15**:252-258.
44. Lemaire P, Brauner N, Hammer P, Trivin C, Souberbielle JC, Brauner R: Improved screening for growth hormone deficiency using logical analysis data. *Med Sci Monit* 2009, **15**:5-10.
45. Smyczyńska J, Lewiński A, Hilczer M, Stawerska R, Karasek M: Partial growth hormone deficiency (GHD) in children has more similarities to idiopathic short stature than to severe GHD. *Endokrynol Pol - Pol J Endocr* 2007, **58**:182-187.
46. Radetti G, Buzi F, Cassar W, Paganini C, Stacul E, Maghnie M: Growth hormone secretory pattern and response to treatment in children with short stature followed to adult height. *Clin Endocrinol (Oxf)* 2003, **59**:27-33.
47. Hilczer M, Smyczyńska J, Lewinski A: Limitations of clinical utility of growth hormone stimulating tests in diagnosing children with short stature. *Endocr Reg* 2006, **40**:69-75.

# 4

# Factors determining the persistence or recurrence of well-differentiated thyroid cancer treated by thyroidectomy and/or radioiodine in the Boston, Massachusetts area: A retrospective chart review

Angela M Leung[1,3*], Shalini Dave[2], Stephanie L Lee[1,3], Francis X Campion[4], Jeffrey R Garber[3,5] and Elizabeth N Pearce[1,3]


## Abstract

**Objective:** To assess predictors of well-differentiated thyroid cancer (WDTC) persistence/recurrence.

**Design:** This was a retrospective chart review of thyroid carcinoma patients seen 1979-2007 in a Boston, Massachusetts-area multispecialty group. Of 1,025 patients, 431 met eligibility criteria. Cox proportional hazards models were used to assess predictors (gender, age, ethnicity, tumor size, surgical histology) of WDTC persistence/recurrence (elevated thyroglobulin levels with negative thyroglobulin-antibodies; or positive imaging). Local extension of disease and lymph node involvement could not be assessed.

**Results:** Mean age at initial surgery (n = 431, 74% women, 79% Caucasian) was 45.8 ± 13.5(SD) years. Mean tumor (papillary, 91%; follicular, 5%; Hurthle cell, 2%; ≥1 type, 2%) size was 2.5 ± 1.6(SD) cm. Most tumors were unifocal (57%) and ≥1 cm (89%). Over 2,600 person-years of follow-up, persistence/recurrence occurred in 52 patients (12%) 4.3 years (median; range 0.2-23.2 years) after surgery. Gender, ethnicity, tumor size, multifocality, and histology were not predictive of persistence/recurrence, while older age was predictive in some models.

**Conclusions:** In WDTC patients treated by total and near total thyroidectomy and radioiodine and analyzed without consideration of local, locoregional, and distant extent of disease, neither size of tumor nor male gender contribute to disease persistence/recurrence. Age at diagnosis seems to have some positive prognostic value even if only patients older than 21 years at diagnosis are considered. Due to the rare occurrence of follicular (also oxyphilic) histotype, this conclusion refers mainly to patients with papillary thyroid cancer.


## Introduction

Many post-operative scoring systems have been proposed to predict outcomes of well-differentiated thyroid cancer (WDTC). The AMES criteria were developed in the late 1980s and examine age, distant metastasis, tumor extent, and tumor size to predict prognosis in patients with differentiated thyroid cancer [1]. Both the AGES system, which scores age, tumor size, histologic grade, tumor extent, and distant metastasis [2] and the MACIS system, which scores distant metastasis, age, completeness of primary tumor resection, local invasion, and tumor size [3] were established by Hay et al. in the late 1980s and early 1990s as prognostic scoring systems for patients with papillary thyroid cancer. In 1998, the Thyroid Cancer Treatment Cooperative Study Registry Group validated a clinicopathologic staging utilizing age at diagnosis, tumor histology, tumor size, intrathyroidal multifocality, extraglandular invasion, metastases, and tumor differentiation [4]. Finally, the TNM scoring system, which utilizes tumor size, lymph node involvement, and distant metastasis, was developed by the American Joint Committee on Cancer to provide a staging system for all malignancies, including differentiated thyroid cancers [5].

* Correspondence: angela.leung@bmc.org
[1]Section of Endocrinology, Diabetes, and Nutrition; Boston University School of Medicine; Boston, MA; USA
Full list of author information is available at the end of the article

The serum thyroglobulin (Tg) concentration is commonly used as a marker of thyroid tissue persistence/recurrence after near-total thyroidectomy in patients with negative Tg-antibody titers, with recombinant human thyroid stimulating hormone (rhTSH)-stimulated Tg levels >2.5 ng/mL as the optimal level for future recurrence [6]. It may remain elevated for several weeks or months after surgery, and its sensitivity is improved with post-operative remnant radioiodine ablation [7]. Although no single scoring system has been clearly superior, in part due to the differences used in the weighting and combinations of independent predictors, distant metastases, age of the patient, and extent of the tumor seem to be the most consistent predictors of persistent or recurrent disease [8].

Several retrospective analyses have assessed outcomes of low-risk thyroid cancer using these and other factors. In what eventually became the Ohio State University staging system for papillary or follicular thyroid carcinomas, Mazzaferri and Jhiang reported that in 1,355 patients with well-differentiated tumors ≥1.5 cm with or without local or lymph node spread followed over 40 years, near-total thyroidectomy followed by radioiodine ablation and TSH suppression therapy improves outcomes [9]. A review summarizing guidelines by the American Thyroid Association, which have recently been revised [8], the European Thyroid Association, and other recent literature has recommended that total or near-total thyroidectomy followed by remnant ablation is acceptable for those with low-risk papillary thyroid cancer, although surgery alone may be sufficient for some tumors removed incidentally during surgery for benign disease, in the absence of other concerning history [10]. Ongoing research is needed to help clarify the factors which best predict persistence or recurrence of well-differentiated thyroid cancer to guide short-term and long-term management.

The objective of this study was to test the hypothesis that certain patient-associated or tumor-associated factors predict well-differentiated thyroid cancer persistence or recurrence in a Boston, Massachusetts-area cohort of well-differentiated thyroid cancer patients treated with thyroidectomy and radioiodine over a 28-year period.

## Methods

### Study sample

A retrospective chart review was conducted of patients with well-differentiated thyroid cancer evaluated at all sites of a large Boston, Massachusetts-area multispecialty group practice (Harvard Vanguard Medical Associates, HVMA) between 1979 and 2007. Patients with ICD-9 code 193 (thyroid carcinoma) had been identified for a previously-created health quality assurance database at all HVMA sites between January 1979 and May 2007. Of the 1,025 individuals in the preexisting database, 65 were incorrectly coded as having thyroid cancer. Of the remaining 960 potentially eligible patients, 431 (45%) met study criteria and were enrolled in the study.

Inclusion criteria were: 1) at least age 21 at the time of thyroid surgery, 2) history of total or near-total thyroidectomy, 3) diagnosis of papillary, follicular, or Hurthle cell carcinoma by surgical pathology, 3) use of radioiodine ablation post-operatively, and 4) follow-up management within HVMA that included at least one serum thyroglobulin measurement, and/or imaging study by either radioiodine scan, neck ultrasonography, CT, MRI, or FDG-PET. Local extension of disease and lymph node involvement were not included due to the absence of these data in many patients who had their thyroid surgery by non-HVMA providers within the cohort. Exclusion criteria were: 1) medullary thyroid cancer, 2) anaplastic thyroid cancer, 3) incorrectly-coded ICD-9 diagnosis of thyroid cancer, 4) no documentation of thyroid cancer pathology, 5) positive thyroglobulin antibody titers (which make thyroglobulin results uninterpretable) without follow-up imaging, and 6) a positive thyroglobulin level within 6 months of thyroid surgery as the last known status. The date of the thyroid surgery was the entry point for the study. The protocol was approved by the Harvard Vanguard Institutional Review Board.

### Assessment of WDTC persistence or recurrence

Various factors assessing patient demographics and tumor characteristics were grouped to assess their predictive effects on WDTC persistence or recurrence. Gender, race, and age in years at thyroid surgery comprised the patient-associated factors. Tumor size in centimeters and histologic tumor type (e.g. papillary, follicular, Hurthle, or a combination of these) by surgical pathology report comprised the tumor-associated factors. Local extension of disease and lymph node involvement could not be assessed.

Based on the chart review, the persistence or recurrence of well-differentiated thyroid cancer, defined as the primary outcome, was determined at the final time point for which their status was known. For the purposes of this study, thyroid cancer persistence or recurrence were considered identical. Recurrence or persistence of tumor, following total thyroidectomy and radioiodine ablation, was defined as serum thyroglobulin levels greater than 0.5 μg/L (unstimulated) or >2 μg/L (following rhTSH stimulation or thyroid hormone withdrawal) with negative thyroglobulin antibodies [8]. Thyroglobulin measurements were performed using a chemiluminescence immunoassay (Immulite 2000, Diagnostics Products Corporation). Because an earlier chemiluminescence immunoassay assay used at HVMA had a lower limit of detection of 0.9 μg/L, an unstimulated thyroglobulin level of 0.9 μg/L or greater was used to define tumor recurrence in individuals whose most recent serum thyroglobulin was obtained prior to the assay change. Imaging modalities also used to define recurrence or persistence were whole body radioiodine scan with any positive uptake, a positive PET scan, and/or a positive neck ultrasound scan with confirmatory fine needle aspiration biopsy or surgical pathology of tissue sampled from the suspected site(s) of recurrence.

### Statistical analysis

This study was a retrospective chart review of a preexisting database, and therefore it was not powered for the primary outcome. Descriptive information is presented as frequencies and percentages for categorical variables and as means ± SD for continuous variables. Age was analyzed as a continuous variable in the primary analysis and dichotomized at 45 years for some of the secondary analyses in the Cox proportional hazard regression models. Tumor size was dichotomized at <1 cm and ≥ 1 cm. Secondary analyses included additional stratifications of tumor size at <1.5 cm and ≥ 1.5 cm, <2 cm and ≥ 2 cm, <3 cm and ≥ 3 cm, <4 cm and ≥ 4 cm; tumor size was also analyzed as a continuous measure. Differences between categorical variables were analyzed using the Chi-square test. Among subjects in whom either the month or date of thyroid surgery was undocumented (but for whom at least the year was recorded), the missing month was assigned as June and the date as the 15th of the month. Study entry was the date of surgery. Follow-up was accrued until the first occurrence of the primary outcome or the date of last contact.

Independent predictors were organized into two conceptual groups (patient-associated and tumor-associated predictors). Separately and together in a comprehensive model, Cox proportional hazards regression models and the appropriate tests for verifying the proportional hazards assumption were constructed to determine the associations of the independent predictors with the time to tumor persistence or recurrence. Person-time was computed to the first recurrence and was censored at the date of last contact. Models were adjusted for sex, race, and subjects' age at surgery. Potential confounders were assessed for as appropriate. A subset analysis of the two conceptual groups, again separately and together in a comprehensive model, was also performed excluding patients who had thyroid surgery prior to the start of the electronic database to minimize any selection bias due to subjects who may have died (from WDTC or otherwise) prior to the start of the study period.

P-values <0.05 were considered statistically significant. All statistical analyses were performed using SAS version 9.1 (SAS Institute, Cary, NC).

## Results

From the database of 1,025 patients, 431 met entry criteria. The 594 excluded patients were comprised of 220 patients who did not have a total or near-total thyroidectomy or postoperative radioiodine ablation (groups in whom Tg levels are difficult to interpret), 152 patients who had no laboratory results or imaging studies for thyroid cancer at least 6 months after thyroid surgery internally at HVMA, 68 patients who had benign thyroid disease or a non-thyroidal cancer, 52 patients who had no surgical pathology results in the HVMA database, 46 patients without a recorded year of surgery, 27 patients who were under age 21 at the time of surgery, 15 patients who had medullary thyroid carcinoma, 5 patients who had anaplastic thyroid carcinoma, 8 patients who had positive Tg-antibody titers without follow-up imaging, and 2 patients who were miscoded with an incorrect medical record number. Descriptive statistics of the study population are given in Table 1.

### Survival analysis

There were 2,600 total person-years of follow-up; 52 subjects (12%) had WDTC persistence/recurrence (Figure 1) at a median of 4.3 years (range 0.2-26.2; mean 6.1 ± 5.6 years) after thyroid surgery.

### Multivariate analyses of the full dataset

The Cox regression model of patient-associated predictors of disease persistence or recurrence was significant (p = 0.02), while that of tumor-associated predictors was not (p = 0.80). In a multivariable analysis (with sex, race, age at diagnosis, number of tumor foci, tumor size, and tumor histology as independent predictors), the comprehensive Cox regression model was predictive (p = 0.04) of disease persistence or recurrence, including older age as a significant independent predictor (p = 0.02). The comprehensive models predicting disease persistence or recurrence were also significant when tumor size was categorized into 4 groups (<1 cm, 1 to <2 cm, 2 to <3 cm, and ≥3 cm) (p = 0.04); dichotomized at 1.5 cm (p = 0.04), 2 cm (p = 0.04), 3 cm (p = 0.04), or 4 cm (p = 0.04); and when analyzed as a continuous measure (p = 0.04). Greater age as a continuous variable was weakly predictive of tumor persistence or recurrence, although this was not consistent across all models. A summary of the Cox regression models is presented in Table 2.

### Multivariate analyses after excluding subjects with thyroid surgery prior to 1979

A subset analysis was also performed to include only patients who had surgery after the start of the study period (January 1979) (n = 415). The Cox regression model of patient-associated factors was predictive (p = 0.03),

**Table 1 Subject demographics, tumor characteristics, and management factors**

| | n |
|---|---|
| ***Gender*** | |
| Male | 110 (26%) |
| Female | 321 (74%) |
| ***Race*** | |
| Caucasian | 280 (79%) |
| Black | 34 (10%) |
| Hispanic | 7 (2%) |
| Asian/Pacific Islander | 12 (3%) |
| Other | 21 (6%) |
| ***Age (years) at surgery*** | 45.8 (mean) ± 13.5 (SD) |
| ***Tumor size (cm)*** | 2.5 (mean) ± 1.6 (SD) (2.2 (median); range, 0.1-10.0 |
| ***Tumor size*** | |
| <1 cm | 39 (11%) |
| ≥1 cm | 329 (89%) |
| ***Tumor histology*** | |
| Papillary (PTC) | 388 (91%) |
| Follicular (FTC) | 20 (5%) |
| Both PTC and FTC | 6 (1%) |
| Hurthle cell carcinoma (HCC) | 9 (2%) |
| Both PTC and HCC | 4 (1%) |
| ***Number of tumor foci*** | |
| 1 | 213 (57%) |
| ≥2 | 161 (43%) |
| ***Thyroid cancer recurrence or persistence*** | |
| Yes | 52 (12%) |
| No | 379 (88%) |
| ***Positive disease on follow-up imaging*** | |
| Yes | 33 (9%) |
| No | 334 (91%) |
| ***Years after surgery at recurrence*** | 6.1 (mean) ± 5.6 (SD) 4.3 (median) 0.2-23.2 (range) |

* Total n for each descriptor may not equal 431 due to missing data, and total percentages may not equal 100 due to rounding.

and male gender was an independent positive significant predictor (HR 0.49; 95% CI, 0.25 to 0.95; p = 0.03). The regression model of tumor-associated factors was not predictive (p = 0.85). Similarly, using this restricted cohort, the multivariable analysis (with sex, race, age at diagnosis, number of tumors, tumor size, and tumor histology as independent predictors) were not predictive of disease persistence or recurrence (p = 0.06).

## Discussion

This retrospective analysis suggests that specific factors may predict disease persistence or recurrence in patients with well-differentiated thyroid carcinoma. The American Thyroid Association has recommended that follow-up treatment varies according to a patient's risk for recurrence [8], yet management, including the extent of surgery, necessity of post-operative ablative radioiodine, and degree of thyroid hormone suppression, has been controversial and practices are not uniform among clinicians.

An analysis of all patients with a history of WDTC in our database, regardless of the extent of surgery or use of radioiodine (n = 651), resulted in a persistence/recurrence rate of 20% (data not shown). While this is virtually identical to what was observed in a similar cohort assessed over 30 years by Mazzaferri and Jhiang (21%) [9], by restricting our analyses to patients who underwent a total or near-total thyroidectomy and radioiodine therapy, the rate dropped to 12%. Our Cox regression model of patient-associated factors and the global model were predictive of well-differentiated thyroid cancer persistence or recurrence, although the regression model of tumor-associated factors was not. Greater age as a continuous variable was a weakly predictive factor, but this was not consistent across all models.

Our analysis included only those who were alive at follow-up, and therefore loss of follow-up due to death [both disease-specific and all-cause mortality) was not ascertained. In addition, some subjects excluded due to the absence of thyroglobulin values or an imaging study within the HVMA database were managed by non-HVMA providers and were not available for this analysis. Finally, the unique demographics and socioeconomic status of this study population (e.g. predominantly Caucasian) may limit generalizability to other populations managed by clinicians experienced in thyroid cancer follow-up.

It is difficult to compare the relative predictive abilities of different models or staging systems, as the components in each are not uniform. Palme et al. reported that male sex, advanced initial stage, and presence of extrathyroidal spread were independent predictors of multiple recurrences of well-differentiated thyroid cancer [11]. In a recent retrospective review of papillary microcarcinoma (≤1 cm), Mercante et al. found that capsular invasion, extrathyroidal tumor extension, and neck lymph node metastasis at presentation were the only independent risk factors for the persistence or recurrence of disease [12]. In contrast to these and other studies [13,14], many of the subjects in our study received their surgery at a non-HVMA site, and thus, information regarding extrathyroidal spread was not codified in a uniform manner and could not be analyzed in our cohort. The inability to capture this information may have introduced a misclassification bias of patients' disease burden, thereby altering our findings. The use of a <1 cm cutoff for tumor size in our study (as compared to ≤1 cm) may also limit direct comparison of our

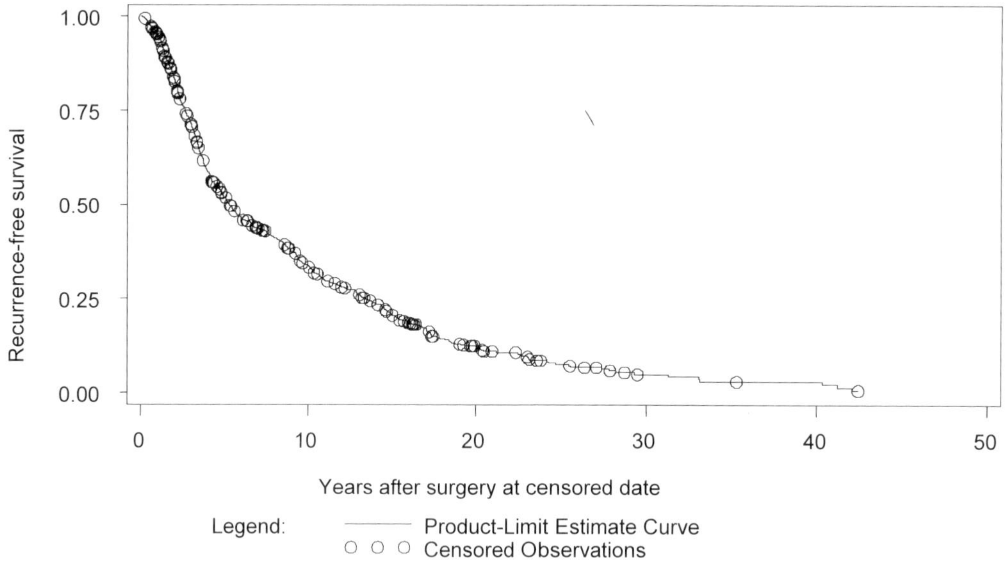


**Figure 1 Kaplan-Meier curve of differentiated thyroid cancer persistence or recurrence (full dataset).**

results to some studies. Finally, although we did not study these specific questions, it was recently reported that recurrence of papillary and follicular thyroid cancer in the first year following thyroid surgery predicts a worse outcome [13], and patients with micropapillary multifocal thyroid cancer have a reduced rate of recurrence following more complete thyroid surgery [15]. The differences between the variables analyzed in this study and those of other investigators do not allow for direct comparison of the predictive models.

There are several strengths of this study, which specifically studied only patients who underwent a total or near-total thyroidectomy and radioiodine ablation to evaluate laboratory and imaging markers of WDTC persistence/recurrence. All sites of a large Boston, Massachusetts-area multispecialty group practice were included, and there was a relatively long period of follow-up of over 28 years. Many subjects contributed substantial person-time toward the primary outcome. Furthermore, this group practice, which consists of

**Table 2 Individual and comprehensive Cox regression models predicting the persistence or recurrence of WDTC**

| | n | number with persistence or recurrence | hazard ratio | 95% CI | p |
|---|---|---|---|---|---|
| ***Patient-associated factors*** | 354 | 44 | | | 0.02 |
| Gender | | | 0.54 | 0.28, 1.03 | 0.06 |
| Age | | | 0.97 | 0.93, 1.01 | 0.09 |
| Ethnicity | | | 1.17 | 0.96, 1.42 | 0.12 |
| Interaction of age and time to persistence or recurrence | | | 1.03 | 1.01, 1.06 | 0.01 |
| ***Tumor-associated factors*** | 368 | 39 | | | 0.80 |
| Size (dichotomized) | | | 0.81 | 0.28, 2.32 | 0.70 |
| Number of foci | | | 0.88 | 0.61, 1.27 | 0.48 |
| Histology | | | 0.89 | 0.53, 1.49 | 0.66 |
| ***Comprehensive model*** | 309 | 37 | | | 0.04 |
| Gender | | | 0.57 | 0.27, 1.21 | 0.14 |
| Age | | | 0.95 | 0.90, 0.99 | 0.02 |
| Ethnicity | | | 1.17 | 0.96, 1.44 | 0.13 |
| Tumor size | | | 0.57 | 0.19, 1.68 | 0.31 |
| Number of foci | | | 0.94 | 0.65, 1.36 | 0.74 |
| Histology | | | 0.68 | 0.32, 1.44 | 0.31 |
| Interaction of age and time to recurrence or persistence | | | 1.04 | 1.02, 1.07 | <0.01 |

14 sites, has utilized an electronic medical record since the late 1970s, thus permitting an easily extractable and long-term comprehensive assessment of patients followed within it with WDTC.

The findings of this study do not confirm previously published data that male gender and larger tumors have a worse prognosis for WDTC persistence/recurrence. We urge the establishment of a comprehensive national registry, created through linkage with electronic health record systems, that would uniformly capture information regarding these and other factors for the long-term monitoring of WDTC outcomes.

### List of Abbreviations

CT: is computed tomography; HVMA: is Harvard Vanguard Medical Associates; MRI: is magnetic resonance imaging; FDG-PET: is positron emission tomography; SD: is standard deviation; rhTSH: is recombinant human thyroid stimulating hormone; Tg: is thyroglobulin; WDTC: is well-differentiated thyroid cancer.

### Acknowledgements and Funding

The previously-created health quality assurance HVMA database was funded in part by Genzyme Corporation. Dr. Jeffrey R. Garber has received fees from Abbott Laboratories and King Pharmaceuticals. Ms. Shalini Dave; Drs. Angela M. Leung, Stephanie L. Lee, Francis X. Campion, and Elizabeth N. Pearce have no conflicts of interest to disclose. These data were presented in poster abstract form at the 80th Annual Meeting of the American Thyroid Association; September 23-25, 2009; Palm Beach, Florida.

### Author details

[1]Section of Endocrinology, Diabetes, and Nutrition; Boston University School of Medicine; Boston, MA; USA. [2]Division of Graduate Medical Sciences; Boston University Medical Center; Boston, MA: USA. [3]Endocrinology; Harvard Vanguard Medical Associates; Boston, MA; USA. [4]Internal Medicine; Harvard Vanguard Medical Associates; Boston, MA; USA. [5]Division of Endocrinology, Diabetes, and Metabolism; Department of Medicine; Beth Israel Deaconess Medical Center; Boston, MA; USA.

### Authors' contributions

AL performed the data analysis and wrote the initial draft of the manuscript. SD obtained approval from the Institutional Review Board and performed the data extraction in preparation for our analysis. SL, FC, and JG helped to establish the creation of the thyroid cancer registry. EP assisted SD in obtaining Institutional Review Board approval and assisted AL in the data analysis and preparation of the manuscript. All authors read and approved the final manuscript.

### Competing interests

The previously-created health quality assurance HVMA database was funded in part by Genzyme Corporation. Dr. Jeffrey R. Garber has received fees from Abbott Laboratories and King Pharmaceuticals. Ms. Shalini Dave; Drs. Angela M. Leung, Stephanie L. Lee, Francis X. Campion, and Elizabeth N. Pearce have no conflicts of interest to disclose.

### References

1. Cady B, Rossi R: **An expanded view of risk-group definition in differentiated thyroid carcinoma.** *Surgery* 1998, **104**:947.
2. Hay ID, Grant CS, Taylor WF, *et al*: **Ipsilateral lobectomy versus bilateral lobar resection in papillary thyroid carcinoma: a retrospective analysis of surgical outcome using a novel prognostic scoring system.** *Surgery* 1987, **102**:1088.
3. Hay ID, Bergstralh EJ, Goellner JR, *et al*: **Predicting outcome in papillary thyroid carcinoma: development of a reliable prognostic scoring system in a cohort of 1779 patients surgically treated at one institution during 1940 through 1989.** *Surgery* 1993, **114**:1050.
4. Sherman SI, Brierley JD, Sperling M, *et al*: **Prospective multicenter study of thyrois]carcinoma treatment: initial analysis of staging and outcome. National Thyroid Cancer Treatment Cooperative Study Registry Group.** *Cancer* 1998, **83**:1012.
5. American Joint Committee on Cancer: *Cancer Staging Manual.* 6 edition. Springer-Verlag; 2002.
6. Kloos RT: **Thyroid Cancer Recurrence in Patients Clinically Free of Disease with Undetectable or Very Low Serum Thyroglobulin Values.** *J Clin Endocrinol Metab* 2010, **12**:5241.
7. Francis Z, Schlumberger M: **Serum thyroglobulin determination in thyroid cancer patients.** *Best Pract Res Clin Endocrinol Metab* 2008, **22**:1039.
8. Cooper DS, Doherty GM, Haugen BR, *et al*: **Revised American Thyroid Association management guidelines for patients with thyroid nodules and differentiated thyroid cancer.** *Thyroid* 2009, **19**:1167.
9. Mazzaferri EL, Jhiang SM: **Long-term impact of initial surgical and medical therapy on papillary and follicular thyroid cancer.** *Am J Med* 1994, **97**:418.
10. Mazzaferri EL: **Management of low-risk differentiated thyroid cancer.** *Endocr Pract* 2007, **13**:498.
11. Palme CE, Waseem Z, Raza SN, *et al*: **Management and outcome of recurrent well-differentiated thyroid carcinoma.** *Arch Otolaryngol Head Neck Surg* 2004, **130**:819.
12. Mercante G, Frasoldati A, Pedroni C, *et al*: **Prognostic factors affecting neck lymph node recurrence and distant metastasis in papillary microcarcinoma of the thyroid: results of a study in 445 patients.** *Thyroid* 2009, **19**:707.
13. Lin HW, Bhattacharyya N: **Survival impact of treatment options for papillary microcarcinoma of the thyroid.** *Laryngoscope* 2009, **119**:1983.
14. Orlov S, Orlov D, Shaytzag M, *et al*: **Influence of age and primary tumor size on the risk for residual/recurrent well-differentiated thyroid carcinoma.** *Head Neck* 2009, **31**:782.
15. Ross DS, Litofsky D, Ain KB, *et al*: **Recurrence after treatment of micropapillary thyroid cancer.** *Thyroid* 2009, **19**:1043.

# 5

# Validity of multiplex biomarker model of 6 genes for the differential diagnosis of thyroid nodules

Kristine Ducena[1*], Arturs Ābols[1,2], Janis Vilmanis[3], Zenons Narbuts[3], Juris Tārs[4], Diana Andrējeva[2], Aija Linē[2] and Valdis Pīrāgs[1,3*]

**Abstract**

**Background:** Currently the cytological examination of fine needle aspiration (FNA) biopsies is the standard technique for the pre-operative differential diagnosis of thyroid nodules. However, the results may be non-informative in ~20% of cases due to an inadequate sampling and the lack of highly specific, measurable cytological criteria, therefore ancillary biomarkers that could aid in these cases are clearly needed. The aim of our study was to evaluate the mRNA expression levels of 8 candidate marker genes as the diagnostic biomarkers for the discrimination of benign and malignant thyroid nodules and to find a combination of biomarkers with the highest diagnostic value.

**Materials and methods:** mRNA expression levels of eight candidate marker genes - *BIRC5, CCND1, CDH1, CITED1, DPP4, LGALS3, MET* and *TFF3* was measured by real-time RT-PCR in paired nodular and surrounding normal thyroid tissue specimens of 105 consecutive patients undergoing thyroid surgery and compared between different types of thyroid lesions.

**Results:** Significant differences in the mRNA expression levels between the normal and malignant thyroid tissues and between benign and malignant nodules were found for *BIRC5, CCND1, CITED1, DPP4, LGALS3, MET* and *TFF3*, but not *CDH1*. On a single gene basis, relative quantity (RQ) of *LGALS3* had the highest diagnostic value for the discrimination of malignant and benign thyroid nodules (AUC = 0.832, $P < 0.0001$ and 90.9% sensitivity and 65.6% specificity at the optimal cut-off on ROC curve). The only two-marker set that outperformed *LGALS3* was RQ sum of *LGALS3* and *BIRC5* (AUC = 0.841, $P < 0.0001$). An application of multivariate logistic regression analysis resulted in the generation of a multiplex biomarker model based on *LGALS3, BIRC5, TFF3, CCND1, MET* and *CITED1* that had considerably higher specificity than a single marker or two marker gene-based models (AUC = 0.895, $P < 0.0001$, 70.5% sensitivity and 93.4% specificity).

**Conclusions:** This study confirmed that mRNA expression levels of 7 out of 8 candidate genes analysed have a diagnostic value for the distinction of benign and malignant thyroid nodules. The multiplex biomarker model based on 6 genes outperformed a single marker or two marker-based models and warrants feasibility studies on FNA biopsies and the validation in a larger cohort of patients.

## Background

Thyroid nodules are a very common clinical finding - the prevalence of palpable nodules ranges from 3 to 7% in the general population but can be as high as 50% based on ultrasonography or autopsy data [1]. Although only less than 5% of the palpable nodules are malignant lesions, thyroid cancers are the most common malignancy of endocrine organs. According to European Cancer Observatory data age-standardised incidence rate was 3.1 cases and 8.8 cases per 100 000 in men and women, respectively in Europe in 2008 and its incidence rates have steadily increased over the recent decades [2,3]. More than 95% of malignant lesions are derived from thyroid follicular cells and are divided into papillary and follicular carcinomas that differ mainly in the mode of metastatic spread (lymphatic and haematogenous spread, respectively) yet both are relatively indolent tumours with 5-year survival rates > 90%, and

* Correspondence: kducena@inbox.lv; pirags@latnet.lv
[1]Faculty of Medicine, University of Latvia, Raina Bulvaris 19, Riga, LV1586, Latvia
Full list of author information is available at the end of the article

undifferentiated or anaplastic carcinoma that is a highly aggressive and lethal cancer with 5-year survival rate below 1-17% [4]. A minority of thyroid carcinomas are derived from parafollicular cells (or C-cells) and are referred to as medullary carcinomas with 5-year survival rate of ~80% [4]. Benign nodules include hyperplasic follicular adenomas, multinodular goiter, thyroiditis and benign cysts [1].

The differential diagnosis of nodular thyroid disease is based on cytological examination of fine needle aspiration (FNA) biopsies, however the results may be non-informative in ~20% of cases due to an inadequate sampling and the lack of highly specific, measurable cytological criteria [4,5]. Furthermore, the principal diagnostic feature for follicular thyroid carcinomas (FTC) is capsular or vascular invasion and therefore it can not be reliably distinguished from follicular adenomas by analysis of FNA smears and the definite diagnosis relies on the histological examination of the postoperative surgical specimens [6]. Hence molecular biomarkers of malignancy that could reliably discriminate between malignant and benign nodules in the grey zone of thyroid FNA and classify tumours into the histological subtypes are clearly needed.

Gene expression profiling using cDNA microarrays or serial analysis of gene expression (SAGE) has revealed several hundreds of genes that are differentially expressed between malignant and benign thyroid nodules [7-9]. A number of them, including *LGALS3, MET* etc have been shown to be functionally involved in the carcinogenic process, have been validated by qRT-PCR and confirmed at protein level by immunohistochemistry [10-12]. However, several studies have demonstrated that none of these genes individually has sufficient sensitivity and specificity to be exploited as an independent diagnostic biomarker [13,14] while using very large panels of genes may not be practical. Therefore the definition of minimal set of marker genes that allows the correct classification of nodules is required in order to develop a clinically applicable biomarker assay. In the current study, we evaluated the diagnostic value of 8 candidate marker genes - *BIRC5, CCND1, CDH1, CITED1, DPP4, LGALS3, MET* and *TFF3* by analysing their mRNA expression levels in nodular and adjacent relatively normal thyroid tissue specimens of 105 consecutive patients with thyroid nodules who underwent thyroidectomy, and developed a multiplex biomarker model for the classification of the nodules.

## Methods

### Patients and tissue specimens

Paired specimens of thyroid nodules and surrounding normal tissues were collected from 105 consecutive patients undergoing total or partial thyroidectomy at the Latvian Centre of Oncology and Pauls Stradi ņš Clinical University Hospital during the period 2009-2010. Tissue samples were macroscopically dissected by histopathologist during the surgery and stored in RNALater® (Applied Biosystems, USA) at -20°C until processing. Tissue sections were evaluated by experienced pathologist and the diagnosis was established according to standard histopathological criteria. Sixty one of the nodules were diagnosed as follicular adenomas (FA), 33 as papillary thyroid carcinomas (PTC), 5 as medullar thyroid carcinomas (MTC), 3 as anaplastic thyroid carcinomas (ATC) and 3 as follicular thyroid carcinomas (FTC). Selected clinical-pathological data of the patient groups are provided in Table 1. The specimens were collected after the patients' informed consent was obtained in accordance with the regulations of Ethics Committee of the University of Latvia Institute of Experimental and Clinical Medicine.

**Table 1 Clinical and pathological characteristics of the patient groups**

| Characteristics | Thyroid cancer n = 44 | Benign nodule n = 61 |
|---|---|---|
| **Gender** | | |
| Male | 9 | 4 |
| Female | 35 | 57 |
| **Age at diagnosis** | | |
| Mean ± SD | 55 ± 17 | 54 ± 15 |
| Median (range) | 55 (24-83) | 57 (25-83) |
| **Family history of cancer** | 37 | 49 |
| **TSH level μIU/mL** | | |
| Mean ± SD | 2,31 ± 1,41 | 0,87 ± 0,74 |
| Median (range) | 1,32 (1,1-4,34) | 0,75 (0,004-2,43) |
| **US criteria** | | |
| Hipoechogenic nodule | 9 | 14 |
| No Halozones | 0 | 1 |
| Irregular frontier (non-homogenic) | 6 | 14 |
| Microcalcinates | 4 | 9 |
| Nodules > 3 cm | 5 | 19 |
| Central vascularization | 3 | 3 |
| Retrosternal | 1 | 7 |
| Swollen lymph nodes | 2 | 0 |
| No data | 18 | 8 |
| **Histopathology** | | |
| PTC | 33 | |
| FTC | 3 | |
| MTC | 5 | |
| ATC | 3 | |
| FA | | 61 |

**RNA extraction and cDNA synthesis**

Tissue specimens were homogenised using the FastPrep-24 instrument and Lysing Matrix D (MP Biomedicals, USA) in 1 ml of Lysis solution® (Ambion, USA) followed by the extraction of total RNA using MirVana® (Ambion, USA) according to manufacturer's instructions. RNA extracted from tissue material was treated with DNAse prior to cDNA synthesis (Ambion, USA) and quantified by NanoDrop ND-100 spectrophotometer. cDNA was synthesized by random hexamer priming from 4 μg of total RNA by using High-Capacity cDNA Reverse Transcription Kit (Applied Biosystems, USA) according to manufacturer's instructions.

**Quantitative RT-PCR**

Quantitative RT-PCR (qPCR) reactions were performed using 2 μl of 1:10 diluted cDNA reaction mixtures, ABSolute Blue™ SYBR green Low ROX (Thermo Scientific, USA) on ABI7500 sequence detection system (Applied Biosystems, USA). Appropriate primer concentrations were established by cDNA 4 log serial dilution curves to ensure amplification efficiency over 95% and the specificity of the amplification products were verified by the melting curve analysis. Sequences of primers used in this study are provided in Table 2. qPCR conditions were as follows: hold for 15 minutes at 95°C, follow by two step PCR for 40 cycles of 95°C for 15 seconds, followed by 60°C for 1 minute. All reactions were performed in duplicates. To choose the appropriate reference genes, a set of seven candidate reference genes (*PGK1, PLA2, TUBA3, ACTB, GAPDH, TBP, POLR2A*) was tested for their mRNA expression stability in 10 thyroid tissue samples from 5 patients (2 PTC, 3 FA, 5 normal) and the two most stable genes (*POLR2A and PGK1*) were determined by using the open-access software GeNorm Win3.4 (http://medgen.ugent.be/~jvdesomp/genorm). Normalisation factor (NF) for each cDNA sample was then calculated by using GeNorm Win3.4 based on *PGK1* and *POLR2A* expression level. Pooled cDNA from 10 thyroid tissue samples was used as a reference sample and included in each experiment to allow the comparison across multiple plates. The expression level of each gene was determined relative to its expression in the sample with the highest expression (lowest Ct value). The analysis of relative gene expression (RQ) data was performed using the $2^{-\Delta CT}$ method and to eliminate variations of cDNA quantity and quality the data were normalised by using NF for each sample ($RQ = (2^{-\Delta CT})/NF$).

**Statistical analysis**

A non-parametric Mann-Whitney *U* test was used to compare the RQ values of each candidate gene between

**Table 2 Primers used for qPCR**

| Name of the gene | Sequence (5'- > 3') | Size of PCR product (bp) | GenBank accession no. |
|---|---|---|---|
| | Candidate genes | | |
| LGALS3 F | CTGATTGTGCCTTATAACCTGC | 100 | NM_002306.3 |
| LGALS3 R | AAGCAATTCTGTTTGCATTGG | | |
| TFF3 F | GTACGTGGGCCTGTCTGC | 121 | NM_003226.3 |
| TFF3 R | GATCCTGGAGTCAAAGCAGC | | |
| DPP4 F | TGATGCTACAGCTGACAGTCG | 164 | NM_001935.3 |
| DPP4 R | CTGAGCTGTTTCCATATTCAGC | | |
| CITED1 F | GCTCTGAAATGCCAACAACG | 174 | NM_001144886.1 |
| CITED1 R | TGGTTCCATTTGAGGCTACC | | |
| MET F | TCTGCCTGCAATCTACAAGG | 153 | NM_001127500.1 |
| MET R | AAGGTGCAGCTCTCATTTCC | | |
| CDH1 F | AGAAACAGGATGGCTGAAGG | 199 | NM_004360.3 |
| CDH1 R | AGCACCTTCCATGACAGACC | | |
| CCND1 F | TGGTGAACAAGCTCAAGTGG | 280 | NM_053056.2 |
| CCND1 R | ATCACTCTGGAGAGGAAGCG | | |
| BIRC5 F | CAGCCCTTTCTCAAGGACC | 152 | NM_001168.2 |
| BIRC5 R | AAGCAGAAGAAACACTGGGC | | |
| | Hausekeeping genes | | |
| PGK1 F | CTTAAGGTGCTCAACAACATGG | 119 | NM_000291.3 |
| PGK1 R | ACAGGCAAGGTAATCTTCACAC | | |
| POLR2A F | GGGTCATCTTCCCAACTGGAG | 164 | NM_000937.4 |
| POLR2A R | CACCAGCTTCTTGCTCAATTCC | | |

F - forward primer, R- reverse primer

two independent groups of samples (benign vs malignant nodules; malignant nodules vs all normal tissue specimens). The statistical significance was set at $p < 0.05$. The receiver operating characteristic (ROC) curve was constructed and the area under the curve (AUC) was calculated to evaluate the diagnostic performance of each marker gene and biomarker model. Youden index (J) was used to define cut-off points on the ROC curves with the maximal sum of sensitivity and specificity. Multivariate logistic regression was used to examine associations between thyroid nodule histopathological status and the gene expression data as described by Laxman B et al [15]. The initial multivariate logistic regression model included all individual genes and all combinations. Stepwise backward elimination based likelihood ratio test was used to drop out insignificant terms from the initial model. The predicted probability for each sample was calculated and used as input to generate ROC curve. Leave one-out cross validation (LOOCV) as described earlier was used to validate biomarkers and combinations of them to eliminate overestimated values [15]. The statistical analyses were performed with SPSS 17.0 (SPSS, USA), Genex (Multid, Sweden) and GraphPadPrism 5 (GraphPad, USA).

## Results and discussion

### Selection of candidate marker genes

The selection of candidate marker genes was based on the functional involvement in various pathways contributing to the acquisition of malignant phenotype and/or previously reported differential expression in the malignant and benign thyroid nodules. Cyclin D1 encoded by *CCND1* is a crucial cell cycle regulator frequently upregulated at protein level in PTC [16]. *CITED1* encodes a cell cycle-dependent transcriptional cofactor involved in TGF-beta and Bmp signalling that may coordinate cellular differentiation and survival signals [17,18] and has been found to be overexpressed in PTC by expression profiling using cDNA microarrays [19], later confirmed as useful marker for FTC [6] and validated at protein level by IHC [20]. Loss of expression or function of E-cadherin - a cell-cell adhesion glycoprotein encoded by *CDH1*, has been demonstrated to contribute to the progression of various cancers, including poorly differentiated thyroid cancers by increasing proliferation, invasion and metastasis [21,22]. Overexpression of dipeptidyl-peptidase 4 encoded by *DPP4* in PTC has been demonstrated at protein level by several groups [23-25], however the mechanism how it may contribute to the development or progression of thyroid malignancies remains unknown. Survivin, an inhibitor of apoptosis encoded by *BIRC5*, has been shown to be overexpressed in a variety of cancers, including thyroid cancer, where it contributes to uncontrolled cancer cell growth and drug resistance [26,27]. Increased expression at the mRNA and protein level of the receptor for hepatocyte growth factor encoded by *MET* has been frequently observed in PTC, follicular variant of PTC and at lesser degree in FTC where it promotes tumour progression by facilitating cell proliferation, survival, migration, invasion, and metastasis [28-30]. However, to our knowledge, so far the diagnostic value of *CDH1*, *DPP4*, *BIRC5* and *MET* mRNA levels has not been established. Galectin 3 encoded by *LGALS3* plays an important role in cell-to-cell adhesion, cell-to-matrix interactions and the regulation of apoptosis and proliferation, and its overexpression correlates with thyroid cancer aggressiveness and metastasis [31,32]. Although *TFF3* mRNA has been shown to be overexpressed in several solid cancers, such as hepatocellular carcinoma, colon and prostate cancer, and suggested to contribute the malignant behaviour and metastasis [33-36], SAGE analysis of thyroid follicular adenomas and carcinomas demonstrated that it is downregulated in FTC [37] and later this finding was confirmed in PTC and ATC by other researchers [14,38], thus validating *TFF3* downregulation as a universal marker of cancers derived from thyroid follicular cells. It encodes a small secreted protein - trefoil factor 3, which is abundantly expressed at mucosal surfaces and promotes regeneration and repair. Interestingly, recent reports demonstrate that both galectin-3 and TFF3 are involved in ciliogenesis, epithelial cell differentiation and polarity [39,40], thus suggesting a yet unexplored role of the deregulation of these processes in the development of thyroid cancer.

### mRNA expression analysis and the diagnostic performance of individual marker genes

mRNA expression analysis of the selected marker genes by RT-qPCR revealed statistically significant differences both between the normal and malignant thyroid tissues and between benign and malignant nodules for all genes except *CDH1*, thus further supporting their role the development and/or progression of thyroid cancer. *LGALS3, DPP4, MET, CITED1, CCND1* and *BIRC5* were found to be significantly upregulated while *TFF3* was downregulated in the malignant tissues (Table 3 and Figure 1). At first, all the genes were tested by ROC curve analysis as individual biomarkers, which demonstrated that *LGALS3* have the highest value for discriminating malignant from benign nodules in our sample set (AUC = 0.832, $P < 0.0001$). The cut-off of *LGALS3* expression level (RQ) that discriminates benign and malignant nodules with the highest accuracy (sensitivity 90.9%, specificity 65.6%) was determined to be 0.019. The sensitivity for the detection of various subtypes of

**Table 3 Relative expression values and the diagnostic performance of the marker genes**

| Gene, protein name | RQ values - Mean ± SEM | | | Mann-Whitney U test - p-values | | ROC curve - AUC (Asimptotic significance) | |
|---|---|---|---|---|---|---|---|
| | Normal | Benign | Malignant | Normal vs Malignant | Benign vs Malignant | Normal vs Malignant | Benign vs Malignant |
| *LGALS3*, Galectin-3 | 0.068 ± 0.013 | 0.035 ± 0.007 | 0.248 ± 0.067 | $2.2 \times 10^{-5}$ | $1 \times 10^{-8}$ | 0.715 (< 0.0001) | 0.832 (< 0.0001) |
| *TFF3*, trefoil factor 3 | 0.115 ± 0.011 | 0.066 ± 0.007 | 0.037 ± 0.008 | $4.1 \times 10^{-8}$ | 0.0003 | 0.782 (< 0.0001) | 0.696 (0.001) |
| *DPP4*, Dipeptidyl peptidase-4 | 0.011 ± 0.002 | 0.0146 ± 0.003 | 0.066 ± 0.016 | 0.0001 | 0.0004 | 0.693 (< 0.0001) | 0.695 (0.001) |
| *MET*, hepatocyte growth factor receptor | 0.048 ± 0.005 | 0.033 ± 0.004 | 0.110 ± 0.021 | 0.01 | 0.0005 | 0.610 (0.037) | 0.689 (0.001) |
| *CITED1*, Cbp/p300-interacting transactivator 1 | 0.010 ± 0.002 | 0.021 ± 0.008 | 0.161 ± 0.048 | 0.001 | 0.001 | 0.654 (0.003) | 0.67 (0.003) |
| *CCND1*, Cyclin D1 | 0.037 ± 0.004 | 0.036 ± 0.007 | 0.084 ± 0.017 | 0.002 | 0.001 | 0.647 (0.005) | 0.67 (0.003) |
| *BIRC5*, Survivin | 0.025 ± 0.011 | 0.009 ± 0.002 | 0.045 ± 0.018 | 0.0001 | 0.001 | 0.694 (< 0.0001) | 0.668 (0.003) |
| *CDH1*,E-cadherin | 0.171 ± 0.013 | 0.117 ± 0.009 | 0.158 ± 0.018 | 0.2 | 0.06 | 0.464 (0.497) | 0.525 (0.697) |

thyroid cancers was mutually comparable (Figure 2C) - 29 out of 33 PTC, 4 of 5 MTC and all FTC and ATC specimens were classified correctly thus confirming that *LGALS3* may serve as a universal diagnostic marker of the thyroid malignancies. However, 22 of 61 benign nodules were misclassified using this cut-off. As the ROC curve was constructed using all the samples, it may lead to overestimation of the AUC, therefore we next used LOOCV to validate it. The AUC for LOOCV *LGALS3* model dropped to 0.783, nevertheless it still outperformed the other marker genes. Although previously the diagnostic utility of *LGALS3* mRNA expression level has been questioned, our data show that the diagnostic accuracy of mRNA quantification is comparable to that reported in immunohistochemical studies [32]. The next marker genes with the highest diagnostic value in our sample set were *TFF3* (AUC = 0.696, P = 0.001) and DPP4 (AUC = 0.695 and P = 0.001). The optimal RQ cut-off for *TFF3* was determined to be 0.011 allowing the discrimination between benign and malignant nodules with sensitivity 54.6% and specificity 90.2%, while for *DPP4* the cut-off was 0.027 with sensitivity 45.6% and specificity 88.5%.

Interestingly, in 3 PTC and 2 MTC cases none or only one of the genes analysed were differentially expressed between cancerous and relatively normal tissues in specimens and they were consistently misclassified as benign nodules. These specimens are likely to represent a distinct molecular subtype of thyroid cancer, in which different molecular pathways predominate and therefore next these samples will be subjected to gene expression profiling using cDNA microarrays.

### Development of multiplex biomarker model

To determine if a combination of markers could outperform the single biomarkers we systematically searched for two-marker ratios or two-marker sums, and determined their diagnostic performance by ROC curve analysis. In total, 27 two-marker combinations were evaluated, however only one of them - *LGALS3* and *BIRC5* RQ sum showed higher AUC for discriminating benign and malignant nodules than the best individual marker gene (AUC = 0.841, P < 0.0001 and AUC = 0.809, P < 0.0001 for the LOOCV model) (Figure 2A,B). At the best cut-off, the sensitivity was 79.5% and specificity was 78.7%. As shown in Figure 2D, this two-gene combination could detect all FTC and ATC cases but failed to detect 7 of 33 PTCs (21%) and 2 of 5 MTCs (40%) thus suggesting it may have lower value for diagnosing MTC, however this finding should be verified in larger cohort of patients. So far, the best reported two-marker set is *TFF3/LGALS3* ratio that has been shown to discriminate follicular carcinomas from follicular adenomas with 72.4% sensitivity and 83.3% specificity (or 80% and 91.5%, when the pathologically questionable cases were excluded) [41]. In our sample set it showed similar performance (AUC = 0.758, P < 0.0001, sensitivity 72.7%, specificity 85.3%). However, although it could improve the specificity, the overall accuracy of *TFF3/LGALS3* ratio was lower than that of *LGALS3* alone. Moreover, as *TFF3* is downregulated in cancer cells, the development of assay that is based on the measurement of its expression level in FNA biopsies consisting of a mixture of different cell types is technically more challenging than the assay

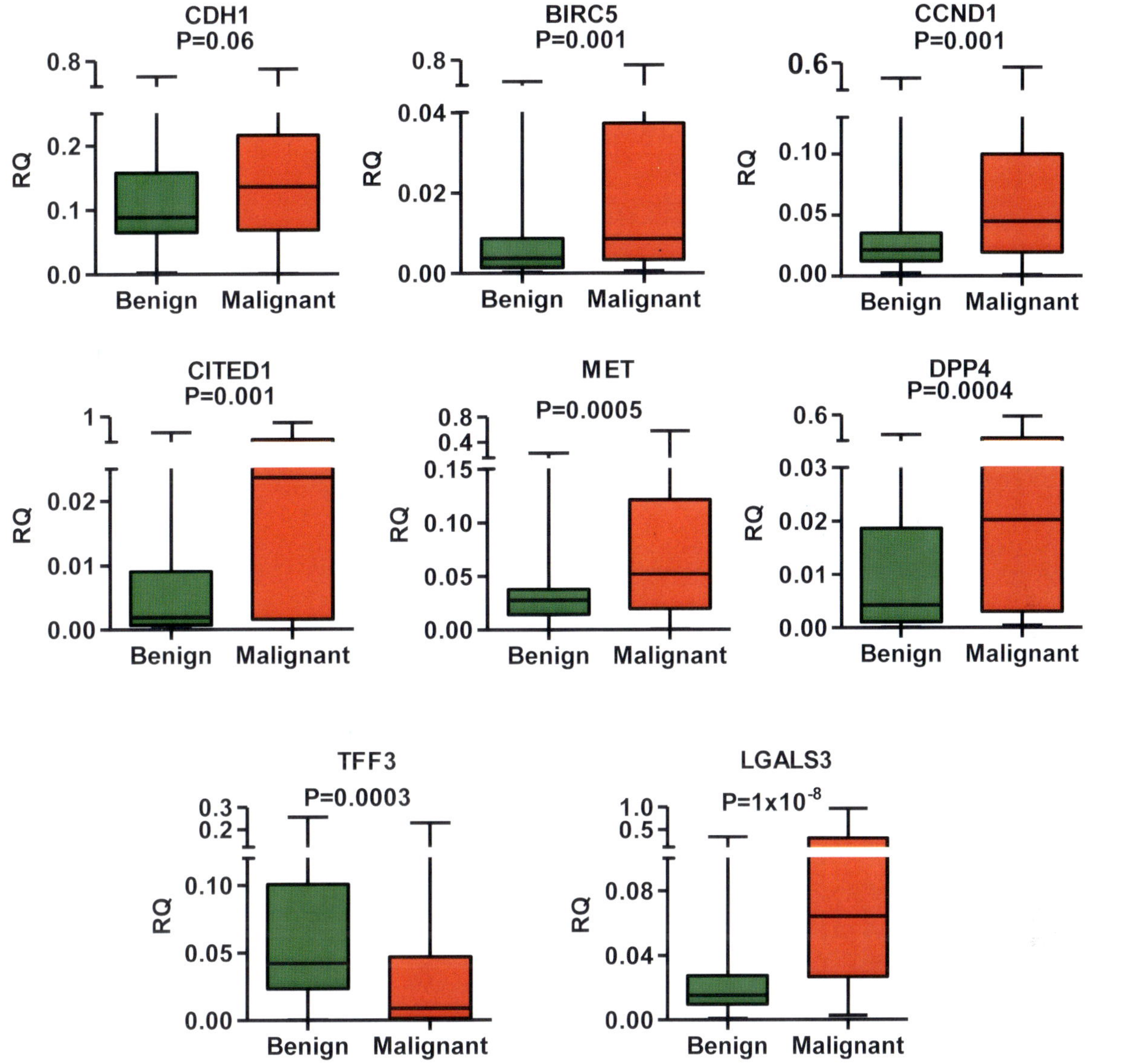


**Figure 1 Median mRNA expression levels of the candidate marker genes in groups of 61 benign and 44 malignant thyroid nodules represented by box plots.** The relative quantity (RQ) of each marker gene in each sample was calculated using $2^{-\Delta CT}$ method and normalised by using normalisation factor obtained by analysis of the two most stable reference genes (RQ = $(2^{-\Delta CT})$/NF). Boxes represent the 25th and 75th percentiles; whiskers represent the minimum and maximum values. Statistical significance was calculated using Mann-Whitney *U* test.

based on overexpressed genes, therefore *LGALS3* and *BIRC5* RQ sum seems to be more suitable for the clinical application.

Next, we applied a multivariate logistic regression analysis to define a multiple marker set that could improve the diagnostic performance over single markers or two-marker combinations. Similar approach has been previously successfully used by Laxman B et al to develop a multiplex biomarker model for the detection of prostate cancer [15]. This resulted in the multiplex model that included LGALS3 and BIRC5 RQ sum, TFF3 and LGALS3 RQ ratio, TFF3 and CCND1 RQ ratio, ratio between TFF3 RQ and MET, CITED1 RQ sum, ratio between TFF3 RQ and MET, BIRC5 RQ sum and ratio between TFF3 RQ and CCND1, BIRC5 RQ sum. Although the overall performance of the model (AUC = 0.895, P < 0.0001 and AUC = 0.823, P < 0.0001 for the LOOCV model) was only slightly improved over *LGALS3* alone or *LGALS3* and *BIRC5* RQ sum, at the best cut-off, this model shows 70.5% sensitivity and 93.4% specificity and as shown in Figure 2A it has considerably higher specificity that is a clear requirement for the development of clinically applicable biomarker assay.

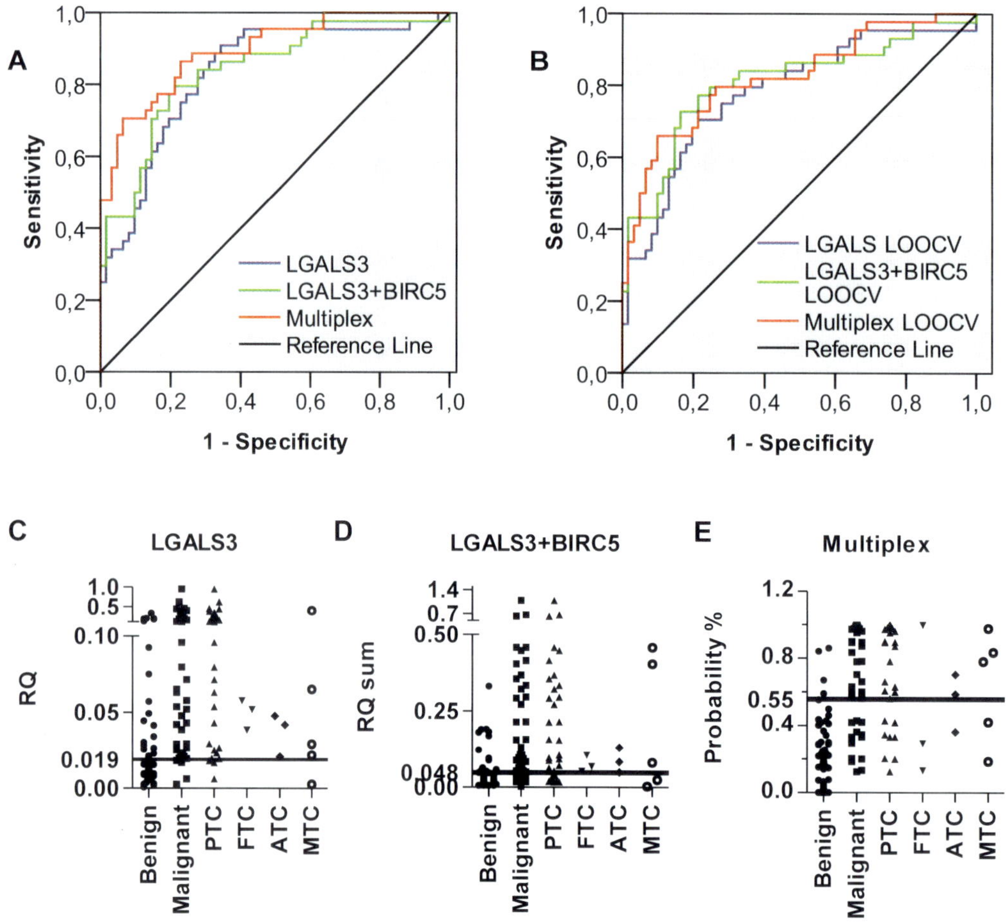


| Test Result Variable(s) | | | | | | Asymptotic 95% Confidence Interval | |
|---|---|---|---|---|---|---|---|
| | Area | Std. Error | Asymptotic Sig. | Sens. | Spec. | Lower Bound | Upper Bound |
| LGALS3 | 0.832 | 0.041 | <0.0001 | 90.9% | 65.6% | 0.752 | 0.913 |
| LGALS3 LOOCV | 0.783 | 0.047 | <0.0001 | 70.5% | 78.7% | 0.691 | 0.875 |
| LGALS3+BIRC5 | 0.841 | 0.04 | <0.0001 | 79.5% | 78.7% | 0.763 | 0.919 |
| LGALS3+BIRC5 LOOCV | 0.809 | 0.046 | <0.0001 | 77.3% | 78.7% | 0.720 | 0.898 |
| Multiplex | 0.895 | 0.031 | <0.0001 | 70.5% | 93.4% | 0.834 | 0.955 |
| Multiplex LOOCV | 0.823 | 0.042 | <0.0001 | 65.9% | 90.2% | 0.74 | 0.906 |

**Figure 2 The diagnostic performance of the best individual marker, two-marker set and multiplex biomarker model.** A and B represents ROC curves of the best individual marker, two-marker set and multiplex model and their LOOCV ROC curves, respectively. C, D, E - Scatter dot plot of LGALS3 RQ, LGALS3 and BIRC5 RQ sum and Multiplex model with the best cut off shows how many benign nodules, malignant nodules and thyroid cancer subtypes are misclassified. In table are the best individual marker, two-marker set and multiplex biomarker model and their LOOCV model ROC curve AUC data and sensitivity and specificity at the best cut-off point.

The future efforts will be focused on adding marker genes to the multiplex model that would enable detecting other molecular subtypes of thyroid cancer, testing the feasibility of the biomarker assay in FNA biopsies and validating the assay in a large multicenter clinical trial.

## Conclusions

mRNA expression analysis of 8 candidate marker genes - *BIRC5, CCND1, CDH1, CITED1, DPP4, LGALS3, MET* and *TFF3* in paired nodular and relatively normal thyroid tissue specimens of 105 consecutive patients undergoing thyroid surgery demonstrated that all of them except *CDH1* are differentially expressed between the normal and malignant thyroid tissues and between benign and malignant nodules, and *LGALS3* had the highest diagnostic value for the discrimination of malignant and benign thyroid nodules on a single gene basis. An application of multivariate logistic regression analysis resulted in the generation of a multiplex biomarker model based on *LGALS3, BIRC5, TFF3, CCND1, MET* and *CITED1* that outperformed a single marker or two marker gene-based models by increasing the specificity, which is a prerequisite for the development of clinically applicable biomarker assay. The next step will be to test the feasibility of this assay on FNA biopsies and to validate it in a larger cohort of patients.

#### Acknowledgements and funding

This study was supported in parts by funds from Latvian Council of Science, grant number 09.1310, European Social Fund project No. 2009/0204/1DP/1.1.1.2.0/09/APIA/VIAA/150 and individual fellowships from European Social Fund No. 10/172/31. The publishing costs are covered by ERDF project No. 2DP/2.1.1.2.0/10/APIA/VIAA/004.

#### Author details

[1]Faculty of Medicine, University of Latvia, Raina Bulvaris 19, Riga, LV1586, Latvia. [2]Department of Molecular Biology, Latvian Biomedical Research and Study Centre, Ratsupites 1,Riga, LV1067, Latvia. [3]Surgery Clinics, Pauls Stradins Clinical University Hospital, Pilsonu 13, Riga, LV1002, Latvia. [4]Oncology department, Riga Eastern Clinical University Hospital, Hipokrata 2, Riga, LV1038, Latvia.

#### Authors' contributions

KD participated in the designing of the study, collecting of clinical data and drafting the manuscript. AA carried out the gene expression analysis, performed the statistical analysis and helped to draft the manuscript. JV, ZN and JT performed thyroid surgery and collected the clinical material. DA participated in the gene expression analysis. AL participated in the design of the study and drafted the manuscript. VP designed and coordinated the study and helped to draft the manuscript. All authors read and approved the final manuscript.

#### Competing interests

The authors declare that they have no competing interests.

#### References

1. Gharib H, Papini E, Valcavi R, Baskin HJ, Crescenzi A, Dottorini ME, *et al*: American Association of Clinical Endocrinologists and Associazione Medici Endocrinologi medical guidelines for clinical practice for the diagnosis and management of thyroid nodules. *Endocr Pract* 2006, **12**:63-102.
2. Liu S, Semenciw R, Ugnat AM, Mao Y: Increasing thyroid cancer incidence in Canada, 1970-1996: time trends and age-period-cohort effects. *Br J Cancer* 2001, **85**:1335-1339.
3. Ferlay J, Parkin DM, Steliarova-Foucher E: Estimates of cancer incidence and mortality in Europe in 2008. *Eur J Cancer* 2010, **46**:765-781.
4. Kondo T, Ezzat S, Asa SL: Pathogenetic mechanisms in thyroid follicular-cell neoplasia. *Nat Rev Cancer* 2006, **6**:292-306.
5. Lloyd RV, Erickson LA, Casey MB, Lam KY, Lohse CM, Asa SL, *et al*: Observer variation in the diagnosis of follicular variant of papillary thyroid carcinoma. *Am J Surg Pathol* 2004, **28**:1336-1340.
6. Foukakis T, Gusnanto A, Au AY, Hoog A, Lui WO, Larsson C, *et al*: A PCR-based expression signature of malignancy in follicular thyroid tumors. *Endocr Relat Cancer* 2007, **14**:381-391.
7. Barden CB, Shister KW, Zhu B, Guiter G, Greenblatt DY, Zeiger MA, *et al*: Classification of follicular thyroid tumors by molecular signature: results of gene profiling. *Clin Cancer Res* 2003, **9**:1792-1800.
8. Finley DJ, Arora N, Zhu B, Gallagher L, Fahey TJ III: Molecular profiling distinguishes papillary carcinoma from benign thyroid nodules. *J Clin Endocrinol Metab* 2004, **89**:3214-3223.
9. Finley DJ, Lubitz CC, Wei C, Zhu B, Fahey TJ III: Advancing the molecular diagnosis of thyroid nodules: defining benign lesions by molecular profiling. *Thyroid* 2005, **15**:562-568.
10. Nardone HC, Ziober AF, LiVolsi VA, Mandel SJ, Baloch ZW, Weber RS, *et al*: c-Met expression in tall cell variant papillary carcinoma of the thyroid. *Cancer* 2003, **98**:1386-1393.
11. Finley DJ, Zhu B, Barden CB, Fahey TJ III: Discrimination of benign and malignant thyroid nodules by molecular profiling. *Ann Surg* 2004, **240**:425-436.
12. Jarzab B, Wiench M, Fujarewicz K, Simek K, Jarzab M, Oczko-Wojciechowska M, *et al*: Gene expression profile of papillary thyroid cancer: sources of variability and diagnostic implications. *Cancer Res* 2005, **65**:1587-1597.
13. Cerutti JM, Delcelo R, Amadei MJ, Nakabashi C, Maciel RM, Peterson B, *et al*: A preoperative diagnostic test that distinguishes benign from malignant thyroid carcinoma based on gene expression. *J Clin Invest* 2004, **113**:1234-1242.
14. Krause K, Eszlinger M, Gimm O, Karger S, Engelhardt C, Dralle H, *et al*: TFF3-based candidate gene discrimination of benign and malignant thyroid tumors in a region with borderline iodine deficiency. *J Clin Endocrinol Metab* 2008, **93**:1390-1393.
15. Laxman B, Morris DS, Yu J, Siddiqui J, Cao J, Mehra R, *et al*: A first-generation multiplex biomarker analysis of urine for the early detection of prostate cancer. *Cancer Res* 2008, **68**:645-649.
16. Lee SH, Lee JK, Jin SM, Lee KC, Sohn JH, Chae SW, *et al*: Expression of cell-cycle regulators (cyclin D1, cyclin E, p27kip1, p57kip2) in papillary thyroid carcinoma. *Otolaryngol Head Neck Surg* 2010, **142**:332-337.
17. Plisov S, Tsang M, Shi G, Boyle S, Yoshino K, Dunwoodie SL, *et al*: Cited1 is a bifunctional transcriptional cofactor that regulates early nephronic patterning. *J Am Soc Nephrol* 2005, **16**:1632-1644.
18. Shi G, Boyle SC, Sparrow DB, Dunwoodie SL, Shioda T, de Caestecker MP: The transcriptional activity of CITED1 is regulated by phosphorylation in a cell cycle-dependent manner. *J Biol Chem* 2006, **281**:27426-27435.
19. Huang Y, Prasad M, Lemon WJ, Hampel H, Wright FA, Kornacker K, *et al*: Gene expression in papillary thyroid carcinoma reveals highly consistent profiles. *Proc Natl Acad Sci USA* 2001, **98**:15044-15049.
20. Liu YY, Morreau H, Kievit J, Romijn JA, Carrasco N, Smit JW: Combined immunostaining with galectin-3, fibronectin-1, CITED-1, Hector Battifora mesothelial-1, cytokeratin-19, peroxisome proliferator-activated receptor-{gamma}, and sodium/iodide symporter antibodies for the differential diagnosis of non-medullary thyroid carcinoma. *Eur J Endocrinol* 2008, **158**:375-384.
21. Mitselou A, Ioachim E, Peschos D, Charalabopoulos K, Michael M, Agnantis NJ, *et al*: E-cadherin adhesion molecule and syndecan-1 expression in various thyroid pathologies. *Exp Oncol* 2007, **29**:54-60.

22. Rocha AS, Soares P, Fonseca E, Cameselle-Teijeiro J, Oliveira MC, Sobrinho-Simoes M: E-cadherin loss rather than beta-catenin alterations is a common feature of poorly differentiated thyroid carcinomas. *Histopathology* 2003, **42**:580-587.
23. de MC, Savchenko V, Giorgi R, Sebag F, Henry JF: Utility of malignancy markers in fine-needle aspiration cytology of thyroid nodules: comparison of Hector Battifora mesothelial antigen-1, thyroid peroxidase and dipeptidyl aminopeptidase IV. *Br J Cancer* 2008, **98**:818-823.
24. Aratake Y, Umeki K, Kiyoyama K, Hinoura Y, Sato S, Ohno A, *et al*: Diagnostic utility of galectin-3 and CD26/DPPIV as preoperative diagnostic markers for thyroid nodules. *Diagn Cytopathol* 2002, **26**:366-372.
25. Kholova I, Ludvikova M, Ryska A, Hanzelkova Z, Cap J, Pecen L, *et al*: Immunohistochemical detection of dipeptidyl peptidase IV (CD 26) in thyroid neoplasia using biotinylated tyramine amplification. *Neoplasma* 2003, **50**:159-164.
26. Cheung CH, Cheng L, Chang KY, Chen HH, Chang JY: Investigations of survivin: the past, present and future. *Front Biosci* 2011, **16**:952-961.
27. Zhang HY, Meng X, Du ZX, Fang CQ, Liu GL, Wang HQ, *et al*: Significance of survivin, caspase-3, and VEGF expression in thyroid carcinoma. *Clin Exp Med* 2009, **9**:207-213.
28. Steffan JJ, Coleman DT, Cardelli JA: The HGF-Met Signaling Axis: Emerging Themes and Targets of Inhibition. *Curr Protein Pept Sci* 2011, **12**:12-22.
29. Ippolito A, Vella V, La Rosa GL, Pellegriti G, Vigneri R, Belfiore A: Immunostaining for Met/HGF receptor may be useful to identify malignancies in thyroid lesions classified suspicious at fine-needle aspiration biopsy. *Thyroid* 2001, **11**:783-787.
30. Wasenius VM, Hemmer S, Kettunen E, Knuutila S, Franssila K, Joensuu H: Hepatocyte growth factor receptor, matrix metalloproteinase-11, tissue inhibitor of metalloproteinase-1, and fibronectin are up-regulated in papillary thyroid carcinoma: a cDNA and tissue microarray study. *Clin Cancer Res* 2003, **9**:68-75.
31. Htwe TT, Karim N, Wong J, Jahanfar S, Mansur MA: Differential expression of galectin-3 in advancing thyroid cancer cells: a clue toward understanding tumour progression and metastasis. *Singapore Med J* 2010, **51**:856-859.
32. Chiu CG, Strugnell SS, Griffith OL, Jones SJ, Gown AM, Walker B, *et al*: Diagnostic utility of galectin-3 in thyroid cancer. *Am J Pathol* 2010, **176**:2067-2081.
33. Babyatsky M, Lin J, Yio X, Chen A, Zhang JY, Zheng Y, *et al*: Trefoil factor-3 expression in human colon cancer liver metastasis. *Clin Exp Metastasis* 2009, **26**:143-151.
34. Okada H, Kimura MT, Tan D, Fujiwara K, Igarashi J, Makuuchi M, *et al*: Frequent trefoil factor 3 (TFF3) overexpression and promoter hypomethylation in mouse and human hepatocellular carcinomas. *Int J Oncol* 2005, **26**:369-377.
35. Yio X, Zhang JY, Babyatsky M, Chen A, Lin J, Fan QX, *et al*: Trefoil factor family-3 is associated with aggressive behavior of colon cancer cells. *Clin Exp Metastasis* 2005, **22**:157-165.
36. Vestergaard EM, Nexo E, Torring N, Borre M, Orntoft TF, Sorensen KD: Promoter hypomethylation and upregulation of trefoil factors in prostate cancer. *Int J Cancer* 2010, **127**:1857-1865.
37. Takano T, Miyauchi A, Yoshida H, Kuma K, Amino N: High-throughput differential screening of mRNAs by serial analysis of gene expression: decreased expression of trefoil factor 3 mRNA in thyroid follicular carcinomas. *Br J Cancer* 2004, **90**:1600-1605.
38. Taniguchi K, Takano T, Miyauchi A, Koizumi K, Ito Y, Takamura Y, *et al*: Differentiation of follicular thyroid adenoma from carcinoma by means of gene expression profiling with adapter-tagged competitive polymerase chain reaction. *Oncology* 2005, **69**:428-435.
39. Koch A, Poirier F, Jacob R, Delacour D: Galectin-3, a novel centrosome-associated protein, required for epithelial morphogenesis. *Mol Biol Cell* 2010, **21**:219-231.
40. LeSimple P, van S, Buisine MP, Copin MC, Hinz M, Hoffmann W, *et al*: Trefoil factor family 3 peptide promotes human airway epithelial ciliated cell differentiation. *Am J Respir Cell Mol Biol* 2007, **36**:296-303.
41. Takano T, Miyauchi A, Yoshida H, Kuma K, Amino N: Decreased relative expression level of trefoil factor 3 mRNA to galectin-3 mRNA distinguishes thyroid follicular carcinoma from adenoma. *Cancer Lett* 2005, **219**:91-96.

6

# *COX-2* expression in papillary thyroid carcinoma (PTC) in cytological material obtained by fine needle aspiration biopsy (FNAB)

Kinga Krawczyk-Rusiecka, Katarzyna Wojciechowska-Durczyńska, Anna Cyniak-Magierska, Zbigniew Adamczewski, Elżbieta Gałecka, Andrzej Lewiński*

**Abstract**

**Background:** COX-2 is an enzyme isoform that catalyses the formation of prostanoids from arachidonic acid. An increased *COX-2* gene expression is believed to participate in carcinogenesis. Recent studies have shown that *COX-2* up-regulation is associated with the development of numerous neoplasms, including skin, colorectal, breast, lung, stomach, pancreas and liver cancers. *COX-2* products stimulate endothelial cell proliferation and their overexpression has been demonstrated to be involved in the mechanism of decreased resistance to apoptosis. Suppressed angiogenesis was found in experimental animal studies as a consequence of null mutation of *COX-2* gene in mice. Despite the role of *COX-2* expression remains a subject of numerous studies, its participation in carcinogenesis or the thyroid cancer progression remains unclear.

**Methods:** Twenty three (23) patients with cytological diagnosis of PTC were evaluated. After FNAB examination, the needle was washed out with a lysis buffer and the obtained material was used for *COX-2* expression estimation. Total RNA was isolated (RNeasy Micro Kit), and RT reactions were performed. β-actin was used as endogenous control. Relative *COX-2* expression was assessed in real-time PCR reactions by an ABI PRISM 7500 Sequence Detection System, using the $\Delta\Delta C_T$ method.

**Results:** *COX-2* gene expression was higher in patients with PTC, when compared to specimens from patients with non-toxic nodular goitre (NTG).

**Conclusions:** The preliminary results may indicate *COX-2* role in thyroid cancer pathogenesis, however the observed variability in results among particular subjects requires additional clinical data and tumor progression analysis.

## Background

The most common thyroid malignancy is papillary thyroid carcinoma (PTC), accounting for approximately 85-90% of all thyroid cancers. PTC usually grows slowly and is clinically indolent, although aggressive forms can also occur. The 10-year survival rate for all PTC patients is estimated at 80-90% [1].

The introduction of fine-needle aspiration biopsy (FNAB) has made PTC identification more accurate, but still the diagnostic tools regarding the differentiation between thyroid benign and malignant lesions are not always reliable. The molecular basis of PTC has been examined and association with variety of molecular prognostic markers has been described, including *RAS, RET, Trk, MET*, and *BRAF* mutations [2].

Cyclooxygenase-2 (COX-2) is an enzyme isoform involved in the conversion of arachidonic acid to prostaglandin $H_2$, the precursor of various molecules, including prostaglandins, prostacyclines and thromboxanes. COX-2 can be expressed in response to various stimuli, such as hormones, mitogens, cytokines, inflammatory mediators and growth factors *via* protein kinase C and RAS-mediated signaling [3,4]. The products of COX-2 activity are believed to be involved in carcinogenesis by promoting angiogenesis, inhibiting apoptosis, increasing

* Correspondence: alewin@csk.umed.lodz.pl
Department of Endocrinology and Metabolic Diseases, Medical University of Lodz, Polish Mother's Memorial Hospital - Research Institute, Lodz, Poland

cell invasion and stimulating cell proliferation. COX-2 also modulates vascular endothelial growth factor (VEGF) production, the factor that promotes angiogenesis and decreases immunity toward cancer cells [5-9].

Recent studies have highlighted the relevance of COX-2 in human carcinogenesis. Increased levels of COX-2 have been reported in numerous tumours, including head and neck squamous cell cancer, as well as colorectal, breast, lung, skin, stomach, liver, pancreas, bladder, ovaries and prostate carcinomas [10-19].

Selective inhibition of COX-2 is a novel therapy under investigation in both the chemoprevention and treatment of solid tumors [20,21]. Experimental animal data indicate that *COX-2* gene may be associated with carcinogenesis of several types of human malignancies.

Whether *COX-2* expression is related to the morphology of PTC remains unclear. In the present study we have investigated *COX-2* expression in 23 cases of PTC diagnosed cytologically following FNAB.

## Methods

45 thyroid specimens were analyzed, i.e. 23 cases of PTC and 22 cases of benign thyroid lesions; 6 men and 39 women participated in the study. Patients ranged in age from 24 to 87 years (median - 48 years in PTC group, 58 years in benign thyroid lesions group). Thyroid aspirates, eligible for the study, were obtained from patients by fine needle aspiration biopsy (FNAB) in the Clinical Hospital No. 3, Medical University of Lodz (2007-2010). Each aspirate was smeared for conventional cytology, while the remaining part of aspirate was immediately washed out of the needle. The cells, obtained from the needle, were used in further investigation. Macroscopically unchanged thyroid tissue, collected from patients treated surgically, was used as an internal control.

The procedures, used in the study, were approved by the Ethical Committee of the Medical University of Lodz (Poland). All patients were informed and agreed to participate in this study.

Total RNA was extracted using RNeasy Micro Kit (Qiagen, Hilden, Germany), based on modified Chomczyński and Sacchi's method [22]. RNA concentration was spectrophotometrically assessed by measuring absorbance at 260 and 280 nm (NanoDrop ND-1000 Spectrophotometer, Thermo Fisher Scientific, USA).

Total RNA was reversely transcribed in a Mastercycler personal thermocycler (Eppendorf, Hamburg, Germany), according to manufacturer's procedures in a total volume of 50 µl including oligo d(T)16 (50 µM), MultiScribe Reverse Transcriptase (50 U/µl), 10 × TaqMan RT Buffer, $MgCl_2$ solution (25 mM), dNTPs mixture (10 mM), RNAse Inhibitor (20 U/µl) and nuclease-free water (TaqMan Reverse Trancriptase Reagents, Applied Biosystems, CA, USA). The reactions were incubated for 10 min in 25°C, 30 min in 48°C, heated for 5 min in 95°C and placed at 4°C.

The relative expression of *COX-2* gene was assessed, using the ABI PRISM 7500 SDS Software (ABI PRISM 7500 Sequence Detection System, Applied Biosystems), according to the manufacturer's protocol. The PCR reactions for COX-2 gene were run with 5 µl of cDNA in a total volume of 50 µl, using TaqMan Universal PCR Master Mix (Applied Biosystems, Foster City, CA, USA) and predesignated primer/probe set (Assays-on-Demand™ Gene Expression assay, Hs 00153133_m1, Applied Biosystems). Amplification reactions were done in triplicate for each examined sample.

Controls with no template cDNA were used with each assay. The reference gene was β-actin (Assays-on-Demand™ Gene Expression assay, Hs 99999903_m1, Applied Biosystems). Samples of cDNA were quantified using a fluorescence based real-time detection method (TaqMan).

Assays-on-Demand Gene Expression product consists of 20 × mix of unlabelled PCR primers and TaqMan MGB probe (5 µM) with FAM™(6-carboxy-fluorescein) at the 5' end as the reporter dye and a non-fluorescent quencher (TAMRA, 6-carboxy-tetramethylrhodamine) at the 3' end. Cycling conditions were 50°C for 2 min and 95°C for 10 minutes, followed by 50 cycles at 95°C and 60°C for 1 minute. A sample of normal thyroid tissue served as a calibrator to compare the relative amount of target in different samples and to adjust for the plate-to-plate variation in amplification efficiency.

### Data and statistical analysis

Relative gene expression - determined by comparing threshold cycle ($C_T$) for gene of interest (COX-2) with $C_T$for the reference gene (β-actin) - was calculated using the $\Delta\Delta C_T$method as described previously [23]. The characteristics, RQ and $\Delta C_T$values of patients groups are shown in Table 1 and Table 2.

Statistical analysis was performed, using a standard parametric Student's t test, followed by non-parametric U Mann-Whitney's test. P values < 0.05 were considered to indicate statistical significance.

## Results

COX-2 mRNA expression was significantly higher in PTC when compared to benign thyroid lesions (Student's t-test, P = 0.021). There was no significant relationship between *COX-2* expression and patients age and sex. The amplification plots of *COX-2* and *β-actin* are shown in Figure. 1 and 2. The statistical analysis of *COX-2* expression by quantitative Real Time PCR in PTC and NTG is presented in Figure. 3 and Figure. 4.

**Table 1 Gender, age, ddCT and RQ values in PTC group**

| No. | Gender | Age | ddCT | RQ |
|---|---|---|---|---|
| 1. | M | 56 | -0.84 | 1.79 |
| 2. | M | 64 | -0.71 | 1.63 |
| 3. | F | 52 | -6.49 | 89.8 |
| 4. | F | 28 | 0.95 | 0.52 |
| 5. | F | 53 | -1.62 | 3.06 |
| 6. | M | 61 | -0.62 | 1.53 |
| 7. | F | 57 | -2.46 | 5.49 |
| 8. | F | 36 | -4.07 | 16.74 |
| 9. | F | 56 | -2.76 | 6.77 |
| 10. | M | 58 | -3.12 | 8.69 |
| 11. | F | 28 | 1.31 | 0.4 |
| 12. | F | 24 | -1.31 | 2.48 |
| 13. | F | 67 | -1.51 | 2.84 |
| 14. | F | no data | 1.24 | 2.36 |
| 15. | F | 39 | -2.0 | 4.01 |
| 16. | F | 49 | -0.75 | 1.68 |
| 17. | F | 28 | 2.86 | 0.14 |
| 18. | F | 45 | -2.75 | 6.73 |
| 19. | F | 50 | -2.11 | 4.31 |
| 20. | F | 63 | -0.86 | 1.82 |
| 21. | M | 53 | -3.98 | 15.8 |
| 22. | F | 39 | -3.44 | 10.84 |
| 23. | F | 49 | -2.22 | 4.66 |

**Table 2 Gender, age, ddCT and RQ values in NTG group**

| No. | Gender | Age | ddCT | RQ |
|---|---|---|---|---|
| 1. | F | 27 | -0.84 | 1.79 |
| 2. | F | 87 | -0.41 | 1.32 |
| 3. | F | 65 | 1.98 | 0.25 |
| 4. | F | 72 | -1.01 | 2.02 |
| 5. | F | 64 | -2.32 | 4.71 |
| 6. | F | 68 | -0.01 | 1.01 |
| 7. | F | 46 | -2.07 | 4.21 |
| 8. | F | 39 | 1.55 | 0.34 |
| 9. | M | 56 | -0.63 | 1.55 |
| 10. | F | 68 | -0.98 | 1.98 |
| 11. | F | 62 | 2.94 | 0.13 |
| 12. | F | 48 | 1.96 | 0.26 |
| 13. | F | 32 | -2.91 | 7.51 |
| 14. | M | 61 | -0.21 | 1.15 |
| 15. | F | 29 | 0.74 | 0.6 |
| 16. | F | 88 | -0.68 | 1.6 |
| 17. | M | 71 | -1.53 | 2.88 |
| 18. | F | 43 | -0.46 | 1.37 |
| 19. | F | 54 | 0.77 | 0.24 |
| 20. | F | 50 | -1.2 | 2.3 |
| 21. | F | 79 | -1.37 | 2.59 |
| 22. | F | 71 | -0.93 | 1.9 |

## Discussion

The relation between *COX-2* activity and carcinogenesis is being examined in variety of human neoplasms. Fine needle aspiration biopsy has become a critical diagnostic tool in management of thyroid nodules. It has allowed to decrease the number of cases inquiring surgical treatment from 67% to 44%; also the percentage of operated carcinomas in those nodules has increased from 14% to 29% [24]. Generally, preoperative discrimination of the thyroid malignancy, using not only cytopathology but also molecular markers, would enhance the proper diagnosis.

In our study, COX-2 expression in both NTG and PTC were examined. *COX-2* expression was significantly higher in PTC group.

All but one of the previously conducted studies found overexpression of COX-2 in cases of PTC and follicular thyroid carcinoma (FTC). In the study of Ito et al. [25], there were 9 COX-2-negative (18,4%) among 49 of PTC cases, studied by immunochemistry. They also suggested significant reduction of COX-2 levels in older patients (over 54 years old), in patients with large tumors and with the advanced disease stages, as well as with the presence of solid, scirrhous or trabecular growth pattern. An association among and age and worse prognosis has been well-recognized in the medical literature. Accordingly, Ito et al. [25] found that the COX-2 levels were significantly reduced in older patients, whereas Siironen et al. [26] demonstrated the older age group of patients, having a much worse prognosis and higher COX-2 levels. However, in our study, we have failed to establish statistical significance between COX-2 expression and patients' age or sex which is similar to results of Garcia-Gonzales et al [27].

The results of Kajita et al. [28] did not show any significant differences in COX-2 expression between normal thyroid tissue and PTC, because of variation in mRNA levels. The authors have also performed the *in vitro* study, with the TPC-1 thyroid carcinoma cell line and a compound NS-398 - a COX-2 enzymatic activity specific inhibitor, showing inhibited growth of tumor cells. They concluded the role of COX-2 in the growth of PTC cell lines.

Cornetta et al. [29] examined a variety of thyroid tissue specimens; COX-2 staining was not observed in none of the 6 specimens obtained from normal or multinodular goiter specimens. Analysis of Hashimoto's thyroiditis revealed COX-2 expression in the follicular epithelium and lymphocytic infiltrates, as well as in cases of FTC and PTC [29].

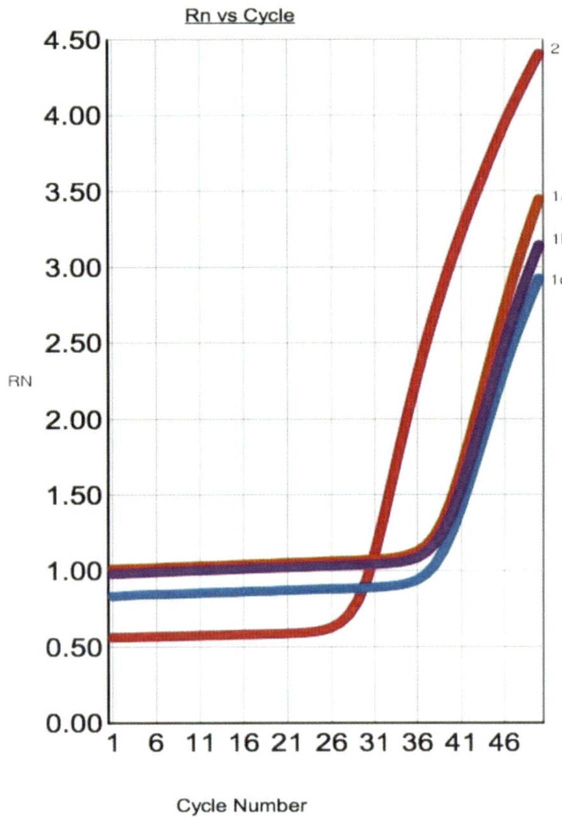


**Figure 1 Representative amplification curves for *COX-2* and *β-actin* genes in real-time PCR in PTC specimen.** 1 a,b,c - amplification curve for *COX-2* gene (mean $C_T$ value - *36.694); 2* - amplification curve for *β-actin* gene (endogenous control) (mean $C_T$ value - 27.071).

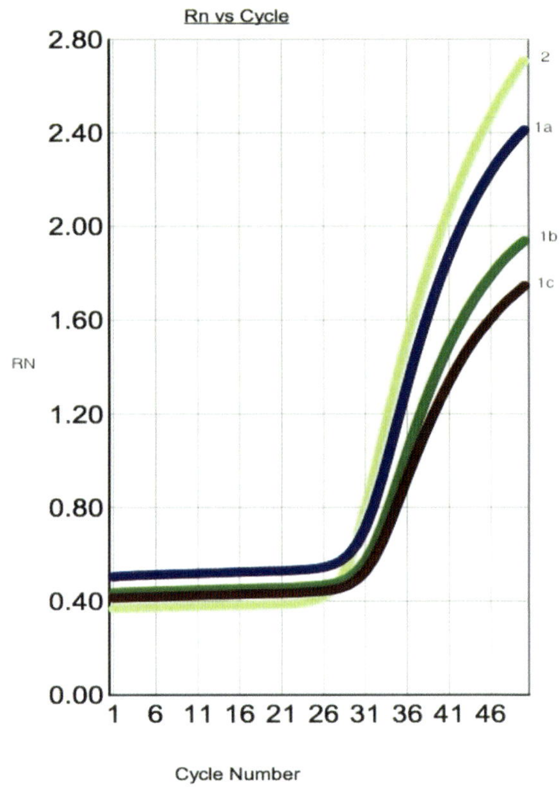


**Figure 2 Representative amplification curves for *COX-2* and *β-actin* genes in real-time PCR in macroscopically unchanged specimen.** 1 a,b,c - amplification curve for *COX-2* gene (mean $C_T$ value - *31.979); 2* - amplification curve for *β-actin gene* (endogenous control) (mean $C_T$ value - 27.250).

The study of Lee et al. [30] showed prominent expression of COX-2 in thyroiditis, benign and malignant thyroid lesions but not in normal thyroid tissues. They also observed no correlation between severity of PTC, regardless of the presence or absence of metastases. Because of the same intensity of COX-2 staining, found in thyroiditis, benign and malignant thyroid lesions the authors concluded that it is unlikely that COX-2 expression is related to the progression of thyroid disease.

The results of study with $Apc^{\Delta 716}$ knockout mice [31], suggested that the induction of *COX-2* was a very early event in colon carcinogenesis. This view has been supported by Garcia-Gonzales et al. [28] who have suggested that even though COX-2 plays an important role in progression of all thyroid cancers, in case of PTC it seems to be more important only in the early stages of disease.

## Conclusions

The usefulness of *COX-2* as a marker of thyroid malignancy has been challenged but its potential role in

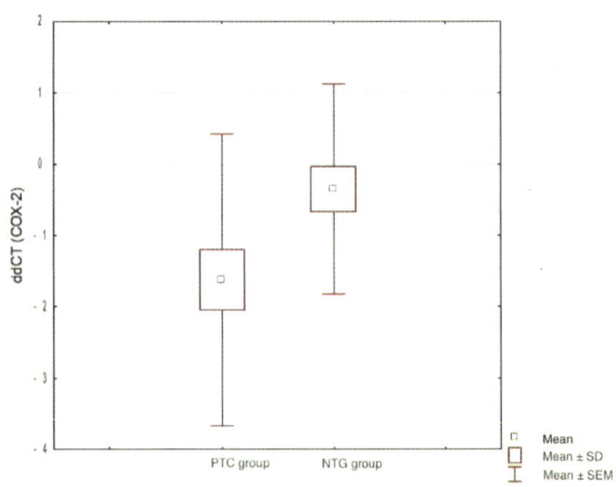


**Figure 3 Box-and-whisker plots representing the COX-2 mRNA expression by quantitative RT-PCR in PTC and NTG groups.** Results are calculated as ddCT values. Whiskers represent means ± SD (standard deviation) for particular groups. Boxes represent means ± SEM (standard error of mean). The results were statistically analyzed, using Student's t test.

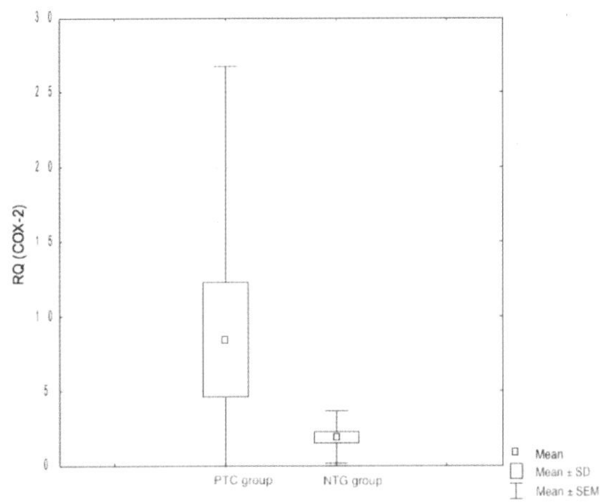


**Figure 4 Box-and-whisker plots representing the COX-2 mRNA expression by quantitative RT-PCR in PTC and NTG groups.** Results are calculated as RQ values. Whiskers represent means ± SD (standard deviation) for particular groups. Boxes represent means ± SEM (standard error of mean). The results were statistically analyzed, using Man-Whitney's U test ($p < 0.05$).

carcinogenesis arouses significant interest. In the present study, *COX-2* expression was found in all studied samples and the elevated level of *COX-2* gene expression was confirmed in PTC genetic material, collected from the fine-needle washout fluids. Thus, *COX-2* gene may play a significant role in the pathogenesis of this cancer type. Furthermore, *COX-2* gene overexpression levels were individually diversified, what may have resulted from their association with different genetic and clinical prognostic factors.

**Acknowledgements**
This study was supported by the funds of the Medical University of Lodz - Grant No. 502-11-843 and of the Ministry of Scientific Research and Information Technology of Poland - Grant No 1296/B/P01/2009/37.
The publication of the above article was financially supported by the Ministry of Science and Higher Education of Poland - the grant of the Polish Thyroid Association.

**Authors' contributions**
KK-R designed and coordinated the study, carried out the molecular genetic studies and drafted the manuscript. KW-D participated in performing molecular studies. AC-M participated in performing molecular studies. ZA and EG participated in coordination of molecular genetic studies. AL, the senior author, wrote the manuscript. All authors read and approved the final manuscript.

**Competing interests**
The authors declare that they have no competing interests.

**References**

1. Sheils O: **Molecular classification and biomarker discovery in papillary thyroid carcinoma.** *Expert Rev Mol Diagn* 2005, **6**:927-946.
2. Lewiński A, Wojciechowska K: **Genetic background of carcinogenesis in the thyroid gland.** *Neuroendocrinol Lett* 2007, **28**:77-105.
3. Wirtschafter A, Schmidt R, Rosen D, Kundu N, Santoro M, Fusco A, Multhaupt H, Atkins JP, Rosen MR, Keane W, Rothstein JL: **Expression of RET/PTC gene as a marker for papillary thyroid carcinoma on Hashimoto's thyroiditis.** *Laryngoscope* 1997, **107**:95-100.
4. Califano D, Rizzo C, D'Alessio A, Colucci-D'Amato GL, Cali G, Bartoli PC, Santelli G, Vecchio G, de Francisis V: **Signaling through Ras is essential for ret oncogene - induced cell differentiation in PC12 cells.** *J Biol Chem* 2000, **275**:19297-19305.
5. Jones DA, Carlton DP, McIntyre TM, Zimmerman GA, Prescott SM: **Molecular cloning of human prostaglandin endoperoxide synthase type II and demonstration of expression in response to cytokines.** *J Biol Chem* 1993, **268**:9049-9054.
6. Tsujii M, DuBois RN: **Alterations in cellular adhesion and apoptosis in epithelial cells overexpressing prostaglandin endoperoxide synthase 2.** *Cell* 1995, **3**:493-501.
7. Fosslien E: **Molecular pathology of cyclooxygenase-2-cancer-induced angiogenesis.** *Ann Clin Lab Sci* 2001, **31**:325-348.
8. Siironen P, Ristimäki A, Narko K, Nordling S, Louhimo J, Andersson S, Haapiainen R, Haglund C: **VEGF-C and COX-2 expression in papillary thyroid cancer.** *Endocr Relat Cancer* 2006, **13**:465-473.
9. Soh EY, Duh Q-Y, Sobhi SA, Young DM, Epstein HD, Wong MG, Garcia YK, Min YD, Grossman RF, Siperstein AE, Clark OH: **Vascular endothelial growth factor expression is higher in differentiated thyroid cancer than in normal or benign thyroid.** *J Clin Endocrinol Metab* 1997, **82**:3741-3747.
10. Hwang D, Scollard D, Byrne J, Levine E: **Expression of cyclooxygenase-1 and cyclooxygenase-2 in human breast cancer.** *J Natl Cancer Inst* 1998, **90**:455-460.
11. van Rees BP, Saukkonen K, Ristimaki A, Polkowski W, Tytgat GN, Drillenburg P, Offerhaus GJ: **Cyclooxygenase-2 expression during carcinogenesis in the human stomach.** *J Pathol* 2002, **196**:171-179.
12. Shirahama T, Sakakura C: **Overexpression of cyclooxygenase-2 in squamous cell carcinoma of the urinary bladder.** *Clin Cancer Res* 2001, **7**:558-561.
13. Soslow RA, Dannenberg AJ, Rush D, Woerner BM, Khan KN, Masferrer J, Koki AT: **COX-2 is expressed in human pulmonary, colonic and mammary tumors.** *Cancer* 2000, **89**:2537-2645.
14. Eberhat CE, Coffey RJ, Radhika A, Giardiello FM, Ferrenbach S, DuBois RN: **Up-regulation of cyclooxygenase-2 gene expression in human colorectal adenomas and adenocarcinomas.** *Gastroenterology* 1994, **107**:1183-1188.
15. Zimmermann KC, Sarbia M, Weber AA, Borchard F, Gabbert HE, Schror K: **Cyclooxygenase-2 expression in human esophageal carcinoma.** *Cancer Res* 1999, **59**:198-204.
16. Koga H, Sakisaka S, Ohishi M, Kawaguchi T, Taniguchi E, Sasatomi K, Harada M, Kusaba T, Tanaka M, Sata M: **Expression of cyclooxygenase-2 in human hepatocellular carcinoma: relevance to tumor dedifferentiation.** *Hepatology* 1999, **29**:688-696.
17. Wolf H, Saukkonen K, Anttila S, Karjalainen A, Vainio H, Ristimaki A: **Expression of cyclooxygenase-2 in human lung carcinoma.** *Cancer Res* 1998, **58**:4997-5001.
18. Sano H, Kawahito Y, Wilder RL, Hashimoto A, Mukai S, Asai K, Kimura S, Kato H, Kondo M, Hla T: **Expression of cyclooxygenase-1 and -2 in human colorectal cancer.** *Cancer Res* 1995, **55**:3785-3789.
19. Okami J, Yamamoto H, Fujiwara Y, Tsujie M, Kondo K, Noura S, Oshima S: **Overexpression of cyclooxygenase-2 in carcinoma of the pancreas.** *Clin Cancer Res* 1999, **5**:2018-2024.
20. Reddy BS, Hirose Y, Lubet R, Steele V, Kelloff G, Paulson S, Seibert K, Rao CV: **Chemoprevention of colon cancer by specific cyclooxygenase-2 inhibitor, celecoxib, administered during different stages of carcinogenesis.** *Cancer Res* 2000, **60**:293-297.
21. Ziegler J: **Early trials probe COX-2 inhibitors' cancer - fighting potential.** *J Natl Cancer Inst* 1999, **91**:1186-1187.
22. Chomczynski P, Sacchi N: **Single-step method of RNA isolation by acid guanidinium thiocyanate-phenol-chloroform extraction.** *Anal Bioch* 1987, **162**:156-159.
23. Brzezianska E, Cyniak-Magierska A, Sporny S, Pastuszak-Lewandoska D, Lewinski A: **Assessment of cyclin D1 gene expression as prognostic factor in benign and malignant thyroid lesions.** *Neuroendocrinol Lett* 2007, **28**:341-350.

24. Hamberger B, Gharib H, Melton LJ, Goellner JR, Zinsmeister AR: **Fine needle aspiration biopsy of thyroid nodules: impact on thyroid practice and cost of care.** *Am J Med* 1982, **73**:381-384.
25. Ito Y, Yoshida H, Nakano K, Takmura Y, Miya A, Kobayashi K, Yokozawa T, Kuma K, Miyauchi A: **Cyclooxygenase-2 expression in thyroid neoplasms.** *Histopathology* 2003, **42**:492-497.
26. Siironen P, Louhimo J, Nordling S, Ristimaki A, Maenpaa H, Haapiainen R, Haglund C: **Prognostic factors in papillary thyroid cancer: an evaluation of 601 consecutive patients.** *Tumor Biol* 2005, **26**:57-64.
27. Garcia-Gonzales M, Abdulkader I, Vazquez Boquete A, Neo XM, Forteza J, Cameselle-Teijeiro J: **Cyclooxygenase-2 in normal, hyperplastic and neoplastic follicular cells of the human thyroid gland.** *Virchows Arch* 2005, **447**:12-17.
28. Kajita S, Ruebel KH, Casey MB, Nakamura N, Lloyd RV: **Role of COX-2, thromboxane A2 synthase, and prostaglandin I2 synthase in papillary thyroid carcinoma growth.** *Mod Pathol* 2005, **18**:221-227.
29. Cornetta AJ, Russell JP, Cunnane M, Keane WM, Rothstein IL: **Cyclooxygenase-2 expression in human thyroid carcinoma and Hashimoto's thyroiditis.** *Laryngoscope* 2002, **112**:238-242.
30. Lee KJ, Jung YS, Kim WH, Yoon TI, Joo HJ, Soh EY: **Cyclooxygenase-2 expression in human thyroid disease.** *J Endocrinol Invest* 2008, **31**:111-118.
31. Oshima M, Dinchuk JE, Kargman SL, Oshima H, Hancock B, Kwong E, Trzaskos JM, Evans JF, Taketo MT: **Suppression of intestinal polyposis in *ApcΔ716* knockout mice by inhibition of cyclooxygenase 2 (COX-2).** *Cell* 1996, **5**:803-809.

7

# Assessment of Japanese iodine intake based on seaweed consumption in Japan: A literature-based analysis

Theodore T Zava and David T Zava*

**Abstract**

Japanese iodine intake from edible seaweeds is amongst the highest in the world. Predicting the type and amount of seaweed the Japanese consume is difficult due to day-to-day meal variation and dietary differences between generations and regions. In addition, iodine content varies considerably between seaweed species, with cooking and/or processing having an influence on iodine content. Due to all these factors, researchers frequently overestimate, or underestimate, Japanese iodine intake from seaweeds, which results in misleading and potentially dangerous diet and supplementation recommendations for people aiming to achieve the same health benefits seen by the Japanese. By combining information from dietary records, food surveys, urine iodine analysis (both spot and 24-hour samples) and seaweed iodine content, we estimate that the Japanese iodine intake–largely from seaweeds–averages 1,000-3,000 μg/day (1-3 mg/day).

**Keywords:** Iodine, iodide, seaweed, algae, kelp, Japanese, thyroid, cancer, life expectancy

## Introduction

Japanese iodine intake exceeds that of most other countries, primarily due to substantial seaweed consumption. Iodine is an essential element required for thyroid hormone synthesis, believed to impart some of its antioxidant and antiproliferative activity in the prevention of cardiovascular disease and cancer [1-8]. Seaweeds have the unique ability to concentrate iodine from the ocean, with certain types of brown seaweed accumulating over 30,000 times the iodine concentration of seawater [9]. The amount of iodine the Japanese consume daily from seaweeds has previously been estimated as high as 13.5 to 45 mg/day by sources that use ambiguous data to approximate intake [10,11], an amount 4.5 to 15 times greater than the safe upper limit of 3 mg/day set by the Ministry of Health, Labor and Welfare in Japan [12]. While high iodine intake from seaweed consumption is believed to have numerous health benefits, it has been reported to negatively affect individuals with underlying thyroid disorders [13-16]. To prevent excessive consumption it is imperative for people seeking health benefits from a high iodine diet to be knowledgeable of the amount of iodine the Japanese consume daily. In this paper we use a combination of dietary records, food surveys, urine iodine analysis, and seaweed iodine content to provide a reliable estimate of Japanese iodine intake, primarily from seaweeds.

## Types of edible seaweeds and their iodine content

In Japan, over 20 species of red, green, and brown algae (seaweed) are included in meals [17]. Iodine content varies depending on species, harvest location and preparation, and is typically highest in fresh cut blades and lowest in sun bleached blades [18]. The three most popular seaweed products in Japan are nori (*Porphyra*), wakame (*Undaria*) and kombu (*Laminaria*). Dried iodine contents range from 16 μg/g in nori to over 8,000 μg/g in kelp flakes; Japanese kombu and wakame contain an estimated 2353 μg/g and 42 μg/g respectively [18,19]. Ten different species of *Laminaria*, a type of kelp commonly labeled as kombu, from around the world were examined for their iodine content and were found to average 1,542 μg/g when dried [17].

* Correspondence: dzava@zrtlab.com
ZRT Laboratory, 8605 SW Creekside Place, Beaverton, 97008, USA

## Japanese seaweed consumption statistics

As the Japanese transitioned from a traditional to a Westernized diet, beginning around the 1950's [20], consumption of certain seaweed species declined while others increased. A decrease in kombu consumption (844 to 685 g/year per household) and an increase in wakame consumption (727 to 1234 g/year per household) can be seen between the years of 1963 and 1973 [21]. Consumption of kombu per Japanese household dropped further to 450 g in 2006 (elders ate up to four times more than those under the age of 29) [19]. Since daily seaweed consumption per person in Japan has remained relatively consistent over the last 40 years (4.3 g/day in 1955 and 5.3 g/day in 1995) [22], it is believed that consumption of wakame and nori have made up for the decline in kombu consumption [23,24]. Both nori and wakame have relatively low iodine contents compared to kombu.

Seaweed consumption frequency differs from person to person in Japan, resulting in a constantly fluctuating iodine intake. Seaweed is served in approximately 21% of Japanese meals [25] with 20-38% of the Japanese male and female population aged 40-79 years consuming seaweed more than five times per week, 29-35% three to four times per week, 25-35% one to two times per week, 6-13% one to two times per month, and 1-2% rarely consuming seaweed [26]. A 2010 food frequency questionnaire on the Japanese Kombu Association website indicates that kelp (assuming kombu) is consumed at a rate of: 27.5% once per week, 25.5% once per month, 18% three or four times per week, and 15.9% once every few months, with only 6.1% of survey respondents stating they consume kelp nearly every day [27].

## Effect of cooking on seaweed iodine content

Seaweed is often cooked to flavor dishes or soup stocks before consumption. When kombu is boiled in water for 15 minutes it can lose up to 99% of its iodine content, while iodine in sargassum, a similar brown seaweed, loses around 40% [28,29]. Processed kelp is often boiled in dye for half an hour ("ao-kombu" or "kizami-kombu") before hanging to dry [21], a process which can reduce seaweed iodine content before it is consumed. When kelp is used to flavor soup stocks the seaweed is often removed after boiling, resulting in soup stock high in iodine. Twenty samples of supermarket soups with kelp or kelp broth were analyzed by Nishiyama et al. to determine iodine content, revealing a minimum concentration of 660 μg/L (0.66 mg/L) and a maximum concentration of 31,000 μg/L (31 mg/L) [16]. Serving size for soup is typically around 0.25 L, resulting in 165 to 7,750 μg (0.165 to 7.75 mg) of iodine per serving.

## Estimating Japanese iodine intake from seaweed consumption

Due to variation of iodine content from one seaweed species to the next, along with confusion stemming from wet and dry weight terminology, many inaccurate assumptions have been made regarding the amount of iodine the Japanese actually consume from seaweed. Not all studies, dietary records or surveys specify whether daily or yearly consumption of seaweeds is recorded using wet weight, dry weight or a combination of the two. In some reports seaweed consumption has been estimated at 4-7 g/day dried weight [17,22,30,31], while other reports claim consumption of 12 g/day using both wet and dry weight [32]. Certain seaweeds have a swelling capacity of nearly ten times their dry volume with moisture content typically over 70% when wet and around 7-20% when dried [33,34]. The difference between wet and dry weight, along with the type of seaweeds being consumed, can result in extreme overestimation (more likely) or underestimation (less likely) of Japanese iodine intake.

Interpreting information to determine Japanese seaweed consumption and resulting iodine intake is a difficult task, and with ever changing diets, a close estimate is all that can be made. Nori and wakame are the most commonly consumed seaweeds in Japan, with nori accounting for 45% and wakame accounting for 30% (75% together) of total seaweed consumption, as stated by the Food and Agriculture Organization of the United Nations [35]. Based on previous estimates and records, dried seaweed consumption of 4-7 g/day [17,22,30,31] results in iodine intakes between 79 and 139 μg/day from nori and wakame when calculated using dried iodine contents of 16 and 42 μg/g respectively [18]. The remainder of iodine intake is derived mainly from kombu consumption, with smaller amounts coming from other seaweeds that have nominal iodine content.

Kombu has the highest iodine content of all seaweeds in the Japanese diet. In 2006 consumption of kombu/household/year was 450 g [19], and with an average of 2.55 members per household in Japan in 2005 [36], 0.48 g kombu/person/day was consumed. When calculated, 0.48 g of kombu with an iodine content of 2,353 μg/g [18] equates to 1,129 μg/day of iodine. Assuming negligible iodine intake from the other seaweeds consumed, daily iodine intake from nori, wakame, and kelp can be estimated at 1,208 to 1,268 μg/day (1.2 to 1.3 mg/day). It is reasonable to assume that iodine intake per day based on seaweed consumption frequency and iodine content averages around 1,000-2,000 μg/day (1-2 mg/day).

## Estimating Japanese iodine intake from diet studies and urine iodine analysis

Seaweed consumption statistics only provide only an estimate of Japanese iodine intake and should be combined with other predictive factors. Fortunately, studies that measure iodine content of single or entire meals are available and are, arguably, the most accurate estimate of Japanese iodine intake from seaweeds. A collection of Japanese diet studies that measure the amount of iodine in 24-hour diet samples or single meals can be seen in Table 1. Daily iodine intake of the Japanese based on 24-hour diet samples generally does not exceed 3,000 μg (3 mg).

Because approximately 97% of dietary iodine is excreted in the urine, urine iodine levels taken from individuals or populations can provide a secondary estimate of Japanese iodine intake from seaweed consumption, when paired with diet studies [37,38]. Urine iodine levels can increase from 100 μg/L to 30,000 μg/L in a single day and return to 100 μg/L within a couple of days, depending on seaweed intake [39]. This is somewhat expected when varying amounts and types of seaweeds are consumed on a day-to-day basis. Urine creatinine levels seen as μg iodine/g creatinine (μg/g Cr) can be used to adjust for an individual's hydration status, correlating well with μg/L in areas of adequate nutrition [40]. Urine iodine levels of the Japanese found in a number of studies are shown in Table 2. Mean and median iodine levels in the Japanese urine collections typically do not exceed 3,000 μg/L (3 mg/L).

**Table 1 Compilation of Japanese diet studies measuring iodine in 24-hour diet samples and single meals**

| Author(s) [source] | Year | Number of Participants | Mean Iodine in 24-Hour Diet Sample (μg) | Lowest Iodine in 24-Hour Diet Sample (μg) | Highest Iodine in 24-Hour Diet Sample (μg) | City/ Region |
|---|---|---|---|---|---|---|
| Katamine et al. [23] | 1986 | 1 | 1023 μg | 45 μg | 1921 μg | Tokyo |
| Katamine et al. [23] | 1986 | 1 | 362 μg | 57 μg | 1244 μg | Tokyo |
| Katamine et al. [23] | 1986 | 1 | 361 μg | 62 μg | 1098 μg | Tokyo |
| Katamine et al. [23] | 1986 | 1 | 429 μg | 52 μg | 1561 μg | Tokyo |
| Katamine et al. [23] | 1986 | 10 (hospital) | 1290 μg | 89 μg | 4746 μg | |
| Katamine et al. [23] | 1986 | 5 (hospital) | 195 μg | 95 μg | 287 μg | |
| Katamine et al. [23] | 1986 | 13 (school) | 113 μg/meal | 47 μg/meal | 203 μg/meal | Ibaraki |
| Katamine et al. [23] | 1986 | 5 (school) | 27 μg/meal | 25 μg/meal | 31 μg/meal | Kanagawa |
| Katamine et al. [23] | 1986 | 5 (school) | 36 μg/meal | 18 μg/meal | 43 μg/meal | Kanagawa |
| Tajiri et al. [48] | 1986 | 1 | 25400 μg est. | | | Kumamoto |
| Tajiri et al. [48] | 1986 | 1 | 43000 μg est. | | | Kumamoto |
| Tajiri et al. [48] | 1986 | 1 | 15000 μg est. | | | Kumamoto |
| Tajiri et al. [48] | 1986 | 1 | 20000 μg est. | | | Kumamoto |
| Tajiri et al. [48] | 1986 | 10 | 2800 μg est. | | | Kumamoto |
| Tajiri et al. [48] | 1986 | 8 | 2300 μg est. | | | Kumamoto |
| Shiraishi et al. [61] | 1999 | 6 | 1770 μg | 545 μg | 4490 μg | Mito |
| Kunachowicz et al. [62] | 2000 | 5 | 1970 μg/kg mean, 550 μg/kg median | 88 μg/kg | 7650 μg/kg | |
| Yoshinaga et al. [25] | 2001 | 29 (476 meals) | 1900 μg/kg | | | All Japan |
| Kucera et al. [63] | 2003 | | 756 μg/kg median | 124 μg/kg | 21660 μg/kg | |
| Nishiyama et al. [16] | 2004 | 5 (pregnant) | | 2280 μg | 3180 μg | Kumamoto |
| Nishiyama et al. [16] | 2004 | 10 (pregnant) | | 820 μg | 1400 μg | Kumamoto |
| Nishiyama et al. [16] | 2004 | 22 (pregnant w/ no kelp) | | 250 μg | 480 μg | Kumamoto |

**Table 2 Compilation of Japanese urine iodine studies**

| Author(s) [source] | Year | Number of participants | Age | Sex | Mean Urine Iodine ( μg/L, μg/g Cr, or μg/24-hour) | Median Urine Iodine ( μg/L) | City/Region |
|---|---|---|---|---|---|---|---|
| Suzuki et al. [50] | 1965 | 2 | | | 1565 μg/24-hour (hospital diet) | | Hokkaido |
| Suzuki et al. [50] | 1965 | 5 | | | 23300 μg/24-hour (seaweed diet) | | Hokkaido |
| Suzuki et al. [50] | 1965 | 7 | | | 175 μg/24-hour (iodine restricted) | | Hokkaido |
| Nagataki et al. [39] | 1967 | 9 | | Both | 3286 μg/24-hour | | Tokyo |
| Suzuki et al. [64] | 1985 | 5 | 19-26 | Male | 357 μg/24-hour | | |
| Suzuki et al. [64] | 1985 | 10 | 19-21 | Male | 149 μg/24-hour | | |
| Yabu et al. [65] | 1986 | 127 | 18-57 | Both | 3238 μg/L | | |
| Yabu et al. [66] | 1988 | 127 | 18-57 | Both | 3022 μg/g Cr | | |
| Yabu et al. [66] | 1988 | 43 | 4-10 | Both | 2756 μg/g Cr | | |
| Yabu et al. [66] | 1988 | 30 | Infant | Both | 1854 μg/g Cr | | |
| Yabu et al. [66] | 1988 | 24 | 11-32 | Female | 1701 μg/g Cr | | |
| Yabu et al. [66] | 1988 | 73 | 18-27 | Female | 2845 μg/g Cr | | |
| Nagataki [67] | 1993 | 14 | | | 660 μg/g Cr | | Tohoku |
| Nagataki [67] | 1993 | 13 | | | 1090 μg/g Cr (hospital diet) | | Tohoku |
| Nagataki [67] | 1993 | 13 | | | 1760 μg/g Cr (hospital diet) | | Tokyo |
| Nagataki [67] | 1993 | 22 | | | 1460 μg/g Cr (hospital diet) | | Shinsyu |
| Nagataki [67] | 1993 | 8 | | | 1370 μg/g Cr (hospital diet) | | Kyoto |
| Nagataki [67] | 1993 | 19 | | | 910 μg/g Cr (hospital diet) | | Nagasaki |
| Konno et al. [49] | 1994 | 4138 | Mean ~45 | Both | 3300 μg/L | | Sapporo |
| Tsuda et al. [68] | 1995 | 84 | | | | 596 μg/L | Nagasaki |
| Nagata et al. [47] | 1998 | 150 | Mean ~52 | Both | 1480 μg/L | | Nishihara |
| Nagata et al. [47] | 1998 | 37 | | | 1470 μg/24-hour | | Nishihara |
| Nagata et al. [47] | 1998 | 20 | Mean ~51 | Both | 1620 μg/L | | Yamagata |
| Nagata et al. [47] | 1998 | 54 | Mean ~49 | Both | 1200 μg/L | | Kobe |
| Nagata et al. [47] | 1998 | 80 | Mean ~50 | Both | 810 μg/L | | Hotaka |
| Ishigaki et al. [69] | 2001 | 250 | 7-14 | Both | | 362 μg/L | Nagasaki |
| Ishigaki et al. [69] | 2001 | 50 | Adult | Both | | 208 μg/L | Hamamatsu |
| Ishigaki et al. [69] | 2001 | 50 | Adult | Both | | 1015 μg/L | South Kayabe |
| Takamura et al. [70] | 2003 | 4 | 18-24 | Male | 406 μg/L | | Nagasaki |
| Zimmermann et al. [71] | 2005 | 302 | 6-12 | Both | 296 μg/L | 292 μg/L | Central Hokkaido |
| Zimmermann et al. [71] | 2005 | 280 | 6-12 | Both | 728 μg/L | 741 μg/L | Costal Hokkaido |
| Tomoda et al. [72] | 2005 | 47 | Mean ~53 | Both | 428 μg/g Cr | | |
| Tomoda et al. [72] | 2005 | 21 | Mean ~56 | Both | 587 μg/g Cr | | |
| Fuse et al. [73] | 2007 | 654 | 6-12 | Both | | 281 μg/L | Tokyo |
| Miyai et al. [74] | 2008 | 6 | Mean ~27 | Both | 560 μg/24-hour | | |
| Miyai et al. [74] | 2008 | 14 | Mean ~27 | Both | 1110 μg/24-hour | | |
| Orito et al. [75] | 2009 | 514 | Adult | Female (pregnant) | | 328 μg/L | Kobe |

When using 1.5 L as an expected 24-hour urine output, urine iodine excretion should rarely exceed an estimated 4,500 μg/24 hr (4.5 mg/24 hr).

## Japanese health statistics linked to high seaweed intake

The Japanese are considered one of the world's longest living people, with an extraordinarily low rate of certain types of cancer. A major dietary difference that sets Japan apart from other countries is high iodine intake, with seaweeds the most common source. Here are some astonishing Japanese health statistics, which are possibly related to their high seaweed consumption and iodine intake:

-Japanese average life expectancy (83 years) is five years longer than US average life expectancy (78 years) [41].

-In 1999 the age-adjusted breast cancer mortality rate was three times higher in the US than in Japan [42].

-Ten years after arriving in the US (in 1991), the breast cancer incidence rate of immigrants from Japan increased from 20 per 100,000 to 30 per 100,000 [43].

-In 2002 the age-adjusted rate of prostate cancer in Japan was 12.6 per 100,000, while the US rate was almost ten times as high [44].

-Heart related deaths in men and women aged 35-74 years are much higher in the US (1,415 per 100,000) as they are in Japan (897 per 100,000) [45].

-In 2004, infant deaths were over twice as high in the US (6.8 per 1,000) as they were in Japan (2.8 per 1,000) [46].

## Negative effects of iodine from seaweed

High iodine intake from seaweed consumption can cause unexpected health problems in a subset of individuals with pre-existing thyroid disorders. Although it is reported that excessive iodine does not cause thyroid antibody positivity, high intake can cause or worsen symptoms for people with previous thyroid autoimmunity or other underlying thyroid issues [47]. Transient hypothyroidism and iodine-induced goiter is common in Japan and can be reversed in most cases by restricting seaweed intake [16,29,48-52]. In Asian cultures, seaweed is commonly cooked with foods containing goitrogens such as broccoli, cabbage, bok choi and soy [18]. The phytochemicals in these foods can competitively inhibit iodine uptake by the thyroid gland (i.e., isothiocyanates from cruciferous vegetables) [53-55], or inhibit incorporation of iodine into thyroid hormone (i.e., soy isoflavones) [56,57].

Certain species of seaweed can concentrate bromine, a halide similar to iodine with no known physiological function, at very high levels [58,59]. If seaweeds with elevated levels of bromine and low levels of iodine are consumed when the body is in an iodine deficient state, inhibition of thyroid hormone synthesis–due to bromine's attachment to tyrosine residues on thyroglobulin in place of iodine–is plausible [60].

## Estimate of daily iodine intake in Japan

We estimate that the average Japanese iodine intake, largely from seaweed consumption–based on dietary records, food surveys, urine iodine analysis and seaweed iodine content–is 1,000-3,000 μg/day (1-3 mg/day). This estimate compares to a recent report claiming that the average iodine intake of the Japanese from kelp is around 1,200 μg/day (1.2 mg/day) [19]. Iodine intake can vary from day-to-day depending on diet, and it is unlikely for a single persons iodine intake to remain constant for an extended period of time. With the multitude of edible seaweeds (each with different iodine content) consumed in the Japanese diet, it is not appropriate to use a single type of seaweed to determine iodine intake, though many estimates do. Although seaweed provides a majority of the Japanese iodine intake, other food sources (containing far less iodine)–such as fish and shellfish–can increase the total amount of iodine consumed daily.

## Conclusions

Japanese iodine intake from seaweed is linked to health benefits not seen in cultures with dissimilar diets. Knowing how much iodine the Japanese consume daily is beneficial for people who wish to consume equivalent amounts of iodine or seaweed supplements while avoiding excessive amounts that may adversely affect health.

### Abbreviations

Cr: Creatinine.

### Authors' contributions

TZ acquired and compiled data shown in this study, interpreted data, and provided intellectual content. DZ provided interpretation of data and intellectual content. All authors read and approved the final manuscript.

### Authors' information

TZ received his Bachelor's degree in Biology from Oregon State University in 2009. He is a Research Associate at ZRT Laboratory in Beaverton, Oregon, where he recently developed a test to measure iodine and creatinine levels in dried urine. His current research focuses on iodine deficiency, Japanese iodine intake, halide competition, thyroid disorders and iodine kinetics in the human body.

DZ received his doctorate in Biochemistry from the University of Tennessee in 1974. He is Laboratory Director and President of ZRT Laboratory, which he founded in 1998. Dr. Zava has developed innovative, simple and cost-effective methods to monitor hormone and other analytes associated with health and disease. His current research focus includes endocrinology, breast cancer, and–most recently–the importance of iodine to optimum health. He is co-author of a landmark book, What Your Doctor May Not Tell You About Breast Cancer: How Hormone Balance Can Help Save Your Life.

### Competing interests

The author declares that they have no competing interests.

## References


1. Cann SA: **Hypothesis: dietary iodine intake in the etiology of cardiovascular disease.** *J Am Coll Nutr* 2006, **25**:1-11.
2. Miller DW: **Extrathyroidal Benefits of Iodine.** *J Am Phys and Surg* 2006, **11**:106-110.
3. Cann SA, van Netten JP, Glover DW, van Netten C: **Iodide accumulation in extrathyroidal tissues.** *J Clin Endocrinol Metab* 1999, **84**:821-822.
4. Yuan YV, Walsh NA: **Antioxidant and antiproliferative activities of extracts from a variety of edible seeweeds.** *Food Chem Toxicol* 2006, **44**:1144-1150.
5. Venturi S: **Is there a role for iodine in breast diseases?** *Breast* 2001, **10**:379-382.
6. Winkler R, Griebenow S, Wonisch W: **Effect of iodide on total antioxidant status of human serum.** *Cell Biochem Funct* 2000, **18**:143-146.
7. Moser M, Buchberger W, Mayer H: **Influence of an iodine-drinking cure on the antioxidative status of diabetes patients.** *Wien Klin Wochenschr* 1991, **103**:183-186.
8. Venturi S, Donati FM, Venturi A, Venturi M, Grossi L, Guidi A: **Role of iodine in evolution and carcinogenesis of thyroid, breast and stomach.** *Adv Clin Path* 2000, **4**:11-17.
9. Küpper FC, Schweigert N, Ar Gall E, Legendre J-M, Vilter H, Kloareg B: **Iodine uptake in Laminariales involves extracellular, haloperoxidase-mediated oxidation of iodide.** *Planta* 1998, **207**:163-671.
10. Abraham GE, Brownstein D: **Validation of the orthoiodosupplementation program: a rebuttal of Dr. Gaby's editorial on iodine.** *The Original Internist* 2005, **12**:184-194.
11. Miller D: **Iodine for health.** 2006 [http://www.lewrockwell.com/miller/miller20.html].
12. The Ministry of Health, Labour, and Welfare, Japan: **Dietary reference intakes for Japanese.** *In the Ministry of Health, Labour, and Welfare* Daiichi Shuppan Publishing. Tokyo; 2005, 189-193.
13. Mussig K, Thamer C, Bares R, Lipp HP, Haring HU, Gallwitz B: **Iodine-induced thyrotoxicosis after ingestion of kelp-containing tea.** *J Gen Intern Med* 2006, **21**:C11-C14.
14. Laurberg P, Pedersen IB, Knudsen N, Ovesen L, Andersen S: **Environmental iodine intake affects the type of non-malignant thyroid disease.** *Thyroid* 2001, **11**:457-469.
15. Markou K, Georgopoulos N, Kyriazopoulou V, Vagenakis AG: **Iodine-induced hypothyroidism.** *Thyroid* 2001, **11**:501-510.
16. Nishiyama S, Mikeda T, Okada T, Nakamura K, Kotani T, Hishinuma : **Transient hypothyroidism or persistent hyperthyrotropinemia in neonates born to mothers with excessive iodine intake.** *Thyroid* 2004, **14**:1077-1083.
17. Arasaki S, Arasaki T: *Vegetables from the sea* Tokyo: Japan Publications Inc; 1983.
18. Teas J, Pino S, Critchley AT, Braverman LE: **Variability of iodine content in common commercially available edible seaweeds.** *Thyroid* 2004, **14**:836-841.
19. Nagataki S: **The average of dietary iodine intake due to the ingestion of seaweeds is 1.2 mg/day in Japan.** *Thyroid* 2008, **18**:667-668.
20. Drewnowski A, Popkin BM: **The nutrition transition: new trends in the global diet.** *Nutr Rev* 1997, **55**:31-43.
21. Naylor J: **Production, trade and utilization of seaweeds and seaweed products.** *FAO Fish Tech Pap 159, FAO, Rome* 1976.
22. Matsumura Y: **Nutrition trends in Japan.** *Asia Pac J Clin Nutr* 2001, **10** S40-S47.
23. Katamine S, Mamiya Y, Sekimoto K, Hoshino N, Totsuka K, Naruse U, Watabe A, Sugiyama R, Suzuki M: **Iodine content of various meals currently consumed by urban Japanese.** *J Nutr Sci Vitaminol* 1986, **32**:487-495.
24. Research Division, Minister's Secretariat, Ministry of Agriculture, Forestry and Fisheries of Japan: *Food balance sheet in 1979* Tokyo; 1981, 107-108.
25. Yoshinaga J, Morita M, Yukawa M, Shiraishi K, Kawamura H: **Certified reference material for analytical quality assurance of minor and trace elements in food and related matrixes based on a typical Japanese diet: interlaboratory study.** *J AOAC Int* 2001, **84**:1202-1208.
26. Iso H, Date C, Noda H, Yoshimura T, Tamakoshi A, JACC Study Group: **Frequency of food intake and estimated nutrient intake among men and women: the JACC Study.** *J Epidemiol* 2005, **15**:S24-S42.
27. Nihon Konbu Kyoukai (Japan Konbu Association) in Konbu-Net: **2nd Kelp Report.** [http://www.kombu.or.jp/btob/data2010-2.pdf].
28. Hou X, Chai C, Qian Q, Yan X, Fan X: **Determination of chemical species of iodine in some seaweeds.** *Sci Total Environ* 1997, **204**:215-221.
29. Ishizuki Y, Yamauchi K, Miura Y: **Transient thyrotoxicosis induced by Japanese kombu.** *Nippon Naibunpi Gakkai Zasshi* 1989, **65**:91-98.
30. Toyokawa H: **Nutritional status in Japan from the view-point of numerical ecology.** *Soc Sci Med* 1978, **12**:517-524.
31. Matsuzaki S, Iwamura K: **Application of seaweeds to human nutrition and medicine.** *In Nahrung aus dem Meer; Food from the sea* New York: Springer; 2001, 162-184.
32. Teas J, Baldeon ME, Chiriboga DE, Davis JR, Sarries AJ, Braverman LE: **Could dietary seaweed reverse the metabolic syndrome?** *Asia Pac J Clin Nutr* 2009, **18**:145-154.
33. Teas J, Hurley TG, Hebert JR, Franke AA, Sepkovic DW, Kurzer MS: **Dietary seaweed modifies estrogen and phytoestrogen metabolism in healthy postmenopausal women.** *J Nutr* 2009, **139**:939-944.
34. Murata M, Nakazoe J: **Production and use of marine algae in Japan.** *Jpn Agr Res Q* 2001, **35**:281-290.
35. Rajadurai MR: **Production, marketing and trade of seaweeds.**Philippines27-31 Aug 1990.
36. Statistics Bureau, Ministry of Internal Affairs and Communications, Government of Japan: *Chapter IX: Household and household status* [http://www.stat.go.jp/english/data/kokusei/2005/poj/pdf/2005ch09.pdf].
37. Hays MT: **Estimation of total body iodine content in normal young men.** *Thyroid* 2001, **11**:671-675.
38. Larsen PR, Davies TF, Hay ID: **The thyroid gland.** In *In Williams textbook of endocrinology.* Edited by: Wilson JD, Foster DW, Kronenberg HM, Larson P. Philadelphia: W.B. Saunders Company; 1998:390-151.
39. Nagataki S, Shizume K, Nakao K: **Thyroid function in chronic excess iodide ingestion: comparison of thyroidal absolute iodine uptake and degradation of thyroxine in euthyroid Japanese subjects.** *J Clin Endocrinol Metab* 1967, **27**:638-647.
40. Caldwell KL, Makhmudov A, Ely E, Jones RL, Wang RY: **Iodine status of the U.S. population, National Health and Nutrition Examination Survey, 2005-2006 and 2007-2008.** *Thyroid* 2011, **21**:419-27.
41. World Health Organization: *World health statistics 2010: Geneva, Switzerland* [http://www.who.int/gho/database/WHS2010_Part2.xls].
42. Mettlin C: **Global breast cancer mortality statistics.** *CA Cancer J Clin* 1999, **49**:138-144.
43. Shimizu H, Ross RK, Bernstein L, Yatani R, Henderson BE, Mack TM: **Cancers of the prostate and breast among Japanese and white immigrants in Los Angeles County.** *Br J Cancer* 1991, **63**:963-966.
44. International Agency for Research on Cancer: *Globocan 2002 Database* [http://www-dep.iarc.fr/].
45. Roger VL, Go AS, Lloyd-Jones DM, Adams RJ, Berry JD, Brown TM, Carnethon MR, Dai S, de Simone G, Ford ES, Fox CS, Fullerton HJ, Gillespie C, Greenlund KJ, Hailpern SM, Heit JA, Ho PM, Howard VJ, Kissela BM, Kittner SJ, Lackland DT, Lichtman JH, Lisabeth LD, Makuc DM, Marcus GM, Marelli A, Matchar DB, McDermott MM, Meigs JB, Moy CS, *et al*: **Heart Disease and Stroke Statistics–2011 Update: A Report From the American Heart Association.** *Circulation* 2011, **123**:e18-e209.
46. National Center for Health Statistics: **Health, United States, 2007. With chartbook on trends in the health of Americans.** Hyattsville, MD; 2007 [http://www.cdc.gov/nchs/data/hus/hus07.pdf#listtables].
47. Nagata K, Takasu N, Akamine H, Ohshiro C, Komiya I, Murakami K, Suzawa A, Nomura T: **Urinary iodine and thyroid antibodies in Okinawa, Yamagata, Hyogo, and Nagano, Japan: the differences in iodine intake do not affect thyroid antibody positivity.** *Endocr J* 1998, **45**:797-803.
48. Tajiri J, Higashi K, Morita M, Umeda T, Sato T: **Studies of hypothyroidism in patients with high iodine intake.** *J Clin Endocrinol Metab* 1986, **63**:412-417.
49. Konno N, Makita H, Yuri K, Iizuka N, Kawasaki K: **Association between dietary iodine intake and prevalence of subclinical hypothyroidism in the central regions of Japan.** *J Clin Endocrinol Metab* 1994, **78**:393-397.
50. Suzuki H, Higuchi T, Sawa K, Ohtaki S, Horiuchi Y: **"Endemic coast goiter" in Hokkaido, Japan.** *Acta Endocrinol (Copenh)* 1965, **50**:161-176.
51. Konno N, Yuri K, Taguchi H, Miura K, Taguchi S, Hagiwara K, Murakami S: **Screening for thyroid diseases in an iodine sufficient area with sensitive thyrotrophin assays, and serum thyroid autoantibody and urinary iodide determinations.** *Clin Endocrinol (Oxf)* 1993, **38**:273-281.

52. Kasagi K, Iwata M, Misaki T, Konishi J: **Effect of iodine restriction on thyroid function in patients with primary hypothyroidism.** *Thyroid* 2003, **13**:561-567.
53. Greer MA, Astwood EB: **The antithyroid effect of certain foods in man as determined with radioactive iodine.** *Endocrinology* 1948, **43**:105-119.
54. Renner R: **More Iodine or Less Perchlorate?** *Environ Health Perspect* 2010, **118**:a289-a289.
55. Zimmermann MB: **Iodine deficiency.** *Endocr Rev* 2009, **30**:376-408.
56. Doerge DR, Sheehan DM: **Goitrogenic and estrogenic activity of soy isoflavones.** *Environ Health Perspect* 2002, **110(suppl 3)**:349-353.
57. Doerge DR, Chang HC: **Inactivation of thyroid peroxidase by soy isoflavones, in vitro and in vivo.** *J Chromatogr B Anal Technol Biomed Life Sci* 2002, **777**:269-279.
58. Saenko GN, Kravtsova YY, Ivanenko VV, Sheludko SI: **Concentration of iodine and bromine by plants in the Seas of Japan and Okhotsk.** *Mar Biol* 1978, **47**:243-250.
59. Rose M, Miller P, Baxter M, Appleton G, Crews H, Croasdale M: **Bromine and iodine in 1997 UK total diet study samples.** *J Environ Monit* 2001, **3**:361-5.
60. Pavelka S, Vobecky M, Babicky A: **Halogen speciation in the rat thyroid: Simultaneous determination of bromine and iodine by short-term INAA.** *J Radioanal Nucl Chem* 2008, **278**:575-579.
61. Shiraishi K, Muramatsu Y, Los IP, Korzun VN, Tsigankov NY, Zamostyan PV: **Estimation of dietary iodine and bromine intakes of Ukrainians.** *J Radioanal Nucl Chem* 1999, **242**:199-202.
62. Kunachowicz H, Stibilj V, Stos K, Gosciniarek R: **Studies on iodine content in daily diets and selected dairy products.** *Eur Food Res Technol* 2000, **211**:229-233.
63. Kucera J, Iyengar GV, Randa Z, Parr RM: **Determination of iodine in Asian diets by epithermal and radiochemical neutron activation analysis.** *J Radioanal Nucl Chem* 2004, **259**:505-509.
64. Suzuki M, Tamura T: **Iodine intake of Japanese male university students: urinary iodine excretion of sedentary and physically active students and sweat iodine excretion during exercise.** *J Nutr Sci Vitaminol* 1985, **31**:409-415.
65. Yabu Y, Miyai K, Hayashizaki S, Endo Y, Hata N, Iijima Y, Fushimi R: **Measurement of iodide in urine using the iodide-selective electrode.** *Endocrinol Jpn* 1986, **33**:905-911.
66. Yabu Y, Miyai K, Endo Y, Hata N, Iijima Y, Hayashizaki S, Fushimi R, Harada T, Nose O, Kobayashi A, Matsuzuka F, Kuma K: **Urinary iodide excretion measured with an iodide-selective ion electrode: studies on normal subjects of varying ages and patients with thyroid diseases.** *Endocrinol Jpn* 1988, **35**:391-398.
67. Nagataki S: **Status of iodine nutrition in Japan.** Nagasaki, Japan: Nagasaki University School of Medicine. IDD Newsltr; 1993:**9**:11.
68. Tsuda K, Namba H, Nomura T, Yokoyama N, Yamashita S, Izumi M, Nagataki S: **Automated measurement of urinary iodine with use of ultraviolet irradiation.** *Clin Chem* 1995, **41**:581-585.
69. Ishigaki K, Namba H, Takamura N, Saiwai H, Parshin V, Ohashi T, Kanematsu T, Yamashita S: **Urinary iodine levels and thyroid diseases in children; comparison between Nagasaki and Chernobyl.** *Endocr J* 2001, **48**:591-595.
70. Takamura N, Hamada A, Yamaguchi N, Matsushita N, Tarasiuk I, Ohashi T, Aoyagi K, Mine M, Yamashita S: **Urinary iodine kinetics after oral loading of potassium iodine.** *Endocr J* 2003, **50**:589-593.
71. Zimmermann MB, Ito Y, Hess SY, Fujieda K, Molinari L: **High thyroid volume in children with excess dietary iodine intakes.** *Am J Clin Nutr* 2005, **81**:840-844.
72. Tomoda C, Kitano H, Uruno T, Takamura Y, Ito Y, Miya A, Kobayashi K, Matsuzuka F, Amino N, Kuma K, Miyauchi A: **Transcutaneous iodine absorption in adult patients with thyroid cancer disinfected with povidone-iodine at operation.** *Thyroid* 2005, **15**:600-603.
73. Fuse Y, Saito N, Tsuchiya T, Shishiba Y, Irie M: **Smaller thyroid gland volume with high urinary iodine excretion in Japanese schoolchildren: normative reference values in an iodine-sufficient area and comparison with the WHO/ICCIDD reference.** *Thyroid* 2007, **17**:145-155.
74. Miyai K, Tokushige T, Kondo M, Iodine Research Group: **Suppression of thyroid function during ingestion of seaweed "Kombu" (Laminaria japonoca) in normal Japanese adults.** *Endocr J* 2008, **55**:1103-1108.
75. Orito Y, Oku H, Kubota S, Amino N, Shimogaki K, Hata M, Manki K, Tanaka Y, Sugino S, Ueta M, Kawakita K, Nunotani T, Tatsumi N, Ichihara K, Miyauchi A, Miyake M: **Thyroid function in early pregnancy in Japanese healthy women: relation to urinary iodine excretion, emesis, and fetal and child development.** *J Clin Endocrinol Metab* 2009, **94**:1683-1688.

# 8

# Influence of dietary iodine deficiency on the thyroid gland in *Slc26a4*-null mutant mice

Tomoyuki Iwata[1,2], Tadao Yoshida[1], Masaaki Teranishi[1], Yoshiharu Murata[3], Yoshitaka Hayashi[3], Yasuhiko Kanou[3], Andrew J Griffith[4] and Tsutomu Nakashima[1*]

**Abstract**

**Background:** Pendred syndrome (PDS) is an autosomal recessive disorder characterized by sensorineural hearing impairment and variable degree of goitrous enlargement of the thyroid gland with a partial defect in iodine organification. The thyroid function phenotype can range from normal function to overt hypothyroidism. It is caused by loss-of-function mutations in the *SLC26A4* (*PDS*) gene. The severity of the goiter has been postulated to depend on the amount of dietary iodine intake. However, direct evidence has not been shown to support this hypothesis. Because *Slc26a4*-null mice have deafness but do not develop goiter, we fed the mutant mice a control diet or an iodine-deficient diet to evaluate whether iodine deficiency is a causative environmental factor for goiter development in PDS.

**Methods:** We evaluated the thyroid volume in histological sections with the use of three-dimensional reconstitution software, we measured serum levels of total tri-iodothyronine (TT3) and total thyroxine (TT4) levels, and we studied the thyroid gland morphology by transmission electron microscopy.

**Results:** TT4 levels became low but TT3 levels did not change significantly after eight weeks of an iodine-deficient diet compared to levels in the control diet animals. Even in *Slc26a4*-null mice fed an iodine-deficient diet, the volume of the thyroid gland did not increase although the size of each epithelial cell increased with a concomitant decrease of thyroid colloidal area.

**Conclusions:** An iodine-deficient diet did not induce goiter in *Slc26a4*-null mice, suggesting that other environmental, epigenetic or genetic factors are involved in goiter development in PDS.

## Background

Pendred syndrome (PDS) is an autosomal recessive disorder characterized by sensorineural hearing impairment, presence of goiter, and a partial defect in iodine organification [1]. The goiter in PDS is variable in its presentation; it can develop at any age (although generally after puberty), but may be totally absent in some affected individuals [2]. Also, there is substantial intrafamilial and regional variation, and nutritional iodine intake may be a significant modifier of the thyroid phenotype [1]. Kopp *et al.* suggested that under conditions of sufficient iodine intake, thyroid enlargement may be very mild or absent, and hence these patients are often simply categorized as having enlarged vestibular aqueduct [1]. Sato *et al.* also suggested that even in patients with impaired iodide transport, high iodine intake may prevent the development of goiter [3].

*Slc26a4*-null (*Slc26a4*$^{-/-}$) mutant mice were generated by Everett *et al.* [2]. *Slc26a4*$^{-/-}$ mice are profoundly deaf with vestibular dysfunction, but they lack goiter and thyroid histological abnormalities. We hypothesized that the absence of goiter and hypothyroidism in *Slc26a4*$^{-/-}$ mice was due to a sufficient iodine intake, and that goiter and hypothyroidism might be induced by iodine deficiency. We, therefore, performed this study to investigate the influence of iodine intake on serum thyroid hormone levels and the histology and volume of the thyroid gland in *Slc26a4*$^{-/-}$ mice.

## Materials and methods

### *Slc26a4*-null mice

An *Slc26a4*-null (*Slc26a4*$^{-/-}$) mouse colony was established and bred with homozygotes and heterozygotes imported from the National Institutes of Health

* Correspondence: tsutomun@med.nagoya-u.ac.jp
[1]Department of Otorhinolaryngology Nagoya University Graduate School of Medicine, 65 Tsurumai-cho, Showa-ku, Nagoya, Aichi 466-8550, Japan
Full list of author information is available at the end of the article

(Rockville, Maryland) [2]. The line was maintained on a 129/SvEv background.

#### Breeding and Diet

Matings were performed between *Slc26a4*$^{-/-}$ and *Slc26a4*$^{-/-}$, and between *Slc26a4*$^{+/-}$ and *Slc26a4*$^{+/-}$ mice. These mice were fed a control diet (CLEA Japan Inc.). F1 offspring at two months of age were paired for mating. The mice were fed iodine-deficient chow (CLEA Japan Inc. T-08514) or control chow (CLEA Japan Inc. T-08513) from the beginning of the mating. Each chow was comprised solely of artificial materials. According to an analysis by the Laboratories for Food & Environmental Science, Tokyo, Japan, the iodine level was less than the sensing threshold (< 0.02 mg%) in iodine-deficient chow (ICD) whereas it was 0.51 mg% in control chow (CCD). F2 offspring were fed with the same diet as their parents for 12 to 16 weeks after weaning. *Slc26a4* genotyping was performed on DNA prepared from tail specimens obtained at the time of sacrifice of the mice. There were six groups comprising one of three different genotypes (*Slc26a4*$^{-/-}$, *Slc26a4*$^{+/-}$, and *Slc26a4*$^{+/}$) and either of ICD or CCD. Thirty-one 12 to 16 week-old males were used for this study (Table 1). Females were not analyzed in order to avoid the effect of menstrual cycles on hormone levels. The experimental protocol was approved by the Experimental Animal Management Committee, Nagoya University, Graduate School of Medicine.

#### Serum thyroid hormones

After deep anesthesia by intraperitoneal injection of pentobarbital sodium, blood was collected from the inferior vena cava. Serum total tri-iodothyronine (TT3) and total thyroxine (TT4) levels were measured by an electrochemiluminescence immunoassay (TT3: DRG® T-3 ELISA, TT4: DRG® T-4 ELISA, DRG International, East Mountainside, New Jersey USA).

#### Thyroid histology and volume

After intracardiac infusion of 4% paraformaldehyde, thyroid glands were excised together with adjacent tracheae and immersed in the same fixative for 24 hours at 4°C. The specimens were placed in 10% EDTA for seven days, washed with phosphate buffered saline (PBS), embedded in paraffin, and sectioned at 4-μm thickness for collection of every fifth section. The sections were stained with hematoxylin-eosin. The serial sections were observed with a light microscope system (BZ-8000, Keyence, Tokyo, Japan) and saved as digital images. A digital image of the whole thyroid was reconstructed and the volume was measured using three-dimensional reconstruction software, ZedView (LEXI, Tokyo, Japan).

#### Ultrastructural evaluation

One mouse was selected randomly for electron microscopic observation of the thyroid gland from each group of *Slc26a4*$^{-/-}$ CCD, *Slc26a4*$^{-/-}$ ICD, *Slc26a4*$^{+/-}$CCD and *Slc26a4*$^{+/-}$ ICD. The electron microscopic observation was done according to the method described previously [4]. Two-mm$^3$ thyroid specimens were excised, fixed in 2.5% glutaraldehyde for 24 hours at 4°C, washed in 0.1M phosphate buffer (pH = 7.0), and fixed again in 1% osmium tetroxide for 3 hours at 4°C. The samples were dehydrated in a graded series of ethanol and embedded in epoxy resin. Ultrathin sections were cut, double stained with uranyl acetate and lead citrate, and examined using a JEOL JEM100S electron microscope (JEOL, Tokyo, Japan).

#### Statistics

Statistical analysis was performed using SPSS Statistics ver.19.0 (SPSS Inc., Chicago, IL). One-way ANOVA and Mann-Whitney U-testing were used for statistical analysis. A *P* value less than 0.05 defined a significant difference.

## Results

#### Volume of thyroid gland

The thyroid volume in each animal is shown in Table 1. Mean thyroid volumes of *Slc26a4*$^{-/-}$, *Slc26a4*$^{+/-}$ and *Slc26a4*$^{+/+}$ mice fed with CCD were 1.8 ± 1.0 mm$^3$, 1.9 ± 0.9 mm$^3$, 1.4 ± 0.2 mm$^3$ respectively. The mean thyroid volumes of *Slc26a4*$^{-/-}$, *Slc26a4*$^{+/-}$ and *Slc26a4*$^{+/+}$ mice fed with ICD were 1.0 ± 0.3 mm$^3$, 1.5 ± 0.6 mm$^3$, 1.1 mm$^3$ respectively. There were no significant differences in mean thyroid volumes between ICD and CCD groups for any genotype. The thyroid images reconstructed by three-dimensional reconstruction software are shown in Figure 1.

#### Histological findings

Figure 2 demonstrates light microscopic observation of the thyroid gland of ICD and CCD groups for the three different *Slc26a4* genotypes. The size and height of epithelial cells increased with a concomitant decrease of colloidal area in ICD thyroid glands as compared to those of CCD animals among all genotypes. Electron microscopic observations in *Slc26a4*$^{-/-}$ and *Slc26a4*$^{+/-}$ thyroid glands were consistent with these findings (Figure 3).

#### Serum thyroid hormone levels

Serum concentrations of TT3 and TT4 in each animal are shown in Table 1. In the CCD group, the average TT3 levels were 1.26 μg/dl, 1.39 μg/dl and 1.53 μg/dl in *Slc26a4*$^{-/-}$, *Slc26a4*$^{+/-}$ and *Slc26a4*$^{+/+}$ mice, respectively. In the ICD group, the average TT3 levels were 0.92 μg/dl, 0.93 μg/dl and 1.07 μg/dl in *Slc26a4*$^{-/-}$, *Slc26a4*$^{+/-}$ and

**Table 1 Total tri-iodothyronine (TT3) and total thyroxine (TT4) levels and thyroid volumes in *Slc26a4*-null mice eating control chow (CCD) or iodine-deficient chow (ICD)**

| Genotype | Diet | Body weight (g) | TT3 (ng/ml) | TT4 (μg/dl) | Volume ($mm^3$) |
|---|---|---|---|---|---|
| *Slc26a4*$^{-/-}$ | CCD | 25.6 | 2.80 | 8.70 | 0.95 |
| | | 22.5 | 1.24 | 5.10 | 1.03 |
| | | 19.8 | 0.74 | 4.68 | EM |
| | | 28.9 | 0.76 | 3.99 | 2.27 |
| | | 29.7 | 0.78 | 3.78 | 2.93 |
| | ICD | 25.4 | 0.87 | 3.60 | 0.67 |
| | | 22.5 | 0.79 | 3.58 | 1.28 |
| | | 21.3 | 0.99 | 2.77 | 0.88 |
| | | 23.0 | 1.01 | 3.52 | 1.28 |
| | | 20.9 | 0.86 | 3.42 | 0.75 |
| | | 25.7 | 1.04 | 3.12 | 1.07 |
| | | 24.6 | 0.88 | 1.79 | EM |
| *Slc26a4*$^{+/-}$ | CCD | 25.6 | 1.30 | 6.30 | 1.48 |
| | | 23.8 | 1.35 | 5.90 | 1.47 |
| | | 23.5 | 1.45 | 4.03 | 1.28 |
| | | 27.4 | 2.40 | 8.10 | 1.03 |
| | | 28.2 | 1.60 | 5.05 | 2.82 |
| | | 25.1 | 0.82 | 3.83 | EM |
| | | 38.0 | 0.81 | 4.13 | 3.22 |
| | ICD | 24.8 | 1.02 | 4.29 | 1.31 |
| | | 23.4 | 0.84 | 3.11 | 0.66 |
| | | 29.2 | 0.87 | 2.64 | EM |
| | | 33.3 | 0.82 | 2.41 | 2.04 |
| | | 31.7 | 1.12 | 2.92 | 1.92 |
| *Slc26a4*$^{+/+}$ | CCD | 26.8 | 1.55 | 3.97 | 1.63 |
| | | 24.5 | 1.60 | 3.88 | 1.44 |
| | | 23.7 | 2.10 | 8.40 | 1.38 |
| | | 25.0 | 1.60 | 5.95 | 1.31 |
| | | 26.7 | 0.79 | 3.45 | 1.24 |
| | ICD | 23.4 | 0.93 | 4.26 | 1.11 |
| | | 23.8 | 1.20 | 4.35 | UM |

EM, examined with electron microscopy.
UM, unmeasurable due to failure to prepare adequate thin sections.

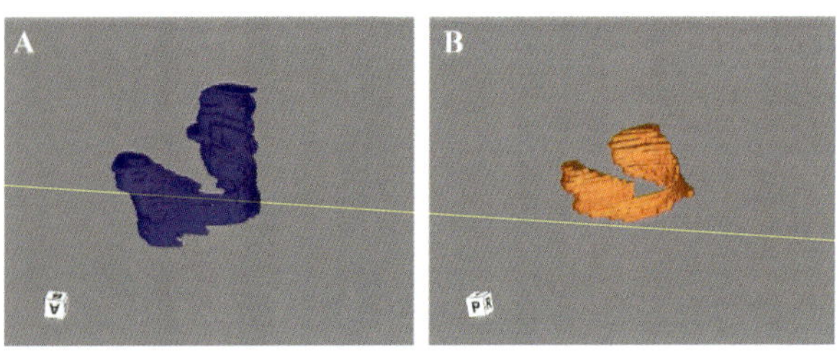


**Figure 1 The thyroid images reconstructed by three-dimensional reconstruction software.** A, *Slc26a4*$^{-/-}$ mouse thyroid with iodine-deficient chow (ICD) (reconstructed with three-dimensional software, Zed View). B, *Slc26a4*$^{-/-}$ mouse thyroid with control chow (CCD) (reconstructed with three-dimensional software, Zed View).

*Slc26a4*$^{+/+}$ mice, respectively. The average TT4 levels in the CCD group were 5.25 μg/dl, 5.33 μg/dl and 5.13 μg/dl in *Slc26a4*$^{-/-}$, *Slc26a4*$^{+/-}$ and *Slc26a4*$^{+/+}$ mice, respectively. The average TT4 levels in the ICD group were 3.11 μg/dl, 3.07 μg/dl and 4.31 μg/dl in *Slc26a4*$^{-/-}$, *Slc26a4*$^{+/-}$ and *Slc26a4*$^{+/+}$ mice, respectively. One-way ANOVA did not reveal a significant difference in TT3 and TT4 levels among the three genotypes.

As shown in Figure 4, Mann-Whitney U-testing revealed that serum TT4 level was lower in the ICD group than in the CCD group both in *Slc26a4*$^{-/-}$ and *Slc26a4*$^{+/-}$ mice ($p$ = 0.004 and $p$ = 0.019, respectively). In *Slc26a4*$^{+/+}$ mice, Mann-Whitney U-testing was not

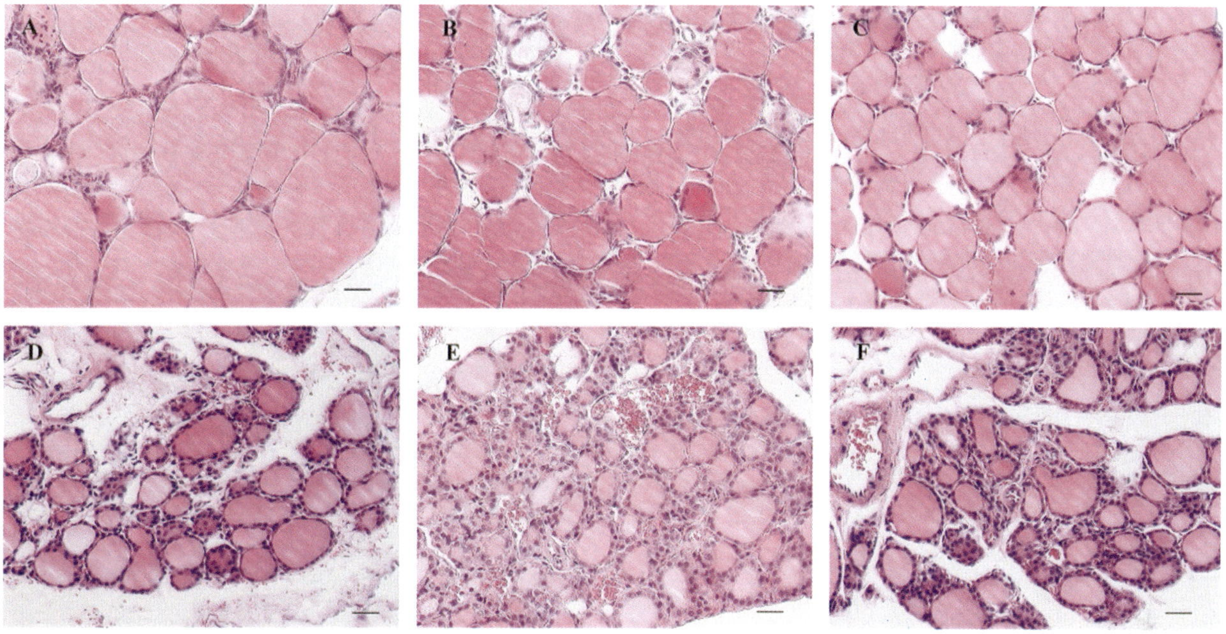


**Figure 2 Light microscopic findings of the thyroid gland**. A, *Slc26a4*$^{-/-}$ control chow (CCD); B, *Slc26a4*$^{+/-}$ CCD; C, *Slc26a4*$^{+/+}$ CCD; D, *Slc26a4*$^{-/-}$ iodine-deficient chow (ICD); E, *Slc26a4*$^{+/-}$ ICD; F, *Slc26a4*$^{+/+}$ ICD. Scale bars: 30 μm.

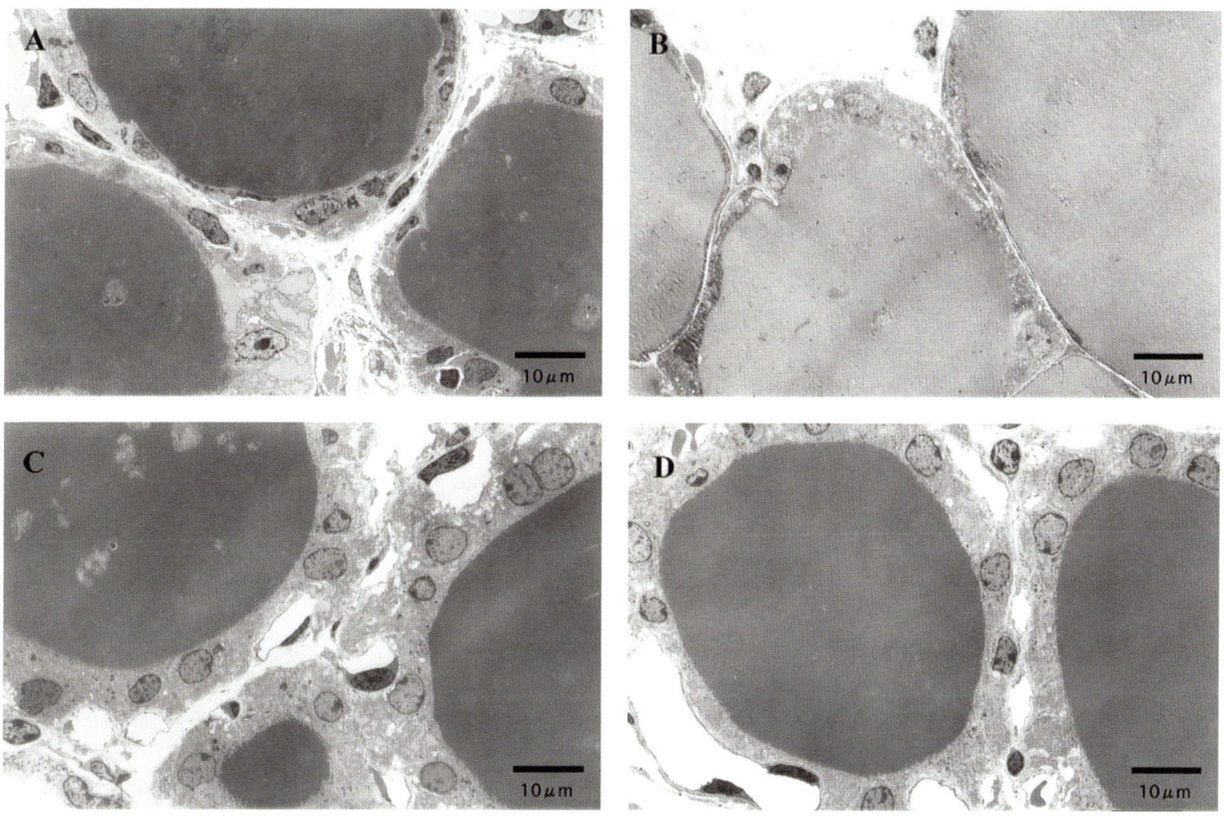


**Figure 3 Electron microscopic findings of the throid gland**. A, *Slc26a4*$^{-/-}$ CCD; B, *Slc26a4*$^{+/-}$ CCD; C, *Slc26a4*$^{-/-}$ ICD; D, *Slc26a4*$^{+/-}$ ICD.

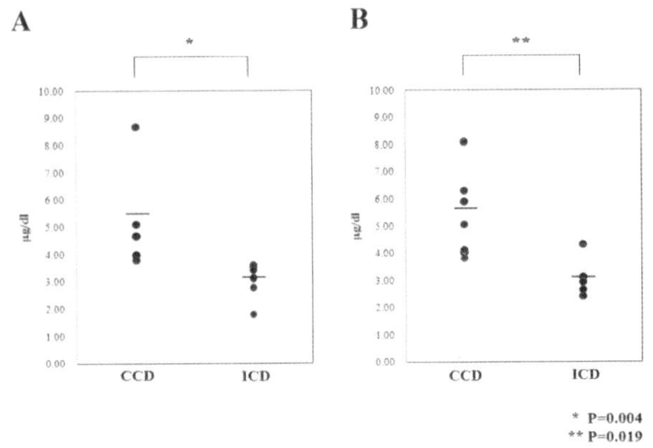


**Figure 4 Effect of iodine deficiency on serum total thyroxine (TT4) levels in Slc26a4$^{-/-}$ and Slc26a4$^{+/-}$ mice.** A, TT4 levels of Slc26a4$^{-/-}$ mice among control chow (CCD) and iodine-deficient chow (ICD) groups. B, TT4 levels of Slc26a4$^{+/-}$ mice among CCD and ICD groups. Mann-Whitney U-testing indicated significant differences for both comparisons.

adequate to compare between ICD group and CCD group because the number of ICD animals was two. On the other hand, the TT3 level was not different significantly between the ICD and CCD groups.

## Discussion

Mutations of the *SLC26A4* (*PDS*) gene can cause sensorineural hearing loss with goiter (PDS) or non-syndromic recessive deafness with enlarged vestibular aqueduct [5,6]. To date, more than 150 mutations in the *SLC26A4* gene have been reported in patients with PDS or nonsyndromic deafness with enlarged vestibular aqueducts (http://www.healthcare.uiowa.edu/labs/pendredandbor/slcMutations.htm). According to previous reports, the H723R missense substitution accounts for up to 75% of *SLC26A4* mutations in Japanese families with EVA [6,7]. There are many cases without goiter associated with the H723R mutation [3]. Madeo *et al.* found that thyroid gland volume is primarily *SLC26A4* genotype-dependent in children but is age-dependent in adults [8]. These reports suggest that the variable degree of thyroid dysfunction and goiter associated with *SLC26A4* mutations may be caused by factors unrelated to *SLC26A4* genotype. It is noteworthy that reported homozygotes for the H723R mutation were mainly from Japan and Korea where daily iodine intake should be comparatively high [3,7,9]. We therefore hypothesized that the amount of iodine intake influences the thyroid phenotype associated with PDS, leading us to study the effect of dietary iodine deficiency on thyroid gland structure and function in *Slc26a4*-null mutant mice.

TT4 levels were lower in the ICD group than in the CCD group. This difference was observed regardless of genotype, and these results suggest the thyroid function of *Slc26a4*$^{-/-}$ mice is approximately the same as of *Slc26a4*$^{+/-}$ and *Slc26a4*$^{+/+}$ mice. While we were preparing the manuscript, we found a similar report by Calebiro *et al* [10]. In their report they also confirmed that dietary iodine restriction did not induce goiter in *Slc26a4*$^{-/-}$ mice. However, Calebiro *et al.* reported that total TT4 levels did not differ significantly between mice fed a low-iodine diet in comparison to those fed a standard diet [10].

The reason why TT3 levels did not decrease might be because incompletely iodinated thyroglobulin (Tg) in the thyroid colloid is accompanied by an increase in monoiodotyrosine (MIT) on Tg molecules, resulting in preferential T3 synthesis [11]. Therefore, TT3 levels may have been maintained despite the decline in TT4 levels in iodine-deficient mice. Another explanation why TT3 was unchanged in mice fed an iodine-deficient diet is an increase of type 1 iodothyronine 5'-deiodinase (D1) activity in the thyroid gland. Pedraza *et al.* reported that thyroidal D1 activity was increased with an iodine-deficient diet [12].

Other factors may compensate for defective iodine transport in both patients with PDS and *Slc26a4*$^{-/-}$ mice. Van den Hove *et al.* have reported that the ClCn5 (chloride channel 5) protein localizes at the apical membrane of thyrocytes. The thyroidal phenotype in ClCn5-deficient mice is similar to that in Pendred syndrome, suggesting that ClCn5 could participate in mediating apical iodine efflux or iodine/chloride exchange [13,14]. Suzuki *et al.* reported that thyroglobulin, by mediating differential expression of several thyroid-specific genes including *TSHR*, *NIS*, and *TPO*, *TG*, *PAX8*, *TTF1*, and *TTF2* regulates the rate of iodide efflux into the follicular lumen and may thus play an important role in regulating thyroid function under constant levels of TSH [13,15].

In conclusion, the ICD did not induce goiter in *Slc26a4*-null mice whereas, in humans, *SLC26A4* mutations sometimes lead to goiter and even hypothyroidism. Mice may be different from humans in their ability to transport iodide into the follicular lumen or mice may respond differently to altered iodine availability. It is also possible that our results result from the use of male experimental animals since goiter and hypothyroidism are more prevalent among human females than males. The genetic strain background may also influence the penetrance and expressivity of the thyroid phenotype associated with *Slc26a4* mutations. These may be some of the factors involved in the development of goiter in PDS.

**Acknowledgements**

This study was supported by research grants from the Ministry of Health, Labor, and Welfare and from the Ministry of Education, Culture, Sports, Science, and Technology of Japan. *Slc26a4*-null mice were kindly provided by NIH. Andrew Griffith was supported by NIH intramural research fund Z01-DC-000060.

**Author details**
[1]Department of Otorhinolaryngology Nagoya University Graduate School of Medicine, 65 Tsurumai-cho, Showa-ku, Nagoya, Aichi 466-8550, Japan. [2]Inazawa City Hospital, 1-1 Gokusho-cho, Inazawa, Aichi 492-8510, Japan. [3]Department of genetics, Research Institute of Environmental Medicine, Nagoya University, Furo-cho, Chikusa-ku, Nagoya, Aichi 464-8601, Japan. [4]National Institute on Deafness and Other Communications Disorders, National Institutes of Health, 5 Research Court, Rockville, MD 20850 USA.

**Authors' contributions**
TI designed and coordinated the study, performed the experiments and drafted the manuscript; TY and MT supervised all experimental procedures, participated in performing experiments, and helped to draft the manuscript; YM participated in coordination of the study and helped to draft the manuscript; YH participated in performing experiments. YK participated in coordination of the study. TN and AJG, the senior author, drafted the manuscript. All authors have read and approved the final manuscript.

**Competing interests**
The authors declare that they have no competing interests.

**References**

1. Kopp P, Pesce L, Solis-S J: **Pendred syndrome and iodide transport in the thyroid.** *Trends Endocrinol Metab* 2008, **19**:260-268.
2. Everett L, Belyantseva I, Noben-Trauth K, Cantos R, Chen A, Thakkar S, Hoogstraten-Miller S, Kachar B, Wu D, Green E: **Targeted disruption of mouse Pds provides insight about the inner-ear defects encountered in Pendred syndrome.** *Hum Mol Genet* 2001, **10**:153-161.
3. Sato E, Nakashima T, Miura Y, Furuhashi A, Nakayama A, Mori N, Murakami H, Naganawa S, Tadokoro M: **Phenotypes associated with replacement of His by Arg in the Pendred syndrome gene.** *Eur J Endocrinol* 2001, **145**:697-703.
4. Kanou Y, Hishinuma A, Tsunekawa K, Seki K, Mizuno Y, Fujisawa H, Imai T, Miura Y, Nagasaka T, Yamada C, Ieiri T, Murakami M, Murata Y: **Thyroglobulin gene mutations producing defective intracellular transport of thyroglobulin are associated with increased thyroidal type 2 iodothyronine deiodinase activity.** *J Clin Endocrinol Metab* 2007, **92**:1451-1457.
5. Everett LA, Glaser B, Beck JC, Idol JR, Buchs A, Heyman M, Adawi F, Hazani E, Nassir E, Baxevanis AD, Sheffield VC, Green ED: **Pendred syndrome is caused by mutations in a putative sulphate transporter gene (PDS).** *Nat Genet* 1997, **17**:411-422.
6. Usami S, Abe S, Weston M, Shinkawa H, Van Camp G, Kimberling W: **Non-syndromic hearing loss associated with enlarged vestibular aqueduct is caused by PDS mutations.** *Hum Genet* 1999, **104**:188-192.
7. Kitamura K, Takahashi K, Noguchi Y, Kuroishikawa Y, Tamagawa Y, Ishikawa K, Ichimura K, Hagiwara H: **Mutations of the Pendred syndrome gene (PDS) in patients with large vestibular aqueduct.** *Acta Otolaryngol* 2000, **120**:137-141.
8. Manichaikul A, Reynolds J, Sarlis NJ, Pryor SP, Shawker T, Griffith AJ: **Evaluation of the thyroid in patients with hearing loss and enlarged vestibular aqueducts.** *Arch Otolaryngol Head Neck Surg* 2009, **135**:670-676.
9. Park H-J, Shaukat S, Liu X-Z, Hahn SH, Naz S, Ghosh M, Kim H-N, Moon S-K, Abe S, Tukamoto K, Riazuddin S, Kabra M, Erdenetungalag R, Radnaabazar J, Khan S, Pandya A, Usami S-I, Nance WE, Wilcox ER, Riazuddin S, Griffith AJ: **Origins and frequencies of SLC26A4 (PDS) mutations in east and south Asians: global implications for the epidemiology of deafness.** *J Med Genet* 2003, **40**:242-248.
10. Calebiro D, Porazzi P, Bonomi M, Lisi S, Grindati A, De Nittis D, Fugazzola L, Marinò M, Bottà G, Persani L: **Absence of primary hypothyroidism and goiter in Slc26a4 (-/-) Mice Fed on a Low Iodine Diet.** *J Endocrinol Invest* 2010.
11. Delange F: **The disorders induced by iodine deficiency.** *Thyroid* 1994, **4**:107-128.
12. Pedraza PE, Obregon MJ, Escobar-Morreale HF, del Rey FE, de Escobar GM: **Mechanisms of adaptation to iodine deficiency in rats: thyroid status is tissue specific. Its relevance for man.** *Endocrinology* 2006, **147**:2098-2108.
13. Bizhanova A, Kopp P: **Genetics and phenomics of Pendred syndrome.** *Mol Cell Endocrinol* 2010, **322**:83-90.
14. van den Hove M, Croizet-Berger K, Jouret F, Guggino S, Guggino W, Devuyst O, Courtoy P: **The loss of the chloride channel, ClC-5, delays apical iodide efflux and induces a euthyroid goiter in the mouse thyroid gland.** *Endocrinology* 2006, **147**:1287-1296.
15. Suzuki K, Kohn LD: **Differential regulation of apical and basal iodide transporters in the thyroid by thyroglobulin.** *J Endocrinol* 2006, **189**:247-255.

# 9

# Pathogenic mechanisms of deregulated microRNA expression in thyroid carcinomas of follicular origin

Juliane Braun, Stefan Hüttelmaier*

**Abstract**

Thyroid cancer is one of the most common malignancies of the endocrine system with increasing incidence. The vast majority of thyroid carcinomas derive from thyroid hormone producing follicular cells. Carcinomas of follicular origin are classified as follicular (FTCs), papillary (PTCs), partially differentiated (PDTCs) or anaplastic (ATCs) thyroid carcinomas. While FTCs and PTCs can be managed effectively, ATCs are considered one of the most lethal human cancers. Despite the identification of various genetic alterations, pathogenic mechanisms promoting the progression of thyroid carcinomas are still largely elusive. Over the recent years, aberrant microRNA expression was revealed in all as yet analyzed human cancers, including thyroid carcinomas. In view of the rapidly evolving perception that deregulated microRNA expression serves a pivotal role in tumor progression, microRNAs provide powerful tools for the diagnosis of thyroid carcinomas as well as the identification of potential therapeutic targets. Here, we summarize recent findings on microRNA signatures in thyroid carcinomas of follicular origin and discuss how deregulated microRNA expression could promote cancer progression.

## Introduction

Thyroid carcinomas represent the most common cancer of the endocrine system [1]. More than 95% of these carcinomas originate from follicular thyroid cells, whereas only 3% are of C-cell origin, referred to as medullary thyroid carcinomas (MTCs) [2]. The most frequent follicular tumors are benign hyperplastic adenomas (FTAs), whereas papillary thyroid carcinomas (PTCs) are the most frequent thyroid carcinoma (approximately 90%) [3]. PTCs are composed of well-differentiated epithelial cells and can be distinguished by visible changes in nuclear morphology and appearance [4]. Follicular thyroid carcinomas (FTCs) with a prevalence of less than 10% are morphological similar to FTAs but capable of vascular invasion [2]. Although some of these well-differentiated carcinomas behave aggressively, the vast majority of PTCs and FTCs can be managed effectively. In contrast, the rare (2-7%) undifferentiated, anaplastic thyroid carcinomas (ATCs) behave very aggressively, rapidly invade adjacent tissues and are thus considered one of the most lethal human cancers [2]. At present there is no effective treatment of ATCs and death usually occurs within six months after diagnosis [5]. ATCs are characterized by partially or completely undifferentiated cells with a high mitosis rate, necrotic areas, spindle-like cell morphologies as well as giant and occasionally squamous cells [5,6]. Poorly differentiated thyroid carcinomas (PDTCs) present an 'intermediate' entity. They appear partially de-differentiated compared to FTCs or PTCs and typically behave more aggressively [5]. Several of these tumors arise *de novo*, whereas others seem to originate from PTCs or FTCs [7].

Thyroid tumors are supposed to be mainly monoclonal malignancies arising based on somatic mutations of progenitor cells. Putative risk factors for genomic instabilities are radiation exposure, active oxygen-species ($H_2O_2$ is necessary for thyroid hormone synthesis) and estrogen. Historical events exhibit radiation exposure as the major risk for PTCs, since atomic bomb survivors and Chernobyl victims frequently developed these tumors [8]. One of the major risks for FTCs is dietary iodine deficiency resulting in thyroid proliferation

* Correspondence: stefan.huettelmaier@medizin.uni-halle.de
Institute of Molecular Medicine, Section for Molecular Cell Biology, Martin Luther University of Halle-Wittenberg, ZAMED Heinrich-Damerow-Str.1, 06120 Halle, Germany
Full list of author information is available at the end of the article

(endemic goiter) as a compensatory mechanism [9]. Genetic predisposition associated thyroid cancers are known for familial polyposis coli (mutations in APC), Cowden disease (mutations in PTEN) and Werner syndrome (mutations in WRN) [2]. Moreover, two sequence variants of *loci* 9q22.33 and 14q13.3 were found to be associated with a higher risk of FTCs and PTCs [10].

Genetic alterations in oncogenes that are involved in the activation of cell signalling pathways have been observed in the vast majority of malignant thyroid carcinomas. Mutation of the BRAF gene is most prominent in PTCs with an appearance up to 50% [2,11,12]. One major gain-of-function mutation of BRAF, a substitution of valine to glutamate at position 600 (V600E), results in constitutive activation of the MAPK pathway [13,14]. RAS gene (KRAS, HRAS, NRAS) mutations instead were found in all thyroid cancers: FTAs (frequency: 20-40%), FTCs (frequency: 40-50%), PDTCs (frequency: 20-55%) and ATCs (frequency: 20-60%) [2,11,12]. Activation of the G-protein RAS stimulates MAPK and other signalling pathways like PI3K/AKT. Less frequent are RET rearrangements (20-40% in PTCs, ~10% in PDTCs) due to inter-chromosomal translocations. In ATCs and PDTCs, CTNNB1 (0-25% in PDTCs, 66% in ATCs) and TP53 mutations (20-38% in PDTCs; 67-88% in ATCs) were observed [2,11,12,15,16]. NTRK1 rearrangements were exclusively identified in PTCs (~10%). The proto-oncogene NTRK1 (also known as TRK) encodes a transmembrane tyrosine-kinase receptor for nerve growth factor and activates ERK, PI3K and phospholipase $\gamma$ (PLC$\gamma$) signalling pathways. Notably, all mutations in PTCs are nearly 100% exclusive. Rearrangements leading to the chimeric protein PAX8-PPAR$\gamma$ were only identified in FTCs (35%) and FTAs (2-10%) [2,3,11]. Additionally, AKT signalling appears most accelerated in ATCs and PTCs due to PTEN mutations and/or PIK3CA amplification [17]. Together the frequency preference of genetic alterations observed in distinct thyroid cancers as well as the observation that well-differentiated thyroid carcinomas precede or co-exist with PDTCs or ATCs supports the view that most undifferentiated thyroid carcinomas evolve by sequential progression (reviewed in: [2]).

In addition to genetic alterations, recent studies indicate that thyroid carcinomas like the majority of as yet analyzed tumors are characterized by aberrant expression of **microRNAs (miRNAs).** These small, non-coding RNAs of 20-24 nucleotides in length are evolutionarily conserved and control gene expression at the post-transcriptional level [18]. At present, 1366 mature human microRNAs are listed in miR-Base (mirbase.org, release 16). The vast majority of identified and characterized microRNAs target the 3'-untranslated region (3' UTR) of mRNAs and modulate target transcript degradation, translation or both [19,20]. Two classes of microRNAs relevant to cancer are distinguished: **'onco-miRs'** with tumor promoting effects versus **'tumor-suppressive'** microRNAs that antagonize cancer progression. In the past years, several studies identified miRNA signatures in thyroid carcinomas aiming to reveal how they modulate thyroid cancer progression and to evaluate their potential for thyroid cancer diagnosis.

## MicroRNA signatures in follicular thyroid carcinomas (FTCs)

Malignant FTCs and benign FTAs share significant similarities at the morphological and molecular level and thus microRNAs could serve as valuable markers to distinguish these tumors. The first study addressing this aspect on the basis of a limited set of human microRNAs (235 distinct human microRNAs) revealed four microRNAs (miR-346, -328, -192, -197) moderately upregulated by 1.34-1.82 fold in FTCs when compared to FTAs [21]. The authors claimed this moderate upregulation sufficed to distinguish FTAs from FTCs in 74% of analyzed patient samples (23 FTCs, 20 FTAs). *In vitro*, the upregulation of miR-197 and -346 was associated with elevated proliferation of HEK293T and two FTC-derived cell lines. This pro-proliferative effect was suggested to correlate with miR-controlled expression of ACVR1 (activin A receptor type 1), TSPAN3 (tetraspanin 3), CFLAR (Caspase 8 and FADD-like apoptosis regulator) and EFEMP2 (fibulin 4), although no direct regulation of these targets by miR-197 or -346 was demonstrated [21]. The abundance of these mRNAs was decreased in the majority of analyzed FTCs and was proposed to distinguish FTAs from FTCs [21]. Notably, previous studies suggested activin signalling to act on growth inhibition of FTC-derived cells *in vitro*, but miRNA-mediated regulation of Activin signalling remains to be shown [22]. TSPAN3 was inversely correlated with the metastatic potential in melanoma and the extracellular matrix (ECM) component EFEMP2 was reported to be over expressed in colon carcinomas but decreased in prostate cancer [23-25].

In comprehensive studies aiming at the identification of microRNA signatures distinguishing thyroid carcinomas from non-transformed thyroid tissue (NT), Nikiforova and colleagues [26] could not confirm the results of Weber et al. [21], except for miR-197. This miRNA showed a higher expression in oncocytic FTCs compared to NTs, whereas expression appeared largely unaffected in conventional FTCs [21,26]. Notably, miR-328 expression, previously suggested being higher in FTCs than in FTAs, was found to be upregulated in FTAs but not in FTCs by Nikiforova et al [26]. The increased expression of miR-221/-222 appears to be a hallmark of thyroid cancers of follicular origin, since both miRNAs were found to be expressed at high levels in FTCs, PTCs, PDTCs and ATCs [26-31] (Figure 1). Accordingly, their expression was largely unaffected in FTAs, hyperplastic nodules and medullary thyroid carcinomas (MTCs) [26]. Compared to non-transformed 'normal' thyroid (NT) and hyperplastic nodules four additional miRNAs were significantly increased in conventional FTCs (miR-187, -224, -155, -146b) as well as in oncocytic FTCs (miR-187, -339, -183, -197). MiR-187 is one of the ten most upregulated microRNAs in PTCs, FTCs and PDTCs but apparently remains unaffected in FTAs. This suggests miR-187 as a useful marker for distinguishing FTCs from FTAs that however is not suitable for discriminating FTCs from other carcinomas of follicular origin. The only few studies addressing miRNA signatures in FTCs focused exclusively on the upregulation of microRNAs. However, by comparing ATC samples with NTs, FTCs and PTCs, we observed a significant reduction in miR-26a/-b and let-7g expression in FTCs. These miRNAs are considered tumor suppressive miRNAs [32-35].

In conclusion, comprehensive miRNA signature analyses in FTCs, in particular with respect to distinct subtypes like oncocytic versus conventional FTCs, are still lacking. Thus, it remains largely elusive if FTCs can be distinguished from other thyroid carcinomas or FTAs by altered miRNA expression profiles at this point.

## MicroRNA signatures in papillary thyroid carcinomas (PTCs)

The upregulation of the miR-221/-222 cluster and miR-181 is the most consistent finding in all studies addressing miRNA signatures in PTCs [26,27,31,36,37]. Moreover, increased expression of miR-146b, -155, -21 and -220 was

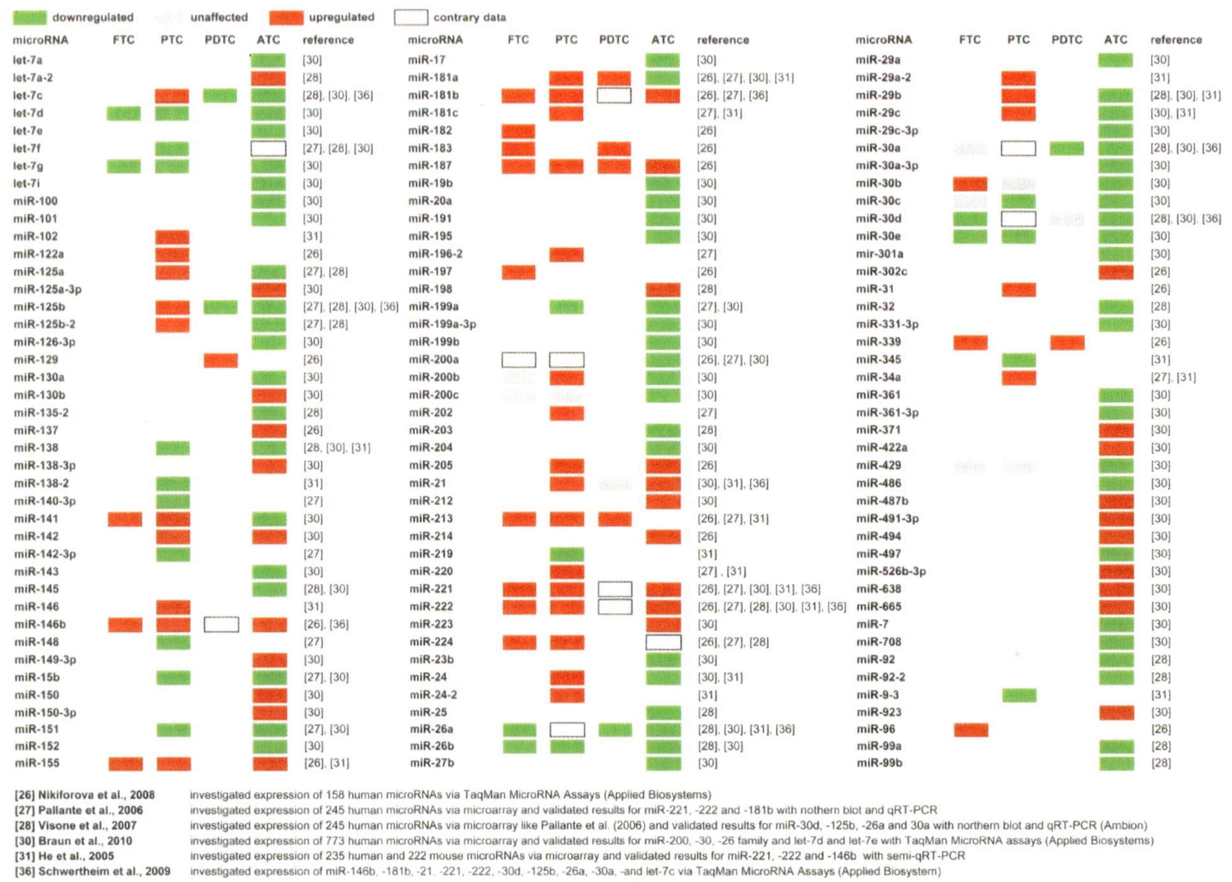
downregulated
unaffected
upregulated
contrary data
microRNA FTC PTC PDTC ATC reference
let-7a [30]
let-7a-2 [28]
let-7c [28], [30], [36]
let-7d [30]
let-7e [30]
let-7f [27], [28], [30]
let-7g [30]
let-7i [30]
miR-100 [30]
miR-101 [30]
miR-102 [31]
miR-122a [26]
miR-125a [27], [28]
miR-125a-3p [30]
miR-125b [27], [28], [30], [36]
miR-125b-2 [27], [28]
miR-126-3p [30]
miR-129 [26]
miR-130a [30]
miR-130b [30]
miR-135-2 [28]
miR-137 [26]
miR-138 [28, [30], [31]
miR-138-3p [30]
miR-138-2 [31]
miR-140-3p [27]
miR-141 [30]
miR-142 [30]
miR-142-3p [27]
miR-143 [30]
miR-145 [28], [30]
miR-146 [31]
miR-146b [26], [36]
miR-148 [27]
miR-149-3p [30]
miR-15b [27], [30]
miR-150 [30]
miR-150-3p [30]
miR-151 [27], [30]
miR-152 [30]
miR-155 [26], [31]
miR-17 [30]
miR-181a [26], [27], [30], [31]
miR-181b [26], [27], [36]
miR-181c [27], [31]
miR-182 [26]
miR-183 [26]
miR-187 [26]
miR-19b [30]
miR-20a [30]
miR-191 [30]
miR-195 [30]
miR-196-2 [27]
miR-197 [26]
miR-198 [28]
miR-199a [27], [30]
miR-199a-3p [30]
miR-199b [30]
miR-200a [26], [27], [30]
miR-200b [30]
miR-200c [30]
miR-202 [27]
miR-203 [28]
miR-204 [30]
miR-205 [26]
miR-21 [30], [31], [36]
miR-212 [30]
miR-213 [26], [27], [31]
miR-214 [26]
miR-219 [31]
miR-220 [27] , [31]
miR-221 [26], [27], [30], [31], [36]
miR-222 [26], [27], [28], [30], [31], [36]
miR-223 [30]
miR-224 [26], [27], [28]
miR-23b [30]
miR-24 [30], [31]
miR-24-2 [31]
miR-25 [28]
miR-26a [28], [30], [31], [36]
miR-26b [28], [30]
miR-27b [30]
miR-29a [30]
miR-29a-2 [31]
miR-29b [28], [30], [31]
miR-29c [30], [31]
miR-29c-3p [30]
miR-30a [28], [30], [36]
miR-30a-3p [30]
miR-30b [30]
miR-30c [30]
miR-30d [28], [30], [36]
miR-30e [30]
mir-301a [30]
miR-302c [26]
miR-31 [26]
miR-32 [28]
miR-331-3p [30]
miR-339 [26]
miR-345 [31]
miR-34a [27], [31]
miR-361 [30]
miR-361-3p [30]
miR-371 [30]
miR-422a [30]
miR-429 [30]
miR-486 [30]
miR-487b [30]
miR-491-3p [30]
miR-494 [30]
miR-497 [30]
miR-526b-3p [30]
miR-638 [30]
miR-665 [30]
miR-7 [30]
miR-708 [30]
miR-92 [28]
miR-92-2 [28]
miR-9-3 [31]
miR-923 [30]
miR-96 [26]
miR-99a [28]
miR-99b [28]
[26] Nikiforova et al., 2008 investigated expression of 158 human microRNAs via TaqMan MicroRNA Assays (Applied Biosystems)
[27] Pallante et al., 2006 investigated expression of 245 human microRNAs via microarray and validated results for miR-221, -222 and -181b with nothern blot and qRT-PCR
[28] Visone et al., 2007 investigated expression of 245 human microRNAs via microarray like Pallante et al. (2006) and validated results for miR-30d, -125b, -26a and 30a with northern blot and qRT-PCR (Ambion)
[30] Braun et al., 2010 investigated expression of 773 human microRNAs via microarray and validated results for miR-200, -30, -26 family and let-7d and let-7e with TaqMan MicroRNA assays (Applied Biosystems)
[31] He et al., 2005 investigated expression of 235 human and 222 mouse microRNAs via microarray and validated results for miR-221, -222 and -146b with semi-qRT-PCR
[36] Schwertheim et al., 2009 investigated expression of miR-146b, -181b, -21, -221, -222, -30d, -125b, -26a, -30a, -and let-7c via TaqMan MicroRNA Assays (Applied Biosystem)

**Figure 1 Deregulated miRNA expression in thyroid carcinomas of follicular origin in comparison to normal thyroid tissue.** Altered expression of miRNAs observed by indicated studies is represented by color coding. Deregulated expression was classified as up- (red), unaffected (grey) or downregulated (green) in comparison to non-transformed thyroid tissue based on individual studies. Contradictory data are indicated by boxes. The presented data base on different thresholds, were quantified using distinct methods and more importantly distinct miRNA sets. Thus, the presented summary of observed miRNA signatures remains incomplete, preliminary and requires substantial further validation. This is particularly important for FTCs and PDTCs for both of which only a very limited set of microRNAs has been analyzed. FTC: Follicular thyroid carcinoma; PTC: Papillary thyroid carcinoma; PDTC: Poorly differentiated thyroid carcinoma, ATC: Anaplastic thyroid carcinoma.

reported in at least two individual studies based on comparing signatures between PTCs and NTs (Figure 1). A comparison of PTCs to hyperplastic nodular tissue from formalin fixed paraffin embedded samples further validated the significance of these findings by identifying altered expression of miR-221/-222, -181, -31, and -224 [38]. Upregulation of miR-31 and -224 was also observed by Nikiforova et al. [26]. However, analyses of 40 fine needle aspirate (FNA) specimen and 84 formalin-fixed paraffin-embedded tissues by Chen et al. identified only the upregulation of miR-146b and -222 as potent markers of PTCs [39].

Most interestingly a significant correlation of increased miRNA expression with genetic alterations was observed in PTCs [26]. For instance, miR-221/-222 were more abundant in PTC samples with RAS and BRAF mutations. RAS-mutations moreover correlated with the most severe upregulation of miR-146b. In contrast, RET-mutations were found to be associated with increased expression of miR-155. *In vitro* analyses using thyroid cancer-derived cells confirmed an 'oncogene connection' for upregulated expression of miR-221 and -181b. The abundance of these microRNAs increased upon overexpression of v-raf, v-ras, RET/PTC1, RET/PTC3, E1-Abl, E1a-v-raf, middle T of polyomavirus and v-mos [27]. PTC cell lines harboring RET/PTC1 or BRAF V600E mutations identified additional microRNAs to be severely increased. The most severe upregulation upon BRAF mutation was observed for the miR-200 family (miR-200a, -200b, 200c and -141), whereas RET/PTC1 rearrangement was correlated with upregulated expression of miR-128a, -128b, -139 and -200a. The most significantly downregulated group of miRNAs in cells with BRAF mutation comprised miR-127, -130a, and -144; with RET/PTC1 rearrangement miR-154*, -181a, -302b and -302c [40,41].

Although there is substantial and consistent data on the upregulation of microRNAs in PTCs, reduced abundance was only reported for a few miRNAs. The three tumor-suppressive miRNA-families miR-26 [31], -30 [38] and let-7 [27] were suggested to be expressed at lower levels in PTCs. Our recent analyses confirmed these observations for the miR-26 and let-7 families [30]. However, expression of the miR-30 family appeared largely unaffected when compared to NT. In contrast, Schwertheim et al. identified an increased expression of miR-30d, -30a, -26a and let-7c in nine analyzed PTCs compared to NTs [36].

In summary, PTCs appear to be well-distinguishable from NT by altered miRNA expression, in particular the upregulation of onco-miRs. However, more comprehensive analyses including FTCs are required to identify miRNAs expressed at distinct levels in these two carcinoma types.

## MicroRNA signatures in anaplastic thyroid carcinomas (ATCs)

The most striking difference between ATCs and all other thyroid carcinomas of follicular origin appears to be a severely decreased expression of various miRNAs (Figure 1) [28,30,36]. Visone et al. observed decreased expression of 20 and elevated abundance of only four miRNAs (miR-222, -198, -let-7f-1, let-7a-2) by comparing ATCs with non-transformed thyroid tissue [28]. The most significant decrease in expression was determined for miR-30d, -125b-1/2, and -26a which could be confirmed by Schwertheim et al [36]. In support of these findings, we identified 62 down- and 21 upregulated miRNAs compared to non-transformed thyroid [30]. Strikingly, the decreased miRNAs comprised 12 miRNA-families and 12 clustered miRNA transcription units. The most significant downregulation was observed for tumor suppressive miRNAs of the let-7, miR-26, -30 and -200 families. Notably, the comparison of miRNA signatures between ATCs, PTCs and FTCs suggested that downregulation of the miR-30 and -200 families is sufficient to unambiguously distinguish ATCs from NT as well as FTCs and PTCs. As observed for PTCs, the miR-138 was found to be severely reduced in ATC samples as well as in ATC-derived cell lines [30,31,42,43]. Consistent with our studies and the analyses of ATC-derived cells, Nikiforova and colleagues observed a severe upregulation of miR-221/-222 [26,43]. Allthough they examined the expression of 158 microRNAs and identified 57 down- and 47 upregulated in the majority of thyroid tumors they only analyzed the ten most upregulated microRNAs in further detail. Finally, the potent onco-miR-21 was found to be highly expressed in ATCs and was observed to promote thyroid tumor growth in mouse [30,44].

In conclusion, ATCs appear to be well-distinguishable from all other thyroid carcinomas by a severe decrease in the expression of various microRNAs. However, future studies have to reveal if altered miRNA profiles suffice to unambiguously distinguish ATCs from PDTCs.

## MicroRNA signatures in poorly differentiated thyroid carcinomas (PDTCs)

PDTCs are poorly defined and show morphological characteristics of both, differentiated and anaplastic thyroid carcinomas. Aiming to distinguish PDTCs from PTCs and ATCs on the molecular level, Schwertheim et al. investigated the expression of two different sets of microRNAs ('set 1': miRNA-146b, -181b, -21, -221 and -222, all upregulated in PTCs; 'set 2': miRNA-30d, -125b, -26a, -30a-5p and let7d, all downregulated in ATC). Abundance of these miRNAs was analyzed in comparison to four NTs in 15 PDTCs, nine PTCs and

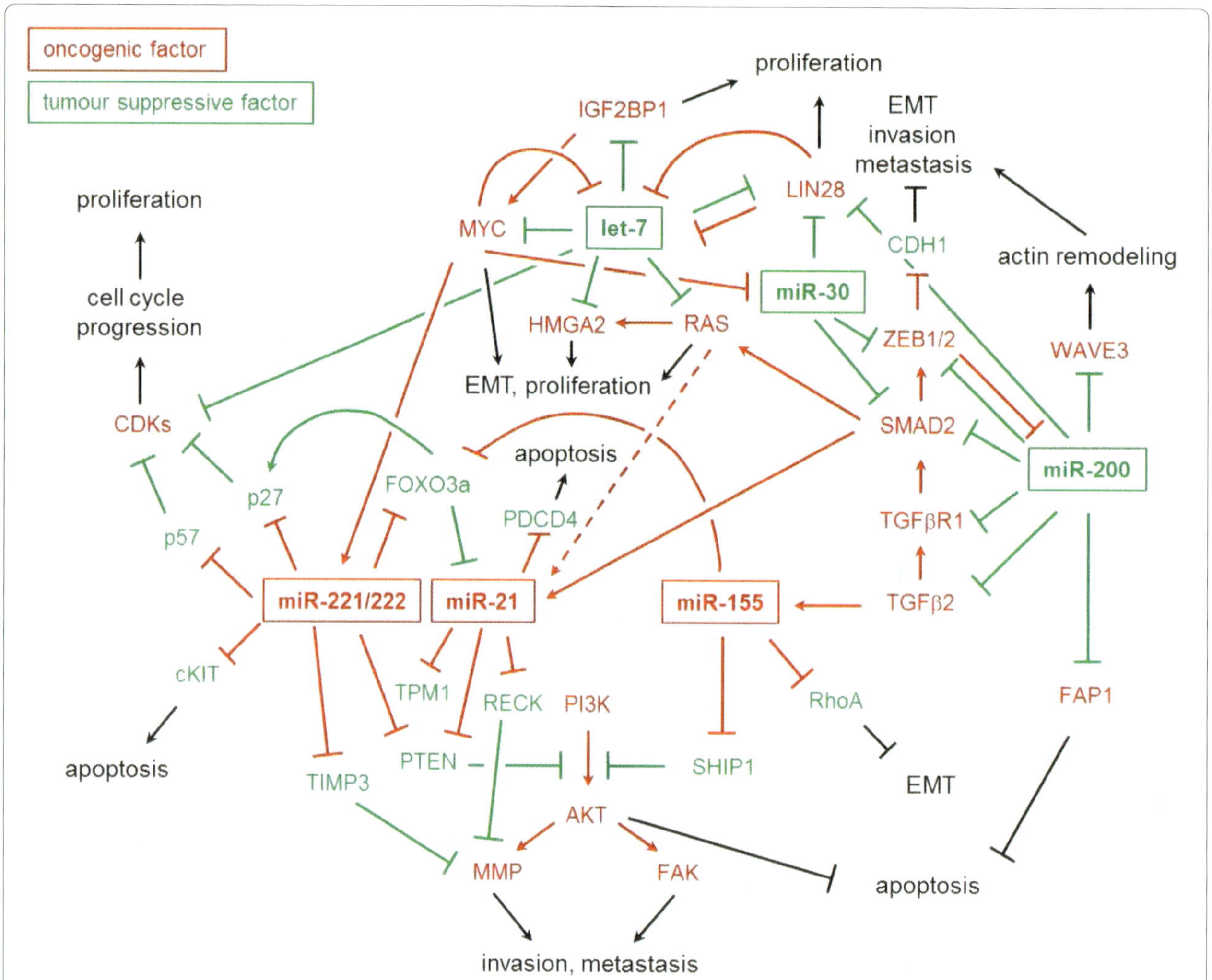


**Figure 2 Regulatory networks facilitated by tumor-suppressive and onco-genic microRNAs / proteins in tumor cells.** Dashed lines indicate indirect regulation.

nine ATCs [36]. 'Set 1' microRNA expression was slightly increased in PDTCs but did not significantly differ from NTs. Since PTCs and ATCs instead showed a more robust upregulation of these microRNAs, the authors suggested 'set 1' microRNAs as a promising diagnostic tool to distinguish PDTCs from PTCs or ATCs. MicroRNAs of 'set 2' instead appear useful to discriminate PDTCs from PTCs, since they were expressed at low levels in PDTCs and ATCs but significantly upregulated in PTCs. Nikiforova et al. investigated the microRNA expression of four PDTCs but did not aim to distinguish PDTCs from PTCs or ATCs [26]. In contrast to Schwertheim et al., Nikiforova and colleagues found miR-181b, -221, -222 and -146b to be upregulated in all four analyzed PDTCs when compared to NTs [26].

Although preliminary evidence indicates that miRNA profiles could be useful molecular markers to identify PDTCs, additional and more comprehensive studies are required.

## Onco-miRs in Thyroid cancer

Onco-miRs are typically classified by an upregulation in cancer and the targeting of transcripts encoding effectors antagonizing tumor progression (Figure 2, red). In the following we discuss validated and suggested phenotypic consequences of aberrant onco-miR expression observed in thyroid cancer.

### miR-221/-222

The overexpression of miR-221/-222 is a hallmark of thyroid malignancies [26-28,30,31]. Moreover, upregulation of both miRNAs was also shown in hepatocellular carcinomas (HCC), glioblastoma and gastric cancer [45-47]. Antagonizing the function of miRs-221/222 in PTC-derived cells interfered with cell proliferation and growth [27]. In subsequent studies it was demonstrated that both miRNAs negatively regulate expression of the cyclin-dependent kinase (CDK) inhibitor $p27^{Kip1}$[29]. This inhibitory role most likely involves miR-221/222 directed control of FOXO3, a key transcriptional activator of $p27^{Kip1}$[48,49]. Notably, FOXO3a mRNA was significantly downregulated in PTCs and FOXO3a represses onco-miR-21 in lung cancer cells [49,50]. An inhibitory role of both miRNAs was also observed for $p57^{Kip2}$ expression [47,51]. Hence, elevated expression of miR-221/-222 presumably indicates aberrant proliferation and cell growth due to their role in antagonizing cell cycle arrest by targeting crucial cell cycle gatekeepers like CDK-inhibitors. Supporting this view, reduced expression of $p27^{Kip1}$ was observed in many primary thyroid tumors as well as thyroid carcinoma-derived cell lines [52].

The expression of the c-kit tyrosine kinase receptor is suppressed or reduced in most tested FTCs and PTCs [53]. Indicating a role of miR-221/-222 in this regulation, it was demonstrated that both miRNAs target c-kit in melanoma-derived cells [54]. Interestingly, 70% of cutaneous melanomas are characterized by BRAF mutations which was also shown to be a precaution of miR-221/-222 upregulation in PTC [26]. Various studies showed that miR-221/-222 downregulate expression of the tumor-suppressive phosphatase PTEN leading to an upregulation of PI3K/AKT signaling [55,56]. This pathway blocks apoptosis and promotes invasion by modulating focal adhesion kinase (FAK) phosphorylation and matrix metalloprotease (MMP) expression levels [57]. PIK3CA amplifications as well as PTEN mutations were reported for many FTCs, PTCs and ATCs suggesting that AKT signaling is sustained by genomic alterations and modified by post-transcriptional control in thyroid carcinomas [17,58,59]. Another pro-apoptotic factor and inhibitor of MMP expression regulated by miR-221/-222 is TIMP3. Reduced expression of PTEN and TIMP3 facilitated by this miRNA-cluster induces TRAIL (tumor necrosis factor (TNF)-related apoptosis inducing ligand) resistance and upregulation of MMPs [55]. *In vivo* evidence for the growth promoting role of elevated miR-221/-222 expression was provided by Xenograft studies in nude mice. The constitutive overexpression of this miRNA cluster resulted in an increased gain of Xenograft weight and volume upon subcutaneous injection of tumor-derived cell lines [47]. Together these findings indicate the overexpression of miR-221/-222 as a key event in thyroid tumor progression. Upregulation of both miRNAs presumably promotes uncontrolled growth and could as well modulate the invasive potential of tumor cell.

#### miR-21

Upregulated expression of miR-21 is observed in multiple types of cancers, such as breast, liver, brain, prostate and myometrial cancers but also in PTCs and ATCs [44,60,61]. Most recently it was shown that oncogenic Ras induces miR-21 expression via activating Raf/MAPK and AKT signaling in rat thyroid cells and in a mouse model of lung tumorigenesis [44]. MiR-21 predominantly acts in an anti-apoptotic manner by interfering with the expression of PTEN and PDCD4 [62-64]. Thus, this miRNA promotes AKT signaling similar to the miR-221/-222 cluster and thereby stimulates its own expression. Elevated AKT signaling and the direct regulation of tropomyosin 1 (TPM1) and maspin (PI5) affects cell morphology, motility and enhances cell invasion [65,66]. By the direct targeting of RECK and the indirect effect on TIMP3 expression, upregulation of miR-21 promotes cell migration and invasiveness but also blocks apoptosis [67]. Hence, the overexpression of miR-21 in thyroid cancers is likely to promote uncontrolled growth and potentially upregulated invasiveness of tumor cells.

#### miR-155

MiR-155 overexpression was observed in FTCs, PTCs and ATCs [26,31]. In leukemia, miR-155 together with miR-21 stimulates PI3K/AKT signaling by blocking expression of SHIP1, another AKT inhibitory phosphatase [68,69]. In addition miR-155 interferes with the expression of RhoA and serves a role in modulating tumor cell invasion as well as epithelial-to-mesenchymal-transition (EMT) [70]. TGFβ induces miR-155 expression and thereby promotes TGFβ-induced EMT and tight junction dissolution involving the depletion of RhoA. Like miR-221/-222, miR-155 also directly targets FOXO3a [71]. Hence, upregulation of miR-155 in thyroid cancers is presumed to promote cell survival, invasiveness and resistance to chemotherapeutics, as for instance demonstrated in breast cancer cells [71].

### Tumor-suppressive miRNAs in thyroid cancer

In contrast to onco-miRs, tumor-suppressive microRNAs are typically downregulated during tumor progression and target transcripts encoding oncogenic factors. The regulatory role of key tumor-suppressive miRNAs in thyroid cancer is discussed in the following (Figure 2, green).

#### miR-200

The miR-200 family (comprising miR-141, -200a, -200b, - 200c and -429) was identified as a potent suppressor of EMT [72-75]. Reduced expression of this miRNA-family was previously reported for stomach, breast and ovarian cancers [76]. Surprisingly, moderately upregulated expression of some miR-200 family members was observed in PTCs and FTCs, whereas a severe downregulation of this microRNA family was found in all ATCs analyzed [30]. This observation supports the view that the miR-200 family serves a key role in preserving an epithelial phenotype or morphology, respectively. Elevated levels of the miR-200 family interfere with the expression of EMT-promoting factors like ZEB1, ZEB2, SNAI2, SMAD2, TGFβR1 and TGFβ2. This antagonizes transcriptional repression of E-cadherin and the miR-200 genomic clusters (miR-141/-200c and miR-200a/-200b/-429) [30,72-74]. In agreement, severely reduced E-cadherin levels have been described as a common characteristic of primary ATCs as well as ATC-derived cells [30,77]. Moreover, elevated expression of TGFβ2 was observed in ATC and PDTC compared to FTC and PTC samples [78]. Beyond the antagonistic role in TGFβ-induced EMT, the miR-200 family presumably also modulates actin dynamics by interfering with the expression of WAVE3, an actin cytoskeleton remodeling protein [79]. Taken together, this provides strong evidence that the loss of miR-200 expression presents a hallmark in the progression of thyroid carcinomas culminating in TGFβ-dependent EMT and elevated invasiveness, as observed for ATCs [30]. The loss of miR-200 expression is probably potentiated by TGFβ-mediated upregulation of miR-155 expression and enhancement of miR-21-maturation, for both of which a pro-metastatic function was proposed [70,80]. More recently, regulation of LIN28B by miR-200 members was identified in prostate cancer-derived cells [81]. LIN28 is a stem cell factor and a powerful inducer of pluripotency [82]. It also represses maturation of the tumor-suppressive let-7 family by binding to the loop region of let-7 precursors [83-85]. Additionally, the miR-200 family apparently promotes apoptosis, as demonstrated in colorectal cancer-derived HCT116 cells. In these cells the repression of FAP1 (Fas-associated phosphatase 1) by the miR-200 family was correlated with elevated susceptibility to TNF-receptor CD95-dependent apoptosis [86]. In summary, these findings indicate reduced expression of the miR-200 family as a key trigger for dedifferentiation and potentiated aggressiveness observed in ATCs.

### let-7

Downregulation of the let-7 family is observed in all thyroid carcinomas of follicular origin [27,28,30]. Let-7 was initially identified as a factor promoting differentiation in C. elegans and was since then validated as a key regulator of gene expression in various organisms [87,88]. The let-7 family is ubiquitously expressed in adult mouse tissue and its reduced expression is considered to be a hallmark in cancer progression [89]. In accord with their tumor-suppressive role, members of the let-7 family target cell cycle regulators and oncogenes like RAS, HMGA1/2, MYC, IGF2BP1 and LIN28 [34,89-93]. Thus it appears likely that the capability to antagonize activating RAS mutations and thus uncontrolled proliferation is severely compromised by reduced levels of the let-7 family. Like activating RAS mutations, the overexpression of MYC is associated with enhanced cell growth and reduced serum dependency in various malignancies [94]. Accordingly, the frequently observed increase of MYC levels in ATCs is likely to correlate with a downregulation of the let-7 family [78,95,96]. Notably, MYC is a key regulator of miRNA transcription and negatively controls expression of various tumor-suppressive miRNA clusters including once again the let-7 family but in addition the miR-30, -26, -34 and -29 families [97,98]. Another layer of post-transcriptional regulation is provided by the control of MYC mRNA degradation via the RNA binding protein IGF2BP1 (Insulin-like growth factor 2 mRNA binding protein 1) [99]. IGF2BP1 shows an oncofetal expression pattern and becomes *de novo* synthesized in various cancers [100]. This is in agreement with a reduction of let-7 expression, since members of this miRNA family interfere with IGF2BP1 expression. Thus, MYC-directed repression of the let-7 family is likely to promote the expression of IGF2BP1 that in turn sustains MYC expression [97]. HMGA1 and HMGA2, two other key factors in tumor progression that are controlled by the let-7 family, support the RAS/MEK-facilitated induction of EMT by enhancing SNAIL expression [101-103]. Moreover, HMGA proteins promote cell growth and HMGA1 depletion induces programmed cells death in ATC-derived cells [104]. In conclusion, loss of the let-7 family is likely to be an early event in the progression of thyroid carcinomas. The sever reduction of this tumor-suppressive miRNA family promotes uncontrolled tumor growth and presumably also affects the invasive potential of tumor cells at later stages.

### miR-30

Significantly reduced expression of the miR-30 family was identified in ATCs. However, moderately reduced expression is also observed in FTCs, PTCs and PDTCs, with the exception of miR-30b in FTCs [28,30]. The first hint of a potential tumor-suppressive role of this miRNA family was revealed by the identification of UBC9 as a direct target [105]. Downregulation of this E2-conjugating enzyme for sumoylation interferes with cell growth and cancer progression. In bladder cancer, reduced expression of the miR-30 family was associated with upregulation of the tumor marker cytokeratin 7, although a functional role of this potential regulation remains elusive [106]. We identified the miR-30 family as an antagonist of TGFβ-induced EMT and *in vitro* invasiveness of ATC-derived cells [30]. This role apparently involves the direct targeting of SMAD2 and ZEB2. In agreement, the forced expression of miR-30 family members interfered with *in vitro* invasiveness of ATC-derived cells and correlated with a downregulation of the mesenchymal marker vimentin. However, in contrast to the miR-200 family, expression of the miR-30 family is apparently controlled in a ZEB-independent manner [30]. Intriguingly, the miR-30 family also targets the stem cell factor LIN28, as previously demonstrated for other key tumor-suppressive miRNA families like miR-200 and let-7 [107]. Hence, the identification of deregulated expression of the miR-30 family in ATCs identified yet another tumor-suppressive miRNA cluster modulating EMT and invasiveness of tumor cells.

## Conclusions

The comprehensive view of distinct miRNA signatures in thyroid carcinomas of follicular origin provides novel insights in the molecular pathologies of these malignancies. However, knowledge of target mRNAs controlled by deregulated miRNAs in thyroid cancers is still sparse at present. To reveal how altered expression of microRNAs promotes or antagonizes thyroid tumor progression it is thus required to identify novel miRNA targets in future studies.

In thyroid carcinomas the most striking observation is that 'less' aggressive FTCs and PTCs (compared to ATCs) are apparently characterized by an upregulation of 'oncogenic' miRNAs (e.g. miR-221/-222 or miR-146b). These miRNAs mainly act in a pro-proliferative and anti-apoptotic manner. In accord with the clonal progression hypothesis, ATCs reveal a severe reduction of tumor-suppressive miRNAs (Figure 1). This decrease presumably promotes dedifferentiation, which morphologically manifests as an epithelial-to-mesenchymal-transition (EMT) driven by reduced expression of the miR-200 and -30 families (see Fig. 1 in [30].). Notably, reduction of these miRNA families is likely to provide a valuable diagnostic tool for distinguishing ATCs from FTC or PTCs. Unresolved aspects of immediate diagnostic and potentially therapeutic importance address the question if miRNA signatures are suitable to distinguish FTAs from FTCs. The presented studies seem to be insufficient to define a subset of microRNAs that unambiguously discriminates these thyroid cancers. Thus, it is required to re-evaluate miRNA signatures in thyroid cancers of follicular origin in a comprehensive manner based on pathologically unambiguously classified primary samples. These studies need to be based on the same evaluation method, for instance miRNA-microarrays, to generate data sets allowing an unbiased direct comparison of miRNA signatures.

Despite their potential as diagnostic tools, miRNAs could also provide promising therapeutic targets based on onco-miR inhibition or restoring levels of tumor suppressive miRNAs. The stage for such approaches was set in rodents already in 2005 by demonstrating that the role of miR-16 as well as -122 could be antagonized by the intravenous injection of anti-miRs [108]. Vice versa, the adenoviral delivery of the tumor-suppressive miR-26 was shown to suppress mouse liver tumorigenesis [33]. However, in clinical practice the specificity of miRNA or anti-miR delivery remains an essential limitation due to off-site effects in non-neoplastic organs.

A third strategy could be envisioned on the level of epigenetic silencing of tumor-suppressive miRNAs. In breast and prostate cancer cell lines methylation of the miR-200 cluster was observed and inhibition of methyltransferases released this transcription block [109]. Moreover, epigenetic silencing might explain the observation that complete miRNA transcription units are downregulated in ATCs (Table1 in [30]). Hence, spatially restricted and cluster specific release of epigenetic silencing could provide a valuable tool in the treatment of cancer but as yet such approaches are not available.

In conclusion the here reviewed findings reveal the potency and current limitations of miRNAs in diagnosis, prognosis and potentially therapeutic strategies for the treatment of thyroid cancer. However, substantial additional work will be required to establish miRNAs in clinical practice and reveal the molecular networks via which altered miRNA expression promotes thyroid cancer progression.

**Acknowledgement and funding**

This work was supported by DFG funding (GRK1591) to SH.

This article has been published as part of *Thyroid Research* Volume 4 Supplement 1, 2011: New aspects of thyroid hormone synthesis and action. The full contents of the supplement are available online at http://www.thyroidresearchjournal.com/supplements/4/S1

**Authors' contribution**

Both authors contributed equally

**Competing interests**

The authors declare that they have no competing interests.

**References**

1. Jemal A, Bray F, Center MM, Ferlay J, Ward E, Forman D: **Global cancer statistics.** *CA Cancer J Clin* **61(2)**:69-90.
2. Kondo T, Ezzat S, Asa SL: **Pathogenetic mechanisms in thyroid follicular-cell neoplasia.** *Nat Rev Cancer* 2006, **6**:292-306.
3. Schmid KW: **Molecular pathology of thyroid tumors.** *Pathologe* 2010, **31(Suppl 2)**:229-233.
4. Williams ED: **Guest Editorial: Two Proposals Regarding the Terminology of Thyroid Tumors.** *Int J Surg Pathol* 2000, **8**:181-183.

5. DeLellis RA, L RV, Heitz PU, Eng C: World Health Organization Classification of Tumours, Pathology and Genetics of Tumours of Endocrine Organs. 2004, 49-133.
6. Ain KB: Anaplastic thyroid carcinoma: a therapeutic challenge. *Semin Surg Oncol* 1999, 16:64-69.
7. Pilotti S, Collini P, Mariani L, Placucci M, Bongarzone I, Vigneri P, Cipriani S, Falcetta F, Miceli R, Pierotti MA, Rilke F: Insular carcinoma: a distinct de novo entity among follicular carcinomas of the thyroid gland. *Am J Surg Pathol* 1997, 21:1466-1473.
8. Williams D: Cancer after nuclear fallout: lessons from the Chernobyl accident. *Nat Rev Cancer* 2002, 2:543-549.
9. Harach HR, Escalante DA, Day ES: Thyroid cancer and thyroiditis in Salta, Argentina: a 40-yr study in relation to iodine prophylaxis. *Endocr Pathol* 2002, 13:175-181.
10. Gudmundsson J, Sulem P, Gudbjartsson DF, Jonasson JG, Sigurdsson A, Bergthorsson JT, He H, Blondal T, Geller F, Jakobsdottir M, *et al*: Common variants on 9q22.33 and 14q13.3 predispose to thyroid cancer in European populations. *Nat Genet* 2009, 41:460-464.
11. Nikiforova MN, Nikiforov YE: Molecular diagnostics and predictors in thyroid cancer. *Thyroid* 2009, 19:1351-1361.
12. Pallante P, Visone R, Croce CM, Fusco A: Deregulation of microRNA expression in follicular-cell-derived human thyroid carcinomas. *Endocr Relat Cancer* 2010, 17:F91-104.
13. Wan PT, Garnett MJ, Roe SM, Lee S, Niculescu-Duvaz D, Good VM, Jones CM, Marshall CJ, Springer CJ, Barford D, Marais R: Mechanism of activation of the RAF-ERK signaling pathway by oncogenic mutations of B-RAF. *Cell* 2004, 116:855-867.
14. Knauf JA, Ma X, Smith EP, Zhang L, Mitsutake N, Liao XH, Refetoff S, Nikiforov YE, Fagin JA: Targeted expression of BRAFV600E in thyroid cells of transgenic mice results in papillary thyroid cancers that undergo dedifferentiation. *Cancer Res* 2005, 65:4238-4245.
15. Garcia-Rostan G, Camp RL, Herrero A, Carcangiu ML, Rimm DL, Tallini G: Beta-catenin dysregulation in thyroid neoplasms: down-regulation, aberrant nuclear expression, and CTNNB1 exon 3 mutations are markers for aggressive tumor phenotypes and poor prognosis. *Am J Pathol* 2001, 158:987-996.
16. Miyake N, Maeta H, Horie S, Kitamura Y, Nanba E, Kobayashi K, Terada T: Absence of mutations in the beta-catenin and adenomatous polyposis coli genes in papillary and follicular thyroid carcinomas. *Pathol Int* 2001, 51:680-685.
17. Paes JE, Ringel MD: Dysregulation of the phosphatidylinositol 3-kinase pathway in thyroid neoplasia. *Endocrinol Metab Clin North Am* 2008, 37:375-387, viii-ix.
18. Ghildiyal M, Zamore PD: Small silencing RNAs: an expanding universe. *Nat Rev Genet* 2009, 10:94-108.
19. Fabian MR, Sonenberg N, Filipowicz W: Regulation of mRNA translation and stability by microRNAs. *Annu Rev Biochem* 2010, 79:351-379.
20. Rigoutsos I: New tricks for animal microRNAS: targeting of amino acid coding regions at conserved and nonconserved sites. *Cancer Res* 2009, 69:3245-3248.
21. Weber F, Teresi RE, Broelsch CE, Frilling A, Eng C: A limited set of human MicroRNA is deregulated in follicular thyroid carcinoma. *J Clin Endocrinol Metab* 2006, 91:3584-3591.
22. Schulte KM, Jonas C, Krebs R, Roher HD: Activin A and activin receptors in thyroid cancer. *Thyroid* 2001, 11:3-14.
23. Boucheix C, Duc GH, Jasmin C, Rubinstein E: Tetraspanins and malignancy. *Expert Rev Mol Med* 2001, 2001:1-17.
24. Gallagher WM, Greene LM, Ryan MP, Sierra V, Berger A, Laurent-Puig P, Conseiller E: Human fibulin-4: analysis of its biosynthetic processing and mRNA expression in normal and tumour tissues. *FEBS Lett* 2001, 489:59-66.
25. Wlazlinski A, Engers R, Hoffmann MJ, Hader C, Jung V, Muller M, Schulz WA: Downregulation of several fibulin genes in prostate cancer. *Prostate* 2007, 67:1770-1780.
26. Nikiforova MN, Tseng GC, Steward D, Diorio D, Nikiforov YE: MicroRNA expression profiling of thyroid tumors: biological significance and diagnostic utility. *J Clin Endocrinol Metab* 2008, 93:1600-1608.
27. Pallante P, Visone R, Ferracin M, Ferraro A, Berlingieri MT, Troncone G, Chiappetta G, Liu CG, Santoro M, Negrini M, *et al*: MicroRNA deregulation in human thyroid papillary carcinomas. *Endocr Relat Cancer* 2006, 13:497-508.
28. Visone R, Pallante P, Vecchione A, Cirombella R, Ferracin M, Ferraro A, Volinia S, Coluzzi S, Leone V, Borbone E, *et al*: Specific microRNAs are downregulated in human thyroid anaplastic carcinomas. *Oncogene* 2007, 26:7590-7595.
29. Visone R, Russo L, Pallante P, De Martino I, Ferraro A, Leone V, Borbone E, Petrocca F, Alder H, Croce CM, Fusco A: MicroRNAs (miR)-221 and miR-222, both overexpressed in human thyroid papillary carcinomas, regulate p27Kip1 protein levels and cell cycle. *Endocr Relat Cancer* 2007, 14:791-798.
30. Braun J, Hoang-Vu C, Dralle H, Huttelmaier S: Downregulation of microRNAs directs the EMT and invasive potential of anaplastic thyroid carcinomas. *Oncogene* 2010, 29:4237-4244.
31. He H, Jazdzewski K, Li W, Liyanarachchi S, Nagy R, Volinia S, Calin GA, Liu CG, Franssila K, Suster S, *et al*: The role of microRNA genes in papillary thyroid carcinoma. *Proc Natl Acad Sci U S A* 2005, 102:19075-19080.
32. Ji J, Shi J, Budhu A, Yu Z, Forgues M, Roessler S, Ambs S, Chen Y, Meltzer PS, Croce CM, *et al*: MicroRNA expression, survival, and response to interferon in liver cancer. *N Engl J Med* 2009, 361:1437-1447.
33. Kota J, Chivukula RR, O'Donnell KA, Wentzel EA, Montgomery CL, Hwang HW, Chang TC, Vivekanandan P, Torbenson M, Clark KR, *et al*: Therapeutic microRNA delivery suppresses tumorigenesis in a murine liver cancer model. *Cell* 2009, 137:1005-1017.
34. Boyerinas B, Park SM, Shomron N, Hedegaard MM, Vinther J, Andersen JS, Feig C, Xu J, Burge CB, Peter ME: Identification of let-7-regulated oncofetal genes. *Cancer Res* 2008, 68:2587-2591.
35. Ricarte-Filho JC, Fuziwara CS, Yamashita AS, Rezende E, da-Silva MJ, Kimura ET: Effects of let-7 microRNA on Cell Growth and Differentiation of Papillary Thyroid Cancer. *Transl Oncol* 2009, 2:236-241.
36. Schwertheim S, Sheu SY, Worm K, Grabellus F, Schmid KW: Analysis of deregulated miRNAs is helpful to distinguish poorly differentiated thyroid carcinoma from papillary thyroid carcinoma. *Horm Metab Res* 2009, 41:475-481.
37. Sheu SY, Grabellus F, Schwertheim S, Worm K, Broecker-Preuss M, Schmid KW: Differential miRNA expression profiles in variants of papillary thyroid carcinoma and encapsulated follicular thyroid tumours. *Br J Cancer* 2010, 102:376-382.
38. Tetzlaff MT, Liu A, Xu X, Master SR, Baldwin DA, Tobias JW, Livolsi VA, Baloch ZW: Differential expression of miRNAs in papillary thyroid carcinoma compared to multinodular goiter using formalin fixed paraffin embedded tissues. *Endocr Pathol* 2007, 18:163-173.
39. Chen YT, Kitabayashi N, Zhou XK, Fahey TJ 3rd, Scognamiglio T: MicroRNA analysis as a potential diagnostic tool for papillary thyroid carcinoma. *Mod Pathol* 2008, 21:1139-1146.
40. Cahill S, Smyth P, Denning K, Flavin R, Li J, Potratz A, Guenther SM, Henfrey R, O'Leary JJ, Sheils O: Effect of BRAFV600E mutation on transcription and post-transcriptional regulation in a papillary thyroid carcinoma model. *Mol Cancer* 2007, 6:21.
41. Cahill S, Smyth P, Finn SP, Denning K, Flavin R, O'Regan EM, Li J, Potratz A, Guenther SM, Henfrey R, *et al*: Effect of ret/PTC 1 rearrangement on transcription and post-transcriptional regulation in a papillary thyroid carcinoma model. *Mol Cancer* 2006, 5:70.
42. Takakura S, Mitsutake N, Nakashima M, Namba H, Saenko VA, Rogounovitch TI, Nakazawa Y, Hayashi T, Ohtsuru A, Yamashita S: Oncogenic role of miR-17-92 cluster in anaplastic thyroid cancer cells. *Cancer Sci* 2008, 99:1147-1154.
43. Mitomo S, Maesawa C, Ogasawara S, Iwaya T, Shibazaki M, Yashima-Abo A, Kotani K, Oikawa H, Sakurai E, Izutsu N, *et al*: Downregulation of miR-138 is associated with overexpression of human telomerase reverse transcriptase protein in human anaplastic thyroid carcinoma cell lines. *Cancer Sci* 2008, 99:280-286.
44. Frezzetti D, Menna MD, Zoppoli P, Guerra C, Ferraro A, Bello AM, Luca PD, Calabrese C, Fusco A, Ceccarelli M, *et al*: Upregulation of miR-21 by Ras in vivo and its role in tumor growth. *Oncogene* 30:275-286.
45. Pineau P, Volinia S, McJunkin K, Marchio A, Battiston C, Terris B, Mazzaferro V, Lowe SW, Croce CM, Dejean A: miR-221 overexpression contributes to liver tumorigenesis. *Proc Natl Acad Sci U S A* 2010, 107:264-269.
46. Ciafre SA, Galardi S, Mangiola A, Ferracin M, Liu CG, Sabatino G, Negrini M, Maira G, Croce CM, Farace MG: Extensive modulation of a set of microRNAs in primary glioblastoma. *Biochem Biophys Res Commun* 2005, 334:1351-1358.

47. Kim YK, Yu J, Han TS, Park SY, Namkoong B, Kim DH, Hur K, Yoo MW, Lee HJ, Yang HK, Kim VN: Functional links between clustered microRNAs: suppression of cell-cycle inhibitors by microRNA clusters in gastric cancer. *Nucleic Acids Res* 2009, **37**:1672-1681.
48. Di Leva G, Gasparini P, Piovan C, Ngankeu A, Garofalo M, Taccioli C, Iorio MV, Li M, Volinia S, Alder H, *et al*: MicroRNA cluster 221-222 and estrogen receptor alpha interactions in breast cancer. *J Natl Cancer Inst* 2010, **102**:706-721.
49. Karger S, Weidinger C, Krause K, Sheu SY, Aigner T, Gimm O, Schmid KW, Dralle H, Fuhrer D: FOXO3a: a novel player in thyroid carcinogenesis? *Endocr Relat Cancer* 2009, **16**:189-199.
50. Wang K, Li PF: Foxo3a regulates apoptosis by negatively targeting miR-21. *J Biol Chem* 2010, **285**:16958-16966.
51. Fornari F, Gramantieri L, Ferracin M, Veronese A, Sabbioni S, Calin GA, Grazi GL, Giovannini C, Croce CM, Bolondi L, Negrini M: MiR-221 controls CDKN1C/p57 and CDKN1B/p27 expression in human hepatocellular carcinoma. *Oncogene* 2008, **27**:5651-5661.
52. Baldassarre G, Belletti B, Bruni P, Boccia A, Trapasso F, Pentimalli F, Barone MV, Chiappetta G, Vento MT, Spiezia S, *et al*: Overexpressed cyclin D3 contributes to retaining the growth inhibitor p27 in the cytoplasm of thyroid tumor cells. *J Clin Invest* 1999, **104**:865-874.
53. Natali PG, Berlingieri MT, Nicotra MR, Fusco A, Santoro E, Bigotti A, Vecchio G: Transformation of thyroid epithelium is associated with loss of c-kit receptor. *Cancer Res* 1995, **55**:1787-1791.
54. Igoucheva O, Alexeev V: MicroRNA-dependent regulation of cKit in cutaneous melanoma. *Biochem Biophys Res Commun* 2009, **379**:790-794.
55. Garofalo M, Di Leva G, Romano G, Nuovo G, Suh SS, Ngankeu A, Taccioli C, Pichiorri F, Alder H, Secchiero P, *et al*: miR-221&222 regulate TRAIL resistance and enhance tumorigenicity through PTEN and TIMP3 downregulation. *Cancer Cell* 2009, **16**:498-509.
56. Chun-Zhi Z, Lei H, An-Ling Z, Yan-Chao F, Xiao Y, Guang-Xiu W, Zhi-Fan J, Pei-Yu P, Qing-Yu Z, Chun-Sheng K: MicroRNA-221 and microRNA-222 regulate gastric carcinoma cell proliferation and radioresistance by targeting PTEN. *BMC Cancer* 2010, **10**:367.
57. Brader S, Eccles SA: Phosphoinositide 3-kinase signalling pathways in tumor progression, invasion and angiogenesis. *Tumori* 2004, **90**:2-8.
58. Hou P, Ji M, Xing M: Association of PTEN gene methylation with genetic alterations in the phosphatidylinositol 3-kinase/AKT signaling pathway in thyroid tumors. *Cancer* 2008, **113**:2440-2447.
59. Hou P, Liu D, Shan Y, Hu S, Studeman K, Condouris S, Wang Y, Trink A, El-Naggar AK, Tallini G, *et al*: Genetic alterations and their relationship in the phosphatidylinositol 3-kinase/Akt pathway in thyroid cancer. *Clin Cancer Res* 2007, **13**:1161-1170.
60. Jazbutyte V, Thum T: MicroRNA-21: from cancer to cardiovascular disease. *Curr Drug Targets* 2010, **11**:926-935.
61. Cho WC: OncomiRs: the discovery and progress of microRNAs in cancers. *Mol Cancer* 2007, **6**:60.
62. Meng F, Henson R, Lang M, Wehbe H, Maheshwari S, Mendell JT, Jiang J, Schmittgen TD, Patel T: Involvement of human micro-RNA in growth and response to chemotherapy in human cholangiocarcinoma cell lines. *Gastroenterology* 2006, **130**:2113-2129.
63. Frankel LB, Christoffersen NR, Jacobsen A, Lindow M, Krogh A, Lund AH: Programmed cell death 4 (PDCD4) is an important functional target of the microRNA miR-21 in breast cancer cells. *J Biol Chem* 2008, **283**:1026-1033.
64. Lu Z, Liu M, Stribinskis V, Klinge CM, Ramos KS, Colburn NH, Li Y: MicroRNA-21 promotes cell transformation by targeting the programmed cell death 4 gene. *Oncogene* 2008, **27**:4373-4379.
65. Asangani IA, Rasheed SA, Nikolova DA, Leupold JH, Colburn NH, Post S, Allgayer H: MicroRNA-21 (miR-21) post-transcriptionally downregulates tumor suppressor Pdcd4 and stimulates invasion, intravasation and metastasis in colorectal cancer. *Oncogene* 2008, **27**:2128-2136.
66. Zhu S, Wu H, Wu F, Nie D, Sheng S, Mo YY: MicroRNA-21 targets tumor suppressor genes in invasion and metastasis. *Cell Res* 2008, **18**:350-359.
67. Gabriely G, Wurdinger T, Kesari S, Esau CC, Burchard J, Linsley PS, Krichevsky AM: MicroRNA 21 promotes glioma invasion by targeting matrix metalloproteinase regulators. *Mol Cell Biol* 2008, **28**:5369-5380.
68. Yamanaka Y, Tagawa H, Takahashi N, Watanabe A, Guo YM, Iwamoto K, Yamashita J, Saitoh H, Kameoka Y, Shimizu N, *et al*: Aberrant overexpression of microRNAs activate AKT signaling via down-regulation of tumor suppressors in natural killer-cell lymphoma/leukemia. *Blood* 2009, **114**:3265-3275.
69. Pedersen IM, Otero D, Kao E, Miletic AV, Hother C, Ralfkiaer E, Rickert RC, Gronbaek K, David M: Onco-miR-155 targets SHIP1 to promote TNFalpha-dependent growth of B cell lymphomas. *EMBO Mol Med* 2009, **1**:288-295.
70. Kong W, Yang H, He L, Zhao JJ, Coppola D, Dalton WS, Cheng JQ: MicroRNA-155 is regulated by the transforming growth factor beta/Smad pathway and contributes to epithelial cell plasticity by targeting RhoA. *Mol Cell Biol* 2008, **28**:6773-6784.
71. Kong W, He L, Coppola M, Guo J, Esposito NN, Coppola D, Cheng JQ: MicroRNA-155 regulates cell survival, growth, and chemosensitivity by targeting FOXO3a in breast cancer. *J Biol Chem* 2010, **285**:17869-17879.
72. Gregory PA, Bert AG, Paterson EL, Barry SC, Tsykin A, Farshid G, Vadas MA, Khew-Goodall Y, Goodall GJ: The miR-200 family and miR-205 regulate epithelial to mesenchymal transition by targeting ZEB1 and SIP1. *Nat Cell Biol* 2008, **10**:593-601.
73. Park SM, Gaur AB, Lengyel E, Peter ME: The miR-200 family determines the epithelial phenotype of cancer cells by targeting the E-cadherin repressors ZEB1 and ZEB2. *Genes Dev* 2008, **22**:894-907.
74. Burk U, Schubert J, Wellner U, Schmalhofer O, Vincan E, Spaderna S, Brabletz T: A reciprocal repression between ZEB1 and members of the miR-200 family promotes EMT and invasion in cancer cells. *EMBO Rep* 2008, **9**:582-589.
75. Korpal M, Lee ES, Hu G, Kang Y: The miR-200 family inhibits epithelial-mesenchymal transition and cancer cell migration by direct targeting of E-cadherin transcriptional repressors ZEB1 and ZEB2. *J Biol Chem* 2008, **283**:14910-14914.
76. Brabletz S, Brabletz T: The ZEB/miR-200 feedback loop–a motor of cellular plasticity in development and cancer? *EMBO Rep* 2010, **11**:670-677.
77. Smallridge RC, Marlow LA, Copland JA: Anaplastic thyroid cancer: molecular pathogenesis and emerging therapies. *Endocr Relat Cancer* 2009, **16**:17-44.
78. Montero-Conde C, Martin-Campos JM, Lerma E, Gimenez G, Martinez-Guitarte JL, Combalia N, Montaner D, Matias-Guiu X, Dopazo J, de Leiva A, *et al*: Molecular profiling related to poor prognosis in thyroid carcinoma. Combining gene expression data and biological information. *Oncogene* 2008, **27**:1554-1561.
79. Sossey-Alaoui K, Bialkowska K, Plow EF: The miR200 family of microRNAs regulates WAVE3-dependent cancer cell invasion. *J Biol Chem* 2009, **284**:33019-33029.
80. Davis BN, Hilyard AC, Lagna G, Hata A: SMAD proteins control DROSHA-mediated microRNA maturation. *Nature* 2008, **454**:56-61.
81. Kong D, Banerjee S, Ahmad A, Li Y, Wang Z, Sethi S, Sarkar FH: Epithelial to mesenchymal transition is mechanistically linked with stem cell signatures in prostate cancer cells. *PLoS One* 2010, **5**:e12445.
82. Yu J, Vodyanik MA, Smuga-Otto K, Antosiewicz-Bourget J, Frane JL, Tian S, Nie J, Jonsdottir GA, Ruotti V, Stewart R, *et al*: Induced pluripotent stem cell lines derived from human somatic cells. *Science* 2007, **318**:1917-1920.
83. Newman MA, Thomson JM, Hammond SM: Lin-28 interaction with the Let-7 precursor loop mediates regulated microRNA processing. *RNA* 2008, **14**:1539-1549.
84. Viswanathan SR, Daley GQ, Gregory RI: Selective blockade of microRNA processing by Lin28. *Science* 2008, **320**:97-100.
85. Rybak A, Fuchs H, Smirnova L, Brandt C, Pohl EE, Nitsch R, Wulczyn FG: A feedback loop comprising lin-28 and let-7 controls pre-let-7 maturation during neural stem-cell commitment. *Nat Cell Biol* 2008, **10**:987-993.
86. Schickel R, Park SM, Murmann AE, Peter ME: miR-200c regulates induction of apoptosis through CD95 by targeting FAP-1. *Mol Cell* 2010, **38**:908-915.
87. Reinhart BJ, Slack FJ, Basson M, Pasquinelli AE, Bettinger JC, Rougvie AE, Horvitz HR, Ruvkun G: The 21-nucleotide let-7 RNA regulates developmental timing in Caenorhabditis elegans. *Nature* 2000, **403**:901-906.
88. Pasquinelli AE, Reinhart BJ, Slack F, Martindale MQ, Kuroda MI, Maller B, Hayward DC, Ball EE, Degnan B, Muller P, *et al*: Conservation of the sequence and temporal expression of let-7 heterochronic regulatory RNA. *Nature* 2000, **408**:86-89.
89. Johnson CD, Esquela-Kerscher A, Stefani G, Byrom M, Kelnar K, Ovcharenko D, Wilson M, Wang X, Shelton J, Shingara J, *et al*: The let-7 microRNA represses cell proliferation pathways in human cells. *Cancer Res* 2007, **67**:7713-7722.

90. Johnson SM, Grosshans H, Shingara J, Byrom M, Jarvis R, Cheng A, Labourier E, Reinert KL, Brown D, Slack FJ: **RAS is regulated by the let-7 microRNA family.** *Cell* 2005, **120**:635-647.
91. Sampson VB, Rong NH, Han J, Yang Q, Aris V, Soteropoulos P, Petrelli NJ, Dunn SP, Krueger LJ: **MicroRNA let-7a down-regulates MYC and reverts MYC-induced growth in Burkitt lymphoma cells.** *Cancer Res* 2007, **67**:9762-9770.
92. Lee YS, Dutta A: **The tumor suppressor microRNA let-7 represses the HMGA2 oncogene.** *Genes Dev* 2007, **21**:1025-1030.
93. Guo Y, Chen Y, Ito H, Watanabe A, Ge X, Kodama T, Aburatani H: **Identification and characterization of lin-28 homolog B (LIN28B) in human hepatocellular carcinoma.** *Gene* 2006, **384**:51-61.
94. Armelin HA, Armelin MC, Kelly K, Stewart T, Leder P, Cochran BH, Stiles CD: **Functional role for c-myc in mitogenic response to platelet-derived growth factor.** *Nature* 1984, **310**:655-660.
95. Kurihara T, Ikeda S, Ishizaki Y, Fujimori M, Tokumoto N, Hirata Y, Ozaki S, Okajima M, Sugino K, Asahara T: **Immunohistochemical and sequencing analyses of the Wnt signaling components in Japanese anaplastic thyroid cancers.** *Thyroid* 2004, **14**:1020-1029.
96. Chang TC, Zeitels LR, Hwang HW, Chivukula RR, Wentzel EA, Dews M, Jung J, Gao P, Dang CV, Beer MA, *et al*: **Lin-28B transactivation is necessary for Myc-mediated let-7 repression and proliferation.** *Proc Natl Acad Sci U S A* 2009, **106**:3384-3389.
97. Chang TC, Yu D, Lee YS, Wentzel EA, Arking DE, West KM, Dang CV, Thomas-Tikhonenko A, Mendell JT: **Widespread microRNA repression by Myc contributes to tumorigenesis.** *Nat Genet* 2008, **40**:43-50.
98. Mott JL, Kurita S, Cazanave SC, Bronk SF, Werneburg NW, Fernandez-Zapico ME: **Transcriptional suppression of mir-29b-1/mir-29a promoter by c-Myc, hedgehog, and NF-kappaB.** *J Cell Biochem* 2010, **110**:1155-1164.
99. Prokipcak RD, Herrick DJ, Ross J: **Purification and properties of a protein that binds to the C-terminal coding region of human c-myc mRNA.** *J Biol Chem* 1994, **269**:9261-9269.
100. Yisraeli JK: **VICKZ proteins: a multi-talented family of regulatory RNA-binding proteins.** *Biol Cell* 2005, **97**:87-96.
101. Watanabe S, Ueda Y, Akaboshi S, Hino Y, Sekita Y, Nakao M: **HMGA2 maintains oncogenic RAS-induced epithelial-mesenchymal transition in human pancreatic cancer cells.** *Am J Pathol* 2009, **174**:854-868.
102. Thuault S, Tan EJ, Peinado H, Cano A, Heldin CH, Moustakas A: **HMGA2 and Smads co-regulate SNAIL1 expression during induction of epithelial-to-mesenchymal transition.** *J Biol Chem* 2008, **283**:33437-33446.
103. Selbach M, Schwanhausser B, Thierfelder N, Fang Z, Khanin R, Rajewsky N: **Widespread changes in protein synthesis induced by microRNAs.** *Nature* 2008, **455**:58-63.
104. Scala S, Portella G, Fedele M, Chiappetta G, Fusco A: **Adenovirus-mediated suppression of HMGI(Y) protein synthesis as potential therapy of human malignant neoplasias.** *Proc Natl Acad Sci U S A* 2000, **97**:4256-4261.
105. Wu F, Zhu S, Ding Y, Beck WT, Mo YY: **MicroRNA-mediated regulation of Ubc9 expression in cancer cells.** *Clin Cancer Res* 2009, **15**:1550-1557.
106. Ichimi T, Enokida H, Okuno Y, Kunimoto R, Chiyomaru T, Kawamoto K, Kawahara K, Toki K, Kawakami K, Nishiyama K, *et al*: **Identification of novel microRNA targets based on microRNA signatures in bladder cancer.** *Int J Cancer* 2009, **125**:345--352.
107. Zhong X, Li N, Liang S, Huang Q, Coukos G, Zhang L: **Identification of microRNAs regulating reprogramming factor LIN28 in embryonic stem cells and cancer cells.** *J Biol Chem* 2010.
108. Krutzfeldt J, Rajewsky N, Braich R, Rajeev KG, Tuschl T, Manoharan M, Stoffel M: **Silencing of microRNAs in vivo with 'antagomirs'.** *Nature* 2005, **438**:685-689.
109. Vrba L, Jensen TJ, Garbe JC, Heimark RL, Cress AE, Dickinson S, Stampfer MR, Futscher BW: **Role for DNA methylation in the regulation of miR-200c and miR-141 expression in normal and cancer cells.** *PLoS One* 2010, **5**:e8697.

# 10

# Hypothyroidism causing paralytic ileus and acute kidney injury - case report

Chaturaka Rodrigo[1*], Champika SSSK Gamakaranage[1], Dhanesha S Epa[1], Ariaranee Gnanathasan[2], Senaka Rajapakse[2]

**Abstract**

We present a patient with severe hypothyroidism complicated by paralytic ileus and acute kidney injury. A 65 year old male patient, diagnosed with hypothyroidism one year ago was transferred to our unit in a state of drowsiness and confusion. He was severely hypothyroid and had paralytic ileus and impaired renal function at the time of transfer. Hypokalaemia was present, and was likely to have contributed to the paralytic ileus and this together with dehydration was likely to have contributed to renal injury. Nonetheless, hypothyroidism is very likely to have been the principal precipitant of both these complications, and both paralytic ileus and acute kidney injury improved with thyroxine replacement. Unfortunately, the patient died unexpectedly eight days after admission to the unit. Hypothyroidism may induce de novo acute kidney injury or it may exacerbate ongoing chronic kidney disease. This rare complication is assumed to be due to the hypodynamic circulatory state created by thyroid hormone deficiency. Paralytic ileus is an even rarer fatal manifestation of hypothyroidism and is thought to be due to an autonomic neuropathy affecting the intestines that is reversible with thyroxine replacement. To our knowledge, both these complications have not been observed in a single patient so far.

It is important that clinicians are aware of these rare manifestations of hypothyroidism as in most occasions, thyroxine deficiency may be missed, and treatment can reverse the complications.

## Background

Hypothyroidism presenting with acute kidney injury is rare, with only few cases reported so far [1,2]. Hypothyroidism may induce de novo acute kidney injury (AKI) or may exacerbate ongoing chronic kidney disease [3] or contribute to the occurrence of AKI in the presence of other renal insults. AKI is life threatening, and identification of possible contributory causes and early treatment is potentially life saving. Paralytic ileus is an even rarer fatal manifestation of hypothyroidism [4]. In this article we discuss a patient presenting with severe hypothyroidism and both these complications.

## Case presentation and discussion

### Case presentation

A 65 year old male patient, diagnosed with hypothyroidism one year ago, was transferred to our unit in a state of drowsiness and confusion. He did not have any other comorbidities and the cause for hypothyroidism was unknown. He had been on thyroxine replacement (150 μg daily) but had defaulted treatment for 3 months. In the months prior to admission, he had complained of constipation, lethargy, coarse skin and family members had noticed mental slowing, hoarse voice and changes in facial appearance. The patient was first admitted to a local hospital in a state of confusion and drowsiness with generalized body swelling, where oral thyroxine replacement was started. Coincidentally, he fell from his bed two days later and became unconscious. CT scan brain showed a small acute subdural haemorrhage over the right parietal lobe and he was transferred to the National Hospital, Colombo, Sri Lanka for neurosurgical opinion. While in the surgical unit, he developed progressive abdominal distension and absent bowel sounds. His urine output progressively declined and the serum creatinine was rising. He was then transferred to the University Medical Unit for medical management.

On admission to our unit, he had typical features of untreated hypothyroidism such as coarse myxoedematous skin, characteristic facial appearance, dry thin hair and oedema. He was not hypothermic but was dehydrated. His heart rate was around 60/min, blood pressure was 150/90 and there were no clinically detectable

* Correspondence: chaturaka.rodrigo@gmail.com
[1]University Medical Unit, National Hospital of Sri Lanka, Colombo, Sri Lanka
Full list of author information is available at the end of the article

pericardial effusions or cardiac murmurs. His respiratory system was clinically normal. His abdomen was grossly distended with absent bowel sounds. There was no palpable organomegaly. He was confused and drowsy (Glasgow coma scale; E-4, M-6, V-4) and had slow-relaxing reflexes.

The records showed that at initial presentation to the local hospital, his TSH (Thyroid Stimulating Hormone) level was 40.5 mIU/μl (normal 0.4-4.0). Serum free thyroxine ($FT_4$ ) level was not available at that time. On admission to our unit (2 weeks after the initial presentation and while on thyroxine replacement), his TSH level had dropped to 29.9 mIU/μl, and the $FT_4$ level was 0.61 ng/dl (0.89-1.76) - thus he was still severely hypothyroid. His serum creatinine had progressively risen from 122 μmol/l to 629 μmol/l with a concomitant drop in urine output (less than 30 ml per hour). He was normotensive throughout. There were no active urinary sediments and ultrasound scan abdomen showed normal sized kidneys with features of acute parenchymal disease together with bilateral fullness in the pelvicalyceal systems. The creatine phosphokinase level was not raised. He was not on any nephrotoxic drugs. At the onset of renal impairment, the patient had hyponatraemia (115-119 meq/l) and later on he was persistently hypokalaemic (2.5 - 3.4 meq/l). Abdominal radiographs showed grossly dilated bowel loops. He had a normal electrocardiogram but the echocardiogram showed grade II mitral regurgitation. There was no pericardial effusion. The patient's inflammatory markers were normal, and clinical features did not support peritonitis. Serum amylase was normal. We considered mechanical bowel obstruction, but found no clinical or investigation findings to support this; surgical opinion was sought, and a surgical acute abdomen was thought to be unlikely. Our diagnosis was paralytic ileus. We were unable to obtain a CT scan abdomen because of the dangers of contrast nephropathy aggravating existing AKI.

The patient was managed on the principles of thyroxine replacement and supportive therapy on the hypothesis that hypothyroidism and its sequalae were responsible for the clinical picture. Thyroxine was replaced (levothyroxine 200 μg/day as standard maintenance dose) via nasogastric tube and dehydration was corrected with carefully administered intravenous fluids with potassium replacement. Intravenous liothyronine was unavailable in our setting. With hydration and thyroxine replacement, the patient's renal functions improved (serum creatinine dropped to 278 μmol/l over 4 days) together with diuresis. Hyponatraemia also normalized without specific treatment. Dialysis was not required. Similarly, the bowel sounds returned and he opened bowels. Oral feeding was initiated with liquid feeds. The overall condition of the patient including the level of consciousness improved with thyroxine replacement. He was conscious, rational and was mobilized. However, on the $8^{th}$ day after transfer to our unit, he suddenly deteriorated and died. The cause for the unexpected death could not be established as the relatives refused a pathological post mortem. The cause of death could not be determined from the available investigation results at the time of death. The serum free T4 level was within normal range although the TSH level was still high (25.6 mIU/μl), and serum creatinine was 209 μmol/l immediately prior to the death. Serum electrolytes were normal for several days prior to death.

#### Discussion

There are several case reports of both acute renal failure [1,5] and paralytic ileus [6,7] occurring in untreated hypothyroidism. However both these complications appearing in the same patient has not been reported.

The exact pathogenesis of acute kidney injury in hypothyroidism is still unclear and thought to be multifactorial. However, the predominant mode of kidney injury is thought to be the reduced plasma flow and glomerular filtration rate due to the hypodynamic circulation [2]. The hypodynamic circulatory state results in a pre-renal insufficiency and this may be aggravated by other multi-systemic effects of hypothyroidism such as reduced cardiac output, low volume status, hyponatraemia with associated haemodynamic changes and increased peripheral resistance due to arterial wall stiffness [2]. However, this alone may not explain the extent of acute kidney injury. Primary glomerular and tubular dysfunction in hypothyroidism has also been observed with supportive histological evidence from biopsy specimens (thickening of glomerular and tubular basement membranes and inclusions in cell cytoplasm) [8]. These were reversible with thyroxine therapy. Rhabdomyolysis, another rare but known manifestation of hypothyroidism can also result in acute kidney injury but it is usually associated with another precipitating factor such as drugs or trauma [5]. Our patient however had no evidence of rhabdomyolysis. The available evidence suggests that renal impairment may start as quickly as two weeks in to the hypothyroid state and it recovers fully with thyroxine replacement [9]. The long term impact (if any) of hypothyroidism on renal function is unknown [5].

Paralytic ileus in hypothyroidism is assumed to be due to an autonomic neuropathy affecting the extrinsic nerves of the colon [10]. There are only a few cases of this complication reported in literature with the first one being reported by Bastenie in 1946 [7]. Bastenie hypothesized that myxoedematous material deposition in the muscle fibers of intestines interfered with their integration with autonomic ganglia. Later in 1969 and 1977, two case reports of death due to paralytic ileus with hypothyroidism were published [11,12]. In the report by Wells et al [11], the patient died after 20 days since presentation and the post mortem at that time gave an insight in to the possible pathogenesis in this unusual complication. Histological sections revealed gross abnormalities in extrinsic nerves entering the intestines while some less prominent changes were also observed in intrinsic plexuses. The authors suggest that the mechanism may be an autonomic neuropathy similar to the peripheral neuropathy frequently observed in hypothyroidism.

Surgical intervention for hypothyroidism induced paralytic ileus is not recommended as the neuropathy is reversible with thyroxine replacement. However, atonia may take time to reverse and the patients can succumb to complications of ileus [4].

In addition to paralytic ileus, patients may also present with urinary retention and this observation is also taken as supportive evidence for the autonomic neuropathy in hypothyroidism [4]. The fullness of the pelvicalyceal systems observed on ultrasound scan of our patient was possibly a result of this. We were unable to find any published data as to how the presence of paralytic ileus would have affected the absorption of thyroxine given via NG tube; the non-availability of intravenous liothyronine was a definite, albeit unavoidable, shortcoming in our management.

In the timeline of events, it is noted that the paralytic ileus preceded the acute kidney injury. The fluid sequestration in the bowels would have led to severe dehydration, hyponatraemia and hypokalaemia. Given the patient's background and sequence of events, it is likely that hypothyroidism was the primary cause of paralytic ileus though subsequent hypokalaemia undoubtedly contributed to making it worse. It is unlikely that hypokalaemia was the primary cause of paralytic ileus since hypokalaemia developed later on. The acute kidney injury in this patient is unlikely to be due to rhabdomyolysis as there was no supportive clinical or laboratory evidence. Instead, it is very likely that reduced renal plasma flow caused by hypothyroidism and the fluid sequestration within the intestines due to paralytic ileus in combination resulted in AKI. The paralytic ileus responded to potassium and thyroxine replacement and the concomitant vigorous fluid management would have improved the renal plasma flow. Both these therapeutic measures would have contributed to the rapid recovery of renal function. The relatively rapid recovery of renal function supports hypothyroidism related AKI rather than acute tubular necrosis due to dehydration.

In this patient, the root cause for paralytic ileus and acute kidney injury was the lack of thyroxine. The patient was managed on thyroxine replacement and supportive therapy leading to clinical improvement without surgery or invasive procedures, thus with hindsight our diagnosis of paralytic ileus was correct. The cause of sudden death in this patient may either be related to hypothyroidism and its complications or caused by an independent factor. Though kidney injury reverses fast with thyroxine replacement, the smooth muscle atonia is believed to take a longer time for recovery, and complications of ileus might have contributed to death [11,12]. Although hyponatraemia and hypokalaemia were present initially, both serum sodium and potassium levels were normal for several days prior to his deterioration, and are hence unlikely to have been responsible for his death. On the other hand, an arrhythmia or pulmonary embolism (the patient was bedridden for over 3 weeks) or possibly an acute rebleed into the existing subdural haemorrhage (with raised intracranial pressure and coning) are possible causes for his death.

## Conclusions

It is important that clinicians are aware of the rare manifestations of hypothyroidism such as acute kidney injury and paralytic ileus. The easily reversible thyroxine deficiency may be missed when patients present with such complications unless there is an obvious past history.

## Consent

Written informed consent was obtained from the patient's relatives for publication of this case report. A copy of the written consent is available for review by the Editor-in-Chief of this journal.

#### List of abbreviations

Abbreviations are explained where they are first used in text

#### Author details

[1]University Medical Unit, National Hospital of Sri Lanka, Colombo, Sri Lanka. [2]Department of Clinical Medicine, Faculty of Medicine, University of Colombo, Sri Lanka.

#### Authors' contributions

CR, CG and DSE collected information on the patient. CR wrote the first draft. SR and CR did the literature searches and wrote the final manuscript and made appropriate revisions. All authors read through and approved the final manuscript.

#### Authors' information

CR and CG (MBBS) are registrars in Internal Medicine attached to the University Medical Unit of the National Hospital of Sri Lanka. DSE (MBBS) is the House Officer of the same unit. AG (MBBS, MD, MPhil, FRCP) is Consultant Physician and Senior Lecturer attached to the Department of Clinical Medicine, Faculty of Medicine, University of Colombo, Sri Lanka. SR (MBBS, MD, FRCP, FCCP, FACP) is Consultant Physician and Professor in the same department.

#### Competing interests

The authors declare that they have no competing interests.

#### References

1. Birewar S, Oppenheimer M, Zawada ET Jr: **Hypothyroid acute renal failure.** *S D J Med* 2004, **57**:109-110.

2. Liakopoulos V, Dovas S, Simopoulou T, Zarogiannis S, Giannopoulou M, Kourti P, Arampatzis S, Eleftheriadis T, Stefanidis I: **Acute renal failure: a rare presentation of hypothyroidism.** *Ren Fail* 2009, **31**:323-326.
3. Makino Y, Fujii T, Kuroda S, Inenaga T, Kawano Y, Takishita S: **Exacerbation of renal failure due to hypothyroidism in a patient with ischemic nephropathy.** *Nephron* 2000, **84**:267-269.
4. Nathan AW, Havard CW: **Paralytic ileus and urinary retention due to hypothyroidism.** *Br Med J (Clin Res Ed)* 1982, **285**:477.
5. Joshi B, Jones D, Rochford A, Giblin L: **Hypothyroidism and associated acute renal failure.** *J R Soc Med* 2009, **102**:199-200.
6. Bentley RJ, Browne RJ: **Paralytic ileus and dementia in a case of myxoedema.** *Postgrad Med J* 1969, **45**:779-781.
7. Bastenie PA: **Paralytic ileus in severe hypothyroidism.** *Lancet* 1946, **1**:413-416.
8. Salomon MI, Di Scala V, Grishman E, Brener J, Churg J: **Renal lesions in hypothyroidism: a study based on kidney biopsies.** *Metabolism* 1967, **16**:846-852.
9. Kreisman SH, Hennessey J: **Consistent reversible elevations of serum creatinine levels in severe hypothyroidism.** *Arch Intern Med* 1999, **159**:79-82.
10. Kumar N, Wheeler MH: **Hypothyroidism presenting as acute abdomen.** *Postgrad Med J* 1997, **73**:373-374.
11. Wells I, Smith B, Hinton M: **Acute ileus in myxoedema.** *BMJ* 1977, **i**:211-212.
12. Chadha JS, Ashby DW, Cowan WK: **Fatal intestinal atony in myxoedema.** *BMJ* 1969, **3**:398.

# 11

# The natural history of interferon-α induced thyroiditis in chronic hepatitis c patients: a long term study

Huy A Tran[1*†], Tracey L Jones[2†], Elizabeth A Ianna[3†], Glenn EM Reeves[4†]

**Abstract**

**Background:** Autoimmune thyroid disease is a common complication of patients with chronic hepatitis C undergoing combination pegylated interferon-α and ribavirin treatment. A small proportion develops interferon-induced thyroiditis of which the long term natural history is unknown and how it compares with de novo thyroiditis. The aim of the study is to determine the natural history of thyroid disease including antibody profile in this particular setting 36 months from the completion of therapy.

**Methods:** A cohort of 18 hepatitis C patients (mean age 45 ± 8 years (standard deviation)) who developed exclusively thyroiditis in this setting was followed every 12 months after the completion of therapy for 36 months. Investigations included thyrotropin, free tetra-iodothyronine, free tri-iodothyronine levels and thyroid autoantibodies.

**Results:** None of the patients developed any long term thyroid disease. Two patients had a prolonged hypothyroid phase of the thyroiditis early after the completion of treatment but recovered fully. The remaining 16 patients remained euthyroid. Similarly, thyroid autoantibodies all declined and returned to reference range.

**Conclusions:** The long term natural history in this small series of interferon induced thyroiditis was benign. If a larger series confirms a similar outcome then there is no long term residual effect on thyroid function and follow-up testing would not be warranted.

## Background

Hepatitis C remains one of the major causes of chronic liver infection and cirrhosis worldwide. The most effective and established treatment available for this condition is the combination ribavirin and pegylated interferon-α (IFN-α). A major and common adverse effect of this treatment is the development of thyroid disease during therapy. A large spectrum of autoimmune thyroid disease (TD) has been described to occur ranging from Graves' disease to thyroiditis to frank primary hypothyroidism [1-3]. As the number of patients undertaking treatment is expected to rise, a proportion of these patients will progress to develop thyroid disease. It is therefore important to understand and fully clarify the natural progression of the disease. This forms a critical part of the long term management and counselling for these patients. It has been reported that ~50% of these patients recover from this complication [4,5]. Furthermore, other reports are retrospective and follow patients in an ad hoc fashion with very variable and unstandardised duration. In addition, some of the studied groups included the use of IFN as monotherapy and regular IFN (rather than pegylated) in combination with ribavirin [6]. In some cases, patients remain permanently thyroxine dependent although no withdrawal trials were attempted. The long term natural history of this condition beyond this time frame remains largely unknown and it is uncertain whether it is different from other forms of thyroiditides arising de novo.

The aim of this report is to follow prospectively the long term natural history of TD 36 months after the completion of treatment in a cohort of patients who

* Correspondence: huy.tran@hnehealth.nsw.gov.au
† Contributed equally
[1]Hunter Area Pathology Service and University of Newcastle, Locked Bag Number 1, Hunter Mail Region Centre, Newcastle, New South Wales 2310, Australia
Full list of author information is available at the end of the article

developed thyroid disease during therapy with pegylated interferon and also to compare the outcome with the natural history of the thyroiditides arising de novo.

## Methods

### Patients

The patients are all recruited from a Hepatitis C service centre in a major tertiary referral hospital. A total of 18 patients were available for study. These were retrieved from a pool of 358 patients over a 5 year period, giving an annual incidence of ~5.0%. All were followed-up over a 36-month period. All were medication naive, i.e. all were undergoing therapy for the first time. All other causes of chronic hepatitis were excluded including hepatitis B and chronic alcoholic liver disease. Baseline characteristics of all studied subjects are summarised in Table 1.

### Thyroid function assessments

All patients were assessed by an endocrinology team and confirmed to have thyroiditis whilst receiving interferon therapy as previously reported [7]. At the end of interferon treatment, all had baseline thyroid function studies and thyroid autoantibodies, at 12, 24 and 36 months post therapy. Follow-ups at 24 and 36 months were performed by mail correspondence and telephone interviews. Patients were recalled and reviewed formally if clinically indicated.

### Laboratory assay characteristics

Third generation serum TSH, serum fT4 and fT3 were determined by two-site sandwich immunoassay using an automated chemiluminescent system (Diagnostic Products Corporation, Immulite 2000). The reference range (RR) for TSH was 0.4-4.0 mU/L, fT4 10.0-26.0 and fT3 3.5-5.5 pmol/L. The coefficients of variation (CV) were 5.0% and 5.1% at TSH concentrations of 4.0 mU/L and 10.0 mU/L respectively. For fT4, the CV was 6.5% at 10.0 pmol/L and fT3 8.9% at 3.5 pmol/L.

Serum autoantibodies to thyroglobulin and thyroperoxidase were measured by agglutination (Serodia-ATG and Serodia-AMC, Fujirebio, Inc., Tokyo, Japan). Titres of less than 1:40 were considered normal for both.

Thyroid Stimulating Immunoglobulin was measured using cell culture and radio-immunoassay. This is an in-house bioassay using Chinese Hamster Ovary (CHO) cells in culture to detect the presence of thyroid stimulating activity. The CHO cells are transfected with the TSH receptor genes and thus are responsive to TSI. Thyroid-stimulating activity is measured by evaluating the intracellular release of cAMP induced by the patient's serum immunoglobulin on the CHO cells. The results are reported as units/mL (U/mL). TSI should be absent in the normal population. A TSI level of <10 is considered negative, 10-50 as weakly, 50-100 as moderately and >100 U/mL as strongly positive.

**Table 1 Baseline characteristics, hepatitic outcomes and thyrotropin outcome profiles in all 18 thyroiditis patients**

| *Subject No.* | *Gender* | *Age* | *Hepatitis C Genotype* | *Duration of Therapy (weeks)* | *SVR* | *End of Rx TSH* | *TSH at 12 months* | *TSH at 24 months* | *TSH at 36 months* |
|---|---|---|---|---|---|---|---|---|---|
| 1 | M | 26 | 1a | 48 | Y | 2.1 | 1.8 | 2.8 | 3.4 |
| 2 | M | 51 | 2 | 24 | Y | 1.7 | 3.2 | 3.1 | 2.7 |
| 3 | M | 54 | 3 | 24 | Y | 3.8 | 2.3 | 2.2 | 3.2 |
| 4 | M | 49 | 4 | 48 | Y | 1.1 | 1.4 | 2.1 | 2.3 |
| 5* | F | 42 | 2 | 24 | Y | 1.6 | 1.8 | 2.1 | 1.9 |
| 6* | F | 34 | 3 | 24 | Y | 2.4 | 2.7 | 2.1 | 2.0 |
| 7 | F | 49 | 4 | 48 | Y | 3.1 | 2.9 | 2.7 | 2.2 |
| 8* | F | 49 | 1 | 48 | Y | 0.03 | 1.5 | 1.2 | 1.3 |
| 9 | F | 50 | 2 | 24 | Y | 2.2 | 2.1 | 2.4 | 2.5 |
| 10* | F | 37 | 4 | 48 | Y | 6.5 | 4.5 | 5.2 | 2.3 |
| 11 | F | 43 | 4 | 48 | Y | 1.8 | 1.9 | 2.3 | 2.1 |
| 12 | F | 42 | 3 | 24 | Y | 2.1 | 2.3 | 1.7 | 2.5 |
| 13* | F | 43 | 1 | 48 | N | 10.5 | 2.3 | 1.8 | 2.4 |
| 14* | F | 51 | 3 | 24 | Y | 8.8 | 4.0 | 3.8 | 2.3 |
| 15 | M | 57 | 1 | 48 | N | 2.2 | 2.7 | 1.9 | 1.2 |
| 16 | F | 38 | 3 | 24 | Y | 1.9 | 2.2 | 2.3 | 3.7 |
| 17 | M | 57 | 1 | 48 | Y | 4.5 | 2.5 | 3.6 | 2.8 |
| 18 | F | 37 | 3 | 24 | Y | 3.4 | 3.3 | 2.5 | 2.8 |

*; Cases 5 and 6 required short-term thyroxine supplement, case 8 progressed to develop post-interferon Graves' like thyrotoxicosis, cases 10 and 14 had subclinical hypothyroidism and case 13 was in the hypothyroid phase at the end of treatment. SVR; Sustained virologic response, Rx; Treatment, TSH; Thyrotropin.

#### Duration of follow-ups

Duration of follow-ups started from the completion of interferon treatment, be it 24 or 48 weeks.

#### Definition of thyroiditis

Thyroiditis is defined as the triad of clinical and/or biochemical thyrotoxicosis followed by a hypothyroid phase, with an initial reduced/negligible thyroid pertechnetate uptake scan. All uptake scans were reviewed by a specialist nuclear physician consultant. Thyroid autoantibodies may be present but are not considered essential to the diagnosis.

### Results

There were 18 cases of thyroiditis available for the study. All recovered from their TD at the end of the study. Cases 5 and 6 required short-term thyroxine supplement but subsequently were successfully withdrawn from thyroxine. Case 8 progressed to developed temporary Graves-like thyrotoxicosis demonstrating the uncommon tri-phasic thyroiditis that had previously been reported [8,9]. In addition, cases 10 and 14 had subclinical hypothyroidism which resolved with time and did not require thyroxine at any stage, Table 2. Similarly, case 13 was in the hypothyroid phase of the thyroiditis at the end of treatment, was treated expectantly and resolved without thyroxine. At 36 months, all cases had normal thyrotropin levels and all thyroid autoantibodies were undetectable. No patient required thyroxine at the end of the study.

With the exception of case 8, thyroid autoantibody titres declined towards normal at the end of treatment and remained unaltered throughout the duration of follow-up.

### Discussion

This is the first report to prospectively investigate the natural history of patients who develop thyroiditis during treatment with pegylated interferon-α and ribavirin for chronic hepatitis C infection. It is reassuring to ascertain that this form of TD is benign and that there is no long term recurrence or hypothyroidism. This benign prognosis is encouraging for both patients and clinicians. There appears to be little need to monitor for associated thyroid condition beyond 36 months after completion of treatment.

This benign outcome also parallels the thyroid autoantibodies which similarly resolved. With the exceptions of one patient (case 8), all thyroid antibodies normalise. In this affected case, autoantibodies persisted at the end of treatment suggesting ongoing immunomodulation but the consequent mild Graves' disease resolved after 12 months.

The involution of thyroid disease after interferon exposure is as expected and is probably due to two reasons. Firstly, it is because of the pharmacokinetics of the

**Table 2 Auto-antibody profiles in 18 thyroiditis patients**

| *Subject No.* | *End of Rx anti-TPO* | *Anti-TPO at 12 months* | *Anti-TPO at 24 months* | *Anti-TPO at 36 months* | *End of Rx anti-Tg* | *Anti-Tg at 12 months* | *Anti-Tg at 24 months* | *Anti-Tg at 36 months* | *End of Rx TSI* | *TSI at 12 months* | *TSI at 24 months* | *TSI at 36 months* |
|---|---|---|---|---|---|---|---|---|---|---|---|---|
| 1 | <1 | <1 | <1 | <1 | <1 | <1 | <1 | <1 | <10 | <10 | <10 | <10 |
| 2 | <1 | <1 | <1 | <1 | <1 | <1 | <1 | <1 | <10 | <10 | <10 | <10 |
| 3 | <1 | <1 | <1 | <1 | <1 | <1 | <1 | <1 | <10 | <10 | <10 | <10 |
| 4 | <1 | <1 | <1 | <1 | <1 | <1 | <1 | <1 | <10 | <10 | <10 | <10 |
| 5* | 1024 | <1 | <1 | <1 | <1 | <1 | <1 | <1 | <10 | <10 | <10 | <10 |
| 6* | 256 | <1 | <1 | <1 | <1 | <1 | <1 | <1 | <10 | <10 | <10 | <10 |
| 7 | <1 | <1 | <1 | <1 | <1 | <1 | <1 | <1 | <10 | <10 | <10 | <10 |
| 8* | 16 | <1 | <1 | <1 | <1 | <1 | <1 | <1 | 19 | 10 | <10 | <10 |
| 9 | <1 | <1 | <1 | <1 | <1 | <1 | <1 | <1 | <10 | <10 | <10 | <10 |
| 10* | <1 | <1 | <1 | <1 | <1 | <1 | <1 | <1 | <10 | <10 | <10 | <10 |
| 11 | <1 | <1 | <1 | <1 | <1 | <1 | <1 | <1 | <10 | <10 | <10 | <10 |
| 12 | <1 | <1 | <1 | <1 | <1 | <1 | <1 | <1 | <10 | <10 | <10 | <10 |
| 13* | <1 | <1 | <1 | <1 | <1 | <1 | <1 | <1 | <10 | <10 | <10 | <10 |
| 14* | 16 | <1 | <1 | <1 | <1 | <1 | <1 | <1 | <10 | <10 | <10 | <10 |
| 15 | <1 | <1 | <1 | <1 | <1 | <1 | <1 | <1 | <10 | <10 | <10 | <10 |
| 16 | <1 | <1 | <1 | <1 | <1 | <1 | <1 | <1 | <10 | <10 | <10 | <10 |
| 17 | <1 | <1 | <1 | <1 | <1 | <1 | <1 | <1 | <10 | <10 | <10 | <10 |
| 18 | <1 | <1 | <1 | <1 | <1 | <1 | <1 | <1 | <10 | <10 | <10 | <10 |

*; see Table 1 legend. Anti-TPO; anti-thyroperoxidase antibody, Anti-Tgl; anti-thyroglobulin antibody, TSI; Thyrotropin stimulating immunoglobulins.

pegylated IFN which is expected to clear within 4 to 6 weeks. As a result, most of the TDs that occur post-therapy tend to do so in this time frame [10]. Secondly, once beyond the 6 month period where sustained virologic response (SVR) had been attained, the immunomodulating effect of the hepatitis C viral particle has been removed and hence its influence on thyroid tissues is no longer pertinent [11].

However our findings are inconsistent with other retrospective reports. Carella et al [12] studied a group of 114 chronic hepatitis C patients after an average of 6.2 years of follow-up and found some persistence of thyroid autoantibodies after 6.2 years of follow-up but without clinical findings of TDs. However, these patients were treated with IFN-α alone for 12 months. However the treatment was monotherapy with regular IFN. Vezali et al [13] described 2 cases which developed thyroiditis within 1 month of treatment completion and another 3 cases at 6, 6.5 and 26 months respectively. No further details were forthcoming. The frequency of thyroid testings was not mentioned during this post-treatment period. Jamil et al [6] looked at 45 cases of thyroid disease over a 12 year period but did not comment on the long-term outcomes of thyroid diseased patients nor the frequency of thyroid monitoring. Generally speaking in other retrospective series, the thyroid follow-ups are often ad hoc as a result and the outcome is not uniform and inconsistent [14,6]. The thyroid surveillance frequency is also inadequate to assess for the thyroid condition.

Most series report hypothyroidism as the commonest thyroid disorder in this setting but our experience has been that of thyroiditis almost exclusively [7]. In this setting, the prevalence of permanent hypothyroidism has been reported at ~50% [13] but where attempts or trials of thyroxine withdrawal were done, none of our patients required long term supplements. This suggests that the thyroid has completely recovered from the interferon-elicited injury and that hypothyroidism occurring in this setting deserved a trial of withdrawal before being committed to life-long therapy and all its potential complications.

The presence of high thyroid autoantibody titres also heavily influences the involution of thyroid diseases. Where they persisted or evolved, clinical diseases appear to follow as evident in cases 5, 6 and 8. However, because of the sporadic nature of post-treatment thyroid diseases, it remains uncertain whether routine thyroid autoantibodies should be performed routinely in this setting.

The major limitation of this study is the small number of subjects due the low prevalence of the condition. The second concern is the testing frequency of 12 month intervals during which it is conceivable that thyroid function may have fluctuated during this time. Regardless, it appears that thyroid disease sustained during interferon therapy for chronic hepatitis C infection is self-limiting and without any long last consequences. All cases recovered, compared with de novo thyroiditis where the progression to hypothyroidism can be as high as 20% in both adults and children [15,16]. Although there is no data beyond 3 years, it can safely be assumed that any development of thyroid conditions beyond this time should be deemed unrelated and treated each on its own merit. Perhaps monitoring for thyroid disease could be safely ceased at 6 months follow-up, coinciding with the SVR review.

## Conclusion

Despite the small number, the long term outcome of interferon induced thyroiditis appears benign. There is no long term risk of hypothyroidism. Larger studies will be needed to confirm this outcome. If this is the case, perhaps there is little need to follow these patients longer than 6 months after the completion of interferon therapy. This is to cover for any immediate thyroid conditions that may occur during this time frame. Follow-ups beyond 3 years appear unwarranted although this time frame is completely arbitrary.

**Acknowledgements**

We would like to sincere thank Geoffrey M Kellerman for his review and constructive comments of this manuscript.

**Author details**

[1]Hunter Area Pathology Service and University of Newcastle, Locked Bag Number 1, Hunter Mail Region Centre, Newcastle, New South Wales 2310, Australia. [2]Hepatitis C Service, Gastroenterology Department, John Hunter Hospital and University of Newcastle, Locked Bag Number 1, Hunter Mail Region Centre, Newcastle, New South Wales 2310, Australia. [3]Hepatitis C Service, Gastroenterology Department, John Hunter Hospital, Locked Bag Number 1, Hunter Mail Region Centre, Newcastle, New South Wales 2310, Australia. [4]Hunter Area Pathology Service and University of Newcastle, Locked Bag Number 1, Hunter Mail Region Centre, Newcastle, New South Wales 2310, Australia.

**Authors' contributions**

HAT conceived the study, participated in its design, assisted with data collection and statistical analysis, and coordinated and helped to draft the manuscript. GEMR contributed to the statistical and meta-analytical methods, and participated in the discussion and drafting of the manuscript. TLJ, EAI gathered, provided the data, and participated in the discussion and drafting of the manuscript. All authors read and approved the final revised manuscript.

**Competing interests**

The authors declare that they have no competing interests.

**References**

1. Tomer Y, Blackard JT, Akeno N: **Interferon alpha treatment and thyroid dysfunction.** *Endocrinol Metab Clin N Am* 2007, **36**:1051-66.
2. Carella C, Mazziotti G, Amato G, Braverman LE, Roti E: **Interferon-α-related thyroid disease: Pathophysiological, epidemiological, and clinical aspects.** *J Clin Endocrinol Metab* 2004, **89**:3656-61.

3. Prummel MF, Laurberg P: **Interferon-α and autoimmune thyroid disease.** *Thyroid* 2003, **13**:547-51.
4. Antonelli A, Ferri C, Fallahi P: **Thyroid dysfunction in patients with hepatitis C on IFN-α therapy.** *Nat Rev Gastroenterol Hepatol* 2009, **6**:633-5.
5. Wong V W-S, Cheng A Y-S, Chan H L-Y: **Interferon-induced thyroid dysfunction - not always transient.** *J Gastroenterol Hepatol* 2009, **24**:933-940.
6. Jamil KM, Leedman PJ, Kontorinis N, Taruinio L, Nazareth S, McInerney M, Connelly C, Flexman J, Burke V, Metcalf C, Cheng W: **Interferon-induced thyroid dysfunction in chronic hepatitis C.** *J Gastroenterol Hepatol* 2009, **24**:1017-23.
7. Tran HA, Reeves GEM, Jones TL: **The natural history of interferon-alpha2b-induced thyroiditis and its exclusivity in a cohorte of patients with chronic hepatitis C infection.** *QJM* 2009, **102**:117-22.
8. Bohbot NL, Young J, Orgiazzi J, Buffet C, Francois M, Bernard-Chabert B, Lukas-Croisier C, Delemer B: **Interferon-alpha-induced hyperthyroidism: a three-stage evolution from silent thyroiditis towards Graves' disease.** *Eur J Endocrinol* 2006, **154**:367-72.
9. Tran HA: **The swinging thyroid in hepatitis C infection and interferon therapy.** *QJM* 2009, **183**:187-191.
10. Tran HA, Reeves GE: **The spectrum of autoimmune thyroid disease in the short to medium term following interferon-alpha therapy for chronic hepatitis C.** *Int J Endocrinol* 2009, **2009**:241786.
11. Akeno N, Blackard JT, Tomer Y: **HCV E2 protein binds directly to thyroid cells and induces IL-8 production: a new mechanism for HCV induced thyroid autoimmunity.** *J Autoimmun* 2008, **31**:339-344.
12. Carella C, Mazziotti G, Morisco F, Manganella G, Rotondi M, Tuccillo C, Sorvillo F, Caporaso N, Amato G: **Long-term outcome of interferon-α-induced thyroid autoimmunity and prognostic influence of thyroid autoantibody pattern at the end of treatment.** *J Clin Endocrinol Metab* 2001, **86**:1925-1929.
13. Vezali E, Elefsiniotis I, Mihas C, Konstantinou E, Saroglou G: **Thyroid dysfunction in patients with chronic hepatitis C: Virus- or therapy-related?** *J Gastroenterol Hepatol* 2009, **24**:1024-1029.
14. Masood N, Shori R, Memon A, Memon S, Memon KI, Memon I, Jaffri M, Baloch GH: **Frequency of thyroid disorders during interferon and ribavirin therapy in chronic hepatitis C infection.** *J Coll Physicians Surg Pak* 2008, **18**:347-351.
15. Demirbilek H, Kandemir N, Gonc EN, Ozon A, Alikasifoglu A: **Assessment of thyroid function during the long course of Hashimoto's thyroiditis in children and adolescents.** *Clin Endocrinol* 2009, **71**:451-454.
16. Bindra A, Braunstein GD: **Thyroiditis.** *Am Fam Physician* 2006, **73**:1769-1776.

# 12

# Cathepsin B trafficking in thyroid carcinoma cells

Sofia Tedelind[1*†], Silvia Jordans[1†], Henrike Resemann[1], Galia Blum[2], Matthew Bogyo[3], Dagmar Führer[4], Klaudia Brix[1]

**Abstract**

**Background:** The cysteine peptidase cathepsin B is important in thyroid physiology by being involved in prohormone processing initiated in the follicle lumen and completed in endo-lysosomal compartments. However, cathepsin B has also been localized to the extrafollicular space in thyroid cancer tissue, and is therefore suggested to promote invasiveness and metastasis in thyroid carcinomas through e.g. extracellular matrix degradation.

**Methods:** Transport of cathepsin B in normal thyroid epithelial and carcinoma cells was investigated through immunolocalization of endogenous cathepsin B in combination with probing protease activity. Transport analyses of cathepsin B-eGFP and its active-site mutant counterpart cathepsin B-C29A-eGFP were used to test whether intrinsic sequences of a protease influence its trafficking.

**Results:** Our approach employing activity based probes, which distinguish between active and inactive cysteine proteases, demonstrated that both eGFP-tagged normal and active-site mutated cathepsin B chimeras reached the endo-lysosomal compartments of thyroid epithelial cells, thereby ruling out alterations of sorting signals by mutagenesis of the active-site cysteine. Analysis of chimeric protein trafficking further showed that GFP-tagged cathepsin B was transported to the expected compartments, i.e. endoplasmic reticulum, Golgi apparatus and endo-lysosomes of normal and thyroid carcinoma cell lines. However, the active-site mutated cathepsin B chimera was mostly retained in the endoplasmic reticulum and Golgi of KTC-1 and HTh7 cells. Hence the latter, as the least polarized of the three carcinoma cell lines analyzed, exhibited severe transport defects in that it retained chimeras in pre-endolysosomal compartments. Furthermore, secretion of endogenous cathepsin B and of other cysteine peptidases, which occurs at the apical pole of normal thyroid epithelial cells, was most prominent and occurred in a non-directed fashion in thyroid carcinoma cells.

**Conclusions:** Transport of endogenous and eGFP-tagged active and inactive cathepsin B in the cultured thyroid carcinoma cells reflected the distribution patterns of this protease in thyroid carcinoma tissue. Hence, our studies showed that sub-cellular localization of proteolysis is a crucial step in regulation of tissue homeostasis. We conclude that any interference with protease trafficking resulting in altered regulation of proteolytic events leads to, or is a consequence of the onset and progression of thyroid cancer.

## Background

Cathepsin B is a cysteine peptidase belonging to the papain clan C1A [1,2]. Cysteine cathepsins in general are homologous with respect to their active-site residues, i.e. cysteine (Cys) and histidine (His) forming the catalytic dyad [3]. Cathepsin B is a ubiquitously expressed member of the family of papain-like cysteine peptidases, but it is exceptional in exhibiting endo- and exopeptidase activities [4]. The main proteolytic function attributed to cathepsin B in physiology is considered in its catabolic action on proteins reaching endo-lysosomal compartments [4-6]. Hence, cathepsin B is considered to predominantly act on its substrates intracellularly, within endocytic compartments. In contrast, the extracellular occurrence of cysteine peptidases like cathepsin B is often considered pathological. Severe conditions of excessive cathepsin B-mediated degradation of extracellular matrix (ECM) components, as it is observed in osteoarthritis [7], is believed to arise when cathepsin B is secreted into the extracellular space in a non-regulated manner. Furthermore, cysteine cathepsins,

* Correspondence: s.tedelind@jacobs-university.de
† Contributed equally
[1]School of Engineering and Science, Research Center for Molecular Life Science, Jacobs University Bremen, 28759 Bremen, Germany
Full list of author information is available at the end of the article

and in particular cathepsin B, are considered to be involved in malignancies and cancer progression due to an increase in expression and activity in cancer cells as well as due to increased secretion from tumor-associated cells [8-12].

Because proteases display their functions by an irreversible mode of substrate cleavage, it is considered crucial to determine (i) time, (ii) location and (iii) extent of proteolytic cleavage in order to understand protease actions in physiology and pathology [1,6,13,14]. Thus, trafficking of proteases and the tight spatiotemporal regulation of proteolysis are decisive for normal or diseased functions of cells or tissues.

In the healthy thyroid gland, cathepsin B bears important functions for maintaining the differentiated state of thyroid epithelial cells in that it contributes to thyroglobulin processing and thyroxine release from the thyroid follicles [15-18]. This role of cathepsin B in thyroid physiology depends on its polarized secretion at the apical plasma membrane domain of differentiated normal thyroid epithelial cells [15,16,19]. However, cathepsin B has also been shown to be localized to the basement membrane of thyroid carcinoma cells *in situ*, where it was proposed to facilitate tumor invasiveness and metastasis through degradation of the extracellular matrix [20]. Recently, we have determined that cathepsin B is the main active cysteine cathepsin present in the human thyroid carcinoma cell lines KTC-1, HTh7 and HTh74 cells [21]. This fact, together with the suggested role of cathepsin B in malignant progression, prompted us to further analyze trafficking of cathepsin B in KTC-1 cells, a poorly differentiated papillary thyroid carcinoma cell line, and in the anaplastic HTh7 and HTh74 thyroid carcinoma cell lines. KTC-1 cells do not express thyroid stimulating hormone (TSH) receptors, thyroid peroxidase (TPO) or the sodium iodide symporter (NIS), but still express thyroglobulin [22]. Thus, these cells are characterized by both, a maintained and a lost expression of key components of the physiological thyroid hormone production machinery. In addition, despite a low expression of thyroglobulin mRNA by HTh74 cells [23], we and others have shown that this cell line still expresses functional TSH receptors [21,24].

Here, we expressed cathepsin B and its active-site mutant counterpart cathepsin B-C29A as chimeric proteins fused to the enhanced green fluorescent protein (eGFP) as visualization tag. Their transport pathways as well as their secretory release into the extracellular space of normal and thyroid carcinoma cell lines were studied with the help of activity based probes that were designed to distinguish between active and inactive cysteine peptidases within the endo-lysosomal compartments of mammalian cells [1,14,25,26]. The results of our investigations led us to conclude that protease trafficking is governed by the thyroid cell type investigated, i.e. transport resulting in polarized secretion is typical for normal, differentiated thyrocytes [1,27] whereas non-polarized transport pathways and non-directed secretion were observed in thyroid carcinoma cells. We therefore propose that cathepsin B transport to the basolateral plasma membrane domain and its secretion into the extrafollicular space as observed in follicular and papillary thyroid carcinoma tissues are features of altered trafficking routes in thyroid cancer.

## Methods

### Cell culture

Fisher rat thyroid (FRT) cells and the human thyroid carcinoma cell lines KTC-1, HTh7 and HTh74 were grown at 37°C and 5% $CO_2$ in a moisturized atmosphere. KTC-1 cells were cultured in RPMI-1640 (Biowhittaker™, Verviers, Belgium), and HTh7 and HTh74 cells in Eagle´s Minimum Essential Medium (Biowhittaker™), all supplemented with 10% fetal calf serum (FCS; PerBio, Aalst, Belgium). The FRT and KTC-1 cells analyzed for the secretion of cathepsin B were grown in Coons F-12 medium (Sigma-Aldrich, Taufkirchen, Germany) containing 2.68 mg/ml sodium bicarbonate and supplemented with 5% FCS. For KTC-1 cells, a mixture consisting of 0.166 mg/ml insulin, 2 μg/ml Gly-His-Lys complex, 0.362 μg/ml hydrocortisone, 0.5 μg/ml transferrin, 1 μg/ml somatostatin and 100 μU/ml TSH (final concentrations; all from Sigma-Aldrich) was added. Barrier function and tightness of the epithelial monolayer of the thyroid carcinoma cell lines grown on permeable filter supports (pore size 0.4 mm) of Transwell inserts (Corning Costar Co., Acton, MA, USA) was estimated by measuring the trans-epithelial electrical resistance with a Millicell ERS ohmmeter (Millipore, Bedford, MA, USA). The values were corrected for background resistance measured across filters without cells.

### Indirect immunofluorescence

KTC-1, HTh7 and HTh74 cells used for indirect immunofluorescence were cultured on cover slips in 6-well plates. The cells were fixed with 4% paraformaldehyde in 200 mM HEPES, pH 7.4, for 30 minutes at room temperature followed by washing 3 times 5 minutes with 200 mM HEPES (pH 7.4) and 3 times 5 minutes with calcium- and magnesium-free PBS (CMF-PBS), i.e. 0.15 M NaCl, 2.7 mM KCl, 1.5 mM $NaH_2PO4$, 8.1 mM $Na_2HPO4$, pH 7.4. Permeabilization was performed with 0.2% Triton X-100 in CMF-PBS for 5 minutes at room temperature. For blocking, 3% bovine serum albumin (BSA; Carl Roth GmbH, Karlsruhe, Germany) in CMF-PBS was used for 1 hour at 37°C. The cells were incubated with an anti-cathepsin B primary antibody (Neuromics, Hiddenhausen, Germany) diluted in 0.1% BSA in CMF-PBS overnight at 4°C. After washing with 0.1% BSA in CMF-PBS, the cells were incubated with Alexa 488-conjugated secondary antibodies (Molecular Probes, Karlsruhe, Germany) for 1 hour at 37°C together with 5 µM of the nuclear counter-stain DRAQ5™ (Biostatus Limited, Shepshed, Leicestershire, UK). After washing with CMF-PBS and de-ionized water, the cover slips were mounted with embedding medium consisting of 33% glycerol, 14% Mowiol in 200 mM Tris-HCl, pH 8.5 (Hoechst AG, Frankfurt, Germany) on microscopic slides. When the thyroid carcinoma cell lines were used for F-actin labelling, they were treated as described above, but instead of antibody immunolabelling, the cells were incubated with FITC-phalloidin (3 µM, Sigma-Aldrich) for 1 hour at 37°C.

Human thyroid tissue was obtained from patients undergoing thyroid surgery and used in compliance with the Helsinki Declaration. The tissue was fixed in paraformaldehyde, embedded in paraffin and sectioned as described [28]. The tissue sections mounted on microscopic slides were de-paraffinated by washing with xylol 4 times 5 minutes followed by 5 minute-washes with decreasing concentrations of ethanol (100% to 30%) and final incubation with freshly prepared sodium borohydride (1%; Carl Roth GmbH) to reduce auto-fluorescence, and de-ionized water for 5 minutes each. Haematoxylin and eosin (0.1%; Sigma-Aldrich) (H&E) staining was performed in order to examine tissue architecture. The protocol for indirect immunofluorescence was performed as described for the cell lines above with the following modifications. Blocking with 3% BSA was performed at 4°C overnight, the permeabilization step was omitted, and the tissue sections were incubated with the secondary fluorophore-conjugated antibody for 2 hours. In addition, DRAQ5™ was used at a concentration of 20 µM. Three tissue samples from each pathological condition, i.e. from papillary and follicular thyroid carcinomas, were prepared as described above and subjected to analysis.

The immunofluorescence samples were viewed with a confocal laser scanning microscope (LSM 510 Meta; Carl Zeiss Jena GmbH, Jena, Germany) and analyzed with the LSM 510 software, Release 3.2 (Carl Zeiss Jena GmbH).

#### Protein precipitation from conditioned media

Conditioned medium was collected from KTC-1 cells and proteins were precipitated with ice-cold trichloroacetic acid (TCA, 10%). The samples were incubated on ice for 30 minutes followed by centrifugation at 10 000 *g* for 10 minutes at 4°C. The supernatant was removed and centrifugation was repeated at the same speed and temperature for another 10 minutes. The remaining supernatant was removed and the pellet was dried in speed vacuum for 20 minutes and re-suspended in sample buffer consisting of 10 mM Tris-HCl (pH 7.6), 0.5% SDS, 25 mM DTT, 10% glycerol and 25 µg/ml bromophenol blue. The sample pH was adjusted using 1.5 M Tris-HCl at pH 8.8 (Carl Roth GmbH) before loading onto SDS-gels.

#### Labelling of active cysteine cathepsins with activity based probes

HTh74 cells cultured in 6-well plates on cover slips were washed with pre-warmed PBS, i.e. 0.9% NaCl, 20 mM $NaH_2PO_4$, pH 6.8, followed by incubation with Yellow-DCG-04 (1 µM) in serum-free growth medium for 30 minutes under standard culture conditions. Washing with PBS 3 times for 5 minutes was followed by a chase period of 1 hour with complete cell culture medium and another set of washes as described above. DRAQ5™ (5 µM) was used as nuclear counter-stain and was added to the medium for the last 10 minutes of the chase period. For live-cell imaging, the cover slips with cells were transferred onto metal slide devices filled with pre-warmed medium supplemented with 20 mM HEPES to maintain neutral pH conditions during microscopy, and analyzed through confocal laser scanning microscopy as described earlier.

Active cysteine cathepsins in FRT cells were visualized using a quenched activity based probe (GB117) [25]. Transfected cells were seeded on cover slips in 6-well plates and cultured until they reached 80-90% confluence. The cells were washed once with pre-warmed PBS followed by addition of DMEM without Phenol Red (Cambrex Bio Science, Wiesbaden, Germany) supplemented with 1 µM GB117 and culturing for 3 hours under normal conditions. The live-cell imaging was performed as described above.

#### SDS-PAGE and immunoblotting

Whole cell lysates of FRT cells transfected with pEGFP-N1 plasmid were obtained as follows: the cells were washed with ice cold PBS, detached with a cell scraper and collected through centrifugation for 10 minutes at 900 *g* and 4°C. The cells were resuspended in lysis buffer consisting of 20 mM $Na_2HPO_4$, 50 mM NaCl, 0.2% Triton X-100, pH 7.4, and supplemented with a protease-inhibitor-mix, i.e. 0.1 mM E64, 0.01 mM Pepstatin, 2 ng/ml Aprotinin, 0.02 M EDTA, followed by incubation for 30 minutes at 4°C on a end-over-end rotor. The supernatants were cleared through centrifugation for 15 minutes at 15 000 *g* and 4°C.

The Bradford assay [29] was used in order to determine the protein concentration of the samples. The proteins and a cathepsin B standard from bovine spleen (Sigma-Aldrich) were separated through SDS-PAGE on 12.5% polyacrylamide gels along with a PageRuler pre-stained protein ladder (Fermentas, St Leon-Rot, Germany) or a See Blue pre-stained standard (Novex, Frankfurt/Main, Germany), and transferred to a nitrocellulose membrane by semi-dry blotting. Unspecific binding sites were blocked with 5% non-fat milk in PBS containing 68 mM NaCl, 63.2 mM $Na_2HPO_4$, 11.7 mM $NaH_2PO_4$, pH 7.2, supplemented with 0.3% Tween (PBS-T) overnight at 4°C. Incubation with goat anti-mouse cathepsin B (Neuromics), rabbit anti-rat cathepsin B (Upstate Biotechnology, Lake Placid, NY, USA), rabbit anti-human cathepsin L (RD Laboratorien GmbH, Diessen, Germany) or rabbit anti-human β-tubulin (Abcam, Cambridge, UK) primary antibodies diluted in PBS-T was for 2 hours at room temperature followed by incubation with horseradish peroxidase-conjugated secondary antibodies (Southern Biotech, Birmingham, Al, USA) for 1 hour at room temperature. Incubation with the peroxidase substrate (ThermoScientific, Bonn, Germany) was followed by visualization through enhanced chemi-luminescence on XPosure films (ThermoScientific).

### Construction of the active site mutant cathepsin B-C29A-eGFP

Cathepsin B cDNA was derived from FRTL-5 cells, a Fisher rat thyroid cell line, as described previously [27]. For site directed mutagenesis and generation of pCathB-C29A-eGFP, the CathB 49-1068 forward primer [27] was combined with a newly designed primer CB-Cys29Ala reverse, 5' – AGA GCC ACA GGA GCC CTG GT – 3', giving rise to the amplification of the first 300 base pairs (bps) of the cathepsin B cDNA. The CB-Cys29Ala reverse primer was constructed such that a codon was changed from TGT to GCT, causing the exchange of cysteine to alanine at amino-acid position 29 of rat cathepsin B. Next, a second PCR reaction was performed using CB-Cys29Ala forward, 5' – GGC TCC TGT GGC TCT GCT TGG GCA TTT G – 3', in combination with the CathB 49-1068 reverse primer [27], giving rise to the last approximately 700 bps from the 3'-end of the *Ctsb* gene. Thereby, two mutations were caused, namely the already mentioned exchange from TGT to GCT (see above) and a 'silent' mutation (GGG to GGC), which would not alter the amino acid composition upon translation, but resulted in the omission of a restriction site for EcoO109I. Thus, the silent mutation allowed for better analysis of cloning success. In addition, the sequences of the primers were designed such that an EcoRI as well as a BamHI cleavage site were inserted at the 5'- and the 3'-ends of the cDNA, respectively, to allow for the insertion of the complete coding sequence of cathepsin B into the pEGFP-N1 vector after fusion PCR was performed as follows and as previously described [27]. The PCR products were separated on 1% agarose gels and the DNA was stained with ethidiumbromide. The 300-bps- and 700-bps-*Ctsb* fragments were cut out, purified from the gel and used as templates for a fusion PCR reaction. Here, the CathB 49-1068 primer pair [27] was used in order to amplify full-length cathepsin B cDNA bearing the above mentioned sequence mutations. This step was repeated and gained the cathepsin B-C29A-fragment with the correct size of 1019 bps, which was excised from the gel, purified and used for subsequent digestion with EcoRI and BamHI restriction enzymes and insertion into pEGFP-N1 as described [27]. The resulting plasmid is schematically illustrated in Figure 1A. Competent *E.coli* JM109 cells were transformed with re-ligated vectors in order to amplify the plasmids. Bacteria were grown using kanamycin as selection antibiotic, and resistant clones were checked for their plasmid content by colony-PCR using CathB 49-1068 forward and reverse primers. Plasmid-DNA was prepared from overnight cultures. Both plasmids were sent for sequencing to verify correct DNA sequences (see Figure 1B).

### Transfection of thyroid cells

Transfection of FRT, KTC-1, HTh7 and HTh74 cells with pEGFP-N1, pCathB-eGFP or pCathB-C29A-eGFP was carried out using jetPEIMan (Qbiogene, Heidelberg, Germany), a mannose-conjugated linear polyethylene imine, which is able to compact DNA into positively charged particles followed by binding of the jetPEI-Man-DNA complexes to cell surface mannose-specific receptors and internalization through endocytosis. FRT and human thyroid carcinoma cells were seeded in 6-well plates on cover slips and transfected at 50-60% confluence. Transfection was performed according to the manufacturers instructions and by mixing jetPEI-Man and plasmid DNA at N/P ratios of 5 based on N-residues of the transfection reagent (7.5 mM) as compared to anionic phosphate of the plasmid DNA (3 nM/μg). The transfected cells were cultured for 24 hours under normal cell culture conditions. On the following day, transfection medium was exchanged for normal medium. The transfected cells were either analyzed directly through live-cell imaging with a confocal laser scanning microscope as described above or, in case of pCathB-C29A-eGFP transfected FRT cells, they were subjected to antibiotic selection with G418 (Merck KGaA, Darmstadt, Germany).

## Results

### Localization of cathepsin B in human thyroid tissue

Human tissue obtained from patients affected by follicular thyroid carcinoma (FTC) or papillary thyroid carcinoma (PTC) was analyzed in order to determine the general tissue architecture and the localization of endogenous cathepsin B. Haematoxylin and eosin-stained

A

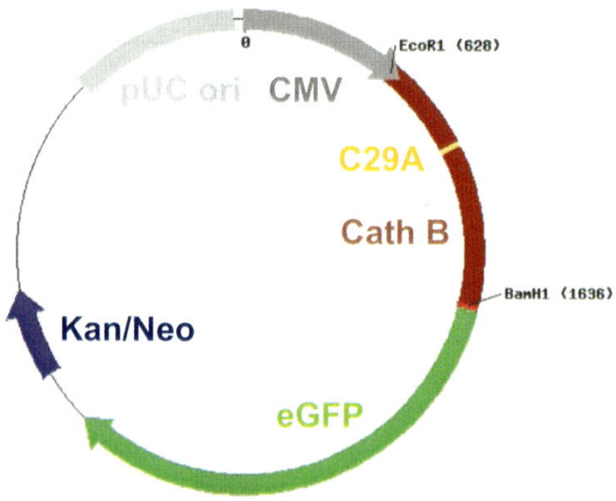


pCathB-C29A-eGFP (5710 bp)

B

```
pCathB-eGFP        GTCGTAACAACTCCGCCCCATTGACGCAAATGGGCGGTAGGCGTGTACGGTGGGAGGTCT
pCathB-C29A-eGFP                                                 TACGGTGGGAGGTCT

pCathB-eGFP        ATATAAGCAGAGCTGGTTTAGTGAACCGTCAGATCCGCTAGCGCTACCGGACTCAGATCT
pCathB-C29A-eGFP   ATATAAGCAGAGCTGGTTTAGTGAACCGTCAGATCCGCTAGCGCTACCGGACTCAGATCT

pCathB-eGFP        CGAGCTCAAGCTTCGAATTCCAGGATGTGGTGGTCCTTGATCCCTCTCTCTTGCCTGCTG
pCathB-C29A-eGFP   CGAGCTCAAGCTTCGAATTCCAGGATGTGGTGGTCCTTGATCCCTCTCTCTTGCCTGCTG

pCathB-eGFP        GCACTGACCAGTGCCCATGACAAGCCTTCCTTTCACCCACTGTCGGACGACATGATTAAC
pCathB-C29A-eGFP   GCACTGACCAGTGCCCATGACAAGCCTTCCTTTCACCCACTGTCGGACGACATGATTAAC

pCathB-eGFP        TATATCAACAAACAGAATACAACATGGCAGGCTGGACGCAACTTCTACAATGTTGACATA
pCathB-C29A-eGFP   TATATCAACAAACAGAATACAACATGGCAGGCTGGACGCAACTTCTACAATGTTGACATA

pCathB-eGFP        AGCTATCTGAAGAAGCTGTGTGGAACTGTCCTGGGTGGACCCAAGCTGCCGGAAAGGGTT
pCathB-C29A-eGFP   AGCTATCTGAAGAAGCTGTGTGGAACTGTCCTGGGTGGACCCAAGCTGCCGGAAAGGGTT

pCathB-eGFP        GGGTTCAGCGAGGACATAAATCTACCTGAATCCTTTGATGCACGGGAACAGTGGTCCAAT
pCathB-C29A-eGFP   GGGTTCAGCGAGGACATAAATCTACCTGAATCCTTTGATGCACGGGAACAGTGGTCCAAT

pCathB-eGFP        TGCCCGACCATCGCACAGATCAGAGACCAGGGGTCCTGTGGCTCTTGTTGGGCATTTGGG
pCathB-C29A-eGFP   TGCCCGACCATCGCACAGATCAGAGACCAGGGCTCCTGTGGCTCTGCTTGGGCATTTGGG

pCathB-eGFP        GCAGTGGAAGCCATGTCTGACCGAATCTGCATTCACACCAATGGCCGAGTCAATGTGGAG
pCathB-C29A-eGFP   GCAGTGGAAGCCATGTCTGACCGAATCTGCATTCACACCAATGGCCGAGTCAATGTGGAG

pCathB-eGFP        GTGTCTGCTGAGGACCTGCTTACCTGCTGTGGTATCCAGTGTGGGGATGGCTGTAATGGT
pCathB-C29A-eGFP   GTGTCTGCTGAGGACCTGCTTACCTGCTGTGGTATCCAGTGTGGGGATGGCTGTAATGGT

pCathB-eGFP        GGCTATCCCTCTGGAGCATGGAACTTCTGGACTAGAAAAGGCCTGGTTTCTGGTGGAGTA
pCathB-C29A-eGFP   GGCTATCCCTCTGGAGCATGGAACTTCTGGACTAGAAAAGGCCTGGTTTCTGGTGGAGTA

pCathB-eGFP        TACAATTCTCATATAGGCTGCTTACCCTACACCATCCCTCCCTGTGAACACCATGTCAAT
pCathB-C29A-eGFP   TACAATTCTCATATAGGCTGCTTACCCTACACCATCCCTCCCTGTGAACACCATGTCAAT

pCathB-eGFP        GGCTCCCGTCCCCCATGCACTGGAGAAGGAGATACTCCCAAGTGCAACAAGATGTGTGAG
pCathB-C29A-eGFP   GGCTCCCGTCCCCCATGCACTGGAGAAGGAGATACTCCCAAGTGCAACAAGATGTGTGAG

pCathB-eGFP        GCTGGCTACTCCACATCCTACAAGGAAGATAAGCACTATGGGTACACTTCCTACAGTGTG
pCathB-C29A-eGFP   GCTGGCTACTCCACATCCTACAAGGAAGATAAGCACTATGGGTACACTTCCTACAGTGTG

pCathB-eGFP        TCTGACAGCGAGAAGGAGATCATGGCGGAAATCTACAAAAATGGCCCAGTGGAGGGTGCT
pCathB-C29A-eGFP   TCTGACAGCGAGAAGGAGATCATGGCGGAAATCTACAAAAATGGCCCAGTGGAGGGTGCT

pCathB-eGFP        TTTACTGTGTTTTCTGACTTCTTGACTTACAAATCAGGCGTATACAAGCATGAAGCCGGT
pCathB-C29A-eGFP   TTTACTGTGTTTTCTGACTTCTTGACTTACAAATCAGGCGTATACAAGCATGAAGCCGGT

pCathB-eGFP        GATGTGATGGGAGGCCATGCCATCCGCATTCTGGGCTGGGGAATAGAGAATGGAGTACCC
pCathB-C29A-eGFP   GATGTGATGGGAGGCCATGCCATCCGCATTCTGGGCTGGGGAATAGAGAATGGAGTACCC

pCathB-eGFP        TACTGGCTGGTAGCAAACTCCTGGAACGTTGACTGGGGTGATAATGGTTTCTTTAAAATC
pCathB-C29A-eGFP   TACTGGCTGGTAGCAAACTCCTGGAACGTTGACTGGGGTGATAATGGTTTCTTTAAAATC
```

**Figure 1 Schematic depiction and sequence of pCathB-C29A-eGFP coding for inactive cathepsin B-eGFP chimeras.** Schematic representation (A) and nucleotide sequence (B) of the mammalian expression vector pCathB-C29A-eGFP that codes for eGFP-tagged cathepsin B containing a cysteine-to-alanine substitution in its active site (yellow) which was introduced by site-directed mutagenesis of the cathepsin B coding sequence inserted into pEGFP-N1 by using EcoR1 and BamH1 restriction sites. The plasmid bears a CMV promotor (dark grey) as well as an origin of replication (pUC ori, light gray). The eGFP coding sequence (green) is located down-stream of the cathepsin B encoding DNA minus the nucleotides encoding the C-terminal pro-peptide extension of the enzyme. In the resulting chimeric protein, cathepsin B will be fused to eGFP by a 6-amino-acids linker peptide (light red). The sequences of pCathB-eGFP [27] and the active-site mutant pCathB-C29A-eGFP were aligned by means of ClustalW (version 1.82) multi alignment tool. The sequences are identical, except for the point mutations inserted through site-directed mutagenesis, and resulting in a GGG to GGC 'silent' mutation (red), as well as a TGT to GCT codon exchange (orange), causing a cysteine to alanine exchange within the active-site of cathepsin B.

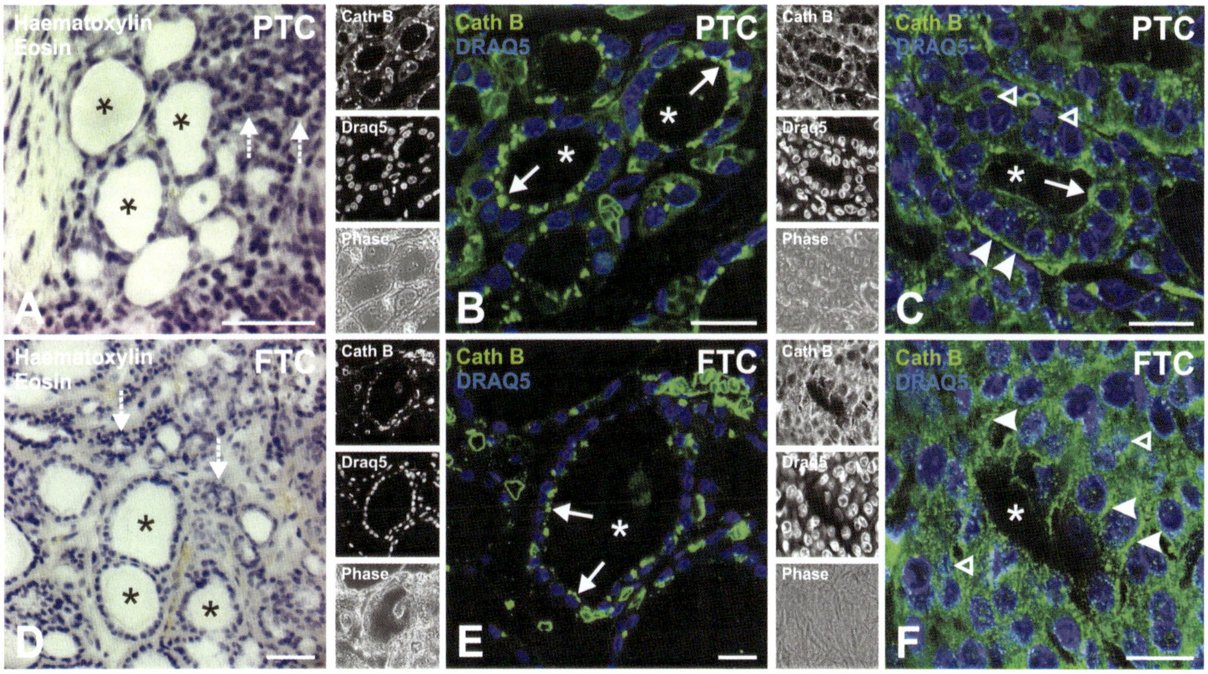


**Figure 2 Tissue architecture and distribution of cathepsin B in thyroid carcinoma *in situ*.** Micrographs of haematoxylin and eosin stained tissue of thyroid tissue derived from patients with papillary (A) and follicular (D) thyroid carcinoma (PTC and FTC, respectively) was inspected by brightfield microscopy. PTC tissue displayed areas with intact follicle structures (A) as well as areas with a disorganized tissue structure (A, dashed arrows). In addition, PTC tissue displayed fibrovascular cores (A). FTC tissue also displayed areas with intact follicle structures as well as areas with a disorganized tissue structure (D, dashed arrows). Merged (B, C, E, F), single channel fluorescence and corresponding phase contrast micrographs (left panels) taken with the confocal laser scanning microscope of thyroid tissue from patients with PTC or FTC showing the endogenous distribution of cathepsin B (green, left panels, top). The nuclei were visualized through DRAQ5™ counter-staining (blue, left panels, middle). Note that cathepsin B was localized to vesicles close to the apical plasma membrane (arrows) in non-neoplastic areas of thyroid carcinoma tissue (B and E, respectively). Cathepsin B distribution was different in the disorganized, neoplastic areas of thyroid carcinoma tissue (C and F). The protease was immunolocalized to vesicles scattered in the cell periphery along the basal and lateral plasma membrane domains as well as scattered throughout the cytosol (C and F, arrowheads). Nuclei of cells in neoplastic areas displayed an abnormal morphology (C and F, open arrowheads). Follicle lumina are denoted by asterisks. Scale bars represent 50 μm in A and D, and 20 μm in B, C, E, and F.

PTC tissue displayed normal thyroid histomorphology with variably sized follicles and colloid-containing lumina that were enclosed by a monolayer of epithelial cells (Figure 2A, follicle lumina denoted with asterisks). In addition, papillary stalks and disorganized neoplastic areas lacking clear follicular structures were abundantly detected in PTC-derived tissue (Figure 2A, dashed arrows). Heterogenous histomorphology was also detectable in haematoxylin and eosin-stained FTC-derived tissue that demonstrated both intact follicles (Figure 2D, follicle lumina denoted with asterisks), microfollicles and disorganized neoplastic areas (Figure 2D, dashed arrows). Cathepsin B was shown by immunostaining to be localized within vesicular structures located close to the apical plasma membrane in the non-altered areas of thyroid carcinoma tissue (Figure 2B and E, arrows). In the areas with altered morphology of the same tissue, however, cathepsin B-positive vesicles were detected only occasionally at the plasma membrane and appeared distributed throughout the cytosol of thyroid follicle cells (Figure 2C and F, arrowheads) that were further characterized by abnormal nuclear morphology and by less polarized states than thyroid cells in normal tissue areas (Figure 2C and F, open arrowheads). In addition, cathepsin B-containing vesicles were localized to the basolateral poles as highlighted by immunostaining of the basal plasma membrane domains of neoplastic cells in PTC (Figure 2C, arrowheads) and of the lateral plasma membrane domains in FTC tissue (Figure 2F, arrowheads), indicating non-directed cathepsin B secretion into the extrafollicular space.

This change in cathepsin B distribution from a prominent apical localization in normal to a basolateral localization in neoplastic areas is therefore not a feature of PTC alone [20], but also observed in FTC. This notion made us to hypothesize that protease trafficking is dramatically altered in thyroid carcinoma, which led us to analyze cathepsin B transport pathways in more detail in different thyroid carcinoma cell lines that are known to exhibit at least some features of differentiated thyrocytes although being transformed and representative of papillary and anaplastic thyroid carcinoma cells. Trafficking of cathepsin B in normal thyroid epithelial cells that are fully differentiated and exhibit a polarized phenotype, i.e. FRT cells, was studied for comparison.

**KTC-1, HTh7 and HTh74 as model cell lines to study cathepsin B trafficking in thyroid carcinoma**

Thyroid carcinoma cells of variable aggressiveness differ in the degree of differentiation and polarization [30,31]. In this study, we have used the papillary thyroid carcinoma cell line KTC-1 as well as the anaplastic thyroid carcinoma cell lines HTh7 and HTh74 [22,23].

KTC-1 and HTh74 cells displayed prominent stress fibers running throughout the cytosol when F-actin was stained with FITC-phalloidin (Figure 3A and C, arrows), whereas HTh7 cells have lost the ability to tightly adhere to the substratum and lacked actin stress fibers (Figure 3B). Thus, KTC-1 and HTh74 cells in particular were polarized and should therefore, in principle, have the ability to establish and maintain an epithelial monolayer, which was analyzed by determination of the trans-epithelial electrical resistance (TER) as a measure of monolayer tightness [32]. KTC-1 cells indeed formed a confluent monolayer but displayed a low TER of 500 $\pm$ 100 $\Omega$ x cm$^2$. In contrast, HTh7 and HTh74 cells were able to hyper-proliferate in culture, thereby forming mono- and multi-layers which were not tight since no TER was measurable. Therefore, KTC-1 cells must be considered to maintain contact-inhibition to some extent, which was clearly lost in HTh74 cells despite their ability to adhere to the substratum in a polarized fashion. In addition, adherens and tight junction proteins such as E-cadherin, claudin-1 and occludin have been detected at the lateral plasma membrane domains of KTC-1 cells (our own unpublished observations; KBr, Laura Panavaite, ST, all Bremen), thus further supporting maintenance of epithelial polarity to some extent in this cell line.

Because of the morphological and functional appearance of KTC-1 cells as well as due to the lack of contact-inhibition in hyper-proliferative HTh7 and HTh74 cells, we considered these cell lines suitable to represent distinct stages in epithelial-to-mesenchymal transition

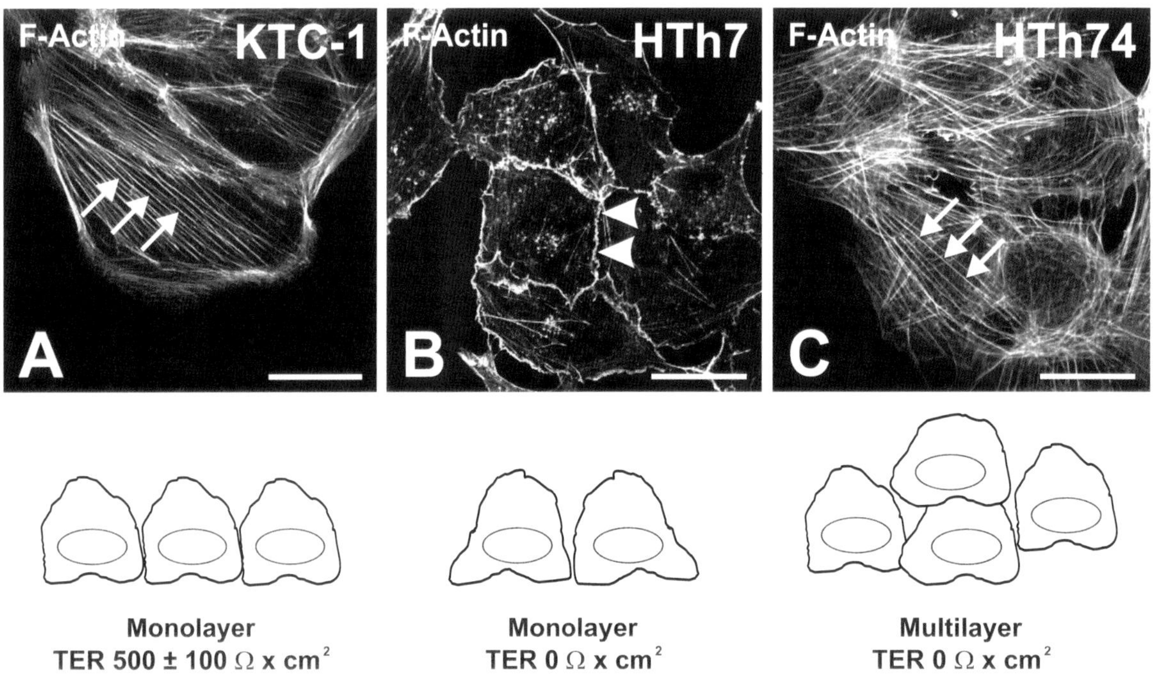


**Figure 3 Thyroid carcinoma cell lines as model systems.** Fluorescence micrographs of the papillary thyroid carcinoma cell line KTC-1 (A) and the anaplastic thyroid carcinoma cell lines HTh7 and HTh74 (B and C, respectively) taken with the confocal laser scanning microscope after fixation and phalloidin staining of the F-actin cytoskeleton. KTC-1 and HTh74 cells displayed stress fibers throughout the cytosol (A and C, arrows) as well as cortical F-actin underneath the plasma membranes. In HTh7 cells stress fibers were largely lacking (B) but cortical F-actin was displayed (B, arrowheads). KTC-1 cells grew in a monolayer fashion and established only a weak barrier as estimated by determination of the trans-epithelial electrical resistance (TER), whereas HTh7 cells formed non-tight monolayers and HTh74 cells grew in multilayers. Scale bars represent 20 μm.

with HTh7 cells being the most progressed toward the mesenchymal phenotype, but HTh74 cells being the most transformed with respect to proliferation and loss of contact inhibition.

**Cathepsin B is secreted from KTC-1 cells**

We have previously shown that cathepsin B is one of the main if not the major cysteine peptidase active in KTC-1, HTh7 or HTh74 cells, and that its predominant expression pattern is vesicular in these thyroid carcinoma cell lines [21]. In this study, we were interested in the investigation of the 3-dimensional distribution of cathepsin B-containing vesicles through optical sectioning by means of confocal laser scanning microscopy in order to approach determination of the transport pathways of the endogenous protease before analyzing trafficking of GFP-tagged chimeras of active and inactive cathepsin B.

Optical sections (xy) were taken at different focal planes of cultured KTC-1 cells in z-direction, i.e. perpendicular to the cellular poles attaching to the substratum. Cathepsin B was detected by immunofluorescence staining within reticular structures and vesicles gathering in the peri-nuclear region (Figure 4A1-A3, arrows) and in a dotted pattern (Figure 4A1-A3, B, D, arrowheads). When the sections of an entire z-stack were compiled and reconstructed in xz, i.e. displayed as side view as schematically indicated in 4C, it became evident that cathepsin B-positive structures were localized in a dotted fashion in close proximity to the cell periphery (Figure 4B and D, arrowheads). This close proximity to the cell surfaces is most probably an indication of cathepsin B being released either towards the apical pole (representative of into the follicle lumen) or towards the basal side (representative of towards the extrafollicular space) and its subsequent re-association with the plasma membrane of KTC-1 cells.

Therefore, we next analyzed the media conditioned by KTC-1 cell cultures for possible occurrence of secreted forms of cathepsin B. In fact, KTC-1 cells were able to secrete mature, proteolytically active cathepsin B, because both, the single chain (SC) and the heavy chain (HC) of the two-chain form of cathepsin B were detectable in the conditioned media (Figure 4E). The levels of both, single and heavy chain cathepsin B increased steadily over time, indicating constant secretion of mature forms of cathepsin B from KTC-1 cells.

**Visualization of active cysteine cathepsins in HTh74 cells**

In order to visualize active cysteine cathepsins in thyroid carcinoma cell lines, we used the activity based probe DCG-04 that binds covalently to active cysteine peptidases in a 1:1 ratio [26]. In HTh74 cells, proteolytically active cysteine peptidases were shown to be distributed throughout the cells in vesicles of various sizes (Figure 5A1-A3 and B, arrows). In addition, active cysteine peptidases were labeled with DCG-04 in differently sized aggregates that were localized in the extracellular space at both poles in between cells throughout the multilayered cultures (Figure 5D, arrowheads). In particular, large DCG-04 positive cysteine peptidase-containing aggregates were found abundantly in association with the surfaces of HTh74 cells of the different layers (Figure 5B and D, arrowheads, schematically depicted in C). It was taken special care to wash the DCG-04 treated cells thoroughly before microscopy to avoid that aggregates would increase in size artificially during mounting for live-cell microscopy. Because the aggregates were visible in all focal planes above, in between, and below the multi-layers of HTh74 cultures (Figure 5D, green signals) and since they were not co-stained with DRAQ5™, we considered these structures as resulting from secretion of active cysteine peptidases rather than being derived from dead cells.

**Construction of a cathepsin B-C29A-eGFP coding vector**

For *in vivo* analyses of cathepsin B-trafficking, vectors coding for different eGFP chimeras were used. As a control for normal trafficking of cathepsin B, the cDNA for cathepsin B from FRTL-5 cells, was cloned into the pEGFP-N1 vector [27]. To test whether the proteolytic activity of cathepsin B would affect its transport to distinct compartments, i.e. whether intrinsic sorting signals of the active enzyme would be a prerequisite of proper trafficking, the cDNA sequence coding for rat cathepsin B was altered by site-directed mutagenesis. The modified cDNA was cloned into pEGFP-N1, thereby constructing a vector coding for an inactive cathepsin B-C29A-eGFP chimera (Figure 1A).

The sequences of the inserted DNA for pCathB-eGFP and pCathB-C29A-eGFP revealed identical nucleotide sequences coding for cathepsin B, except the specifically inserted mutations, i.e. the codon exchange at position 421-423 for the cysteine to alanine exchange (Figure 1B, sequence 1) as well as a restriction site omission at position 406-408. The so-called C-terminal extension of cathepsin B, normally at amino acid positions 334-339, which is not needed for protease function [33] was lacking in both constructs, because both were linked to the eGFP portion by a 6-amino-acid spacer peptide instead.

**Expression of eGFP-tagged active and inactive cathepsin B in rat thyroid cells**

FRT cells, a thyroid epithelial cell line derived from Fisher rats, form monolayers with tight and adhesive junctions separating apical and basolateral plasma membrane domains from each other. Therefore, they are an excellent model system to study the morphological

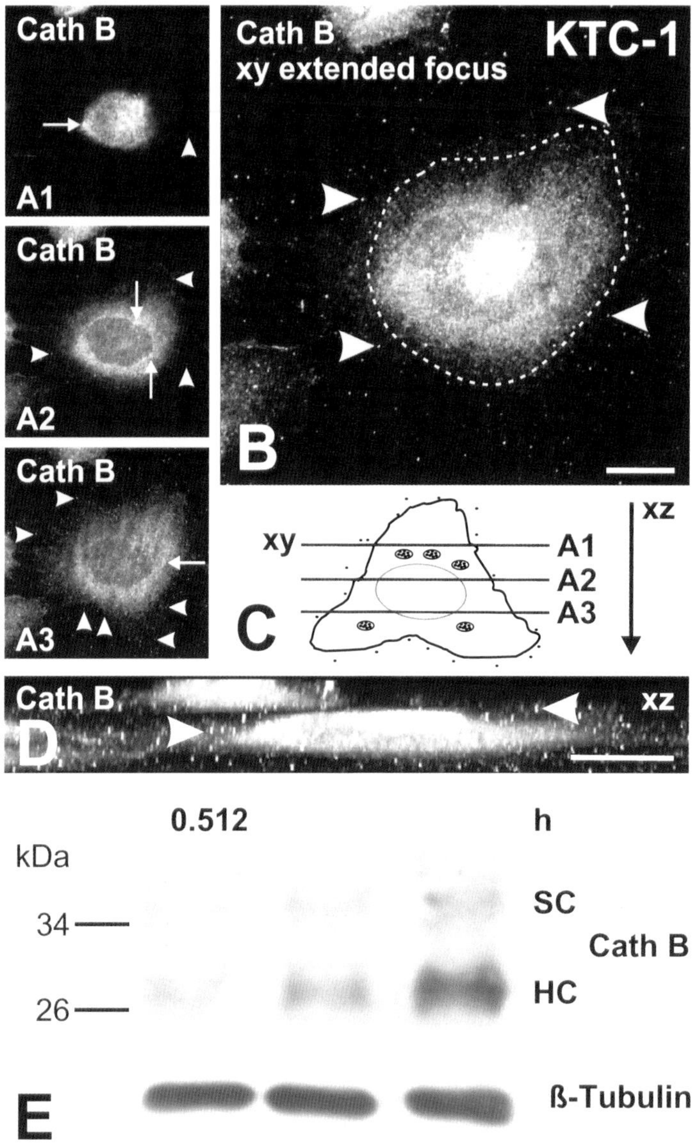


**Figure 4 Secretion of endogenous cathepsin B from KTC-1 cells.** Single channel fluorescence micrographs of cathepsin B localization in KTC-1 cells as detected by immunolabelling and confocal laser scanning microscopy (A, B, D). Three-dimensional distribution of cathepsin B representative signals is sketched in C. Single optical sections taken in xy were obtained in different focal planes (A1-A3, cf. lines in C) and compiled in a zero-projection as an extended focus (B) as well as in xz-direction as a side view (D). Cathepsin B displayed a reticular and vesicular staining pattern throughout the cell, and it appeared extracellularly in a dotted fashion due to its re-association with the plasma membrane (A-D, arrowheads). Note that cathepsin B secretion was non-directional. The dashed line in B denotes the cell circumference. Scale bars represent 10 μm. (E) TCA-precipitated and SDS-PAGE separated proteins from conditioned media of KTC-1 cells were immunoblotted with anti-cathepsin B antibodies. Note the presence of mature forms of cathepsin B, i.e. single chain (SC) and heavy chain (HC) cathepsin B in conditioned media and their increasing amounts with time. Immunoblotting of beta-tubulin in the corresponding whole cell lysates were used as loading controls.

properties of thyrocytes, which are highly polarized *in situ*[27,34]. FRT cells were transfected with pCathB-eGFP and pCathB-C29A-eGFP by means of jetPEI-Man. The expression of cathepsin B-eGFP as well as of the active-site mutant cathepsin B-C29A-eGFP showed prominent signals of the chimeric proteins within numerous vesicles that were reminiscent of endo-lysosomal compartments because of their accumulation within the peri-nuclear regions of FRT cells (Figure 6A and B, arrows). Importantly, the cathepsin B-eGFP chimeric protein has been shown not to be over-expressed in these cells [27]. Hence, in normal rat thyroid epithelial

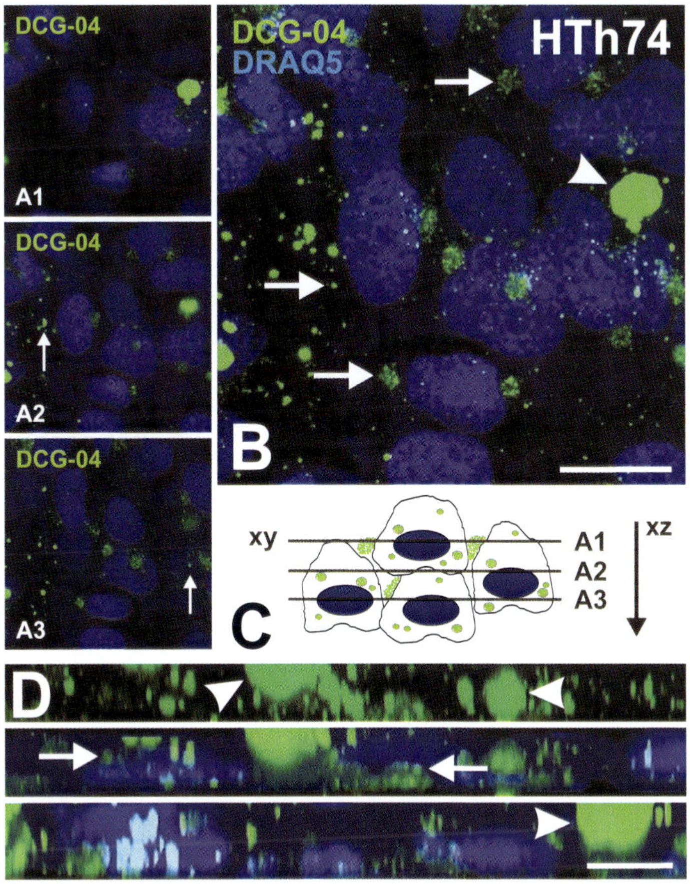


**Figure 5 Visualization of active cysteine cathepsins in HTh74 cell cultures.** Merged fluorescence micrographs of HTh74 cells growing in multilayers as detected after incubation with the fluorophore-conjugated activity based probe DCG-04 (green signals), counter-staining of nuclear DNA with DRAQ5™ (blue signals), and confocal laser scanning microscopy (A, B, D). The activity based probe DCG-04 binds to the active site of mature cysteine peptidases in a 1:1 ratio and visualizes proteolytically active cysteine proteases, only. Three-dimensional distribution of cysteine peptidase representative signals is sketched in C. Single optical sections taken in xy were obtained in different focal planes (A1-A3, cf. lines in C) and compiled in a zero-projection as an extended focus (B) as well as in xz-direction as a side view (D). Active cysteine peptidases were localized to variably sized vesicles throughout the cell (arrows). In addition, active cysteine peptidases were secreted from HTh74 cells and associated in aggregates with the plasma membrane (arrowheads). Note that active cysteine peptidases were secreted in a non-directional fashion at all poles of HTh74 thyroid carcinoma cells (D, arrowheads). Scale bars represent 10 μm.

cells, eGFP-tagged cathepsin B and its active-site mutant were destined to endo-lysosomes, thereby ruling out that the active site mutation affected the structure and folding of cathepsin B in such a way that it would induce major alterations in its cellular transport pathways.

However, by eGFP-tagging alone it could not be determined whether identical vesicles contained both, the active protease cathepsin B (or any other active cysteine cathepsin) and its inactive counterpart cathepsin B-C29A-eGFP. Therefore and in order to directly visualize active cysteine cathepsins versus inactive cathepsin B, pCathB-C29A-eGFP-transfected FRT cells were additionally labeled with activity based probes as reporters of proteolytic activity of cysteine peptidases. In this case we used GB117, a quenched Activity Based Probe (qABP) that reacts primarily with the active forms of cysteine cathepsins B, L, and S [25]. The big advantage of using a qABP is that it contains a fluorescence donor- and a quencher group keeping it non-fluorescent before binding to and reacting with an active cysteine peptidase [6,25]. Upon covalent attachment of the qABP by reacting with the active-site residues of an active protease molecule, the quencher is released and fluorescence is exhibited. Hence, GB117 provides a tool to analyze whether inactive cathepsin B-C29A-eGFP is transported to vesicles that also contain active proteases, or, instead, whether the active site mutant counter-part of cathepsin B displayed sorting signals that would enable transport to a different vesicle population which would not contain any active cysteine proteases.

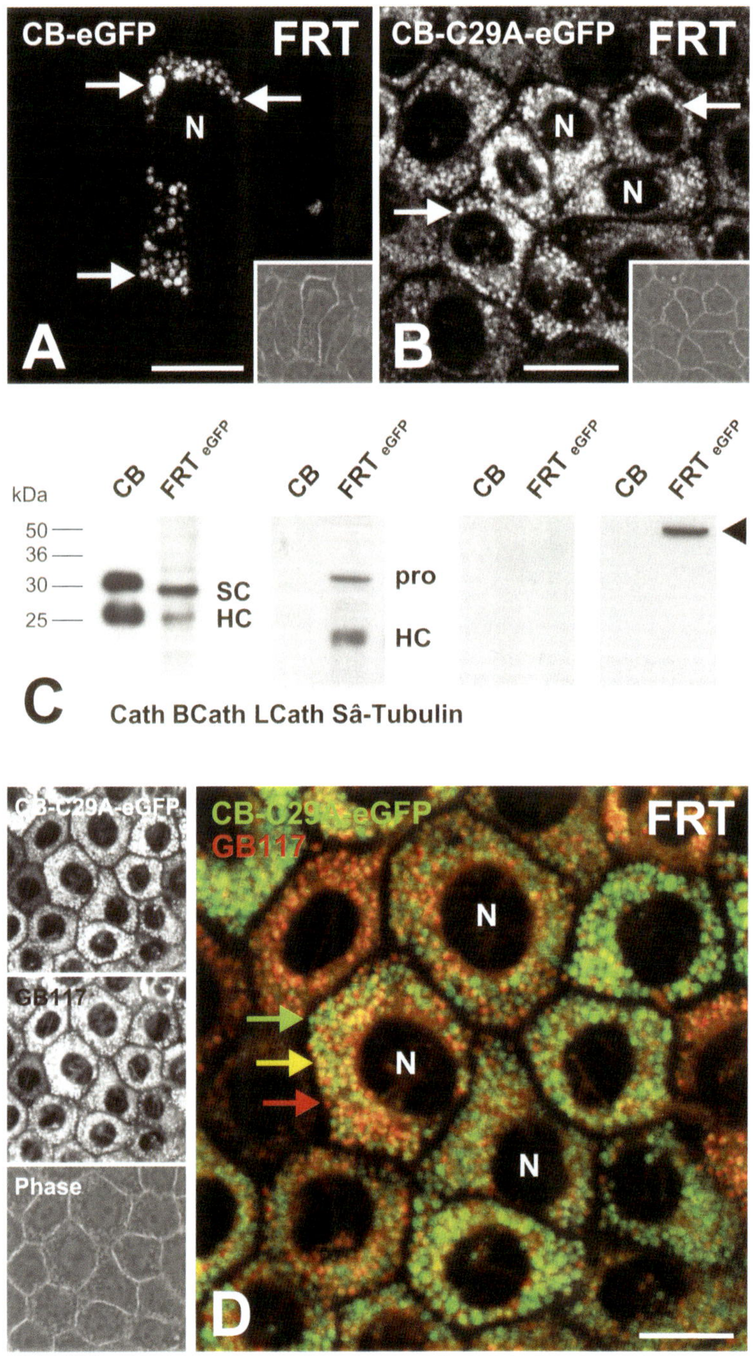


**Figure 6 Expression of cathepsin B-eGFP and cathepsin B-C29A-eGFP chimeras in normal thyroid epithelial cells.** Single channel fluorescence (A and B, left panels in D), merged (D) and corresponding phase contrast micrographs (insets in A and B, left panel, bottom, in D) taken with the confocal laser scanning microscope of FRT cells after transfection with plasmids coding for eGFP-tagged active (A) and inactive cathepsin B (B and D) as indicated. The expression pattern of both chimeric proteins was vesicular in FRT cells (arrows in A and B, green signals in D). The endogenous levels of mature cathepsins B, L and S (SC – single chain, HC – heavy chain) were estimated through immunoblotting and densitometry analysis and the cathepsins B:L:S ratio was shown to be 7:3:0 (C). The cathepsin levels were normalized against β-tubulin (C, arrowhead) that was used as a control for equal loading. The quenched activity based probe GB117 became fluorescent upon reaction with active cysteine peptidases and exhibited a vesicular staining indicative of active cysteine cathepsins in endo-lysosomal compartments (red signals in D). Note that the inactive cathepsin B-C29A-eGFP protein was localized within the same (yellow signals) or different vesicles (green signals) of normal rat thyroid epithelial cells (D), ruling out the existence of sorting signals intrinsic in cathepsin B's primary structure. N denotes nuclei. Scale bars represent 20 μm.

However, since GB117 has been shown to have a relative selectivity for cathepsin L over cathepsins B and S [25], we analyzed the amounts of these three cathepsins in whole cell fractions of FRT cells transfected with pEGFP-N1 vectors, i.e. lacking the cDNA coding for active or inactive cathepsin B, by immunoblotting. The amounts of mature cathepsin B (single chain plus heavy chain normalized to ß-tubulin) exceeded those of cathepsin L by more than 2-fold while cathepsin S was not detectable at all (Figure 6C). We can therefore conclude that GB117 evoked signals in FRT cells would derive primarily from its interaction with cathepsin B.

Next, cathepsin B-C29A-eGFP expressing FRT cells were analyzed by live-cell imaging after incubation with GB117 for 3 hours at normal cell culture conditions. The labelling of active cysteine peptidases with GB117 in FRT cells expressing inactive cathepsin B-eGFP chimeras resulted in a vesicular staining pattern, indicative for the presence of active cysteine proteases in endo-lysosomal compartments (Figure 6D, red signals). Furthermore, the GB117-labeled molecules co-localized with cathepsin B-C29A-eGFP chimeras within these vesicular structures, as was obvious from the yellow signals resulting from overlapping of red and green signals (Figure 6D, yellow signals). However, some vesicles were positive for cathepsin B-C29A-eGFP but lacked the signal for GB117 (Figure 6D, green signals). Thus, eGFP-tagging of the inactive cathepsin B mutant form as well as qABP-tagging of active cysteine proteases resulted in the notion that most endosomes and lysosomes of normal, polarized thyroid epithelial cells contained mixtures of active and inactive cysteine proteases thereby ruling out that active and inactive cathepsin B were sorted into distinct vesicle populations. These results indicated that sorting signals are unlikely to exist in the vicinity of the active site cleft of cathepsin B.

#### Localization of active and inactive cathepsin B fused to eGFP in thyroid carcinoma cell lines

Next, we were interested to determine whether cathepsin B trafficking is altered in thyroid carcinoma cells in comparison to normal thyroid epithelial cells. The active cathepsin B-eGFP chimeric protein was localized to vesicular structures in KTC-1 and HTh74 cells (Figure 7A and C), i.e. in a similar distribution pattern as that observed for endogenous cathepsin B. Thus, cathepsin B-eGFP is likely following the same transport pathway as endogenous cathepsin B. HTh7 cells, on the other hand, displayed an accumulation of CB-eGFP in the endoplasmic reticulum (ER) and was retained even more prominent in the Golgi apparatus (Figure 7B). This localization pointed to a transport defect of this thyroid carcinoma cell line, because the cathepsin B pattern observed by expression of the GFP-tagged protease was reminiscent to the predominant reticular staining pattern with only few vesicular structures that were immunolabeled in KTC-1 cells with cathepsin B-specific antibodies (see, Figure 4).

When the inactive cathepsin B-C29A-eGFP chimeras were expressed in KTC-1 and HTh7 cells, the green fluorescence was abundant in the endoplasmic reticulum (Figure 7D and E, arrowheads) but mostly absent from endo-lysosomes. In contrast, HTh74 cells expressing the inactive cathepsin B-C29A-eGFP chimeric protein still displayed a vesicular staining pattern resembling the peri-nuclear pattern of endo-lysosomal compartments (Figure 7F).

### Discussion

Cathepsin B processes thyroglobulin under physiological conditions in the extracellular follicle lumen as well as in endo-lysosomal compartments which is followed by the release of thyroid hormones from the thyroid gland [15-17]. Hence, transport of cathepsin B to the apical plasma membrane domain of normal thyroid epithelial cells is a prerequisite for its TSH-stimulated secretion into the follicle lumen in order to maintain thyroid homeostasis [19]. In pathological conditions, however, such as papillary thyroid carcinoma, cathepsin B has been localized to the basement membrane [20]. Here we provide evidence that such re-routing of cathepsin B transport from apical-to-basolateral poles is a hallmark also of neoplastic cells in FTC (see Figure 2). Therefore, we propose that cathepsin B transport towards basal poles is characteristic for cells in both, papillary and follicular thyroid carcinoma, whereas an apical-directed transport that is characteristic for thyrocytes of normal thyroid tissue, is also still displayed in cells of PTC and FTC-derived tissue areas with intact follicle structures. This notion motivated us to analyze the pathways resulting in altered cathepsin B trafficking and leading to its secretion into the extrafollicular space, which most probably enhances the invasive potential of thyroid carcinoma cells due to cathepsin B's ability to degrade ECM components [1,10-12,35,36].

The data achieved by 3-dimensional immunolocalization of endogenous cathepsin B and experiments employing activity based probes indicated that the thyroid carcinoma cell lines investigated in this study were characterized by cathepsin B trafficking that is destined to endo-lysosomes and, in addition, that cathepsin B is secreted into the extracellular space in a proteolytically active form (see Figures 4 and 5). Moreover, secretion of cathepsin B and related cysteine peptidases from KTC-1 and HTh74 cells was non-directed. We conclude that active cysteine peptidases are likely to reach extrafollicular locations in thyroid carcinoma tissue.

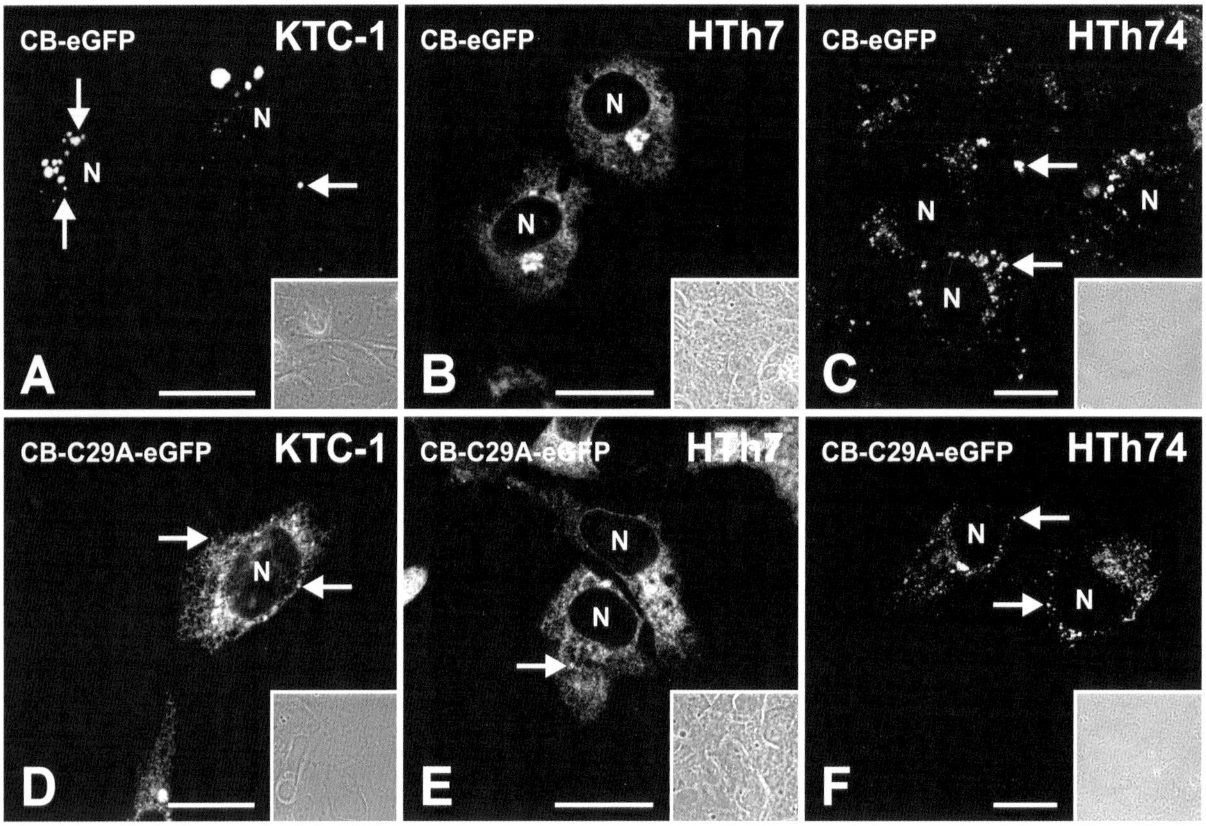


**Figure 7 Expression of cathepsin B-eGFP and cathepsin B-C29A-eGFP chimeras in thyroid carcinoma cells.** Single channel fluorescence (A-F) and corresponding phase contrast micrographs (insets) taken with the confocal laser scanning microscope of KTC-1 (A and D), HTh7 (B and E) and HTh74 cells (C and F) after transfection with plasmids coding for eGFP-tagged active (A-C) and inactive cathepsin B (D-F) as indicated. The localization of the eGFP-tagged cathepsin B was vesicular in KTC-1 and HTh74 cells (A and C, arrows), whereas it was retained in the Golgi of HTh7 cells (B). In contrast, the eGFP-tagged active site mutant counter-part of cathepin B was localized within reticular structures, the Golgi apparatus and a few vesicles (arrows) of KTC-1 (D) and HTh7 cells (E), while it was mainly localized to vesicles of HTh74 cells (F), indicating that the inactive mutant form of cathepsin B is transport-competent in principle. N denotes nuclei. Scale bars represent 10 μm.

From the trafficking studies with GFP-tagged chimeras, it can be deduced that the active site mutant of cathepsin B, which is transport competent and reaches endo-lysosomes of FRT and HTh74 cells, is retained in the endoplasmic reticulum of KTC-1 and HTh7 cells (see Figures 6 and 7). Furthermore, eGFP-tagged wild type cathepsin B was retained in the Golgi of HTh7 cells. Hence, trafficking of cathepsin B is largely independent of signals intrinsic in the primary structure of the protease, rather transport pathways differ in the thyroid cell lines tested with trafficking defects being more prominent in the thyroid carcinoma cell lines KTC-1 and HTh7, while HTh74 cells remained transport competent and sorted cathepsin B into endo-lysosomes. This is likely to be the prerequisite for the massive secretion of cysteine peptidases like cathepsin B into the extracellular space of HTh74 cell cultures (see Figure 5) and it is likely to explain, why this cell line in particular has lost its contact inhibition and acquired an invasive phenotype.

### Protease transport in mammalian cells

The molecular mechanisms underlying protease trafficking to their points-of-action have been studied in a variety of tissues and cell types [6,27,37-39]. However, the transport of proteases in mammalian cells is still not fully understood up until today [1]. Cysteine cathepsins, i.e. endo-lysosomal proteases that may also act extracellularly, are synthesized as inactive pre-pro-enzymes at the rough ER (rER). There, the signal peptide is cleaved-off co-translationally. In the oxidizing milieu of the ER lumen, disulfide bridges are formed with the help of protein disulfide isomerase (PDI), an ER-resident enzyme, assisting in the correct folding of the proteins. Further, N-glycosylation of the synthesized proteases may be performed upon recognition of an Asn-X-Ser/

Thr-Y motif (amino-acids given in three-letter code, with 'X' indicating any amino-acid, and 'Y' indicating any amino-acid except proline) by means of oligosaccharyl transferase. The pro-forms of cysteine cathepsins are further transported to the Golgi apparatus, where the zymogenes are modified in terms of N-linked oligosaccharide processing resulting in the addition of mannose-6-phosphate residues by a phosphotransferase and a phosphodiesterase. The mannose-6-phosphate tags are recognized in the *trans*-Golgi network (TGN) by highly specific mannose-6-phosphate receptors (M6P-R), which sort the pro-forms of cysteine proteases directly to the endo-lysosomal compartments [40]. However, some M6P-tagged proteins like for instance thyroglobulin or the aspartic lysosomal protease cathepsin D, escape endo-lysosomal targeting in thyroid epithelial cells and become secreted instead [41,42].

These results are similar to observations made in lysosomal storage diseases, such as I-cell disease, where it was shown that transport pathways of lysosomal enzymes may differ tremendously with respect to the cell type. For instance, I-cell disease patients lack an enzyme responsible for the addition of the M6P-tag, i. e. phosphotransferase, thus the lysosomal enzymes are not transported to the endo-lysosomal compartments, but become secreted [39]. The mis-routing of lysosomal enzymes was also examined in fibroblasts isolated from mice deficient in M6P-receptors and displaying an I-cell disease-like phenotype [43]. Interestingly, isolated hepatocytes from the same mice exhibited the complete set of enzymes within their endo-lysosomal compartments [44] highlighting that alternative pathways of endo-lysosomal targeting exist. Furthermore, it has been shown that cathepsin B can reach peripherally located vesicles in cancer cells by a pathway that is independent of M6P and most probably driven by sorting signals located within the pro-peptide region of the enzyme [45].

Hence, even though compelling evidence for alternative trafficking mechanisms has been published, the underlying sorting signals or alternative transport routes were not fully elucidated until today (for review see [46]). An excellent model system for the study of transport differences are cells which are characterized by distinct plasma membrane domains thus polarized into a basolateral and an apical plasma membrane domain. In order to elucidate the mechanisms that trigger apically or basolaterally-directed transport, Madin-Darby canine kidney cells (MDCK) or the thyroid epithelial cell line FRT have been intensively studied. Interestingly, FRT cells transport plasma membrane proteins to opposite cell poles as MDCK cells, even though both cell lines are polarized and display apparently morphological features of differentiated epithelial cells [27,34,47,48]. Interestingly, the precise mechanisms that explain why e.g. transmembrane proteins are inserted into either the basolateral or the apical plasma membrane domain of MDCK or FRT cells, respectively, remain elusive. However, because thyrocytes are able to perform vesicular protein transport to opposite cell poles, they qualify as excellent models in order to study protein trafficking in epithelial cells.

### GFP-tagging and activity based probes as tools to study protease trafficking in thyroid epithelial and carcinoma cells

Previously, we have constructed a mammalian expression vector encoding cathepsin B-eGFP that proved suitable for trafficking studies of cathepsin B in the fully differentiated and polarized rat thyroid epithelial cell line FRT as well as in TSH-responsive FRTL-5 cells [27]. This vector can also be used to analyze cathepsin B transport in Chinese Hamster Ovary cells and in a number of other cell types indicating that eGFP tagging of cathepsin B does not grossly alter its trafficking in mammalian cells. More recently, our original pCathB-eGFP vector has been modified in the eGFP portion in order to improve signal-to-noise ratios [49] and it was sub-cloned into a modified plasmid for tissue-specific expression under the control of the A33-antigen promoter [50]. In these cases, the cathepsin B-encoding sequence of the original vector was not altered.

In contrast, here we describe the construction of a vector coding for an inactive mutant counter-part of cathepsin B, in which the active site cysteine was substituted for an alanine. It was taken care to exchange cysteine with alanine instead of the more likely exchange of cysteine with serine (sulfhydryl side chain would then be exchanged by hydroxyl group), because we wanted to exclude the possibility of creating a serine protease-like protein by site directed mutagenesis of the cDNA coding for the cysteine peptidase cathepsin B. A serine exchange could have meant to create a catalytic dyad consisting of serine and histidine. Hence, our site-directed mutagenesis and cloning strategy aimed at the generation of an inactive enzyme with subtle changes in the active site cleft. The goal was to modify the primary structure of cathepsin B in such a way that the protein would still fold properly and thus, would not induce an unfolded protein response due to mis-folding and retention in the ER. In fact, these aims were achieved as is obvious from the observation that cathepsin B-C29A-eGFP chimeras proved fully transport-competent in the normal thyroid epithelial cell line FRT (see Figure 6), where it reached endo-lysosomes. In addition, the active site mutant counterpart of cathepsin B was sorted into endocytic compartments of the thyroid carcinoma cell line HTh74 (see Figure 7).

The cathepsin B-eGFP and cathepsin B-C29A-eGFP chimeric proteins were not only expressed in normal thyrocytes and in thyroid carcinoma cells, rather cathepsin trafficking was also investigated in combination with the activity based probe GB117 [13,25] in order to specify its sorting into transport vesicles. Hence, several aspects of protease transport were addressed in this study. (i) We analyzed whether active cysteine proteases are directed to vesicles different from those that are reached by inactive proteases. Thus, mature enzymes would display specific sorting signals to direct them into distinct sub-cellular compartments. (ii) As an alternative explanation of re-routing of cathepsin B transport in thyroid carcinoma cells, it was tested whether cathepsin B can be transported differently when expressed in normal epithelial cells versus tumor-transformed cells. Thus, assuming that sorting of proteases is governed by the features of the different cell-types themselves.

We provide evidence for the notion that HTh74 cells, although representing anaplastic thyroid carcinoma cells, maintain transport competence and directed cathepsin B-eGFP in both versions, active and inactive, to endo-lysosomes. In this respect, HTh74 cells clearly resembled normal, non-transformed FRT cells that transported both chimeric proteins to identical destinations. However, the non-TSH receptor bearing anaplastic thyroid carcinoma cell line HTh7 and the papillary thyroid carcinoma cell line KTC-1 exhibited trafficking defects. Here inactive cathepsin B was retained within the ER and only the active cathepsin B-eGFP was transported further, i.e. up to the Golgi apparatus and to the endo-lysosomes, respectively.

## Conclusions

In this study, we showed that specific transport signals within the sequence of cathepsin B are unlikely to exist that would explain why thyroid carcinoma cells transport the cysteine protease differently than normal thyroid epithelial cells. Hence, future studies have to show differences between benign and malignant or highly invasive thyroid carcinoma cells. We propose that the differences reside in expression of e.g. distinct members of the Rab-protein family which are known to co-determine the directionality of protein transport in epithelial and carcinoma cells of non-thyroid origin [51-53].

In summary, we conclude that protease trafficking requires tight regulation in order to ensure proper physiological functions. In a pathological context, mis-routed proteases can cleave in a non-regulated manner, because they reach new locations and perform their actions under conditions different from what is considered 'normal'. Finally, re-routing of proteases in cancer may well lead to altered proteolytic potencies in that proteases will encounter a variety of substrates which they would not have been able to interact with under physiological conditions. Hence, the action of proteases is decisive for normal and diseased functions of cells or tissues in many respects. In turn, the understanding of transport pathways of proteases in normal versus tumor cells still provides clues for elucidating drug targets in new therapeutic approaches.

**Acknowledgements and funding**

The authors would like to thank Ruth Hunegnaw, Martin Linke and Maren Rehders for excellent technical contributions and Nils-Erik Heldin as well as Junichi Kurebayashi for providing the thyroid carcinoma cell lines. This work was supported by Jacobs University Bremen, Foundation Blanceflor and The Royal Society of Arts and Sciences in Göteborg.

This article has been published as part of *Thyroid Research* Volume 4 Supplement 1, 2011: New aspects of thyroid hormone synthesis and action. The full contents of the supplement are available online at http://www.thyroidresearchjournal.com/supplements/4/S1

**Author details**

[1]School of Engineering and Science, Research Center for Molecular Life Science, Jacobs University Bremen, 28759 Bremen, Germany. [2]School of Pharmacy, Faculty of Medicine, The Hebrew University, 91120 Jerusalem, Israel. [3]Departments of Pathology and Microbiology and Immunology, Stanford University School of Medicine, Stanford, California 94305-5324, USA. [4]Universitätsklinikum Leipzig Medizinische Klinik III, 04103 Leipzig, Germany; as of June 2011: Klinik für Endokrinologie, Zentrum für Innere Medizin, Bereich Forschung und Lehre im Zentrallabor, 45147 Essen, Germany.

**Authors' contributions**

ST performed the *in situ* analysis, the cathepsin immunoblotting, the characterization and trafficking studies of the human carcinoma cells and contributed in drafting the manuscript. SJ performed the cloning and the trafficking studies of the rat thyroid cells and contributed in drafting the manuscript. HR performed the studies with activity based probes in carcinoma cells. GB and MB provided the activity based probes and gave advice on data interpretation. DF provided the human thyroid tissue and gave advice on data interpretation. KBr devised the study and its design and drafted the manuscript. All authors read and approved the manuscript.

**Competing interests**

The authors declare that they have no competing interests.

**References**

1. Brix K, Dunkhorst A, Mayer K, Jordans S: **Cysteine cathepsins: cellular roadmap to different functions.** *Biochimie* 2008, **90**:194-207.
2. Rawlings ND, Barrett AJ: **MEROPS: the peptidase database.** *Nucleic Acids Res* 1999, **27**:325-331.
3. Rawlings ND, Tolle DP, Barrett AJ: **Evolutionary families of peptidase inhibitors.** *Biochem J* 2004, **378**:705-716.
4. Mort JS, Buttle DJ: **Cathepsin B.** *Int J Biochem Cell Biol* 1997, **29**:715-720.
5. Kirschke H, Wiederanders B: **Lysosomal proteinases.** *Acta Histochem* 1987, **82**:2-4.
6. Brix K, Jordans S: **Watching proteases in action.** *Nat Chem Biol* 2005, **1**:186-187.
7. Baici A, Lang A, Horler D, Kissling R, Merlin C: **Cathepsin B in osteoarthritis: cytochemical and histochemical analysis of human femoral head cartilage.** *Ann Rheum Dis* 1995, **54**:289-297.
8. Sloane BF, Honn KV: **Cysteine proteinases and metastasis.** *Cancer Metastasis Rev* 1984, **3**:249-263.
9. Joyce JA, Baruch A, Chehade K, Meyer-Morse N, Giraudo E, Tsai FY, Greenbaum DC, Hager JH, Bogyo M, Hanahan D: **Cathepsin cysteine proteases are effectors of invasive growth and angiogenesis during multistage tumorigenesis.** *Cancer Cell* 2004, **5**:443-453.

10. Gocheva V, Zeng W, Ke D, Klimstra D, Reinheckel T, Peters C, Hanahan D, Joyce JA: **Distinct roles for cysteine cathepsin genes in multistage tumorigenesis.** *Genes Dev* 2006, **20**:543-556.
11. Mohamed MM, Sloane BF: **Cysteine cathepsins: multifunctional enzymes in cancer.** *Nat Rev Cancer* 2006, **6**:764-775.
12. Vasiljeva O, Turk B: **Dual contrasting roles of cysteine cathepsins in cancer progression: apoptosis versus tumour invasion.** *Biochimie* 2008, **90**:380-386.
13. Fonovic M, Bogyo M: **Activity-based probes as a tool for functional proteomic analysis of proteases.** *Expert Rev Proteomics* 2008, **5**:721-730.
14. Blum G: **Use of fluorescent imaging to investigate pathological protease activity.** *Curr Opin Drug Discov Devel* 2008, **11**:708-716.
15. Brix K, Lemansky P, Herzog V: **Evidence for extracellularly acting cathepsins mediating thyroid hormone liberation in thyroid epithelial cells.** *Endocrinology* 1996, **137**:1963-1974.
16. Brix K, Linke M, Tepel C, Herzog V: **Cysteine proteinases mediate extracellular prohormone processing in the thyroid.** *Biol Chem* 2001, **382**:717-725.
17. Friedrichs B, Tepel C, Reinheckel T, Deussing J, von Figura K, Herzog V, Peters C, Saftig P, Brix K: **Thyroid functions of mouse cathepsins B, K, and L.** *J Clin Invest* 2003, **111**:1733-1745.
18. Jordans S, Jenko-Kokalj S, Kuhl NM, Tedelind S, Sendt W, Bromme D, Turk D, Brix K: **Monitoring compartment-specific substrate cleavage by cathepsins B, K, L, and S at physiological pH and redox conditions.** *BMC Biochem* 2009, **10**:23.
19. Linke M, Jordans S, Mach L, Herzog V, Brix K: **Thyroid stimulating hormone upregulates secretion of cathepsin B from thyroid epithelial cells.** *Biol Chem* 2002, **383**:773-784.
20. Shuja S, Murnane MJ: **Marked increases in cathepsin B and L activities distinguish papillary carcinoma of the thyroid from normal thyroid or thyroid with non-neoplastic disease.** *Int J Cancer* 1996, **66**:420-426.
21. Tedelind S, Poliakova K, Valeta A, Hunegnaw R, Yemanaberhan EL, Heldin NE, Kurebayashi J, Weber E, Kopitar-Jerala N, Turk B, *et al*: **Nuclear cysteine cathepsin variants in thyroid carcinoma cells.** *Biol Chem* 2010, **391**:923-935.
22. Kurebayashi J, Tanaka K, Otsuki T, Moriya T, Kunisue H, Uno M, Sonoo H: **All-trans-retinoic acid modulates expression levels of thyroglobulin and cytokines in a new human poorly differentiated papillary thyroid carcinoma cell line, KTC-1.** *J Clin Endocrinol Metab* 2000, **85**:2889--2896.
23. Heldin NE, Westermark B: **The molecular biology of the human anaplastic thyroid carcinoma cell.** *Thyroidology* 1991, **3**:127-131.
24. Heldin NE, Cvejic D, Smeds S, Westermark B: **Coexpression of functionally active receptors for thyrotropin and platelet-derived growth factor in human thyroid carcinoma cells.** *Endocrinology* 1991, **129**:2187-2193.
25. Blum G, Mullins SR, Keren K, Fonovic M, Jedeszko C, Rice MJ, Sloane BF, Bogyo M: **Dynamic imaging of protease activity with fluorescently quenched activity-based probes.** *Nat Chem Biol* 2005, **1**:203-209.
26. Greenbaum D, Medzihradszky KF, Burlingame A, Bogyo M: **Epoxide electrophiles as activity-dependent cysteine protease profiling and discovery tools.** *Chem Biol* 2000, **7**:569--581.
27. Linke M, Herzog V, Brix K: **Trafficking of lysosomal cathepsin B-green fluorescent protein to the surface of thyroid epithelial cells involves the endosomal/lysosomal compartment.** *J Cell Sci* 2002, **115**:4877-4889.
28. Krause K, Karger S, Sheu SY, Aigner T, Kursawe R, Gimm O, Schmid KW, Dralle H, Fuhrer D: **Evidence for a role of the amyloid precursor protein in thyroid carcinogenesis.** *J Endocrinol* 2008, **198**:291-299.
29. Bradford MM: **A rapid and sensitive method for the quantitation of microgram quantities of protein utilizing the principle of protein-dye binding.** *Anal Biochem* 1976, **72**:248-254.
30. Krohn K, Fuhrer D, Bayer Y, Eszlinger M, Brauer V, Neumann S, Paschke R: **Molecular pathogenesis of euthyroid and toxic multinodular goiter.** *Endocr Rev* 2005, **26**:504-524.
31. Sequeira MJ, Morgan JM, Fuhrer D, Wheeler MH, Jasani B, Ludgate M: **Thyroid transcription factor-2 gene expression in benign and malignant thyroid lesions.** *Thyroid* 2001, **11**:995-1001.
32. Tedelind S, Ericson LE, Karlsson JO, Nilsson M: **Interferon-gamma down-regulates claudin-1 and impairs the epithelial barrier function in primary cultured human thyrocytes.** *Eur J Endocrinol* 2003, **149**:215-221.
33. Hasnain S, Huber CP, Muir A, Rowan AD, Mort JS: **Investigation of structure function relationships in cathepsin B.** *Biol Chem Hoppe Seyler* 1992, **373**:413-418.
34. Nitsch L, Tramontano D, Ambesi-Impiombato FS, Quarto N, Bonatti S: **Morphological and functional polarity of an epithelial thyroid cell line.** *Eur J Cell Biol* 1985, **38**:57-66.
35. Büth H, Luigi Buttigieg P, Ostafe R, Rehders M, Dannenmann SR, Schaschke N, Stark HJ, Boukamp P, Brix K: **Cathepsin B is essential for regeneration of scratch-wounded normal human epidermal keratinocytes.** *Eur J Cell Biol* 2007, **86**:747-761.
36. Vreemann A, Qu H, Mayer K, Andersen LB, Stefana MI, Wehner S, Lysson M, Farcas AM, Peters C, Reinheckel T, *et al*: **Cathepsin B release from rodent intestine mucosa due to mechanical injury results in extracellular matrix damage in early post-traumatic phases.** *Biol Chem* 2009, **390**:481-492.
37. De Duve C, Wattiaux R: **Functions of lysosomes.** *Annu Rev Physiol* 1966, **28**:435-492.
38. Mach L, Mort JS, Glossl J: **Maturation of human procathepsin B. Proenzyme activation and proteolytic processing of the precursor to the mature proteinase, in vitro, are primarily unimolecular processes.** *J Biol Chem* 1994, **269**:13030-13035.
39. von Figura K: **Molecular recognition and targeting of lysosomal proteins.** *Curr Opin Cell Biol* 1991, **3**:642-646.
40. Lodish H, Berk A, Matsudaira P, Kaiser C, Krieger M, Scott M, Zipursky L, Darnell J: **Molecular Cell Biology.** W. H. Freeman & Co.;, 5 2003.
41. Herzog V, Berndorfer U, Saber Y: **Isolation of insoluble secretory product from bovine thyroid: extracellular storage of thyroglobulin in covalently cross-linked form.** *J Cell Biol* 1992, **118**:1071-1083.
42. Lemansky P, Brix K, Herzog V: **Iodination of mature cathepsin D in thyrocytes as an indicator for its transport to the cell surface.** *Eur J Cell Biol* 1998, **76**:53-62.
43. Pohlmann R, Boeker MW, von Figura K: **The two mannose 6-phosphate receptors transport distinct complements of lysosomal proteins.** *J Biol Chem* 1995, **270**:27311-27318.
44. Dittmer F, Ulbrich EJ, Hafner A, Schmahl W, Meister T, Pohlmann R, von Figura K: **Alternative mechanisms for trafficking of lysosomal enzymes in mannose 6-phosphate receptor-deficient mice are cell type-specific.** *J Cell Sci* 1999, **112(Pt 10)**:1591-1597.
45. Moin K, Demchik L, Mai J, Duessing J, Peters C, Sloane BF: **Observing proteases in living cells.** *Adv Exp Med Biol* 2000, **477**:391-401.
46. Collette J, Bocock JP, Ahn K, Chapman RL, Godbold G, Yeyeodu S, Erickson AH: **Biosynthesis and alternate targeting of the lysosomal cysteine protease cathepsin L.** *Int Rev Cytol* 2004, **241**:1-51.
47. Zurzolo C, Le Bivic A, Quaroni A, Nitsch L, Rodriguez-Boulan E: **Modulation of transcytotic and direct targeting pathways in a polarized thyroid cell line.** *Embo J* 1992, **11**:2337-2344.
48. Zurzolo C, Rodriguez-Boulan E: **Delivery of Na+,K(+)-ATPase in polarized epithelial cells.** *Science* 1993, **260**:550-552.
49. Katayama H, Yamamoto A, Mizushima N, Yoshimori T, Miyawaki A: **GFP-like proteins stably accumulate in lysosomes.** *Cell Struct Funct* 2008, **33**:1-12.
50. Mayer K, Iolyeva ME, Meyer-Grahle U, Brix K: **Intestine-specific expression of green fluorescent protein-tagged cathepsin B: proof-of-principle experiments.** *Biol Chem* 2008, **389**:1085-1096.
51. Wang X, Kumar R, Navarre J, Casanova JE, Goldenring JR: **Regulation of vesicle trafficking in madin-darby canine kidney cells by Rab11a and Rab25.** *J Biol Chem* 2000, **275**:29138-29146.
52. Zerial M, McBride H: **Rab proteins as membrane organizers.** *Nat Rev Mol Cell Biol* 2001, **2**:107-117.
53. Chavrier P, Gorvel JP, Stelzer E, Simons K, Gruenberg J, Zerial M: **Hypervariable C-terminal domain of rab proteins acts as a targeting signal.** *Nature* 1991, **353**:769-772.

# 13

# Thyroid storm associated with Graves' disease covered by diabetic ketoacidosis: A case report

Erika Osada, Naoki Hiroi*, Mariko Sue, Natsumi Masai, Ryo Iga, Rika Shigemitsu, Reiko Oka, Masahiko Miyagi, Kaoru Iso, Koji Kuboki and Gen Yoshino

**Abstract**

**Background:** Thyroid storm is a condition in which multiple organ dysfunction results from failure of the compensatory mechanisms of the body owing to excessive thyroid hormone activity induced by some factors in patients with thyrotoxicosis. While diabetic ketoacidosis (DKA) is an important trigger for thyroid storm, simultaneous development of DKA and thyroid storm is rare.

**Case presentation:** A 59-year-old woman with no history of either diabetes mellitus or thyroid disease presented to our hospital because of developing nausea, vomiting and diarrhea for 2 days. Physical examination showed mild disturbance of consciousness, fever, and tachycardia. There were no other signs of thyrotoxicosis. Laboratory studies revealed elevation of random blood glucose and glycosylated hemoglobin, strongly positive of urine acetone, and metabolic acidosis. Since DKA was diagnosed, we initiated the patient on treatment with administration of insulin and adequate fluid replacement. Although the hyperglycemia and acidosis were immediately relieved, the disturbance of consciousness and tachycardia remained persistent. Levels of FT3 and FT4 were extremely high and TSH was below the detectable limit. TRAb was positive. The thyroid storm score of Burch & Wartofsky was 75/140, and the thyroid storm diagnostic criteria of the Japan Thyroid Association were satisfied. Oral administration of thiamazole, potassium iodide and propranolol resulted in immediate relief of the tachycardia.

**Discussion:** We encountered a case of thyroid storm associated with Graves' disease covered by DKA. Thyroid storm and DKA are both potentially fatal, and the prognosis varies depending on whether or not these conditions are detected and treated sufficiently early. The thyroid storm diagnostic criteria prepared in 2008 by the Japan Thyroid Association are very simple as compared to the Burch & Wartofsky scoring system for thyroid storm. The Japanese criteria may be useful in the diagnosis of this condition since they enable clinicians to identify a broad range of cases with thyroid storm. When dealing with cases of DKA or thyroid storm, it seems essential to bear in mind the possibility of the coexistence of these two diseases.

## Introduction

Thyroid storm is a condition involving failure of multiple organs arising from collapse of the compensatory mechanism for excessive thyroid hormone activity triggered by factors associated with thyrotoxicosis. The incidence of thyroid storm is reported to be less than 10% in patients hospitalized for thyrotoxicosis, but the fatality rate is reportedly 20 - 30%, if this disease is not treated promptly [1,2]. Diabetic ketoacidosis (DKA) is a severe metabolic disorder arising from deficient insulin activity. It is reported that DKA develops in 5 out of 1000 diabetic patients annually from Taiwan [3]. If this disease follows a severe course due to lack of appropriate diagnosis and treatment, the patient may die in the comatose state, with the death rate reported to be 2% or less [4]. We recently encountered a case in which thyroid storm and DKA developed simultaneously.

* Correspondence: n-hiroi@med.toho-u.ac.jp
Division of Diabetes, Metabolism and Endocrinology, Department of Internal Medicine (Omori), Toho University School of Medicine, Tokyo, Japan

## Case report

The patient was a 59-year-old woman with chief complaints of nausea and vomiting. Four months prior to presentation, malaise and anorexia manifested but were left untreated. She had been free of signs of diabetes, eg, thirst, polydipsia, and polyuria, and signs of Graves' disease, eg, hyperhidrosis, tremor, neck swelling, and exophthalmos. Two days before presentation, she developed nausea, vomiting and diarrhea. At that time, acute gastroenteritis was suspected, and oral medication was prescribed. However, frequent vomiting persisted thereafter. At that time, a high blood glucose level and positive urinary acetone were noted. She was thus suspected of having DKA and was brought by ambulance to our hospital. When first examined at our hospital, the patient was 159 cm in height, weighed 64.0 kg, and had a body mass index of 25.3 kg/m$^2$, blood pressure 140/62 mm Hg, heart rate 170/min (regular), and temperature 38.2°C. Consciousness level was E3, V3, M6 and total 12 points according to the Glasgow Coma Scale. The skin showed low turgor and was not moist. No tremor was observed. Upper eyelid edema was present, but there was no marked exophthalmos. Slight erosive swelling of the thyroid was noted. There were no chest abnormalities. Borborygmus was enhanced but no other abnormalities were noted in the abdomen. There were no neurological abnormalities.

Biochemically, blood glucose and glycosylated hemoglobin were markedly elevated (336 mg/dL, 10.9%), while total cholesterol (126 mg/dL) and neutral fat (72 mg/dL) were at the lower limits of their normal ranges. Mild hepatic dysfunction, hyperuricemia, and mild hypoproteinemia were noted. Urine acetone was strongly positive. On blood gas analysis, acidosis (pH 7.257) was noted, accompanied by an expanded anion gap, and blood ketone body elevation (predominantly β-hydroxybutyric acid) was also seen (β-hydroxybutyric acid 5920 mmol/L, acetoacetic acid 2101 mmol/L). Anti-glutamic acid decarboxylase antibody and anti-insulinoma-associated protein-2 antibody were negative, and normal reaction of insulin was observed to glucagon loading. Chest X-ray disclosed only mild cardiomegaly, and electrocardiography revealed sinus tachycardia. After heart rate improvement, echocardiography disclosed no evident abnormalities.

### Clinical course

Based on the diagnosis of DKA, the patient was fasted and received a massive physiological saline infusion for correction of dehydration, accompanied by initiation of insulin therapy. Her blood glucose level dropped rapidly, but the slightly reduced consciousness level (the Glasgow Coma Scale: E4, V4, M6 and total 14 point), tachycardia (150/min), and fever (38.0°C) persisted. Because tachycardia could not be explained by DKA-associated dehydration alone, thyroid disease was added to the differential diagnosis. Free triiodothyronine (FT3) and free thyroxin (FT4) were 26.28 pg/mL and >7.77 ng/dL, respectively, and thyroid stimulating hormone (TSH) was below the detectable limit. TSH receptor antibody (TRAb) was positive (24.9 IU/L). Thyroid ultrasonography revealed diffuse swelling of the thyroid gland, a reduced internal echo level, and increased internal blood flow. Although the patient had DKA as a complication, the thyroid storm score of Burch & Wartofsky [5] was 75/140, and the thyroid storm diagnostic criteria of the Japan Thyroid Association (JTA) [6] were satisfied. Thyroid storm associated with Graves' disease was thus considered highly probable in this case, and treatment with 15 mg/day of thiamazole, 100 mg/day of potassium iodide and 30 mg/day of propranolol was started. The following day, the fever subsided to approximately 37°C and tachycardia also showed alleviation.

Two months later, thyroid function had been normalized. The patient is still being managed with oral thiamazole therapy. Regarding diabetes, this case initially required a maximum insulin aspart dose of 52 units/day. Blood glucose control was achieved with 14 units of insulin aspart plus 16 units of insulin glargine. The patient was suspected of having type 2 diabetes mellitus because all islet-related antibodies were negative and delta C-peptide (CPR) level after glucagon loading (6 min after glucagon loading - before glucagon loading) was 1.1 ng/mL. However, the honeymoon phenomenon in the type 1 diabetes mellitus could not be ruled out. One year later, the dosage of insulin was decreased gradually to 12 units in total, and the improvement in ability of insulin secretion was assessed by glucagon loading (delta CPR: 1.6 ng/mL). Therefore, the patient was finally diagnosed as having type 2 diabetes mellitus although insulin administration was required.

## Discussion

Our present case had thyroid storm associated with Graves' disease covered by DKA. She lacked signs of thyrotoxicosis and was strongly suspected of having DKA on the basis of clinical findings and test data. Upon admission to the hospital, she was diagnosed as having DKA and was treated accordingly. Although it has been reported that detection of thyroid storm tends to be delayed in patients with DKA because of suppression of fever [4,7,8], relatively low thyroid hormone levels [9], in the present case, none of these findings was obtained. In this case, the diagnosis of thyroid storm was probably delayed because the symptoms of DKA resembled those of thyroid storm and because no symptoms of Graves' disease were observed before the onset of thyroid storm. However, the presence of thyrotoxicosis was suspected in a relatively early stage in this case based on the following findings: (1) symptoms of central nervous system involvement, as well as tachycardia and fever, not alleviated despite correction of the dehydration associated with DKA; and (2) a relatively low total cholesterol level. Thus, treatment with an iodine preparation, β-blocker, and thiamazole was initiated relatively quickly, and this early treatment probably accounts for the favorable outcome of our patient. Generally, large amounts of thiamazole, potassium iodide, and prednisolone are required for the treatment of thyroid crisis; however, thyroid function was restored with a few doses of these medications in our case. This could be one of the reasons why DKA could deteriorate the thyroid storm symptoms.

An interesting point in this case is whether or not the patient really had thyrotoxicosis at the time of admission. When initially examined, she showed laboratory data of thyrotoxicosis and was given a score of 75 according to the thyroid storm score of Burch & Wartofsky [5]. Thus, the patient seemed to satisfy the thyroid storm diagnostic criteria. Furthermore, this patient also apparently satisfied the thyroid storm diagnostic criteria prepared by the JTA (Table 1) [6], because she had signs of thyrotoxicosis, accompanied by a reduced consciousness level (a central nervous system symptom), tachycardia, fever, and gastrointestinal symptoms. Even after correction of dehydration and blood glucose level, the Burch & Wartofsky score was 45 and symptoms of central nervous system involvement, fever, and tachycardia persisted, thus satisfying the Japanese diagnostic criteria. Treatment with potassium iodide rapidly alleviated clinical symptoms, suggesting that thyroid storm had already been present on admission. The thyroid storm diagnostic criteria prepared in 2008 by the JTA are very simple as compared to the thyroid storm score of Burch & Wartofsky. Thyroid storm has a high fatality rate if it is not appropriately diagnosed and treated. The Japanese criteria may be useful in the diagnosis of this condition since they enable clinicians to identify a broad range of cases with thyroid storm.

The malaise and anorexia, which this patient had been experiencing for 4 months, were not inconsistent with the symptoms of diabetes mellitus. However, whether or not Graves' disease was present 4 months prior to presentation is unknown. Which developed earlier, the diabetes or Graves' disease, also remains unknown. Regarding the influence of Graves' disease on diabetes mellitus, there is a general agreement that the deterioration of glucose intolerance, including diabetes mellitus, is observed under a hyperthyroid state [10]. Graves' disease has been reported to increase the intestinal absorption of carbohydrates [11] and production of hepatic glucose from glycogen due to hepatic insulin resistance [12,13]. Hyperthyroid patients show marked insulin resistance to oral glucose tolerance test that resolves with the treatment of hyperthyroidism [14]. Glucose uptake in the skeletal muscle is known to be lower in hyperthyroid patients than in euthyroid patients; this difference is also attributable to insulin resistance [15,16]. The ability of insulin to suppress hormone-sensitive lipase –an enzyme responsible for adipocyte fatty acid release, which facilitates β-oxidation and ketone body production in the liver– is also known to be affected by hyperthyroidism-induced insulin resistance [15]. The increase in the glomerular filtration rate in hyperthyroidism leads to an increased insulin clearance and hence a decreased insulin level [17]. In the hyperthyroid state, the ratio of C-peptide to proinsulin is low [18], suggesting an increase in the rate of biologically inactive insulin precursor release. These findings suggest that thyroid hormones are associated with the onset and aggravation of diabetes mellitus. In addition, β-cell function is known to be lower in Japanese individuals than in other ethnic groups [19], and age-related β-cell dysfunction and/or reduction of insulin sensitivity were usually observed [20,21]. It seems probable that

**Table 1 Diagnostic criteria for thyroid storm of Japan Thyroid Association and Japan Endocrine Society**

| | |
|---|---|
| Essential criterion | Presence of thyrotoxicosis (elevation of free T3 and/or T4) |
| Symptoms | 1. Symptoms involving the central nervous system |
| | 2. Fever (≥ 38°C) |
| | 3. Tachycardia (≥ 130/min) |
| | 4. Symptoms of heart failure |
| | 5. Gastrointestinal symptoms |
| Cases definitely diagnosed as having thyroid storm | |
| Satisfaction of the essential criterion and at least one of the following criteria | |
| | a. Central nervous system symptoms + one or more of the other systems, or |
| | b. 3 or more symptoms other than those of central nervous system. |
| Cases suspected of having thyroid storm | |
| | a. Satisfaction of essential criterion + 2 symptoms other than those of the central nervous system, or |
| | b. Satisfaction of essential criterion is not confirmed, but positive history of thyroid disease + exophthalmos + goiter are present and criterion a or b for definite cases is satisfied. |

these factors aggravated the underlying abnormal glucose metabolism (ie, diabetes mellitus) and intensified insulin deficiency, serving as a factor responsible for the onset of DKA in this case. Meanwhile, thyroid storm is usually precipitated by infection, trauma and surgical emergencies, or operations and less commonly by radiation thyroiditis, DKA, toxemia of pregnancy, or parturition [22,23]. Therefore DKA cannot be ignored as a factor triggering the onset of thyroid storm [24]. It seems likely that DKA aggravated her underlying Graves' disease, triggering the onset of thyroid storm.

As illustrated above, we recently encountered a DKA case with Graves' disease complicated by thyroid storm. DKA and thyroid storm are both potentially fatal, and the prognosis varies depending on whether or not these conditions are detected and treated with sufficient earliness. When dealing with cases of DKA or thyroid storm, it seems essential to bear in mind the possibility of the coexistence of these two diseases. The present report is presented from this perspective.

## Consent

Written informed consent was obtained from the patient's relatives for publication of this case report. A copy of the written consent is available for review by the Editor-in-Chief of this journal.

### Authors' contributions

EO wrote the first draft. NM, RI, RS and RO collected information on the patient. MS, MM and KI did the literature searches. NH wrote the final manuscript and made appropriate revisions. NH, KK and GY were in a position of leadership for the patient. All authors read through and approved the final manuscript.

### Competing interests

The authors declare that they have no competing interests.

### References


1. Jameson L, Weetman A: **Disorders of the thyroid gland.** In *Herrison' principles of internal medicine.*. 15 edition. Edited by: Brawnwald E, Fauci A, Kasper D. New York: McGraw-Hill; 2001:2060-2084.
2. Tietgens ST, Leinung MC: **Thyroid storm.** *Med Clin North Am* 1995, **79**:169-184.
3. Liu CC, Chen KR, Chen HF, Huang HL, Ko MC, Li CY: **Trends in hospitalization for diabetic ketoacidosis in diabetic patients in Taiwan: analysis of national claims data, 1997-2005.** *J Formos Med Assoc* 2010, **109**:725-734.
4. Kitabchi AE, Umpierrez GE, Murphy MB: **Diabetes ketoacidosis and hyperglycemic hyperosmolar state.** In *International textbook of diabetes mellitus.*. 3 edition. Edited by: DeFronzo RA, Ferrannini E, Keen H, Zimmet P. Chichester, UK: John Wiley, Sons, Ltd; 2004:1101-1119.
5. Burch HB, Wartofsky L: **Life-threatening thyrotoxicosis. Thyroid storm.** *Endocrinol Metab Clin North Am* 1993, **22**:263-277.
6. **The Guideline Committee for Thyroid Storm of Japan Thyroid Association and Japan Endocrine Society (2008) Diagnostic criteria for thyroid storm (1stedition).** [http://thyroid.umin.ac.jp/rinsyo/crise1.pdf], (In Japanese).
7. Troen LP, Taymor RC, Goldberg BI: **Thyroid crisis associated with diabetic come.** *N Engl J Med* 1951, **244**:394-398.
8. Kunishige M, Sekimoto E, Komatsu M, Bando Y: **Thyrotoxicosis masked by diabetic ketoacidosis.** *Diabetes care* 2001, **24**:171.
9. Mouradian M, Abourizk N: **Diabetes mellitus and thyroid disease.** *Diabetes care* 1983, **6**:512-520.
10. Cooppan R, Kozak GP: **Hyperthyroidism and diabetes mellitus. An analysis of 70 patients.** *Arch Intern Med* 1980, **140**:370-373.
11. Middleton WR: **Thyroid hormones and the gut.** *Gut* 1971, **12**:172-177.
12. Bratusch-Marrain PR, Komjati M, Waldhäusl WK: **Glucose metabolism in noninsulin-dependent diabetic patients with experimental hyperthyroidism.** *J Clin Endocrinol Metab* 1985, **60**:1063-1068.
13. Dimitriadis GD, Leighton B, Vlachonikolis IG, Parry-Billings M, Challiss RA, West D, Newsholme EA: **Effects of hyperthyroidism on the sensitivity of glycolysis and glycogen synthesis to insulin in the soleus muscle of the rat.** *Biochem J* 1988, **253**:87-92, [Erratum in: Biochem J 255: 1988].
14. Al-Shoumer KA, Vasanthy BA, Al-Zaid MM: **Effects of treatment of hyperthyroidism on glucose homeostasis, insulin secretion, and markers of bone turnover.** *Endocr Pract* 2006, **12**:121-130.
15. Potenza M, Via MA, Yanagisawa RT: **Excess thyroid hormone and carbohydrate metabolism.** *Endocr Pract* 2009, **15**:254-262.
16. Shen DC, Davidson MB, Kuo SW, Sheu WH-H: **Peripheral and hepatic insulin antagonism in hyperthyroidism.** *J Clin Endocrinol Metab* 1988, **66**:565-569.
17. Gonzalo MA, Grant C, Moreno I, Garcia FJ, Suárez AI, Herrera-Pombo JL, Rovira A: **Glucose tolerance, insulin secretion, insulin sensitivity and glucose effectiveness in normal and overweight hyperthyroid women.** *Clin Endocrinol (Oxf)* 1996, **45**:689-697.
18. Beer SF, Parr JH, Temple RC, Hales CN: **The effect of thyroid disease on proinsulin and C-peptide levels.** *Clin Endocrinol (Oxf)* 1989, **30**:379-383.
19. Kuroe A, Fukushima M, Usami M, Ikeda M, Nakai Y, Taniguchi A, Matsuura T, Suzuki H, Kurose T, Yasuda K, Yamada Y, Seino Y: **Impaired beta-cell function and insulin sensitivity in Japanese subjects with normal glucose tolerance.** *Diabetes Res Clin Pract* 2003, **59**:71-72.
20. Chang AM, Halter JB: **Aging and insulin secretion.** *Am J Physiol Endocrinol Metab* 2003, **284**:E7-12.
21. Kanauchi M, Kanauchi K, Inoue T, Kimura K, Saito Y: **Insulin sensitivity and beta-cell function in older Japanese adults without diabetes.** *Age Ageing* 2008, **37**:330-333.
22. Davies TF, Larsen PR: **Thyroid storm (Accelerated Hyperthyroidsm), Thyrotoxicosis.** In *Williams Text Book of Endocrinology.*. 11 edition. Edited by: Kronenberg HM, Melmed S, Polonsky KS, Larsen PR. Philadelphia, PA, Sounders; 2008:357-358.
23. Kearney T, Dang C: **Diabetic and endocrine emergencies.** *Postgrad Med J* 2007, **83**:79-86.
24. Goldberg PA, Inzucchi SE: **Critical issues in endocrinology.** *Clin Chest Med* 2003, **24**:583-606.

# 14

# Increased expression of *PIN1* gene in papillary thyroid carcinoma

Andrzej Lewiński[1,2*], Ewa Brzeziańska[3], Karolina Czarnecka[3], Joanna Latek[2], Włodzimierz Koptas[4], Anna Cyniak-Magierska[1,2]

**Abstract**

**Background:** Peptidyl-prolyl *cis/trans* isomerase (Pin1), encoded by *PIN1* gene with *locus* in chromosome 19p13, is an enzyme that catalytically induces conformational changes in proteins after phosphorylation on serine or threonine residues preceding proline (pSer/Thr-Pro motifs); in this way, it has an influence on protein interactions and intracellular localizations of proteins. The aim of the study were: 1) an assessment of *PIN1* gene expression level in benign and malignant thyroid lesions; 2) the evaluation of possible correlations between gene expression and histopathological variants of papillary thyroid carcinoma (PTC) or tumour size, classified according to TNM classification of primary tumours (in case of PTC only); 3) the estimation of possible relationships between expression of the gene in question and patients' sex or age.

**Methods:** Seventy (70) tissue samples were analyzed: 32 cases of PTC, 7 cases of medullary thyroid carcinoma (MTC), 7 cases of follicular adenoma (FA), and 24 cases of nodular goitre (NG). In real-time polymerase chain reaction (real-time PCR), two-step RT-PCR (reverse transcriptase-polymerase chain reaction) in an ABI PRISM 7500 Sequence Detection System was employed. The *PIN1* gene expression level was assessed, calculating the mean relative quantification rate (RQ rate) increase for each sample.

**Results:** The level of *PIN1* gene expression (compared to that in macroscopically unchanged thyroid tissue) was higher in PTC group than those in FA, MTC and/or NG groups, but the statistical significance was noted for difference between PTC and NG groups only. On the other hand, the differences of RQ rate value between different PTC variants were statistically insignificant. No correlations were found between RQ values and tumour size, as well as between RQ values and patients' sex or age in PTC group.

**Conclusions:** The *PIN1* gene expression may have - in future - an important meaning in the diagnostics of PTC and in understanding its pathogenesis. However, our results - mostly due to the small number of cases - do not yet allow considering *PIN1* gene as a prognostic molecular PTC marker.

## Background

The *PIN1* gene encodes an essential peptidyl-prolyl *cis/trans* isomerase (PPIase; EC 5.2.1.8) which has a profound impact on key proteins involved in the regulation of cell cycle [1]. The human *PIN1* gene is mapped to chromosome 19p13 [2]. Catalyzing conformational changes in substrates after phosphorylation, Pin1 recognizes phospho-serine or phospho-threonine bonds followed by proline (pSer/Thr-Pro motifs) and plays a vital role in protein folding or refolding [3]. Through isomerization Pin1 can modulate the conformation of protein substrates, changing their enzymatic activity which leads to alteration in different cell function [1].

Pin1 enzyme activity is important for oncogenic and cell-signalling pathways *via* conformational changes following phosphorylation of many molecules (e.g. Bcl-2, p53, c-Jun, beta-catenin, cyclin D1 and RAF kinase) [4-7]. The Pin1-regulated alteration in protein interactions and stability have been shown to be associated with cell transformation and progression of certain types of human tumours (e.g., prostate, colon, lung, ovary and breast cancers, and lymphoma) [8-10]. It has also been reported that inhibition of Pin1 function in human tumour cells, using Pin1 antisense RNA, induces mitotic

* Correspondence: alewin@csk.umed.lodz.pl
[1]Department of Endocrinology and Metabolic Diseases, Medical University of Lodz, Poland
Full list of author information is available at the end of the article

arrest and apoptosis [11]. Further studies indicate that Pin1 plays a critical role in cell restriction points - particularly in G1/S phase; Pin1 modulates some important regulators of that cell cycle point, e.g. cyclin D1 and its upstream transcriptional factors. The increased Pin1 expression correlates significantly with overexpression of cyclin D1 mRNA and protein. Interestingly, Pin1 binds phosphorylated c-Jun, influencing the increase of its transcriptional activity towards cyclin D1 - by activating c-Jun/AP-1 and beta-catenin/T-cell factor (TCF) and, in this way it cooperates with Ras signalling pathway [4].

Pin1 is involved not only in the pathogenesis of human cancer, but - presumably - also in the pathogenesis of asthma and Alzheimer's disease [12].

Recently, in some reports - including the study on thyroid tumours - strong correlation between Pin1 and cyclin D1 immunoexpression and/or cyclin D1 mRNA and *PIN1* expression *via* interaction with Wnt signalling pathway has been observed [13]. Moreover, it has been suggested that Pin1 may promote cyclin D1 overexpression directly or through accumulation of beta-catenin in thyroid cancer cells [13].

There are rather scarce reports which are focused on evaluation of PIN1 mRNA expression in thyroid tumours. Therefore, in order to recognize the Pin1 role in the pathogenesis of thyroid gland, we have compared the levels of *PIN1* gene expression in benign and malignant thyroid lesions. We have assessed *PIN1* gene expression in real-time polymerase chain reaction (real-time PCR), two-step RT-PCR (reverse transcriptase-polymerase chain reaction) and we have evaluated the possible correlations between the gene expression and the histopathological variant of examined PTCs (classic, tall-cell, follicular), tumour size grouped according to TNM classification of primary tumours (pT1, pT2, pT3, pT4). We have also decided to estimate the possible relationships between expression of the gene in question and patients' sex or age.

## Materials and methods

The Ethical Committee of the Medical University of Lodz approved the studies reported in the present article.

### Thyroid tissue samples

Tumour tissue samples (100-150 mg) were obtained from 70 patients who had undergone surgery treatment at the Centre of Oncology, the Maria Skłodowska-Curie Institute in Gliwice, at the Holy Family Municipal Hospital in Lodz and at the Department of General and Colorectal Surgery, Medical University of Lodz, Poland during the years 2002-2007. Total tumour tissue samples, immediately after resection, were collected into lysis buffer (Buffer RLT, Qiagen Sciences, USA).

Among the studied samples 32 cases of primary papillary thyroid carcinoma - PTC (26 females, 6 males; mean age 41.8 ± 15.7; mean ± SD) were used. Histopathological variants of PTC were as follows: PTC classic variant (20 cases: 17 females, 3 males; mean age 36.5 ± 14.4), PTC follicular variant (9 cases: 6 females, 3 males; mean age 49.9 ± 16.0), PTC tall-cell variant (3 cases: 3 females; mean age 53.3 ± 5.1) (Table 1). Seven (7) cases of medullary thyroid carcinoma - MTC (6 females, 1 male; mean age 56.0 ± 17.6) and 7 cases of follicular adenoma - FA (6 females, 1 male; mean age 49.4 ± 14.8) were also included in the study. The control group consisted of 24 cases of nodular goitre - NG (22 females, 2 males; mean age 48.9 ± 14.7) (Table 2).

The whole study cohort comprised 70 persons: 60 females and 10 males, the mean age was 46.4 ± 15.8 years (age ranged from 16 to 75 years). Histopathological diagnoses for malignant thyroid lesions, according to WHO Classification of Tumours [14], have been obtained from pathomorphological reports and are presented in Table 1, together with TNM classification and AJCC stage groupings [15].

In the study design, macroscopically unchanged thyroid tissue served for the reference standard (calibrator).

### Isolation of total RNA and reverse transcription (RT)

Total RNA was extracted from fresh tisssues, using RNeasy Protect Midi Kit, (Qiagen, Hilden, Germany), according to the manufacturer's recommendations. RNA concentration was spectrophotometrically assessed by measuring absorbance at 260 and 280 nm (Ultraspec 2000 UV/Visible Spectrophotometer, Pharmacia Biotech, Sweden).

Afterwards the reverse transcription (RT) was performed in a Personal Thermocycler (Eppendorf, Germany), using 1 μg of total RNA in the presence of 50 μM of oligo d(T)16 and Reverse Transcriptase MultiScribe™ (50 U/μl) in a total volume of 30 μl, including also: 10× TaqMan RT Buffer (containing 100 mM Tris-HCL pH 8.3, 500 mM KCL), $MgCl_2$ solution (25 mM), dNTPs mixture (10 mM), RNAse Inhibitor (20 U/μl), and nuclease-free water (TaqMan Reverse Transcriptase Reagents, Applied Biosystems, Foster City, CA, USA). The reactions were conducted for 10 minutes at 25°C, followed by 30 minutes at 48°C, afterwards the samples were heated for 5 min to 95°C, and next placed at 4°C. The cDNA concentration and purity were spectrophotometrically assessed by measuring absorbance at 260 and 280 nm (Ultraspec 2000 UV/Visible Spectrophotometer, Pharmacia Biotech, Sweden).

### Quantitative analysis of the relative amount of PIN1 mRNA by real-time PCR

An established Relative Quantification Polymerase Chain Reaction (RQ-PCR) assay for PIN1 mRNA expression

**Table 1 Sex, age, histopathological diagnosis of malignant thyroid tumours in the studied patients**

| Case number | Sex | Age | Histopathological diagnosis | TNM staging system | American Joint Committee on Cancer (AJCC) grouping system |
|---|---|---|---|---|---|
| 1 | F | 23 | PTC, classic variant | pT1bNxM0 | I |
| 2 | F | 38 | PTC, classic variant | pT1N0M0 | I |
| 3 | F | 52 | PTC, classic variant | pT2N0M0 | II |
| 4 | F | 71 | PTC, classic variant | pT2N0Mx | II |
| 5 | F | 47 | PTC, classic variant | pT1aN0M0 | I |
| 6 | F | 24 | PTC, classic variant | pT1N0Mx | I |
| 7 | F | 33 | PTC, classic variant | pT2aNxMx | II |
| 8 | F | 28 | PTC, classic variant | pT1bNxMx | I |
| 9 | F | 40 | PTC, classic variant | pT4N0Mx | IVA |
| 10 | F | 17 | PTC, classic variant | pT2bN1aM0 | III |
| 11 | M | 47 | PTC, classic variant | pT2aN1aM0 | III |
| 12 | M | 31 | PTC, classic variant | pT2aN0M0 | II |
| 13 | F | 16 | PTC, classic variant | pT2aN0M0 | II |
| 14 | F | 61 | PTC, classic variant | pT2aN0M0 | II |
| 15 | F | 48 | PTC, classic variant | pT4N1aM0 | IVA |
| 16 | M | 30 | PTC, classic variant | pT4N1bM0 | IV |
| 17 | F | 31 | PTC, classic variant | pT1NxMx | I |
| 18 | F | 40 | PTC, classic variant | pT1aNxMx | I |
| 19 | F | 28 | PTC, classic variant | pT1aNxMx | I |
| 20 | F | 25 | PTC, classic variant | pT1aN1aMx | I |
| 21 | F | 49 | PTC, tall-cell variant | pT2bN0M0 | II |
| 22 | F | 52 | PTC, tall-cell variant | pT4N0M0 | IVA |
| 23 | F | 59 | PTC, tall-cell variant | pT4bN1Mx | IV |
| 24 | F | 36 | PTC, follicular variant | pT2aNxMx | II |
| 25 | M | 28 | PTC, follicular variant | pT2N1aMx | II |
| 26 | M | 52 | PTC, follicular variant | pT3NxMx | III |
| 27 | F | 62 | PTC, follicular variant | pT1aNxMx | I |
| 28 | F | 26 | PTC, follicular variant | pT4N1aM0 | IVA |
| 29 | F | 56 | PTC, follicular variant | pT3aN0M0 | III |
| 30 | F | 68 | PTC, follicular variant | pT2bN1aM0 | II |
| 31 | M | 66 | PTC, follicular variant | pT4aN0M0 | IVA |
| 32 | F | 55 | PTC, follicular variant | pT2aN0M0 | II |
| 33 | M | 74 | MTC | pT4N0M0 | IVA |
| 34 | F | 32 | MTC | pT1NxMx | I |
| 35 | F | 32 | MTC | pT1NxMx | I |
| 36 | F | 59 | MTC | pT3N1bM0 | III |
| 37 | F | 56 | MTC | pT3N0M0 | III |
| 38 | F | 71 | MTC | pT4N1aM0 | IVA |
| 39 | F | 68 | MTC | pT3aN0M0 | III |

was conducted in ABI PRISM 7500 Sequence Detection System (Applied Biosystems), according to the manufacturer's protocol. The PCR reactions for *PIN1* gene were run with 50 ng of cDNA in a total volume of 50 µl, using TaqMan® Universal PCR Master Mix (Applied Biosystems, Foster City, CA, USA) and the predesigned and labelled primer/probe set (Assays-on-Demand™ Gene Expression assay mix, Hs01598309_ml, Applied Biosystems). After initial incubation at 50°C for 2 min to allow uracil-N-glycosylase (UNG) digestion, and at 95°C for 10 min to activate the AmpliTaq Gold®DNA polymerase, both of them were provided by the

**Table 2 Sex, age, histopathological diagnosis of benign thyroid lesions in the studied patients**

| Case number | Sex | Age | Histopathological diagnosis |
|---|---|---|---|
| 1 | F | 49 | FA |
| 2 | F | 52 | FA |
| 3 | M | 75 | FA |
| 4 | F | 29 | FA |
| 5 | F | 41 | FA |
| 6 | F | 41 | FA |
| 7 | F | 59 | FA |
| 8 | F | 40 | NG |
| 9 | F | 42 | NG |
| 10 | F | 30 | NG |
| 11 | F | 48 | NG |
| 12 | F | 42 | NG |
| 13 | F | 64 | NG |
| 14 | F | 69 | NG |
| 15 | F | 72 | NG |
| 16 | F | 50 | NG |
| 17 | F | 51 | NG |
| 18 | F | 63 | NG |
| 19 | F | 49 | NG |
| 20 | F | 49 | NG |
| 21 | F | 38 | NG |
| 22 | M | 52 | NG |
| 23 | F | 31 | NG |
| 24 | F | 29 | NG |
| 25 | M | 75 | NG |
| 26 | F | 28 | NG |
| 27 | F | 30 | NG |
| 28 | F | 72 | NG |
| 29 | F | 50 | NG |
| 30 | F | 40 | NG |
| 31 | F | 59 | NG |

Universal PCR Master Mix, the samples were amplified through 40 biphasic cycles of 95°C for 15 sec and 60°C for 1 min (Table 3).

Macroscopically unchanged thyroid tissue was used as a calibrator (standard sample). Amplification reactions were done in triplicate for each sample (cDNA from the same PCR reaction but in separate wells). Controls with no template cDNA were used with each assay (negative control).

The expression levels of *β-actin* gene (*ACTB*) were measured, as endogenous control (reference gene), using the appropriate Assays-on-Demand™ Gene Expression product (Hs99999903_ml, Applied Biosystems Foster City, CA, USA).

**Table 3 Real-time PCR conditions for *PIN1* gene amplification**

| Times and temperatures | | | |
|---|---|---|---|
| Initial setup | | Each of 40 cycles | |
| | | Denaturation | Annealing/ Elongation |
| HOLD | HOLD | CYCLE | |
| UNG activation 2 min, 50°C | 10 min, 95°C | 15 s, 95°C | 1 min, 60°C |

Both gene expressions were measured for each thyroid lesion sample in the same PCR reaction but in separate wells.

Assays-on-Demand™ Gene Expression product consists of 20 × mix of unlabelled PCR primers (18 μM for each) and TaqMan® MGB probes (5 μM) with FAM™ (6-carboxy-fluorescein) at the 5' end as the reporter dye, and a non-fluorescent quencher (TAMRA, 6-carboxy-tetramethylrhodamine) at the 3' end. The two-minute, 50°C step was required for optimal AmpErase® UNG activity when TaqMan® Universal PCR Master Mix (P/N 4304437) was used.

The fluorescence signal was measured in real-time PCR in the extension phase of the PCR reaction, and the measurement, proportional to the quantity of sample cDNA in the reaction, was plotted as an amplification curve against cycle number. A threshold value of fluorescence in the exponential part of the amplification curve was selected, and - for each sample - the number of cycles was measured, which was needed by the signal to reach the threshold (threshold cycle, $C_T$). The larger were the quantities of the starting material, the lower were $C_T$ values.

### Data analysis

Data analysis of relative gene expression was performed with the Taq-Man SDS analysis software on an ABI PRISM 7500 Sequence Detection System (Applied Biosystems), and the results were exported to Excel sheets for further processing.

Fluorescence emission data were determined as $C_T$ values for each reaction and, for each sample, triplicate $C_T$ values were averaged. The average $C_T$ value for *β-actin* was subtracted from the average *PIN1* $C_T$ value to yield the $\Delta C_T$ value ($\Delta C_T$ = $C_T$ target - $C_T$ reference). Normalization to the reference gene (*β-actin*) has been necessary to account for the variabilities in sample quantity and quality, and for the variabilities in PCR efficiency among samples. The assay, described in this report, involves the determination of a $\Delta\Delta C_T$ value. This is calculated by: $\Delta\Delta C_T$ = $\Delta C_T$ test sample - $\Delta C_T$ calibrator sample. The higher is the $\Delta\Delta C_T$ value, the lower is the expression of *PIN1* in the specimen. Fold-differences, representing relative expression results, are calculated using the following equation: relative fold increase = $2^{-\Delta\Delta C_T}$. In order to evaluate the analytical sensitivity, specificity, and accuracy of the assay, serial dilutions were performed.

### Statistical analysis

The data were statistically analyzed, using Newman-Keuls' multiple comparison test followed by Kruskal-Wallis' test, in order to compare the level of expression values (RQ) among the four studied independent groups (PTC, MTC, FA, NG). Basic measures of location (i.e. mean, median), measures of dispersion (SD, SEM), and minimum and maximum values were calculated to provide detailed descriptions of gene expressions in selected groups. Additionally, box-and-whiskers plots were introduced to display the difference in gene expressions levels in different samples.

The Kruskal-Wallis' test was used to compare the level of expression values (RQ) among three variants of PTC (PTC v. classic, PTC v. tall-cell, PTC v. follicular). The Spearman's rank correlation coefficient and U Mann-Whitney's test were performed in order to correlate the level of expression of *PIN1* gene (RQ values) with examined parameters (age, sex, tumour size, classified according to TNM definition of primary tumours - pT1, pT2, pT3, pT4).

The accepted level of statistical significance was at $p < 0.05$. The results are presented as means ± SEM and means ± SD values.

Statistica for Windows 7.0 program was applied for calculations.

## Results

The specimens were amplified in the ABI PRISM 7500 Sequence Detection System in reaction, containing primers and probes for *PIN1* gene and a control gene, *β-actin*. The Sequence Detection System software, provided with the instrument, analyses the fluorescence data, generated during the reaction, and calculates the cycle number at which fluorescence crosses the threshold value ($C_T$). Triplicate amplifications of the sample produced nearly identical, overlapping curves, from which $C_T$ values were calculated.

In our experiment low $C_T$ values for *PIN1* gene in all malignant thyroid tissues (PTC - 32 and MTC - 7 specimens) were observed.

The assay, described in this paper, was based on the determination of a $\Delta\Delta C_T$ value ($\Delta\Delta C_T$ method) for each sample (the greater was the $\Delta\Delta C_T$ value, the lower was the expression of *PIN1* gene) and on calculating the difference in *PIN1* expression level between tumour sample and calibrator (RQ value). The results for calculated RQ in the studied groups (PTC, MTC, FA, NG) are presented in Table 4. The RQ value for PTC, classic variant, ranged from 0.441 to 52.279 (the mean RQ was 8.43); for PTC, follicular variant, ranged from 0.804 to 9.124 (the mean RQ was 3.03) and for PTC, tall-cell variant, ranged from 0.363 to 12.616 (the mean RQ was 6.42).

**Table 4 The expression level (RQ) of *PIN1* gene, calculated by the $\Delta\Delta C_T$ method in the studied groups**

| Group | No. of cases | Mean RQ | Range of RQ values |
|---|---|---|---|
| PTC | 32 | 6.72 | 0.363-52.279 |
| MTC | 7 | 5.55 | 0.917-19.408 |
| FA | 7 | 2.79 | 0.511-8.207 |
| NG | 24 | 2.15 | 0.322-13.153 |

Kruskal-Wallis' test, applied for RQ comparison between the four studied groups (PTC, MTC, FA, NG), showed statistically significant differences ($p = 0.0233$) among them (Figure 1). The results of Newman-Keuls' multiple comparison test revealed statistically significant differences in RQ values only between the PTC group (higher RQ values) and the control group - NG ($p = 0.031977$). In cases of other groups, the differences in RQ values were not significant ($p > 0.05$) (Table 5). Similarly, the results of Kruskal-Wallis' test did not show any significant differences among the particular variants of PTC (PTC v. classic, PTC v. tall-cell, PTC v. follicular) ($p = 0.9501$) (Figure 2). Additionally, in the whole studied group of PTCs, no correlations were

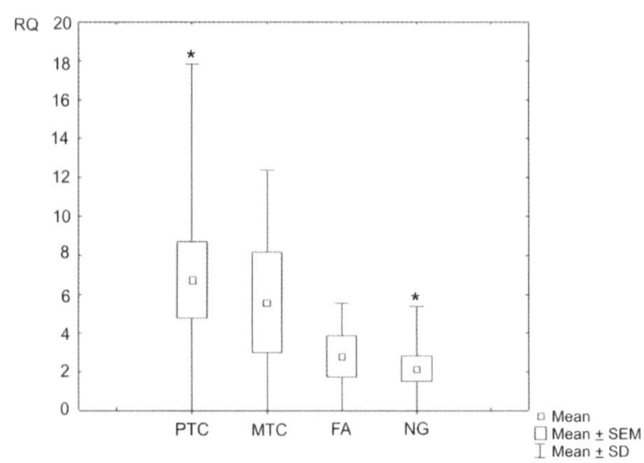


**Figure 1 Box-and-whisker plots, representing the expression of *PIN1* gene in the studied groups (PTC, MTC, FA, NG).** Results are calculated as RQ values. Whiskers represent means ± SD (standard deviation) for particular groups. Boxes represent means ± SEM (standard error of mean). The data were statistically analyzed, using Newman-Keuls' multiple comparison test, followed by Kruskal-Wallis' test, in order to compare the level of expression values (RQ) among the four studied independent groups, $p < 0.05$; * - $p < 0.031977$ (Neuman-Keuls' test).

**Table 5 Statistical analysis of results - comparison of RQ value among the four studied groups (PTC, MTC, FA, NG). Newman-Keuls' test, p - level of significance**

| | PTC | MTC | FA | NG |
|---|---|---|---|---|
| PTC | | 1.000000 | 1.000000 | **0.031977** |
| MTC | 1.000000 | | 1.000000 | 0.154248 |
| FA | 1.000000 | 1.000000 | | 1.000000 |
| NG | **0.031977** | 0.154248 | 1.000000 | |

found between *PIN1* expression level and patients' sex, age or tumour size ($p > 0.05$). The results of Mann-Whitney's U test confirmed no significant differences in RQ values between the PTC group and MTC group ($p = 0.6873$) (Figure 3).

## Discussion

The molecular pathogenesis of thyroid cancer is very complex and still unclear. Recent molecular studies on thyroid carcinogenesis have proved that many specific genetic alterations in protooncogenes are associated with development of thyroid cancer [16,17]. The mutational activation of MAPK/ERK signalling pathway is crucial to understand the carcinogenesis in the thyroid. The mutations of genes coding effectors of MAPK/ERK pathway (*RET, RAS, NTRK1, BRAF*) which rarely overlap, may be identified in more than 70% of PTC cases [18-20]. Additionally, the chromosomal rearrangements (*RET/PTC* or *Trk*) appear to be of crucial importance in activation of MAPK/ERK pathway [21,22].

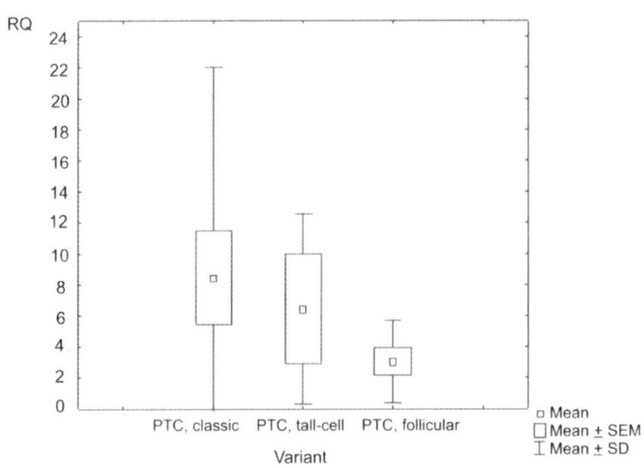


**Figure 2 Box-and-whisker plots, representing the difference in the expression of *PIN1* gene in the variants of PTC (PTC v. classic, PTC v. tall-cell, PTC v. follicular)**. Results are calculated as RQ values; no significant differences among studied groups are shown. Whiskers represent means ± SD (standard deviation) for particular groups. Boxes represent means ± SEM (standard error of mean). The results were statistically analyzed using Kruskal-Wallis' test, $p = 0.9501$.

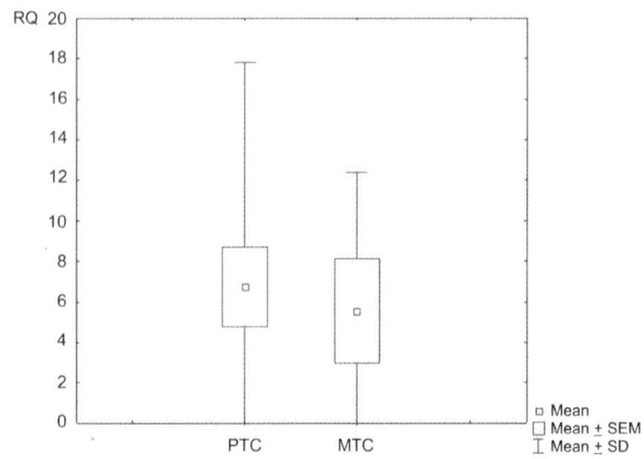


**Figure 3 Box-and-whisker plots, representing the difference in the expression of *PIN1* gene between the PTC group and the MTC group**. Results are calculated as RQ values; no significant differences between studied groups are demonstrated. Whiskers represent means ± SD (standard deviation) for particular groups. Boxes represent means ± SEM (standard error of mean). The results were statistically analyzed using Mann-Whitney's U test, $p = 0.6873$.

Despite the fact that constitutive activation of the above mentioned pathway is a very important for the development of thyroid cancer, many other molecular regulatory mechanisms, involved in thyroid cancer transformation, are recognized.

In our study, we have examined whether the *PIN1* gene participates in thyroid carcinogenesis.

The phosphorylation of proteins on serine or threonine residues preceding proline (pSer/Thr-Pro motifs), catalized by the peptidyl-prolyl *cis/trans* isomerase Pin1, has been confirmed as a major cell transformation mechanism activating different oncogenic pathways in many types of human tumours (including thyroid cancer) [9,13,23,24]. In immunohistochemical studies of thyroid tumours, as well as of other types of cancers (e.g., oral squamous carcinoma), high Pin1 expression promotes cyclin D1 overexpression, directly or through accumulation of beta-catenin [13,25]. It has been reported that *PIN1* expression is regulated by the transcription factor E2F and Neu/Ras signalling. The enhanced expression and stability of cyclin D1 by transcriptional activation and/or posttranslational stabilization by *PIN1* gene or Pin1 protein may lead to cell proliferation and transformation. Therefore, *PIN1* might be a crucial factor in modulating upregulation of cyclin D1 level by *Neu/Ras* oncogenic signalling [7,26].

Bearing in mind all these facts, in our present study, we have assessed *PIN1* gene expression level in benign and malignant thyroid lesions. In our earlier study, we demonstrated that *cyclin D1* gene expression levels were higher in malignant thyroid tumours (PTC, MTC), when compared to those in NG or FA groups [27]. Our present results have revealed statistically significant differences in expression of PIN1 mRNA between PTC group and benign thyroid lesions (FA, NG) (higher RQ value in PTC). It should be stressed that our data are in accordance with observations of other authors [13]. Nakashima et al. [13] have observed overexpression of cyclin D1 mRNA in PTC (thyroid tumours from a radiocontaminated area), taking course with high expression of *PIN1* gene. In the quoted paper, correlation between high Pin1 protein level and cyclin D1 immunoexpression level in PTC has also been confirmed [13]. It is important that Pin1 can promote cyclin D1 overexpression directly or through beta-catenin stabilization [6,13]. Our present results, which have focused on PIN1 mRNA expression, as well as our earlier data, concerning cyclin D1 mRNA overexpression in thyroid malignancy, may suggest that one of the major regulatory mechanisms in cell transformation in thyroid carcinogenesis is *PIN1* gene activity [27]. It is tempting to speculate that *PIN1* gene positively regulates *cyclin D1* gene function not only through posttranslational stabilization but also by an effect on transcriptional level.

In our present study, we have applied real-time relative quantification PCR assay for PIN1 mRNA expression and, employing this extremely sensitive and precise method, we have confirmed overexpression of *PIN1* gene in PTC. These results may suggest a diagnostic utility of PIN1 mRNA expression - as a malignant lesion marker - for thyroid PTC. However, the results should be confirmed in larger number of PTC cases. The utility of *PIN1* gene may be - in future - very crucial for diagnostics and treatment of thyroid cancer (especially of PTC), based on the facts that overexpression of Pin1 has been found to be an excellent prognostic marker in some other human cancers (e.g., prostate, breast, colorectal cancers) [8,10,23]. In these immunohistochemical studies, strong relationship between Pin1 protein level and clinical outcome has been observed [8,10,23]. Unfortunately, it is difficult to discuss the relationship between PIN1 mRNA and prognosis in PTC, because - according to our knowledge - there were no reported studies, focusing on the evaluation of *PIN1* gene expression in association with pathological features and clinical outcome of PTC, so far. Our present data have not documented any significant differences in the expression level of PIN1 mRNA among the particular variants of PTC (classic vs. tall-cell, vs. follicular variants). Moreover, no correlations were found between *PIN1* expression level and patients' sex, age or tumour size in PTC group.

In summary, *PIN1* gene expression may have - in future - certain significance in PTC diagnostics and in understanding its pathogenesis. However, our results - due to the small number of cases - do not yet allow considering *PIN1* gene as a prognostic molecular PTC marker.

**Acknowledgements**
This study was supported by the funds from the Medical University of Lodz, Poland (project no. 502-11-570).

**Author details**
[1]Department of Endocrinology and Metabolic Diseases, Medical University of Lodz, Poland. [2]Department of Endocrinology and Metabolic Diseases, Polish Mother's Memorial Hospital - Research Institute, Lodz, Poland. [3]Department of Molecular Basis of Medicine, Medical University of Lodz, Poland. [4]Department of General and Colorectal Surgery, Medical University of Lodz, Poland.

**Authors' contributions**
AL designed and coordinated the study and wrote the manuscript; EB and KC carried out the molecular genetic studies; JL participated in performing molecular studies; WK coordinated the collection of tissue samples; AC-M participated in performing molecular studies and drafted the manuscript.

**Competing interests**
The authors declare that they have no competing interests.

**References**

1. Joseph JD, Yeh ES, Swenson KI, Means AR, Winkler KE: The peptidyl-prolyl isomerase Pin1. *Prog Cell Cycle Res* 2003, 5:477-487.
2. Campbell HD, Webb GC, Fountain S, Young IG: The human PIN1 peptidyl-prolyl cis/trans isomerase gene maps to human chromosome 19p13 and the closely related PIN1L gene to 1p31. *Genomics* 1997, 44:157-162.
3. Stukenberg PT, Kirschner MW: Pin1 acts catalytically to promote a conformational change in Cdc 25. *Mol Cell* 2001, 7:1071-1083.
4. Wulf GM, Ryo A, Wulf GG, Lee SW, Niu T, Petkova V, Lu KP: Pin1 is overexpressed in breast cancer and cooperates with Ras signaling in increasing the transcriptional activity of c-Jun towards cyclin D1. *EMBO J* 2001, 20:3459-3472.
5. Wulf GM, Liou YC, Ryo A, Lee SW, Lu KP: Role of Pin1 in the regulation of p53 stability and p21 transactivation, and cell cycle checkpoints in response to DNA damage. *J Biol Chem* 2002, 277:47976-47979.
6. Ryo A, Nakamura M, Wulf G, Liou YC, Lu KP: Pin1 regulates turnover and subcellular localization of beta-catenin by inhibiting its interaction with APC. *Nat Cell Biol* 2001, 3:793-801.
7. Ryo A, Liou YC, Wulf G, Nakamura M, Lee SW, Lu KP: PIN1 is an E2F target gene essential for Neu/Ras-induced transformation of mammary epithelial cells. *Mol Cell Biol* 2002, 22:5281-5295.
8. Ayala G, Wang D, Wulf G, Frolov A, Li R, Sowadski J, Wheeler TM, Lu KP, Bao L: The prolyl isomerase Pin1 is a novel prognostic marker in human prostate cancer. *Cancer Res* 2003, 63:6244-6251.
9. Bao L, Kimzey A, Sauter G, Sowadski JM, Lu KP, Wang DG: Prevalent overexpression of prolyl isomerase Pin1 in human cancers. *Am J Pathol* 2004, 164:1727-1737.
10. Wulf G, Ryo A, Liou YC, Lu KP: The prolyl isomerase Pin1 in breast development and cancer. *Breast Cancer Res* 2003, 5:76-82.
11. Rippmann JF, Hobbie S, Daiber C, Guillard B, Bauer M, Birk J, Nar H, Garin-Chesa P, Rettig WJ, Schnapp A: Phosphorylation-dependent proline isomerization catalyzed by Pin1 is essential for tumor cell survival and entry into mitosis. *Cell Growth Differ* 2000, 11:409-416.
12. Takahashi K, Uchida C, Shin RW, Shimazaki K, Uchida T: Prolyl isomerase, Pin1: new findings of post-translational modifications and physiological substrates in cancer, asthma and Alzheimer's disease. *Cell Mol Life Sci* 2008, 65:359-375.
13. Nakashima M, Meirmanov S, Naruke Y, Kondo H, Saenko V, Rogounovitch T, Shimizu-Yoshida Y, Takamura N, Namba H, Ito M, Abrosimov A, Lushnikov E, Roumiantsev P, Tsyb A, Yamashita S, Sekine I: Cyclin D1 overexpression in thyroid tumours from a radio-contaminated area and its correlation with Pin1 and aberrant beta-catenin expression. *J Pathol* 2004, 202:446-455.

14. DeLellis RA, Lloyd RV, Heitz PU, Eng C, (eds): **World Health Organization classification of tumours: Pathology and genetics of tumours of endocrine organs.** IARC Press, Lyon; 2004.
15. American Joint Committee on Cancer: **Thyroid.** *AJCC Cancer Staging Manual.* 6 edition. New York, NY: Springer; 2002, 77-87.
16. Lewiński A, Ferenc T, Sporny S, Jarząb B: **Thyroid carcinoma: diagnostic and therapeutic approach; genetic background.** *Endocr Regul* 2000, **34**:99-113.
17. Lewiński A, Wojciechowska K: **Genetic background of carcinogenesis in the thyroid gland.** *Neuroendocrinol Lett* 2007, **28**:77-105.
18. Kimura ET, Nikiforova MN, Zhu Z, Knauf JA, Nikiforov YE, Fagin JA: **High prevalence of BRAF mutations in thyroid cancer: genetic evidence for constitutive activation of the RET/PTC-RAS-BRAF signaling pathway in papillary thyroid carcinoma.** *Cancer Res* 2003, **63**:1454-1457.
19. Soares P, Trovisco V, Rocha AS, Lima J, Castro P, Preto A, Maximo V, Botelho T, Seruca R, Sobrinho-Simoes M: **BRAF mutations and RET/PTC rearrangements are alternative events in the pathogenesis of PTC.** *Oncogene* 2003, **22**:4578-4580.
20. Frattini M, Ferrario C, Bressan P, Balestra D, De Cecco L, Mondellini P, Bongarzone I, Collini P, Gariboldi M, Pilotti S, Pierotti MA, Greco A: **Alternative mutations of BRAF, RET, and NTRK1 are associated with similar but distinct gene expression patterns in papillary thyroid cancer.** *Oncogene* 2004, **23**:7436-7440.
21. Santoro M, Melillo RM, Fusco A: **RET/PTC activation in papillary thyroid carcinoma: European Journal of Endocrinology Prize Lecture.** *Eur J Endocrinol* 2006, **155**:645-653.
22. Brzeziańska E, Karbownik M, Migdalska-Sęk M, Pastuszak-Lewandoska D, Włoch J, Lewiński A: **Molecular analysis of the RET and NTRK1 gene rearrangements in papillary thyroid carcinoma in the Polish population.** *Mutat Res* 2006, **599**:26-35.
23. Kuramochi J, Arai T, Ikeda S, Kumagai J, Uetake H, Sugihara K: **High Pin1 expression is associated with tumor progression in colorectal cancer.** *J Surg Oncol* 2006, **94**:155-160.
24. Zhou CX, Gao Y: **Aberrant expression of beta-catenin, Pin1 and cyclin D1 in salivary adenoid cystic adenoma: relation to tumor proliferation and metastasis.** *Oncol Rep* 2006, **16**:505-511.
25. Leung KW, Tsai CH, Hsiao M, Tseng CJ, Ger LP, Lee KH, Lu PJ: **Pin1 overexpression is associated with poor differentiation and survival in oral squamous cell carcinoma.** *Oncol Rep* 2009, **21**:1097-1104.
26. Liou YC, Ryo A, Huang HK, Lu PJ, Bronson R, Fujimori F, Uchida T, Hunter T, Lu KP: **Loss of Pin1 function in the mouse causes phenotypes resembling cyclin D1-null phenotypes.** *Proc Natl Acad Sci USA* 2002, **99**:1335-1340.
27. Brzeziańska E, Cyniak-Magierska A, Sporny S, Pastuszak-Lewandoska D, Lewiński A: **Assessment of *cyclin D1* gene expression as a prognostic factor in benign and malignant thyroid lesions.** *Neuroendocrinol Lett* 2007, **28**:341-350.

# 15

# Histological subtype is the most important determinant of survival in metastatic papillary thyroid cancer

Alexandra Chrisoulidou[1†], Maria Boudina[1†], Athanasios Tzemailas[2], Eleni Doumala[1], Pashalia K Iliadou[1], Frideriki Patakiouta[3] and Kalliopi Pazaitou-Panayiotou[1*]

**Abstract**

**Background:** Papillary thyroid cancer (PTC) comprises the commonest type of thyroid cancer and carries the highest rate of survival. However, when metastatic disease occurs, survival is significantly affected.

**Methods:** We aimed to identify prognostic histopathological and clinical factors that modify survival in metastatic PTC. All cases of metastatic PTC treated at our department in the last 20 years were reviewed and analyzed.

**Results:** Histological subtype was the most important determinant of survival, as classic PTC demonstrated clearly improved survival compared to follicular subtype of PTC and other less frequently seen histological subtypes. The instant risk of death for the other histological subtypes was 4.56 times higher than the risk for the classic papillary type. Overall, a 10-year survival of 76.6% in our patients was seen.

**Conclusions:** Patients with aggressive variants of PTC are more at risk for the development of metastatic disease. In these patients, established treatment modalities (surgery, radioiodine therapy) should be offered promptly, as well as close follow-up.

**Keywords:** papillary thyroid carcinoma, distant metastases

## Background

Differentiated thyroid cancer, comprising papillary and follicular thyroid cancer, generally carries a good prognosis. Papillary thyroid cancer (PTC) is the most frequent type of thyroid malignancy and its metastases are usually lymphatic [1]. The risk of distant metastases, usually to the lung, mediastinal lymph nodes and bone, is greater in follicular than in papillary carcinoma [2]. Distant metastases from PTC may occur with a frequency ranging from 1.73-8.4% in most studies [3,4]. The most common site of distant metastases from PTC is the lung followed by mediastinal lymph nodes [5]. Less often, distant metastases may appear in bones [6], central nervous system [7,8], liver [9], pericardium and pleura [10], kidney [11], pancreas [12], skin and muscle [13], gastrointestinal tract [14]. As effective treatment may not exist for many of these patients, it is of paramount importance to identify, if possible, those who are at greater risk for developing metastatic disease.

A limited number of retrospective studies have analyzed the prognostic factors, which affect clinical outcome in metastatic PTC. Prognostic factors as sex and age, tumor size, histologic type, tumor infiltration, vascular or lymphatic invasion, have been shown to affect survival in these patients [15]. However, most studies looked into prognostic factors in differentiated thyroid cancer, including both papillary and follicular thyroid cancer in the analysis. In recent years, marked differences in prognostic factors, clinicopathologic features and treatment necessitate the distinction of these two entities [4]. Even in patients with metastatic disease, the overall survival in papillary thyroid cancer is higher than in follicular cancer [16].

In this retrospective study we aimed to investigate patients with metastatic PTC only in order to delineate

* Correspondence: kpazaitou@in.gr
† Contributed equally
[1]Department of Endocrinology & Endocrine Oncology, Theagenio Cancer Hospital, Thessaloniki 54007, Greece
Full list of author information is available at the end of the article

specific prognostic factors affecting survival in this rare entity. Within this group, we subdivided patients according to histologic subtype, and studied the clinical and histological characteristics and the received treatment modalities during a mean follow-up of 9 years. Using multivariate analysis, we estimated the factors that significantly affect survival in metastatic PTC.

## Patients and methods

We retrospectively reviewed the records of 1550 patients who had PTC. From this cohort, we identified 52 patients (29 females and 23 males) who presented with or developed (during follow up) distant metastatic disease. For all patients we collected data regarding histological features, age at diagnosis, site of distant metastases, treatment modalities and outcome of the disease. All patients were followed up at the Department of Endocrinology & Endocrine Oncology of Theagenio Cancer Hospital from 1988-2009. Patients' characteristics are shown in Table 1. Tumor, lymph nodes and metastases (TNM) staging at the time of diagnosis is shown in table 2.

The diagnosis of distant metastases was based on whole body scan findings and elevated thyroglobulin levels and was verified by computed tomography or MRI. Whenever feasible, biopsy of the metastatic lesions confirmed the diagnosis. Upper mediastinal metastases were not considered as distant. Metastases were classified according to the site of involvement. Histological classification was in accordance with WHO classification 2004 [17].

In all patients work-up included 1) measurements of thyroglobulin, TSH and free thyroxine on suppressive therapy and 2) neck ultrasound annually. Diagnostic

**Table 1 Characteristics of the 52 patients with metastatic PTC**

| | Number of patients | Number of deaths (%) |
|---|---|---|
| **Age (years)** | | |
| > 19 | 7 (4F/3M) | 1 (1M) (14.3%) |
| 19-45 | 10 (6F/4M) | 4 (3F/1M) (40.0%) |
| < 45 | 35 (19F/16M) | 16 (6F/10M) (45.7%) |
| **Sex** | | |
| Males | 23 | 12 |
| Females | 29 | 9 |
| **Histology** | | |
| Classic papillary | 24 | |
| Follicular variant | 20 | |
| Papillary with low differentiation of the cells | 6 | |
| Insular | 1 | |
| Columnar | 1 | |
| **Size of tumor (mm)** | 33 (7-80) | |
| **Multifocal tumors** | 27 (15F/12M) | |
| **Bilateral tumors** | 25 (13F/12M) | |
| **Invasion of tumor capsule** | 4 | |
| **Absence of tumor capsule** | 34 | |
| **Thyroid capsule invasion** | 43 | |
| **Extrathyroidal invasion** | 38 | |
| **Vascular infiltration** | 17 | |
| **Presence of metastases** | | |
| At diagnosis | 17 | |
| During follow-up | 35 | |
| **Years of follow-up (years)** | 8 (1-29) | |
| **Thyroidectomy** | | |
| TT | 46 | |
| NTT | 6 | |
| **Total RAI dose (mCi)** | 360 (100-1500) | |
| **Thyroglobulin at 1st RAI** | 121 (1.9-4000) | |

Data as median (range); F: female, M: male, TT: total thyroidectomy, NTT: near total thyroidectomy.

**Table 2 TNM staging of patients at initial diagnosis**

| | N0 (n = 20) | | | N1 (n = 32) | | | Total (n = 52) |
|---|---|---|---|---|---|---|---|
| | n | | n | n | | n | n |
| *T1* | | M0 | 2 | | M0 | 1 | |
| | 3 | M1 | 1 | 3 | M1 | 2 | 6 |
| T2 | | M0 | 1 | | M0 | 2 | |
| | 1 | M1 | 0 | 3 | M1 | 1 | 4 |
| T3 | | M0 | 10 | | M0 | 9 | |
| | 12 | M1 | 2 | 16 | M1 | 7 | 28 |
| T4 | | M0 | 2 | | M0 | 3 | |
| | 4 | M1 | 2 | 10 | M1 | 7 | 14 |

T: tumor, N: lymph nodes, M: metastases, n represents the number of patients in each category

According to AJCC Cancer Staging Manual, Sixth Edition (2002) published by Springer-Verlag, Inc., New York.

**Table 3 Factors considered for prediction of survival**

| Factor | Significance |
|---|---|
| Sex | 0.523 |
| Age | 0.132 |
| Histology | 0.004 |
| Multifocality | 0.887 |
| Bilaterality | 0.292 |
| Type of surgery | 0.603 |
| Size of tumor | 0.392 |
| Lymph node metastases at operation | 0.263 |
| Thyroid parenchyma invasion | 0.502 |
| Thyroid capsule invasion | 0.095 |
| Extrathyroidal invasion | 0.863 |
| Vessel invasion | 0.058 |
| Metastatic disease from diagnosis | 0.180 |
| First site of metastasis | 0.874 |
| Uptake at ablation | 0.568 |
| TSH on T4 withdrawal | 0.782 |
| Thyroglobulin on T4 withdrawal | 0.799 |
| Total 131 I mCi | 0.426 |
| Years to metastasis | 0.115 |

whole body scans and thyroglobulin after thyroxine withdrawal were performed at 9-12 months after treatment with $^{131}$I and when necessary thereafter. The Institutional Review Board approved the study.

### Statistical analysis

The Cox proportional hazards model was used for the assessment of possible predictors of survival. Variables with $p < 0.20$ in the univariate analysis were included in the multivariate analysis. Forward stepwise methodology was used for the multivariate analysis. Variables with $p < 0.05$ were considered statistically significant in this step. Kaplan-Meier plots were constructed in order to depict survival. PASW 18.0 (IBM-SPSS Inc., Chicago, IL) was used for data analysis. Factors considered for prediction of survival were summarised in Table 3.

## Results

Fifty-two patients (29 females and 23 males) were found to have distant metastases. Most patients were above 45 years of age (35 out of 52 patients). Twenty-two patients (42.3%) had distant metastases at the time of diagnosis (11 women and 11 men) and 30 patients (57.7%) developed metastatic disease during follow-up. Tumor size was ≥ 2 cm in 39 patients. Regional lymph node metastases were present in 30 patients. All patients had total or near total thyroidectomy. Clinical characteristics of the patients and specific characteristics of the tumors are shown in Table 1.

Twenty-four patients had classic papillary thyroid cancer, 20 patients follicular variant of papillary cancer, 1 had papillary carcinoma with insular components and 1 patient had columnar cell variant of papillary carcinoma. The remaining 6 cases exhibited papillary cancer with low differentiation of the cells (with focal follicular elements in 2 patients).

The commonest sites of metastatic disease were lung (32 patients), followed by bone (13 patients), lower mediastinum (6 patients) extracervical soft tissue (4 patients), central nervous system (4 patients), pleura (4 patients), liver (1 patient), and oeshophagus (1 patient). Multiple site metastases were found in 14 patients.

Table 3 indicates the factors affecting survival in our series: histology comprised the most significant factor in the analysis, the classic papillary type carrying significantly improved survival than follicular and other subtypes of papillary thyroid cancer. The instant risk of death for the other histological subtypes was 4.56 times higher than the risk for the classic papillary type. The other parameters tested did not affect survival significantly.

Mortality ranged according to age (table 1), with the worst outcome in patients above 45 years of age. Overall 5-year survival in metastatic papillary thyroid cancer was 88.2%, 10-year 76.6% and 15-year survival 35.8% (for 10 patients). Cumulative survival is shown in Figure 1.

## Discussion

Only a few studies so far examined specific factors affecting survival in patients with PTC, as in most studies patients with papillary and follicular thyroid cancer were included. The striking finding in this study was that histological variant plays the most significant role in patient's survival in metastatic PTC. The classic papillary type of PTC demonstrated improved prognosis compared to other papillary cancer variants.

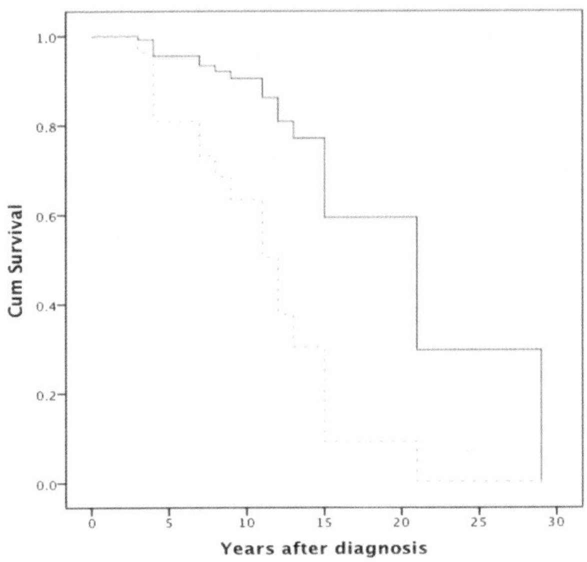


**Figure 1 Survival over time in patients with classic PTC** (continuous line) and PTC variants (dotted line).

Although papillary thyroid carcinoma carries the most favorable prognosis amongst all types of thyroid cancer, distant metastatic disease may occur with subsequent compromise in patient's survival. Even in the presence of metastatic disease, papillary thyroid cancer in our series has an overall 10-year survival of 76.6%. In general, disease-related mortality varies greatly in PTC: papillary microcarcinomas exhibit no mortality at all [18], even in the presence of distant metastases [19]. In other series with larger PTCs, 10-year survival ranged from 14-80% [20-22], with limited survival in older patients. Old age is a predictor of worse prognosis, although an exact cut off point was not uniformly identified [23]. In this study, we did not observe statistical differences in survival according to age, although we also observed an increase in mortality in patients above 45 years of age.

Previous studies indicated many factors, as capsular infiltration, extrathyroidal extension and lymph node metastases at diagnosis as unfavorable prognostic factors for persistent disease or recurrences [24]. Cervical lymph node metastases have been related to poor prognosis occurring synchronously or metachronously to diagnosis [25], although this was not seen in the present study. Extranodal invasion and perithyroidal invasion to muscles and soft tissues showed a higher incidence of distant metastases and death [26]. The presence of vessel invasion was associated, as in other reports, with poor prognosis, although in our series this association had a marginal significance (Table 2).

Although differentiated thyroid cancer is frequently seen in women, in patients with metastatic PTC the female: male ratio was 1.26:1, in accordance with the general notion that male gender adversely affects outcome in differentiated thyroid cancer. In the studied group 52% of males and 31% of females died during follow-up, however this was not significant probably due to small numbers. Histology increased nearly 5-fold the risk of death in patients with PTC variants other than the classic papillary type.

In keeping with other reports, we observed lung as the primary metastatic site, followed by bone, multiple site involvement and other, less frequently seen, affected organs. The development of rare metastases, as CNS, liver and extracervical soft tissue metastases, indicates the importance of close clinical follow-up in these patients.

In conclusion, the histological subtype in metastatic PTC determines survival in a significant way. As a result, patients with follicular and other uncommon subtypes of PTC that present with or develop distant metastatic disease should be vigorously treated with surgery, where appropriate, radioiodine therapy and should also be considered for inclusion to studies concerning new therapies, like tyrosine kinase inhibitors.

**Author details**

[1]Department of Endocrinology & Endocrine Oncology, Theagenio Cancer Hospital, Thessaloniki 54007, Greece. [2]Department of Nuclear Medicine, Theagenio Cancer Hospital, Thessaloniki 54007, Greece. [3]Department of Pathology, Theagenio Cancer Hospital, Thessaloniki, Greece.

**Authors' contributions**

KPP conceived and coordinated the study. MB, PKI, ED gathered the data. MB and AT prepared the database and inserted the relevant data. FP examined the histological material. AC did the statistical analysis and drafted the tables. KPP and AC wrote the manuscript. All authors read and approved the final manuscript.

**Competing interests**

The authors declare that they have no competing interests.

**References**

1. Salter KD, Andersen PE, Cohen JI, Schuff KG, Lester L, Shindo ML, Sauer D, Gross ND: Central node metastases in papillary thyroid carcinoma based on tumor histologic type and focality. *Arch Otolaryngol Head Neck Surg* 2010, **136**:692-696.
2. Maxon HR, Smith HS: Radioiodine-131 in the diagnosis and treatment of metastatic well-differentiated thyroid cancer. *Endocrinol Metab Clin North Am* 1990, **19**:685-671.
3. Sugitani I, Fujomoto Y, Yamamoto N: Papillary thyroid cancer with distant metastases:survival predictors and the importance of local control. *Surgery* 2008, **143**:35-42.
4. Lang BH-H, Lo CY, Chan WF, Lam AK, Wan KY: Classical and follicular variant of papillary thyroid carcinoma: a comparative study on clinicopathologic features and long-term outcome. *World J Surg* 2006, **30**:752-758.
5. Lin JD, Chao TC, Chou SC, Hsueh C: Papillary thyroid carcinomas with lung metastases. *Thyroid* 2004, **14**:1091-1096.
6. Do MY, Rhee Y, Kim DJ, Kim CS, Nam KH, Ahn CW, Cha BA, Kim KR, Lee HC, Park CS, Lim SK: Clinical features of bone metastases resulting from thyroid cancer: a review of 28 patients over a 20-year period. *Endocr J* 2005, **52**:701-707.

7. Parker LN, Wu SY, Kim DD, Kollin J, Prasasvinichai S: Recurrence of papillary thyroid carcinoma presenting as focal neurologic deficit. *Arch Intern Med* 1986, **146**:1985-1987.
8. Holmquest DL, Lake P: Sudden hemorrhage in metastatic thyroid carcinoma of the brain during treatment with iodine-131. *J Nucl Med* 1976, **17**:307-309.
9. Agriantonis DJ, Hall L, Wilson MA: Utility of SPECT/CT as an adjunct planar whole body I-131 imaging: liver metastases from papillary thyroid cancer. *Clin Nucl Med* 2009, **34**:247-248.
10. Mizukami Y, Michigishi T, Nonomura A, Hashimoto T, Terahata S, Nogushi M, Hisada K, Matsubara F: Distant metastases differentiated thyroid carcinomas: a clinical and pathologic study. *Hum Pathol* 1990, **21**:283-290.
11. Sardi A, Agnone DM, Pellegrini A: Renal metastasis from papillary thyroid cancer. *J Louisiana State Med Soc* 1992, **144**:416-420.
12. Borschitz T, Eichhorn W, Fottner C, Hansen T, Schad A, Schadmand-Fischer S, Weber MM, Schreckenberger M, Lang H, Musholt TJ: Diagnosis and treatment of pancreatic metastases of a papillary thyroid carcinoma. *Thyroid* 2010, **20**:93-98.
13. Bruglia M, Palmonella G, Silvetti F, Rutigliano P, Criante P, Marmorale C, Boscaro M, Taccaliti A: Skin and thigh muscle metastasis from papillary thyroid carcinoma. *Singapore Med J* 2009, **50**:61-64.
14. Klubo-Gwiezdzinska J, Morowitz D, Van Nortrand D, Burman KD, Vasko V, Chia S, Deng T, Kulkarni K, Wartofsky L: Metastases of well-differentiated thyroid cancer to the gastrointestinal tract. *Thyroid* 2010, **20**:381-387.
15. Showalter TN, Siegel BA, Moley JF, Baranski TJ, Grisby PW: Prognostic factors in patients with well-differentiated thyroid cancer presenting with pulmonary metastasis. *Cancer Biother Radiopharm* 2008, **23**:655-659.
16. Benbassat CA, Mechlis-Frish S, Hirsch D: Clinicopathological characteristics and long-term outcome in patients with distant metastases from differentiated thyroid cancer. *World J Surg* 2006, **30**:1088-1095.
17. De Lellis RA, Lloyd RV, Heinz PU, Eng C, editors: World Health Organization Classification of Tumours.Pathology and Genetics-Tumours of Endocrine Organs. *IARC Press* Lyon; 2004.
18. Roti E, Rossi R, Trasforini G, Bertelli F, Ambrosio MR, Busutti L, Pearce EN, Braverman LE, Degli Uberti EC: Clinical and histological characteristics of papillary thyroid microcarcinoma: results of a retrospective study in 243 patients. *J Clin Endocrinol Metab* 2006, **91**:2171-2178.
19. Pellegriti G, Scollo C, Lumera G, Regalbuto C, Vigneri R, Belfiore A: Clinical behaviour and outcome of papillary thyroid cancers smaller than 1.5 cm in diameter: study of 299 cases. *J Clin Endocrinol Metab* 2004, **89**:3713-3720.
20. Dinneen SF, Valimaki MJ, Bergstralh EJ, Goellner JR, Gorman CA, Hay ID: Distant metastases in papillary thyroid carcinoma: 100 cases observed at one institution during 5 decades. *J Clin Endocrinol Metab* 1995, **80**:2041-2045.
21. Durante C, Haddy N, Baudin E, Leboulleux S, Hartl D, Travagli JP, Caillou B, Ricard M, Lumbroso JD, De Vathaire F, Schlumberger M: Long-term outcome of 444 patients with distant metastases from papillary and follicular thyroid carcinoma:benefits and limits of radioiodine therapy. *J Clin Endocrinol Metab* 2006, **91**:2892-2899.
22. Ito Y, Masuoka H, Fukushima M, Inoue H, Kihara M, Tomoda C, Higashiyama T, Takamura Y, Kobayashi K, Miya A, Miyauchi A: Prognosis and prognostic factors of patients with papillary carcinoma showing distant metastasis at surgery. *Endocr J* 2010, **57**:523-531.
23. Kakudo K, Tang W, Ito Y, Nakamura Y, Yasuoka H, Morita S, Miyauchi A: Papillary carcinoma of the thyroid in Japan: subclassification of common type and identification of low risk group. *J Clin Pathol* 2004, **57**:1041-1046.
24. Mercante G, Frasoldati A, Pedroni C, Formisano D, Renna L, Piana S, Gardini G, Valcani R, Barbieri V: Prognostic factors affecting neck lymph node recurrence and distant metastasis in papillary microcarcinoma of the thyroid:results of a study in 445 patients. *Thyroid* 2009, **19**:707-716.
25. Baek SK, Jung KY, Kang SM, Kwon SY, Woo JS, Cho SH, Chung EJ: Clinical risk factors associated with cervical lymph node recurrence in papillary thyroid carcinoma. *Thyroid* 2010, **20**:147-152.
26. Sebastian SO, Gonzalez JM, Paricio PP, Perez JS, Flores DP, Madrona AP, Romero PR, Tebar FJ: Papillary thyroid carcinoma:prognostic index for survival including the histologic variety. *Arch Surg* 2000, **135**:272-277.

# 16

# Assessment of *RET/PTC1* and *RET/PTC3* rearrangements in fine-needle aspiration biopsy specimens collected from patients with Hashimoto's thyroiditis

Anna Cyniak-Magierska[1,2], Katarzyna Wojciechowska-Durczyńska[1,2], Kinga Krawczyk-Rusiecka[1,2], Arkadiusz Zygmunt[1,2], Andrzej Lewiński[1,2*]

**Abstract**

**Background:** *RET/PTC* rearrangements are the most frequent molecular changes in papillary thyroid carcinoma (PTC). So far, 15 main *RET/PTC* rearrangements have been described, among which *RET/PTC1* and *RET/PTC3* are the most common in PTC - especially in radiation-induced tumours. *RET/PTC1* and *RET/PTC3* are the result of intrachromosomal paracentric inversions in chromosome 10, where *RET* and the activating genes (*H4* and *ELE1*, respectively) are located. Recently, *RET/PTC* rearrangements have been shown not only in PTC but also in benign thyroid lesions, including Hashimoto's thyroiditis (HT). The aim of study was an assessment of *RET/PTC1* and *RET/PTC3* rearrangements in patients with Hashimoto's thyroiditis.

**Materials and methods:** Thyroid aspirates, eligible for the study, were obtained from 26 patients with Hashimoto's thyroiditis by fine-needle aspiration biopsy (FNAB). Each aspirate was smeared for conventional cytology, while its remaining part was immediately washed out of the needle. The cells, obtained from the needle, were used in further investigation. Total RNA from FNAB was extracted by use of an RNeasy Micro Kit, based on modified Chomczynski and Sacchi's method and reverse transcription (RT-PCR) was done. Quantitative evaluation of *RET/PTC1* and *RET/PTC3* rearrangements by real-time PCR was performed by an ABI PRISM® 7500 Sequence Detection System. In the study, PTC tissues with known *RET/PTC1* and *RET/PTC3* rearrangements served as a reference standard (calibrator), while *β-actin* gene was used as endogenous control.

**Results:** Amplification reactions were done in triplicate for each examined sample. No *RET/PTC1* and *RET/PTC3* rearrangements were found in the examined samples.

**Conclusions:** Our results indicate that *RET/PTC1* and *RET/PTC3* rearrangements in Hashimoto's thyroiditis, if any, are rather rare events and further investigations should be conducted in order to determine molecular changes, connecting Hashimoto's thyroiditis with PTC.

## Background

Chromosomal rearrangements involving *RET* receptor tyrosine kinase (TK) protooncogene (*RET/PTC*) are a specific feature of papillary thyroid carcinoma (PTC). The *RET* protooncogene is activated by fusion of 3'-terminal portion of *RET*, coding for TK domain, with the 5' terminal region of different unrelated genes, leading to constitutive activation of the *RET* TK [1]. There are - at least -15 different *RET/PTC* rearrangements [2], but the two: *RET/PTC1* and *RET/PTC3* are the most common ones [3]. *RET/PTC1* is formed by fusion with the *H4* gene [1], and *RET/PTC3* by fusion with the *ELE1* (also designed *NCOA4*, *RFG* or *ARA70*) gene [4]. However, apart from *RET/PTC1* and *RET/PTC3*, all the other variants of rearrangements do not seem to have

* Correspondence: alewin@csk.umed.lodz.pl
[1]Department of Endocrinology and Metabolic Diseases, Medical University of Lodz, Poland
Full list of author information is available at the end of the article

an important role in the pathogenesis of PTC since they have been isolated just in rare cases [5].

Chromosomal rearrangements of *RET* in PTC were found with different frequency, depending on geographic variability and studied population. The reported frequency of *RET/PTC* in PTC varies from 0 to 87% [6]. It is interesting that the frequency of *RET/PTC* rearrangements not only depends on geographical region but also on applied technique of identification [6].

The relatively high prevalence of *RET/PTC* rearrangements was described in tumours associated with radiation exposure [7]. The higher prevalence of *RET/PTC3* activation in PTC was observed in the contaminated areas after Chernobyl explosion [7]. The analysis of PTC, which developed after a long latency period after explosion showed higher prevalence of *RET/PTC1* rearrangements [8]. This can suggest that *RET/PTC3* rearrangements may be typical for radiation-induced childhood PTC with a short latency period, while *RET/PTC1* rearrangements may be a marker for later-occurring PTC of radiation-exposed children and adults [8]. *RET/PTC* rearrangements have not been found in follicular thyroid carcinomas and anaplastic thyroid carcinomas [9].

Recently, *RET/PTC* rearrangements have been shown not only in PTC but also in Hürthle thyroid adenomas and carcinomas and also in Hashimoto's thyroiditis (HT) [10,11].

The prevalence of *RET/PTC* rearrangements in HT is still controversial. The study aimed at estimating the frequency of rearrangements of *RET* protooncogene in HT in the Polish population.

**Table 1 Characteristics of HT patients involved in the study**

| Case number | Sex | Age | Diagnosis |
|---|---|---|---|
| 1 | F | 68 | HT |
| 2 | F | 67 | HT |
| 3 | F | 48 | HT |
| 4 | F | 45 | HT |
| 5 | F | 37 | HT |
| 6 | F | 68 | HT |
| 7 | F | 18 | HT |
| 8 | F | 53 | HT |
| 9 | F | 31 | HT |
| 10 | F | 52 | HT |
| 11 | F | 63 | HT |
| 12 | F | 54 | HT |
| 13 | F | 83 | HT |
| 14 | F | 88 | HT |
| 15 | F | 39 | HT |
| 16 | F | 50 | HT |
| 17 | F | 51 | HT |
| 18 | F | 41 | HT |
| 19 | F | 41 | HT |
| 20 | F | 49 | HT |
| 21 | F | 38 | HT |
| 22 | F | 65 | HT |
| 23 | F | 51 | HT |
| 24 | F | 54 | HT |
| 25 | F | 63 | HT |
| 26 | M | 57 | HT |

## Materials and methods

The Ethical Committee of the Medical University of Lodz approved the studies in this paper.

### Patients

Thyroid aspirates, eligible for this study, were obtained from patients undergoing FNAB for Hashimoto's thyroiditis. All tissue samples were taken after patients' informed consent was obtained. FNAB specimens from 26 patients (25 women, 1 man) were examined. Data characterising the patients involved in the study are presented in Table 1. The mean age of patients was 52.8 ± 15.4 years (mean ± SD), ranging from 18 to 88 years.

Thyroiditis was diagnosed, according to clinical symptoms and signs, together with data of hormonal and immunological tests and the results of cytological evaluation of FNAB specimens, collected under ultrasound guidance.

Ultrasound-guided FNAB was performed with the use of a 22-gauge needle and each aspirate was smeared for conventional cytology, while the remaining material was immediately washed out of the needle with 350 μl of RLT lysis buffer, containing β-mercaptoethanol and guanidine thiocyanate, used for RNA isolation (Qiagen, Germany). The samples were immediately frozen at -70°C and, thus, stored until total RNA isolation. The samples, containing visible blood contamination, were disqualified from further investigations.

### RNA extraction from FNAB

Total RNA from FNAB was extracted with the use of RNeasy Micro Kit (Qiagen, Germany). The manufacturer's instructions were followed, except that the cell lysate was applied for the second time to the column before the wash-step was carried out. The quality and quantity of total RNA was spectrophotometrically measured and - for some samples - with an Agilent 2100 Bioanalyzer.

### Reverse transcription

Reverse transcription (RT) was performed, using the whole RNA, extracted with TaqMan® Reverse Transcripton Reagents (Applied Biosystems, Branchburg,

New Jersey, USA). RT reaction mixture contained 5 μl of 10 × TaqMan RT Buffer (100 mM Tris-HCl pH 8.3, 500 mM KCl), 11.0 μl 25 mM $MgCl_2$, 1.25 μl Multi Scribe™ reverse transcriptase (50 U/μl), 2.5 μl 50 μM oligo$(dT)_{16}$, 1.0 μl RNase Inhibitor - RI (20 U/μl), and 10 μl 10 mM dNTPs in a total volume of 50 μl. RNAs were incubated for 10 minutes at 25°C, followed by 30 minutes at 48°C and 5 minutes at 95°C to inactivate reverse transcriptase (Multi Scribe™). Negative controls were performed simultaneously to eliminate a possible genomic DNA contamination (no reverse transcriptase reactions), as well as to eliminate a possible contamination of RT reagents (no RNA-added reactions).

### Real-time quantitative PCR

An established Relative Quantification Polymerase Chain Reaction (RQ-PCR) assay for *RET/PTC1* and *RET/PTC3* mRNA expressions, using the relative quantification method ($\Delta\Delta C_T$) were conducted in ABI PRISM 7500 Sequence Detection System (Applied Biosystems), according to the manufacturer's protocol. The PCR reactions for *RET/PTC1* and *RET/PTC3* rearrangements of genes were run with 50 ng of cDNA in a total volume of 50 μl, using TaqMan® Universal PCR Master Mix (Applied Biosystems, Foster City, CA, USA) and the predesigned and labelled primer/probe set (Applied Biosystems, Foster City, CA, USA). Sequences of primers and probes used for this study were reported and validated according to Rhoden's *et al.* protocol (Table 2) [12]. After initial incubation at 50°C for 2 min to allow uracil-N-glycosylase (UNG) digestion, and at 95°C for 10 min to activate the AmpliTaq Gold®DNA polymerase, both of them were provided by the Universal PCR Master Mix, the samples were amplified through 45 biphasic cycles of 95°C for 15 sec and 60°C for 1 min (Table 3).

In the study, PTC tissues with known *RET/PTC1* and *RET/PTC3* rearrangements served as a reference standard (calibrator) [13]. Amplification reactions were done in triplicate for each sample (cDNA from the same PCR reaction but in separate wells). Controls with no template cDNA were used with each assay (negative control).

The expression levels of *β-actin* gene (*ACTB*) were measured, as endogenous control (reference gene), using the appropriate Assays-on-Demand™ Gene Expression product (Hs99999903_ml, Applied Biosystems Foster City, CA, USA).

**Table 3 Amplification conditions for *RET/PTC1* and *RET/PTC3* rearrangements using real-time PCR**

| Times and temperatures | | | |
|---|---|---|---|
| | | Each of 45 cycles | |
| Initial setup | | Denaturation | Annealing/ Elongation |
| HOLD | HOLD | CYCLE | |
| UNG activation 2 min, 50°C | 10 min, 95°C | 15 s, 95°C | 1 min, 60°C |

Both gene expressions were measured for each thyroid lesion sample in the same PCR reaction but in separate wells.

Results were presented as Rn (normalized receptor) versus cycle graph, where Rn is the fluorescence of the receptor dye, divided by fluorescence of a passive reference dye (Figure 1 and 2).

## Results

The specimens were amplified in the ABI PRISM 7500 Sequence Detection System in reaction, containing primers and probes for *RET/PTC1* and *RET/PTC3* rearrangements and a control gene, *β-actin*. The Sequence Detection System software, provided with the instrument, analyses the fluorescence data, generated during the reaction, and calculates the cycle number at which fluorescence crosses the threshold value ($C_T$). Amplification reactions were done in triplicate for each examined sample.

No *RET/PTC1* and *RET/PTC3* rearrangements were found in the examined HT specimens (for *RET/PTC1* - see Figure 1 and 2; for *RET/PTC3* - data not shown).

## Discussion

The prevalence of *RET/PTC* rearrangements in Hashimoto's thyroiditis remains a subject of controversy. Some authors have described activation of *RET* protooncogene in the majority number of HT patients. Sheils *et al.* [14] have shown the presence of *RET/PTC1* rearrangement in a significant number of HT cases (95%). The majority of specimens have shown no evidence of concomitant PTC [14]. Wirtschafter *et al.* also have documented the presence of transcripts of *RET/PTC1* and *RET/PTC3* in 95% cases of HT [15]. Their study has suggested that multiple, independent occult PTCs exist in patients with HT at high frequency and *RET/PTC1* and *RET/PTC3* are early molecular markers of

**Table 2 The sequences of probes and primers of *RET/PTC1* and *RET/PTC3* gene rearrangements [12]**

| Gene | Amplicon (bp) | Forward primer | Reverse primer | Probe sequence |
|---|---|---|---|---|
| *RET/PTC1* | 66 | CGCGACCTGCGCAAA | CAAGTTCTTCCGAGGGAATTCC | *6FAM*-CAAGCGTAACCATCGAGGATCCAAAGT-*TAMRA* |
| *RET/PTC3* | 81 | CCCCAGGACTGGCTTACCC | CAAGTTCTTCCGAGGGAATTCC | *6FAM*-AAAGCAGACCTTGGAGAACAGTCAGGAGG-*TAMRA* |

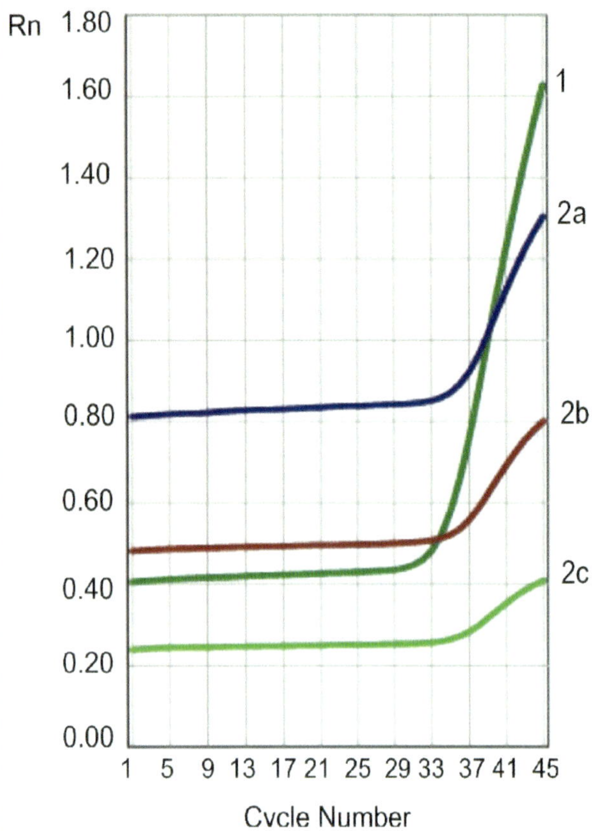


**Figure 1** Representative amplification curves for *β-actin* gene (curve no. 1) and *RET/PTC1* rearrangement (curves nos. 2a, 2b, 2c) in PTC specimen.

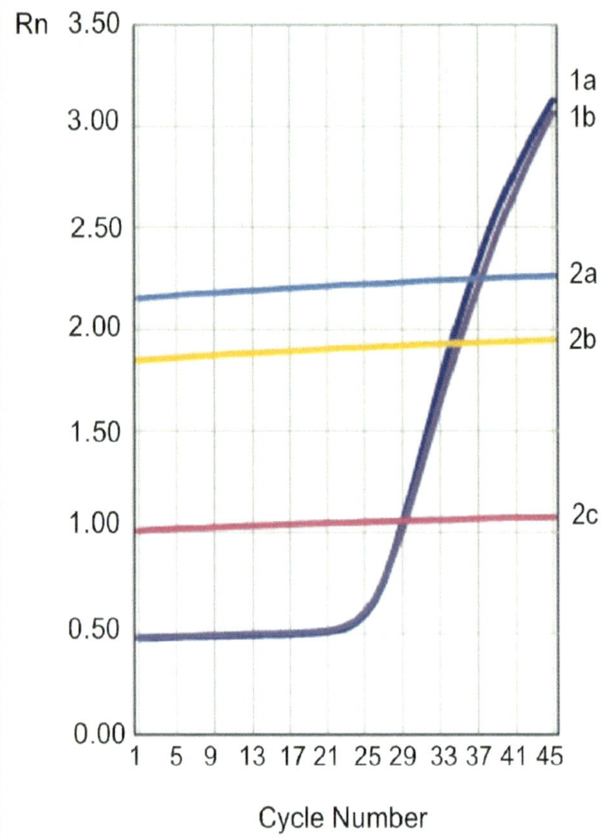


**Figure 2** Representative amplification curves for *β-actin* gene (curves nos. 1a, 1b) and *RET/PTC1* rearrangement (curves nos. 2a, 2b, 2c) in HT specimen.

microcarcinoma. However, both of these studies had technical limitations, the authors used highly degraded RNA which was isolated from formalin-fixed and paraffin-embedded tissues. Kang *et al.* [16] have investigated the expression of RET, RAS and ERK proteins in oxyphilic cells in HT. They have shown greatly enhanced immunoexpression of these proteins, suggesting a molecular link between oxyphilic cell metaplasia in HT and the progression of PTC [16].

Rhoden *et al.* [11] have analyzed *RET/PTC* oncogenic activation in HT, PTC, oncocytic tumours and in normal thyroid samples using three independent techniques: real-time RT-PCR, laser capture microdissection (LCM) RT-PCR, and fluorescence *in situ* hybridization (FISH) method. In their study, normal samples have not shown *RET* protooncogene rearrangement. Sixty eight percent of HT were positive by FISH analysis, whereas only 17% HT have shown *RET/PTC* activation by real-time PCR. It is interesting that these conflicting results depended only on the method used in the study [11]. Despite some technical controversies (RT-PCR should be typically more sensitive method of detection than FISH), the importance of this paper is expressed through providing additional evidence for the possibility of presence *RET/PTC* rearrangements in a subpopulation of cells within the thyroid gland affected by HT.

On the other hand, other groups have not detected *RET* rearrangements in histologically benign thyroid tissue with HT. Moreover, they have not shown *RET/PTC* activation in PTCs arising on the background of HT, in contrast to PTC not associated with that disease [17]. Also, Sadow *et al.* have not identified *RET/PTC1* and *RET/PTC3* in dominant nodules from Hashimoto's goitre, supporting the notion that these nodules are neither malignant nor precursor lesions of PTC [18].

In our study, we have performed real-time relative PCR assay for *RET/PTC1* and *RET/PTC3* rearrangements, based on fluorescent TaqMan methodology and using the ABI PRISM 7500 Sequence Detection System (Applied Biosystems). Real-time PCR is a sensitive, precise technique for detection of nucleic acids. Unfortunately, we have not found *RET/PTC1* and *RET/PTC3* rearrangements in the examined samples of patients with HT. On one hand, it could be a result of the limited number of cases of HT in our study, on the other, it could suggest that the association between Hashimoto's thyroiditis and follicular cell-derived thyroid tumours, as well as *RET/PTC* rearrangements as a putative link between them, remain still controversial.

In summary, the results of our study indicate that *RET/PTC1* and *RET/PTC3* rearrangements in Hashimoto's thyroiditis, if any, are rather rare events and further investigations seem to be necessary to determine molecular changes associating Hashimoto's thyroiditis with PTC.

**Acknowledgements**
This study was supported financially by funds from the Medical University of Lodz, Poland (project no. 502-11-569).

**Author details**
[1]Department of Endocrinology and Metabolic Diseases, Medical University of Lodz, Poland. [2]Polish Mother's Memorial Hospital - Research Institute, Lodz, Poland.

**Authors' contributions**
AC-M designed and coordinated the study, carried out the molecular genetic studies and drafted the manuscript. KW-D and KR-K participated in performing molecular studies. AZ participated in coordination of the study. AL, the senior author, wrote the manuscript. All authors have read and approved the final manuscript.

**Competing interests**
The authors declare that they have no competing interests.

**References**

1. Grieco M, Santoro M, Berlingieri MT, Melillo RM, Donghi R, Bongarzone I, Pierotti MA, Della Porta G, Fusco A, Vecchio G: **PTC is a novel rearranged form of the ret proto-oncogene and is frequently detected in vivo in human thyroid papillary carcinomas.** *Cell* 1990, **60**:557-563.
2. Tallini G, Asa SL: **RET oncogene activation in papillary thyroid carcinoma.** *Adv Anat Pathol* 2001, **8**:345-354.
3. Nikiforov YE: **RET/PTC rearrangement in thyroid tumors.** *Endocr Pathol* 2002, **13**:3-16.
4. Santoro M, Dathan NA, Berlingieri MT, Bongarzone I, Paulin C, Grieco M, Pierotti MA, Vecchio G, Fusco A: **Molecular characterization of RET/PTC3; a novel rearranged version of the RET proto-oncogene in a human thyroid papillary carcinoma.** *Oncogene* 1994, **9**:509-516.
5. Fusco A, Santoro M: **20 years of RET/PTC in thyroid cancer: clinicopathological correlations.** *Arq Bras Endocrinol Metabol* 2007, **51**:731-735.
6. Zhu Z, Ciampi R, Nikiforova MN, Gandhi M, Nikiforov YE: **Prevalence of RET/PTC rearrangements in thyroid papillary carcinomas: effects of the detection methods and genetic heterogeneity.** *J Clin Endocrinol Metab* 2006, **91**:3603-3610.
7. Bounancer A, Wicker R, Caillou B, Cailleux AF, Sarasin A, Schlumberger M, Suarez HG: **High prevalence of activating *RET* proto-oncogene rearrangements in thyroid tumors from patients who had received external radiation.** *Oncogene* 1997, **15**:1263-1273.
8. Smida J, Salassidis K, Hieber L, Zitzelsberger H, Kellerer AM, Demidchik EP, Negele T, Spelsberg F, Lengfelder E, Werner M, Bauchinger M: **Distinct frequency of ret rearrangements in papillary thyroid carcinomas of children and adults from Belarus.** *Int J Cancer* 1999, **80**:32-38.
9. Tallini G, Santoro M, Helie M, Carlomagno F, Salvatore G, Chiappetta G, Carcangiu ML, Fusco A: **RET/PTC oncogene activation defines a subset of papillary thyroid carcinomas lacking evidence of progression to poorly differentiated or undifferentiated tumor phenotypes.** *Clin Cancer Res* 1998, **4**:287-294.
10. Chiappetta G, Toti P, Cetta F, Giuliano A, Pentimalli F, Amendola I, Lazzi S, Monaco M, Mazzuchelli L, Tosi P, Santoro M, Fusco A: **The RET/PTC oncogene is frequently activated in oncocytic thyroid tumors (Hürthle cell adenomas and carcinomas), but not in oncocytic hyperplastic lesions.** *J Clin Endocrinol Metab* 2002, **87**:364-369.
11. Rhoden KJ, Unger K, Salvatore G, Yilmaz Y, Vovk V, Chiappetta G, Qumsiyeh MB, Rothstein JL, Fusco A, Santoro M, Zitzelsberger H, Tallini G: **RET/papillary thyroid cancer rearrangement in nonneoplastic thyrocytes: follicular cells of Hashimoto's thyroiditis share low-level recombination events with a subset of papillary carcinoma.** *J Clin Endocrinol Metab* 2006, **91**:2414-2423.
12. Rhoden KJ, Johnson C, Brandao G, Howe JG, Smith BR, Tallini G: **Real-time quantitative RT-PCR identifies distinct c-RET, RET/PTC1 and RET/PTC3 expression patterns in papillary thyroid carcinoma.** *Lab Invest* 2004, **84**:1557-1570.
13. Brzeziańska E, Karbownik M, Migdalska-Sęk M, Pastuszak-Lewandoska D, Włoch J, Lewiński A: **Molecular analysis of the RET and NTRK1 gene rearrangements in papillary thyroid carcinoma in the Polish population.** *Mutat Res* 2006, **599**:26-35.
14. Sheils OM, O'Leary JJ, Uhlmann V, Lüttich K, Sweeney EC: **ret/PTC-1 activation in Hashimoto thyroiditis.** *J Surg Pathol* 2000, **8**:185-189.
15. Wirtschafter A, Schmidt R, Rosen D, Kundu N, Santoro M, Fusco A, Multhaupt H, Atkins J, Rosen MR, Keane W, Rothstein JL: **Expression of the *RET/PTC* fusion gene as a marker for papillary carcinoma in Hashimoto's thyroiditis.** *Laryngoscope* 1997, **107**:95-100.
16. Kang DY, Kim KH, Kim JM, Kim SH, Kim JY, Baik HW, Kim YS: **High prevalence of RET, RAS, and ERK expression in Hashimoto's thyroiditis and in papillary thyroid carcinoma in the Korean population.** *Thyroid* 2007, **11**:1-7.
17. Nikiforova MN, Caudill CM, Biddinger P, Nikiforov YE: **Prevalence of *RET/PTC* rearrangements in Hashimoto's thyroiditis and papillary thyroid carcinomas.** *Int J Surg Pathol* 2002, **10**:15-22.
18. Sadow PM, Heinrich MC, Corless CL, Fletcher JA, Nosé V: **Absence of BRAF, NRAS, KRAS, HRAS mutations, and RET/PTC gene rearrangements distinguishes dominant nodules in Hashimoto thyroiditis from papillary thyroid carcinomas.** *Endocr Pathol* 2010, **21**:73-79.

# 17

# Hypothyroidism and mood disorders: integrating novel insights from brain imaging techniques

Maximilian Pilhatsch, Michael Marxen, Christine Winter, Michael N Smolka, Michael Bauer*

**Abstract**

Thyroid hormones play a critical role in brain development but also in the adult human brain by modulating metabolic activity. Hypothyroid states are associated with both functional and structural brain alterations also seen in patients with major depression. Recent animal experimental and preclinical data indicate subtle changes in myelination, microvascular density, local neurogenesis, and functional networks. The translational validity of such studies is obviously limited. Clinical evidence for neurobiological correlates of different stages and severities of hypothyroidism and effects of pharmacological intervention is lacking but may be achieved using advanced imaging techniques, e.g. functional and quantitative MRI techniques applied to patients with hypothyroidism before and after hormone replacement therapy.

## Introduction

The profound influence of thyroid hormones on brain development in humans has been studied extensively [1-6]. Hypothyroidism is a clinical condition which is either characterized only by elevated levels of the thyroid stimulating hormone (TSH; "subclinical hypothyroidism") or additional low levels of trijodothyronine (T3) and thyroxin (T4) respectively (overt hypothyroidism). Taken together overt (0.4%) and subclinical (9%) hypothyroisism is prevalent in about 9.4 % of the adult population [7] and commonly affects brain function. Conversely, 15% of patients with depression display hypothyroid states including subclinical hypothyroidism [8], and about 25-30% of depressed patients show a pathological response to the thyreotropine releasing hormone (TRH) stimulation test [9].

The concepts of thyroid hormone action in the adult brain have changed dramatically along with rapid advances in basic science and methodological techniques over the past decades [10]. Particularly brain imaging techniques evaluating cerebral metabolism, perfusion, and anatomy enabled encouraging insights into the thyroid-brain relationship. As a result, it is now widely accepted that thyroid hormones play a critical role in the adult brain impacting mood and cognition. Even if crucial details of the underlying mechanisms still remain unknown [11], the therapeutic use of thyroid hormones in the clinical treatment of mood disorders has already been established in predominantly open trials with sometimes limited numbers of patients.

Thyroid hormone treatment has been shown to accelerate and augment antidepressant pharmacotherapy and to support maintenance therapy of bipolar affective disorders, even in patients with euthyroid hormonal state [10,12]. Specifically, there is good evidence that trijodthyronine ($T_3$) can accelerate [13] and augment [14] the therapeutic response to tricyclic antidepressants and selective serotonin reuptake inhibitors (SSRIs) in depression.

Adjunctive treatment with supraphysiological doses of Levothyroxine ($T_4$) was found to be effective in open clinical studies of patients with affective disorders [15-18]. In a subset of 21 patients with treatment-resistant affective disorder, very high doses of up to 600 µg per day L-$T_4$ were required to achieve therapeutic response with a good tolerability even over mean treatment periods of up to 51 month [16].

In the first double-blind randomized placebo-controlled trial (RCT) to evaluate efficacy and tolerability of supraphysiological doses of L-T4 in 63 patients, we found that bipolar depressed women treated with L-T4 showed a better improvement in depression scores than those treated with placebo. However including both genders, the study failed to detect an overall

* Correspondence: michael.bauer@uniklinikum-dresden.de
Department of Psychiatry and Psychotherapy, University Hospital Carl Gustav Carus, Technische Universität Dresden, Dresden, Germany
Full list of author information is available at the end of the article

statistically significant treatment effect (Stamm et al., in preparation).

## Brain imaging methods

Principal brain imaging techniques mentioned in this article are single photon emission computed tomography (SPECT), positron emission tomography (PET), and different methods of magnetic resonance imaging (MRI). PET and SPECT are nuclear imaging methods that require the injection of radioactive tracers into the circulatory system. Those tracers bind to molecular structures like transporters and receptors in the human brain. Measuring of the local distribution of the bound tracers allows an estimation of regional brain activation or availability of receptors. The glucose analog [$^{18}$F]-Fluor-2-Desoxy-D-Glucose (FDG) is by far the most commonly used PET tracer and its metabolism reflects the amount of brain activity in different brain regions.

In contrast to these nuclear imaging methods, MRI is non-invasive and uses magnetic fields and radio waves instead of ionizing radiation. Structural MRI methods allow creating images of anatomical structures in an excellent spatial resolution (less than 1 mm). Diffusion tensor imaging (DTI) characterizes the mobility of water molecules and, thus, the directionality and integrity of white matter tracts. Magnetization transfer (MT) is sensitive to myelin content and is therefore useful in detecting early demyelination processes.

Functional magnetic resonance imaging (fMRI) has become the tool of choice to study functional aspects of the human brain. This method detects local increases of blood flow and the following decrease of deoxygenated hemoglobin during task related brain activity. The signal measured directly relies on the so-called BOLD (blood oxygen level dependent) effect. It is based on the different magnetic properties of oxygenated and deoxygenated hemoglobin. The origin of the BOLD signal is still a matter of discussion as it is also based on the complex interaction of neuronal metabolism, neuronal activity, blood flow and blood volume. Nevertheless fMRI enables the monitoring of active neuronal networks during the performance of specific paradigms, e.g. a memory task. Related to affective disorders, MRI allows the investigation of functional and structural deficits associated with neuropsychiatric symptoms as well as treatment effects.

Major advantages of neuroimaging methods are that brain structure and function as well as molecular and neurochemical processes can be studied in the living human. An important limitation of the mentioned brain imaging techniques refers to temporal resolution. While neuronal activities occur in the range of milliseconds, processes detected by imaging methods currently ranges between seconds (fMRI) and minutes (PET). Additionally, all methods measure brain activity indirectly through changes in blood flow or glucose uptake. Consequently, alterations in baseline perfusion and metabolic rate of oxygen may affect the results. Moreover it is currently not possible to reliably distinguish between inhibitory and excitatory neuronal activities. Nevertheless, given the rapid developments in neuroimaging methods; many limitations may hopefully be overcome in the next decades [19].

## Mechanisms of action

On the molecular level, thyroid hormones act via genomic and non-genomic effects. As part of the nuclear superfamily of ligand-modulated transcription factors, thyroid hormones bind to intracellular nuclear receptors [20]. Genomic actions of $T_3$ are mediated through the control and usually increase of gene expression [12,21,22]. Genes that are regulated by thyroid hormones are known to encode for proteins such as myelin, neurotrophins, and proteins that are involved in intracellular signaling pathways [23].

Non-genomic actions of thyroid hormones have been described in the brain and peripheral tissues. After binding to cytoplasmic thyroid hormone receptors, $T_3$ appears to be able to rapidly activate the phosphatidylinositol-3-kinase protein pathway and thereby achieves vasodilatory and neuroprotective effects [24]. Additionally, an increase in serotonergic neurotransmission is mediated by a thyroid hormone induced reduction of the sensitivity of 5-HT1A autoreceptors in the raphe nuclei and increase in 5-HT2 receptor sensitivity [25,26]. The exact role of these non-genomic signaling mechanisms, their regulation, and interaction with the slower genomic pathways remains to be elucidated.

Thyroid hormone homeostasis in the brain underlies a complex interaction of different autoregulative mechanisms [27,28]. The activity of specific thyroid hormone transporters (MCT8, LAT2) and the carrier transthyretin determines intracellular concentration of thyroid hormones via mediating their cellular influx and efflux under consideration of overall circulating levels of $T_4$ and $T_3$[27]. The activity of deiodinases [29,30] controls local bioavailability of T3 in concert with other less understood mechanisms, e.g. the local distribution of the different nuclear thyroid hormone receptors (TR$\alpha$ and TR$\beta$ in diverse isoforms) [31]. Thyroid hormone receptors are widely distributed in the brain with highest concentrations in cerebral cortex, hippocampus, amygdala, plexus choroideus and olfactory bulb [31].

Interestingly, the limbic structures, where thyroid hormone receptors are prevalent, have repeatedly been shown to be implicated in the pathogenesis of mood disorders [32]. However, the neuropharmacological basis and the functional pathways for the modulatory effects of thyroid hormones on mood are yet to be understood, even though several studies revealed interactions with different neurotransmitter systems, which are generally believed to play a major role in the regulation of mood and behaviour, i.e norepinephrine or serotonine [26,33].

**Structural changes induced by hypothyroidism**

Thyroid hormones are known to affect neuronal differentiation, migration, myelination, synaptogenesis, and dendritic branching [8,9,34,35]. Therefore, hypothyroidism will change brain structure and the changes will depend on the onset time of the condition. Hypothyroid rodents display a loss of neurons in several brain regions. Next to the visual cortex [36] and cerebellum [37], the hippocampal formations were studied repeatedly. The number of granule cells in the dentate gyrus was reduced [38] with a more severe effect of hypothyroidism during development than during adulthood [39]. Rats treated with methimazole, a hypothyroidism inducing drug, showed a reduced count of pyramidal neurons in the CA3 hippocampal region [40]. This was found even if methimazole was administered in adulthood. Animals could be fully protected with T4 replacement and partially protected with T3 replacement [41]. It is speculated that this protective potency is mediated through the activation of hippocampal progenitor cells of the supraventricular zone and the dentate gyrus [42]. Mice with a heterozygous mutation of the thyroid hormone receptor alpha 1 showed a reduced density of GABAergic inhibitory interneurons in the CA1 hippocampal region [40]. On the behavioural side, these mice show increases in markers for depression and anxiety [43,44]. Both the behavioural measures as well as the neuronal density normalized with high levels of T3 administered in adulthood. In contrast to the above findings, hypothyroid rats treated at age 0-30 days with propylthiouracil (PTU) showed a loss of pyramidal neurons in CA1, which did not ameliorate after withdrawal of the drug and approximate normalization of serum T4 levels [45]. A thyroidectomy at day 30 also reduced the number of neurons. The same study reported in CA3 a volume decrease of the pyramidal layer combined with an increase in neuronal density and no loss in the total number of pyramidal neurons. Only one study is known in this context that applied MRI in rodents [46]. Using manual segmentation, perinatal hypothyroidism induced with methimazole administered to mother rats was found to reduced total brain size of the litter but not the relative size of the hippocampus.

Effects of T3 and T4 have also been reported in the process of myelination or remyelination in mice [47,48] and rats [49,50]. Harsan et al. [48] used Diffusion Tensor Imaging (DTI) in combination with histology to serve as a marker for remyelination in mice and found that cuprizone induced demyelination in adulthood was reversable through treatment with T3, which increased the number of oligodendrocyte progenitor cells. Using histology and electronmicroscopy, Franklin and Gilson [51] found that Schwann cell remyelination was decreased in thyroidectomized rats but not oligodendrocyte remyelination.

While the efficacy of thyroid hormone treatments is generally accepted, human data on structural changes in the brain is sparse. Using proton MRS, Jagannathan et al. [52] found that abnormalities related to myelin maturation were reversible under T4 therapy in three mentally disabled patients with congential hypothyroidism. A more recent investigation [53] using similar MRS and MRI methodology demonstrated general atrophy and signs of demyelination in two children with monocarboxylate transporter 8 (MCT8) gene deficiency, which is associated with a syndrome combining thyroid and severe neurological abnormalities.

Systematic group studies of structural brain changes due to hypothyroidism and thyroid hormone therapy are needed both during development and in adulthood. In addition to MRS, recent advances in structural MRI, quantitative MRI, and image analysis techniques could be utilized to test hypotheses derived from animal studies in human. Structural changes related to myelin can now be studied with quantitative T2 or quantitative magnetization transfer (MT) imaging [54]. Diffusion tensor imaging (DTI) can reveal information on white matter integrity. Changes in grey matter density [55] or cortical thickness [56,57] can be studied with T1-weighted images.

**Vascular Changes and Perfusion**

Thyroid hormones are known to affect the vascular system. Hypothyroidism is associated with impaired fibrinolysis and blood coagulation resulting in cerebrovascular diseases [58]. It also compromises protective endothelial [59] and thrombocyte functions as well as lipid metabolism [60].

In the rat forebrain, a significant reduction in blood vessel density was observed in untreated rats thyroidectomised shortly after birth compared to euthyroid control animals and thyroidectomized rats treated with T4 or the thyroid hormone analog 3,5-diiothyroprionic acid (DITPA) [61]. Treatment induced angiogenesis and improved functioning of endothelial cells with secondary impact on local oxygen consumption and metabolic activity.

PET and SPECT measurements of cerebral blood flow under consideration of the thyroid system revealed partially conflicting results. Most consistently hypothyroidism was associated with global, diffuse hypoperfusion [62,63]. Several studies pointed to more regional effects including perfusion deficits pronounced in posterior brain regions [64-66] or in the parietal lobe [63].

Interpretation of the findings regarding reversibility of perfusion abnormalities under treatment is especially challenging. Whereas several studies report partial normalization of perfusion [17,62,67], others demonstrate [64-66] ongoing regional hypoperfusion under hormone replacement therapy. In contrast to the hypoperfusion pattern reported for hypothyroidism by Kraus et al. [64] in otherwise healthy subjects with posterior hypoperfusion and slight hyperperfusion anteriorly, depressed patients showed hypoperfusion in limbic, subcortical and frontal brain regions [32], which normalized under therapy with supraphysiological dosages (300 mcg/day) of $T_4$.

Differences in the studied populations may be the reason for such variable findings. Published results refer either to severe cases of hypothyroidism [62,63] or mild cases [66,68]. Some studies excluded patients with comorbid psychiatric diseases like depression [64,68], while other studies included also depressed patients [17,69]. In addition, the duration of the disease was variable. Only one study examined populations with varying severity and duration of the disease [17]. Taken together the existing data may indicate that long and severe hypothyroidism, presumably leading to irreversible structural neuronal and vascular changes, is associated with chronic perfusion and functional alterations, which may be ameliorated by treatment but not fully restored. In contrast, shorter and milder courses of hypothyroidism, presumably not being paralleled by irreversible structural changes, seem to be more accessible to substitution treatment.

## Glucose metabolism

In line with findings that general glucose metabolism is tightly coupled to perfusion [3], preclinical studies generally reported alterations of glucose metabolism in hypothyroid conditions [63,69]. More specifically, Bauer et al. related depressive symptoms in hypothyroidism to regionally decreased glucose metabolism, particularly in the peri-genual anterior cingulate cortex region and the hippocampus [17] in a glucose-PET study. After 3 months of T4 substitution therapy, activity patterns normalized. Circulating TSH levels before initiation of therapy showed a significant positive correlation with glucose metabolism in the right ACC and negative correlations in the hippocampus. Interestingly, these two regions express TSH receptors very densely according to topographic studies in rat and human [70], whereby suggesting a direct and relevant effect of elevated TSH levels on the limbic system is of course highly speculative.

## Cognitive and emotional functional changes

In line with the wide range of metabolic, perfusional and structural implications of the thyroid system, the literature on functional alterations related to thyroid diseases is large. Disturbances of the thyroid system, particularly if leading to a hypothyroid state, may profoundly alter mental functions influencing cognition and emotions. Severe hypothyroidism may lead to both severe depression and dementia [71] especially if left untreated [72].

Neuropsychologically, several cognitive defects in general intelligence, psychomotor speed, visual-spatial skills, working and long-term memory have been observed ranging from minimal to severe [73-75]. It was suggested that hypothyroid-related memory defects are not attributable to an attention deficit but rather to specific retrieval deficits [73,76]. Motor skills, language, inhibitory efficiency, and sustained attention appear to be less impacted by hypothyroidism [73,75]. Older adults were more vulnerable to cognitive changes due to hypothyroidism [75].

It is still a matter of discussion as to whether subclinical hypothyroidism is associated with cognitive impairments. In some studies, patients with subclinical hypothyroidism performed worse than controls on well established neuropsychological tests such as the Wechsler Adult Intelligence Scale or the Wechsler Memory scale [77,78], while other studies found no association between subclinical hypothyroidism and several aspects of cognition [75,79,80]. A consistent finding among many studies was a specific deficit in working memory tasks [73]. These neuropsychological findings were additionally underlined by a functional MRI (fMRI) study by Zhu et al. [68] who found that working memory was impaired in patients with subclinical hypothyroidism but not other memory functions. These impairments were reversible with l-thyroxine ($L\text{-}T_4$) treatment.

Despite clinical evidence of an increased vulnerability for affective disorders coming along with hypothyroid states, neurobiological correlates of this disposition are not systematically investigated yet. This is of particular interest because a study by Maheu et al. [81] demonstrated that fMRI could detect greater hippocampal and amygdala activation in 12 non-depressed adolescent patients with Cushing's syndrome, when encoding affective stimuli (i.e. emotional faces) compared to 22 healthy controls. A similar pattern of brain activation has previously been demonstrated in adolescents suffering from manifest depression in an equivalent paradigm [82]. CushingÂ´s syndrome is defined by hypercortisolemia and highly associated with prevalence of depressive symptoms in adults [83] and shows in this respect distinct parallels to hypothyroidism.

## Conclusions

Hypothyroid states have a multitude of effects on structure, perfusion and function of the central nervous system. Recent research aims to combine modern brain imaging techniques with years of experience in neuropsychological and clinical evaluations of thyroid dysfunctions. The results are encouraging, and the description of the interactions between thyroid and affective disorders is taking on a new dimension. Nonetheless, the potential of modern techniques has hardly been exhausted. For example, non invasive measurements of brain perfusion like arterial-spin-labeling (ASL) – already established in characterisation of different cerebrovascular diseases [84] – would be suitable for transferring hypotheses about the influence of angiogenesis [85] from animal models into humans. fMRI in patients with thyroid diseases of different length and severity could help to identify functional aberrations such as memory impairments or altered emotional processing, which has long been suggested from animal studies. Structural changes related to myelin, which have been observed in various animal models, can now be studied with quantitative T2 or quantitative magnetization transfer (MT) imaging [86]. Finally diffusion tensor imaging (DTI) [54] can reveal information on white matter integrity.


### Acknowledgements
This article has been published as part of *Thyroid Research* Volume 4 Supplement 1, 2011: New aspects of thyroid hormone synthesis and action. The full contents of the supplement are available online at http://www.thyroidresearchjournal.com/supplements/4/S1


### Authors' contributions
MP participated in the design and the preparation of the manuscript. MM participated in the preparation and revision of the manuscript. MNS, CW and MB participated in its design, revisions and coordination. All authors read and approved the final manuscript.

### Competing interests
The authors declare that they have no competing interests.

### References

1. Bernal J, Nunez J, Gjessing R: **Thyroid-Hormones and Brain-Development.** *European Journal of Endocrinology* 1995, **133**:390-398.
2. Ahmed OM, El Gareib AW, El Bakry AM, Abd El-Tawab SM, Ahmed RG: **Thyroid hormones states and brain development interactions.** *Int J Dev Neurosci* 2008, **26**:147-209.
3. Gur RC, Ragland JD, Reivich M, Greenberg JH, Alavi A, Gur RE: **Regional Differences in the Coupling between Resting Cerebral Blood Flow and Metabolism may Indicate Action Preparedness as a Default State.** *Cerebral Cortex* 2009, **19**:375-382.
4. Horn S, Heuer H: **Thyroid hormone action during brain development: more questions than answers.** *Mol Cell Endocrinol* 2010, **315**:19-26.
5. Koibuchi N, Chin WW: **Thyroid hormone action and brain development.** *Trends Endocrinol Metab* 2000, **11**:123-128.
6. Koibuchi N: **Effects of thyroid hormone on function and development of the brain.** *Nippon Rinsho* 2005, **63(Suppl 10)**:78-83.
7. Canaris GJ, Manowitz NR, Mayor G, Ridgwa EC: **The Colorado thyroid disease prevalence study.** *Arch Intern Med* 2000, **160(4)**:526-24.
8. Gold MS, Pottash ALC, Extein I: **Hypothyroidism and Depression - Evidence from Complete Thyroid-Function Evaluation.** *JAMA* 1981, **245(19)**:1919-1922.
9. Loosen PT: **The Trh-Induced Tsh Response in Psychiatric-Patients - A Possible Neuro-Endocrine Marker.** *Psychoneuroendocrinology* 1985, **10**:237-260.
10. Oppenheimer JH: **Evolving concepts of thyroid hormone action.** *Biochimie* 1999, **81**:539-543.
11. Bauer M, Goetz T, Glenn T, Whybrow PC, Gjessing R: **The thyroid-brain interaction in thyroid disorders and mood disorders.** *Journal of Neuroendocrinology* 2008, **20**:1101-1114.
12. Bernal J: **Action of thyroid hormone in brain.** *Journal of Endocrinological Investigation* 2002, **25**:268-288.
13. Aronson R, Offman HJ, Joffe RT, Naylor CD: **Triiodothyronine augmentation in the treatment of refractory depression - A meta-analysis.** *Archives of General Psychiatry* 1996, **53**:842-848.
14. Cooper-Kazaz R, Apter JT, Cohen R, Karagichev L, Muhammed-Moussa S, Grupper D, Drori T, Newman ME, Sackeim HA, Glaser B, *et al*: **Combined treatment with sertraline and liothyronine in major depression - A randomized, double-blind, placebo-controlled trial.** *Archives of General Psychiatry* 2007, **64**:679-688.
15. Bauer M, Hellweg R, Graf KJ, Baumgartner A: **Treatment of refractory depression with high-dose thyroxine.** *Neuropsychopharmacology* 1998, **18**:444-455.
16. Bauer M, Berghofer A, Bschor T, Baumgartner A, Kiesslinger U, Hellweg R, Adli M, Baethge C, Muller-Oerlinghausen B: **Supraphysiological doses of L-thyroxine in the maintenance treatment of prophylaxis-resistant affective disorders.** *Neuropsychopharmacology* 2002, **27**:620-628.
17. Bauer M, Silverman DH, Schlagenhauf F, London ED, Geist CL, Van Herle K, Rasgon N, Martinez D, Miller K, Van Herle A, *et al*: **Brain glucose metabolism in hypothyroidism: a positron emission tomography study before and after thyroid hormone replacement therapy.** *J Clin Endocrinol Metab* 2009, **94**:2922-2929.
18. Baumgartner A, Bauer M, Hellweg R: **Treatment of Intractable Non-Rapid Cycling Bipolar Affective-Disorder with High-Dose Thyroxine - An Open Clinical-Trial.** *Neuropsychopharmacology* 1994, **10**:183-189.
19. Kobiella A, Smolka M: **Neuroimaging of nicotine and tobacco smoking in humans.** *Encyclopedia of Addictive Behaviours* 2011, Chapter 261.
20. Lechan RM, Toni R: **Thyroid hormones in neural tissue.** 2002.
21. Koenig RJ: **Thyroid hormone receptor coactivators and corepressors.** *Thyroid* 1998, **8**:703-713.
22. Yen PM: **Physiological and molecular basis of thyroid hormone action.** *Physiological Reviews* 2001, **81**:1097-1142.
23. Bauer M, London ED, Silverman DH, Rasgon N, Kirchheiner J, Whybrow PC: **Thyroid, brain and mood modulation in affective disorder: insights from molecular research and functional brain imaging.** *Pharmacopsychiatry* 2003, **36(Suppl 3)**:S215-S221.
24. Hiroi Y, Kim HH, Ying H, Furuya F, Huang ZH, Simoncini T, Noma K, Ulek K, Nguyen NH, Scanlan TS, *et al*: **Rapid nongenomic actions of thyroid hormone.** *Proceedings of the National Academy of Sciences of the United States of America* 2006, **103**:14104-14109.
25. Bauer M, Baur H, Berghofer A, Strohle A, Hellweg R, Muller-Oerlinghausen B, Baumgartner A: **Effects of supraphysiological thyroxine administration in healthy controls and patients with depressive disorders.** *Journal of Affective Disorders* 2002, **68**:285-294.
26. Whybrow PC, Prange AJ: **A Hypothesis of Thyroid-Catecholamine-Receptor Interaction - Its Relevance to Affective-Illness.** *Archives of General Psychiatry* 1981, **38**:106-113.
27. Hennemann G, Docter R, Friesema ECH, De Jong M, Krenning EP, Visser TJ: **Plasma membrane transport of thyroid hormones and its role in thyroid hormone metabolism and bioavailability.** *Endocrine Reviews* 2001, **22**:451-476.
28. Schreiber G: **The evolutionary and integrative roles of transthyretin in thyroid hormone homeostasis.** In *J Endocrinol. Volume 175.* ; 2002:(1):61-73.
29. Visser TJ: **Thyroid hormone transporters.** *Hormone Research* 2007, **68**:28-30.
30. Baqui M, Botero D, Gereben B, Curcio C, Harney JW, Salvatore D, Sorimachi K, Larsen PR, Bianco AC: **Human type 3 iodothyronine selenodeiodinase is located in the plasma membrane and undergoes**

rapid internalization to endosomes. *Journal of Biological Chemistry* 2003, **278**:1206-1211.
31. Williams GR: **Neurodevelopmental and neurophysiological actions of thyroid hormone.** *Journal of Neuroendocrinology* 2008, **20**:784-794.
32. Bauer M, London ED, Rasgon N, Berman SM, Frye MA, Altshuler LL, Mandelkern MA, Bramen J, Voytek B, Woods R, *et al*: **Supraphysiological doses of levothyroxine alter regional cerebral metabolism and improve mood in bipolar depression.** *Mol Psychiatry* 2005, **10**:456-469.
33. Marwaha J, Prasad KN: **Hypothyroidism Elicits Electro-Physiological Noradrenergic Subsensitivity in Rat Cerebellum.** *Science* 1981, **214**:675-677.
34. Surks MI, Ortiz E, Daniels GH, Sawin CT, Col NF, Cobin RH, Franklyn JA, Hershman JM, Burman KD, Denke MA, *et al*: **Subclinical thyroid disease - Scientific review and guidelines for diagnosis and management.** *JAMA* 2004, **291(2)**:228-238.
35. Joffe RT, Marriott M: **Thyroid hormone levels and recurrence of major depression.** *American Journal of Psychiatry* 2000, **157**:1689-1691.
36. Ruizmarcos A, Sancheztoscano F, Obregon MJ, Delrey FE, Deescobar GM: **Thyroxine Treatment and Recovery of Hypothyroidism-Induced Pyramidal Cell-Damage.** *Brain Research* 1982, **239**:559-574.
37. Madeira MD, Azevedo FP, Paula-Barbosa MM: **Effects of long-term hypothyroidism in the morphology and synaptic organization of cerebellar ectopic granule cells.** *Histol Histopathol* 1988, **3**:351-359.
38. Ambrogini P, Cuppini R, Ferri P, Mancini C, Ciaroni S, Voci A, Gerdoni E, Gallo G: **Thyroid hormones affect neurogenesis in the dentate gyrus of adult rat.** *Neuroendocrinology* 2005, **81**:244-253.
39. Madeira MD, Cadete-Leite A, Andrade JP, Paula-Barbosa MM: **Effects of hypothyroidism upon the granular layer of the dentate gyrus in male and female adult rats: a morphometric study.** *J Comp Neurol* 1991, **314**:171-186.
40. Alva-Sanchez C, Ortiz-Butron R, Pacheco-Rosado J: **Kainic acid does not affect CA3 hippocampal region pyramidal cells in hypothyroid rats.** *Brain Research Bulletin* 2004, **63**:167-171.
41. Alva-Sancheza C, Sanchez-Huerta K, Arroyo-Helquera O, Anquiano B, Aceves C, Pacheco-Rosado J: **The maintenance of hippocampal pyramidal neuron populations is dependent on the modulation of specific cell cycle regulators by thyroid hormones.** *Brain Research* 2009, **1271**:27-35.
42. Panagiotakos G, Alshamy G, Chan B, Abrams R, Greenberg E, Saxena A, Bradbury M, Edgar M, Gutin P, Tabar V: **Long-Term Impact of Radiation on the Stem Cell and Oligodendrocyte Precursors in the Brain.** *PLoS One* 2007, **2(7)**:e588.
43. Venero C, Guadano-Ferraz A, Herrero AI, Nordstrom K, Manzano J, de Escobar GM, Bernal J, Vennstrom B: **Anxiety, memory impairment, and locomotor dysfunction caused by a mutant thyroid hormone receptor alpha 1 can be ameliorated by T3 treatment.** *Genes & Development* 2005, **19**:2152-2163.
44. Pilhatsch M, Winter C, Nordström K, Vennström B, Bauer M, Juckel G: **Increased depressive behaviour in mice harboring the mutant thyroid receptor alpha 1.** *Behav Brain Res* 2010, **214(2)**:187-192.
45. Madeira MD, Sousa N, Lima-Andrade MT, Calheiros F, Cadete-Leite A, Paula-Barbosa MM: **Selective vulnerability of the hippocampal pyramidal neurons to hypothyroidism in male and female rats.** *J Comp Neurol* 1992, **322**:501-518.
46. Hasegawa M, Kida I, Wada H: **A volumetric analysis of the brain and hippocampus of rats rendered perinatal hypothyroid.** *Neuroscience Letters* 2010, **479**:240-244.
47. Baas D, Legrand C, Samarut J, Flamant F: **Persistence of oligodendrocyte precursor cells and altered myelination in optic nerve associated to retina degeneration in mice devoid of all thyroid hormone receptors.** *Proceedings of the National Academy of Sciences of the United States of America* 2002, **99**:2907-2911.
48. Harsan LA, Steibel J, Zaremba A, Agin A, Sapin R, Poulet P, Guignard B, Parizel N, Grucker D, Boehm N, *et al*: **Recovery from Chronic Demyelination by Thyroid Hormone Therapy: Myelinogenesis Induction and Assessment by Diffusion Tensor Magnetic Resonance Imaging.** *Journal of Neuroscience* 2008, **28**:14189-14201.
49. Fernandez M, Giuliani A, Pirondi S, D'Intino G, Giardino L, Aloe L, Levi-Montalcini R, Calza L: **Thyroid hormone administration enhances remyelination in chronic demyelinating inflammatory disease.** *Proceedings of the National Academy of Sciences of the United States of America* 2004, **101**:16363-16368.
50. Franco PG, Silvestroff L, Soto EF, Pasquini JM: **Thyroid hormones promote differentiation of oligodendrocyte progenitor cells and improve remyelination after cuprizone-induced demyelination.** *Experimental Neurology* 2008, **212**:458-467.
51. Franklin RJM, Gilson JM: **Remyelination in the CNS of the hypothyroid rat.** *Neuroreport* 1996, **7**:1526-1530.
52. Jagannathan NR, Tandon N, Raghunathan P, Kochupillai N: **Reversal of abnormalities of myelination by thyroxine therapy in congenital hypothyroidism: localized in vivo proton magnetic resonance spectroscopy (MRS) study.** *Developmental Brain Research* 1998, **109**:179-186.
53. Sijens PE, Rodiger LA, Meiners LC, Lunsing RJ: **H-1 magnetic resonance spectroscopy in monocarboxylate transporter 8 gene deficiency.** *Journal of Clinical Endocrinology & Metabolism* 2008, **93**:1854.
54. Basser PJ, Jones DK: **Diffusion-tensor MRI: theory, experimental design and data analy.** *NMR Biomed* 2002, **15**:456-467.
55. Ashburner J, Friston KJ: **Voxel-based morphometry–the methods.** *Neuroimage* 2000, **11**:805-821.
56. Fischl B, Dale AM: **Measuring the thickness of the human cerebral cortex from magnetic resonance images.** *Proc Natl Acad Sci U S A* 2000, **97**:11050-11055.
57. Hutton C, De Vita E, Ashburner J, Deichmann R, Turner R: **Voxel-based cortical thickness measurements in MRI.** *Neuroimage* 2008, **40**:1701-1710.
58. Lass P, Slawek J, Derejko A, Rubello D: **Neurological and psychiatric disorders in thyroid dysfunctions. The role of nuclear medicine: SPECT and PET imaging.** *Minerva Endocrinologica* 2008, **33**:75-84.
59. Napoli R, Apuzzi V, Bosso G, D'Anna C, De Sena A, Pirozzi C, Marano A, Lupoli GA, Cudemo G, Oliviero U, *et al*: **Recombinant Human Thyrotropin Enhances Endothelial-Mediated Vasodilation of Conduit Arteries.** *Journal of Clinical Endocrinology & Metabolism* 2009, **94**:1012-1016.
60. Erikci AA, Karagoz B, Ozturk A, Caglayan S, Ozisik G, Kaygusuz I, Ozata M: **The effect of subclinical hypothyroidism on platelet parameters.** *Hematology* 2009, **14**:115-117.
61. Schlenker EH, Hora M, Liu Y, Redetzke RA, Morkin E, Gerdes AM: **Effects of thyroidectomy, T-4, and DITPA replacement on brain blood vessel density in adult rats.** *American Journal of Physiology-Regulatory Integrative and Comparative Physiology* 2008, **294**:R1504-R1509.
62. Kinuya S, Michigishi T, Tonami N, Aburano T, Tsuji S, Hashimoto T: **Reversible cerebral hypoperfusion observed with Tc-99m HMPAO SPECT in reversible dementia caused by hypothyroidism.** *Clinical Nuclear Medicine* 1999, **24**:666-668.
63. Constant EL, De Volder AG, Ivanoiu A, Bol A, Labar D, Seghers A, Cosnard G, Melin J, Daumerie C: **Cerebral blood flow and glucose metabolism in hypothyroidism: A positron emission tomography study.** *Journal of Clinical Endocrinology and Metabolism* 2001, **86**:3864-3870.
64. Krausz Y, Freedman N, Lester H, Newman JP, Barkai G, Bocher M, Chisin R, Bonne O: **Regional cerebral blood flow in patients with mild hypothyroidism.** *Journal of Nuclear Medicine* 2004, **45**:1712-1715.
65. Nagamachi S, Jinnouchi S, Nishii R, Ishida Y, Fujita S, Futami S, Kodama T, Tamura S, Kawai K: **Cerebral blood flow abnormalities induced by transient hypothyroidism after thyroidectomy–analysis by tc-99m-HMPAO and SPM96.** *Ann Nucl Med* 2004, **18**:469-477.
66. Krausz Y, Freedman N, Lester H, Barkai G, Levin T, Bocher M, Chisin R, Lerer B, Bonne O: **Brain SPECT study of common ground between hypothyroidism and depression.** *International Journal of Neuropsychopharmacology* 2007, **10**:99-106.
67. Forchetti CM, Katsamakis G, Garron DC: **Autoimmune thyroiditis and a rapidly progressive dementia: Global hypoperfusion on SPECT scanning suggests a possible mechanism.** *Neurology* 1997, **49**:623-629.
68. Zhu DF, Wang ZX, Zhang DR, Zhuang J, Zhou JN: **The effects of subclinical hypothyroidism on working memory: An FMRI study.** *Brain* 2006, **192(11)**:2923-2930.
69. Marangell LB, Ketter TA, George MS, Pazzaglia PJ, Callahan AM, Parekh P, Andreason PJ, Horwitz B, Herscovitch P, Post RM: **Inverse relationship of peripheral thyrotropin-stimulating hormone levels to brain activity in mood disorders.** *American Journal of Psychiatry* 1997, **154**:224-230.
70. Crisanti P, Omri B, Hughes EJ, Meduri G, Hery C, Clauser E, Jacquemin C, Saunier B: **The expression of thyrotropin receptor in the brain.** *Endocrinology* 2001, **142**:812-822.
71. Whybrow P, Bauer M: **Behavioural and psychiatric aspects of hypothyroidism.** 2005.

72. Haupt M, Kurz A: **Reversibility of Dementia in Hypothyroidism.** *Journal of Neurology* 1993, **240**:333-335.
73. Burmeister LA, Ganguli M, Dodge HH, Toczek T, DeKosky ST, Nebes RD: **Hypothyroidism and cognition: Preliminary evidence for a specific defect in memory.** *Thyroid* 2001, **11**:1177-1185.
74. Haggerty JJ, Prange AJ: **Borderline Hypothyroidism and Depression.** *Annual Review of Medicine* 1995, **46**:37-46.
75. Osterweil D, Syndulko K, Cohen SN, Pettlerjennings PD, Hershman JM, Cummings JL, Tourtellotte WW, Solomon DH: **Cognitive Function in Nondemented Older Adults with Hypothyroidism.** *Journal of the American Geriatrics Society* 1992, **40**:325-335.
76. Miller K, Parsons T, Rasgon N, Van Herle K, Whybrow P, Bauer M: **Hypothyroidism and specific memory deficits.** *Archives of Clinical Neuropsychology* 2003, **18**:729-730.
77. Monzani F, Delguerra P, Caraccio N, Pruneti CA, Pucci E, Luisi M, Baschieri L: **Subclinical Hypothyroidism - Neurobehavioral Features and Beneficial Effect of L-Thyroxine Treatment.** *Clinical Investigator* 1993, **71**:367-371.
78. Baldini IM, Vita A, Mauri MC, Amodei V, Carrisi M, Bravin S, Cantalamessa L: **Psychopathological and cognitive features in subclinical hypothyroidism.** *Progress in Neuro-Psychopharmacology & Biological Psychiatry* 1997, **21**:925-935.
79. Gussekloo J, van Exel E, de Craen AJM, Meinders AE, Frolich M, Westendorp RGJ: **Thyroid status, disability and cognitive function, and survival in old age.** *JAMA* 2004, **292(21)**:2591-2599.
80. Jorde R, Waterloo K, Storhaug H, Nyrnes A, Sundsfjord J, Jenssen TG: **Neuropsychological function and symptoms in subjects with subclinical hypothyroidism and the effect of thyroxine treatment.** *Journal of Clinical Endocrinology & Metabolism* 2006, **91**:145-153.
81. Maheu FS, Mazzone L, Merke DP, Keil M, Stratakis CA, Pine DS, Ernst M: **Altered amygdala and hippocampus function in adolescents with hypercortisolemia: A functional magnetic resonance imaging study of Cushing syndrome.** *Development and Psychopathology* 2008, **20**:1177-1189.
82. Roberson-Nay R, McClure EB, Monk CS, Nelson EE, Guyer AE, Fromm SJ, Charney DS, Leibenluft E, Blair J, Ernst M, Pine DS: **Increased amygdala activity during successful memory encoding in adolescent major depressive disorder: An FMRI study.** *Biol Psychiatry* 2006, **60(9)**:966-73.
83. Wolkowitz OM, Burke H, Epel ES, Reus VL: **Glucocorticoids. Mood, memory, and mechanisms.** *Ann N Y Acad Sci* 2009, **1179**:19-40.
84. Paiva FF, Tannus A, Silva AC: **Measurement of cerebral perfusion territories using arterial spin labelling.** *Nmr in Biomedicine* 2007, **20**:633-642.
85. Barrett T, Brechbiel M, Bernardo M, Choyke PL: **MRI of tumor angiogenesis.** *Journal of Magnetic Resonance Imaging* 2007, **26**:235-249.
86. Laule C, Vavasour IM, Kolind SH, Li DK, Traboulsee TL, Moore GR, Mackay AL: **Magnetic resonance imaging of myelin.** *Neurotherapeutics* 2007, **4**:460-484.

# Serum calcitonin estimation in medullary thyroid cancer: basal or stimulated levels?

Chantal Daumerie[1*], Dominique Maiter[1], Damien Gruson[2]

*From* 9th Meeting of the European Thyroid Association Cancer Research Network (ETA-CRN)
Lisbon, Portugal.

**Abstract**

Calcitonin (Ct) is a tumour marker essential for the diagnosis and follow-up of medullary thyroid cancer (MTC). Accurate and consistent measurements of serum Ct are of critical importance. Ct measurements by different methods can differ, leading to difficulties in the interpretation of results. Second generation assays for Ct have been developed and are now available in clinical laboratories. However, the lack of standardization for Ct assays remains a common problem with Ct assays. The reference interval and reliability should be carefully defined.

The role of stimulated Ct for the diagnosis and follow-up of MTC should also be pointed out as the pentagastrin test is no more available in all countries. However, the stimulated test remains very useful to exclude MTC if the basal Ct serum level is in the grey zone (15-20 ng/L), after surgery to confirm the complete cure. A residual response after surgery could indicate a need for aggressive surgery or - in case of metastatic disease - could suggest the prognosis.

High-dose Ca test (2.5mg/kg) seems to be a reliable and effective test for the diagnosis and follow-up of MTC. It seems more potent than pentagastrin with fewer side effects. The threshold able to discriminate healthy subjects from C-cell hyperplasia (CCH) cases for the stimulated Ct concentration is 184 ng/L for women and 1620 ng/L for men.

As stimulated Ca test will eventually replace the pentagastrin test, there is a need to confirm or to modify the threshold identified for each assay individually.

## Introduction

Medullary thyroid carcinoma (MTC) originates from thyroid C cells, which secrete calcitonin (Ct).

Routine measurement of Ct in patients with nodular goitre allows for the preoperative diagnosis of unsuspected MTC, often at a very precocious stadium.

Ct is a 32 amino- acid- polypeptide, in which the disulphide bridges are essential for biological activity. The physiological role of Ct is unknown. The C cells use the same calcium receptor as do parathyroid cells [1], and high calcaemia is their physiological stimulant. Non physiological stimulants include glucagon, β-adrenergic agonists, alcohol, and gastrin [2].

* Correspondence: chantal.daumerie@uclouvain.be
[1]Department of Endocrinology, Université Catholique de Louvain, Cliniques Universitaires Saint-Luc, Avenue Hippocrate 10, 1200 Brussels, Belgium
Full list of author information is available at the end of the article

### Basal calcitonin

Accurate and consistent measurements of serum Ct are of critical importance. Ct values measured by different methods can differ, leading to difficulties in interpretation of results

Since 1988, RIA with polyclonal antibodies that recognised both mature Ct monomer and other circulating forms lacking specificity and sensibility, have been used. Second generation automated immunoassays with more specific antibodies are now available for clinical laboratories.

Minimal and mild elevations in serum Ct may be seen in C-Cells hyperplasia, renal failure, autoimmune thyroiditis, and hypercalcaemia. Elevated Ct levels may result from non thyroid neuroendocrine tumours. Falsely low Ct levels may occur in the setting of heterophilic antibodies and from a "hook effects". Optimally, an individual should be followed using the same Ct assay over time and the laboratory should report which Ct assay is being used. Ct values should also be interpreted in the setting of gender specific reference intervals. Moreover, caution has to be taken in interpreting values in children younger than 3 years.

The effort of standardization for some thyroid related assays is on-going; nevertheless Ct assays remain yet not standardized [3]. Table 1 summarizes the Ct assay performances and data provided by the manufactures. Therefore, the reference interval for a healthy population as well as the reliability should be clearly defined for every Ct assay. The American Thyroid association guidelines do not specify any reference range for Ct but several recent reports have proposed some cut-off points for Ct testing.

Doyle reported [4] that the basal Ct (measured by a two-site automated chemiluminescent immunometric assay) was 5 ng/L for men and 5.7 ng/L for women (95$^{th}$ percentile). Rink [5] found that the basal Ct level was 32.9 ng/L for men and 14.6 ng/L for women.

An upper limit of 15 ng/L should be able to rule out MTC and reduce false positive cases [5]. In the range between 15-50 ng/L, the predictive value for detection of MTC was 4%. d'Herbomez et al. [6] suggested a 20 ng/L threshold to limit false positive results and a second control. Colombo et al. [7] demonstrated that the best levels of basal Ct (assayed by chemiluminescence, Immulite 2000) to separate healthy subjects and CCH cases from MTC patients were above 18.7 ng/L in females and above 68 ng/L in males.

However, the question arises whether the decision-making can be reliably based on a single basal Ct measurement for diagnosis in patients with a genetic susceptibility to develop MTC (i.e., activated *RET* oncogene-carriers) or for the follow-up after surgery for a known MTC. This strategy was recently recommended by the American thyroid association as the pentagastrin is now unavailable in many countries [8]. However, even if the ultrasensitive Ct assay will reduce the false negative rate of basal Ct measurements when diagnosing familial MTC and in post-operative follow-up, compared to previously used assays, it has recently been shown that its sensitivity to detect C-cell disease remains lower than a stimulation test [9].

### Indications of calcitonin stimulation tests

The role of stimulated Ct for the diagnosis and follow-up of MTC has recently been pointed out since the classical pentagastrin test is no more available in some European countries.

The stimulation test remained very useful to exclude an MTC in an unaffected individual when basal Ct was in the grey zone (15-50 ng/L) as observed in autoimmune thyroiditis with CCH or in neuroendocrine tumours. Another indication for the stimulation test was to detect residual disease or recurrence after surgery for MTC in patients with low basal Ct levels. Patients who have non-detectable and non-stimulable post-operative Ct at two consecutive follow-up visits are considered disease-free, although they still require yearly follow-up assessments as late recurrence of disease can occur, and there might thus be a need for future complementary surgery. However, it must be remembered that the volume of residual disease is usually very low when only the stimulated Ct level is detectable, and unlikely to be found by imaging until basal Ct is over 150 ng/L [10]. In case of metastatic disease, the response and the peak value could also be indicative of the prognosis. Finally, in genetically predisposed patients with intermediate or low-risk *RET* proto-oncogene mutations, a prophylactic thyroidectomy is usually advised if basal Ct is lower than 10 ng/L and peak Ct (following pentagastrin stimulation test) is between 50 and 100 ng/L.

### Pentagastrin stimulation test

The pentagastrin stimulation test uses a slow intravenous injection of pentagastrin (0.5 µg/kg body weight) over three minutes. Blood samples are obtained at baseline, and two and five minutes after pentagastrin injection.

The cut-off of the pentagastrin-stimutated Ct is still not clear in the literature and depends on the assay

**Table 1 Calcitonin assays performances**

| Assay | Format | Sample volume | Pretreatment | Within-run CV | Between-run CV | Measuring range | LLD |
|---|---|---|---|---|---|---|---|
| **Cis-bio** | RIA | 200µl | 30 min 56°C | 6.7% at 10.9 ng/L | 5.2% at 21.1 ng/L | 1.5 -1530 ng/L | 1.5 ng/L |
| **Diasorin** | Automated chemiluminescent | 150µl | NO | 2. 5% at 25 ng/L 3.1% at 160 ng/L | 5% at 25 ng/L 4.7% at 160 ng/L | 1.0 – 2000 ng/L | 4 ng/L |
| **Siemens** | Automated chemiluminescent | 200 µl | NO | 3.4% at 29 ng/L 2.3% at 200 ng/L | 4.2% at 29 ng/L 5.5% at 260 g/L | 2.0 – 2000 ng/L | 2 ng/L |
| **IBL** | ELISA | 100 µl | NO | 2.8% at 37 ng/L 2.4% at 260 ng/L | 8.6% at 41 ng/L 6.3% at 167 ng/L | 1.3 – 790 ng/L | 1.3 ng/L |
| **DSL** | IRMA | 150 µL | NO | 2.4% at 27 ng/L 5.1% at 390 ng/L | 9.0% at 24.3 ng/L 7.8% at 391 ng/L | 5 – 500 ng/L | 5 ng/L |

used. Verga et al. [11] showed that a peak above 50ng/L indicated a risk of CCH and MTC, while Scheuba et al. [12] found that the probability of having an MTC was 100% if the peak value was higher than 560 ng/L; finally, Elisei et al. [13] determined the lowest peak of Ct for MTC to be 118 ng/L. In chronic renal disease, the peak may reach 400 ng/L. In 2002, the National Academy of Clinical Biochemistry (NACB) has documented that 80% of healthy subjects have a Ct peak lower than 10 ng/L, 15% have a peak between 10 and 30 ng/L and 5% may have a peak between 30 and 50 ng/L [14]. When the peak stimulated Ct was between 50 and 100 ng/L, the risk of diagnosis of C-cell pathology is intermediate and a peak higher than 100 ng/L likely indicates CCH or MTC.

In a recent study, a peak Ct of 275 ng/L determined by IRMA after pentagastrin was able to clearly distinguish patients with MTC from patients with CCH with 100% sensitivity and 89% specificity [15].

It therefore appeared that if stimulated Ct (sCt) values were higher than 200 ng/L, MTC was likely and thyroidectomy and lymphadenectomy required. If sCt reached values between 100 and 200 ng/L, the risk was uncertain. Such values could be indicative of C cell hyperplasia or microscopic MTC. Some would advise surgery, others preferred observation.

### The calcium stimulation test

Due to the unavailability of pentagastrin in many countries, there is a growing interest in the calcium stimulation test.

This test uses an infusion of calcium gluconate (2.5 mg elemental calcium/kg body weight) over 30 seconds administered in fasting state. Blood samples for Ct are obtained at baseline and two and five minutes after the stimulus. High-dose calcium is more effective and a better-tolerated Ct stimulator than pentagastrin.

There are very few data using the calcium stimulation as a confirmatory test in patients with C-cell disease. Cut-off points for the discrimination of healthy subjects, C cell hyperplasia and MTC cases have not been standardized yet. In one study [4] the levels of Ct stimulated after either pentagastrin or calcium were significantly correlated. In this study, calcium stimulated Ct levels above 32.6 ng/L (females) and 192 ng/L (males) had the best accuracy to differentiate normal subjects from patients with C cell hyperplasia and MTC and values above 184 ng/mL in females and above 1620 ng/L in males had the highest accuracy to distinguish healthy subjects and CCH cases from the patients with MTC.

The criteria for abnormal Ct values may vary according to Ct assays and reference values must be defined for every assay. Provided these references ranges are clearly assessed, the indications and usefulness of the high-dose calcium stimulation test should be very similar to the now "old " pentagastrin test.

## Conclusions

Evaluation of both basal and stimulated Ct may be useful in the diagnosis and follow-up of MTC. Even though ultrasensitive Ct assays have greatly reduced the false negative rate of a basal Ct measurement when diagnosing C-cell disease, its sensitivity remains lower than a stimulation test. The calcium stimulation test may be used in this setting, in particular when basal Ct is in the grey zone or to detect residual disease or early recurrence after surgery for MTC in patients with low basal Ct levels. However, each Ct assay must be evaluated and each laboratory has to define its own reference ranges for basal and stimulated values. Further studies are clearly needed to optimize the Ct thresholds to be used to distinguish patients with C-cell pathology from normal, and to better define the patterns of response in particular conditions, such as in thyroid autoimmune disease and in renal insufficiency.

#### List of abbreviations used

Ct: Calcitonin; CCH: C-cell hyperplasia; MTC: medullary thyroid carcinoma; IRMA: immuno radiometric assay; RIA: radio immuno assay.

#### Competing interests

No competing interests exist for me and my co-authors.

#### Declarations

This article has been published as part of *Thyroid Research* Volume 6 Supplement 1, 2013: European comments on Medullary Thyroid Cancer Management Guidelines of the American Thyroid Association. The full contents of the supplement are available online at http://www.thyroidresearchjournal.com/supplements/6/S1. Publication of this supplement has been supported by the European Thyroid Association-Cancer Research Network.

#### Author details

[1]Department of Endocrinology, Université Catholique de Louvain, Cliniques Universitaires Saint-Luc, Avenue Hippocrate 10, 1200 Brussels, Belgium. [2]Department of Biochemistry, Université Catholique de Louvain, Cliniques Universitaires Saint-Luc, Avenue Hippocrate 10, 1200 Brussels, Belgium.

#### References

1. Garrett JE, Tamir H, Kifor O, Simin RT, Rogers KV, Mithal A, Gagel RF, Brown EM: **Calcitonin-secreting cells of the thyroid express an extracellular calcium receptor gene.** *Endocrinology* 1995, **136**:5202-211.
2. Erdogan MF, Gursoy A, Kulalaksizoglu M: **Long-term effects of elevated gastrin levels on calcitonin secretion.** *J Endocrinol Invest* 2006, **29**:771-775.
3. Thienpont LM, Van Uyfanghe K, Van Houcke S, IFCC Working Group for Standardization of Thyroid Function Tests (WG-STFT): **Standardization activities in the field of thyroid function tests: a status report.** *Clin Chem Lab Med* 2010, **48**:1577-1583.
4. Doyle P, Düren C, Nerlich K, Verburg FA, Grelle I, Jahn H, Fassnacht M, Mäder U, Reiners C, Luster M: **Potency and tolerance of calcitonin stimulation with high dose calcium versus pentagastrin in normal adults.** *J Clin Endocrinol Metab* 2009, **94**:2970-2974.
5. Rink T, Truong PN, Schroth HJ, Diener J, Zinny M, Diener J, Zimny M, Grünwald F: **Calculation and validation of a plasma calcitonin limit for**

early detection of medullary thyroid carcinoma in nodular disease. *Thyroid* 2009, **19**:327-332.
6. d'Herbomez M, Caron P, Bausters C, Do Cao C, Schlienger JL, Sapin R, Baldet L, Carnaille B, Wemeau JL: Reference range of serum calcitonin levels in humans: influence of calcitonin assays, sex, age and cigarette smoking. *Eur J Endocrinol* 2007, **157**:749-755.
7. Colombo C, Verga U, Mian C, Ferrero S, Perrino M, Vicentini L, Dazzi D, Opocher G, Pelizzo MR, Beck-Peccoz P, Fugazzola L: Comparison of Calcium and Pentagastrin for the diagnosis and Follow-up of Medullary Thyroid cancer. *J Clin Endocrinol Metab* 2012, **97**:905-913.
8. Kloos RT, Eng C, Evans DB, Francis GL, Gharib H, Moley JF, Pacini F, Ringel MD, Schlumberger M, Wells SA: Medullary thyroid cancer: management guidelines of the American Thyroid Association. *Thyroid* 2009, **19**:565-612.
9. Pina G, Dubois S, Murat A, Berger N, Niccoli P, Peix JL, Cohen R, Guillausseau C, Charrie A, Chabre O, Cornu C, Borson-Chazot F: Is basal ultrasensitive of calcitonin capable of substituting for the pentagastrin-stimulation test? *Clin Endocrinol (Oxf)* 2013, **78**:358-364.
10. Costante G, Durante C, Francis Z, Schlumberger M, Filetti S: Determination of calcitonin levels in C-cell disease: clinical interest and potential pitfalls. *Nat Clin Pract Endocrinol Metab* 2009, **5**:35-44.
11. Verga U, Ferrrero S, Vincentini L, Brambilla T, Cirello V, Muzza M, Beck-Peccoz P, Fugazzola L: Histopathological and molecular studies in patients with goiter and hypercalcitoninemia: reactive or neoplastic C-cell hyperplasia? *Endocr Relat Cancer* 2007, **14**:393-403.
12. Scheuba C, Kaserer K, Moritz A, Drosten R, Vierhapper H, Bieglmayer C, Haas OA, Niederle B: Sporadic hypercalcitonemia: clinical and therapeutic consequences. *Endocr Relat Cancer* 2009, **16**:243-253.
13. Elisei R, Bottici V, Luchetti F, Di Coscio G, Romei C, Grasso L, Miccoli P, Iacconi P, Basolo F, Pinchera A, Pacini F: Impact of routine measurement of serum calcitonin on the diagnosis and outcome of medullary thyroid cancer: experience in 10,864 patients with nodular thyroid disorders. *J Clin Endocrinol Metab* 2004, **89**:163-168.
14. Baloch Z, Carayon P, Conte-Devolx B, Demers LM, Feldt-Rasmussen U, Henry JF, Livolsi VA, Nicolli-Sire P, John R, Ruf J, Smyth PP, Spencer CA, Stockigt JR, Guidelines Committee, National Academy of Clinical Biochemistry: Laboratory medicine practice guidelines. Laboratory support for the diagnosis and monitoring of thyroid disease. *Thyroid* 2003, **13**:3-126.
15. Milone F, Ramundo V, Chlofalo MG, Severino R, Paciolla I, Pezzullo L, Lombardi G, Colao A, Faggiano A: Predictive value of pentagastrin test for preoperative differential diagnosis between C-cell hyperplasia and medullary thyroid carcinoma in patients with moderately elevated basal calcitonin levels. *Clin Endocrinol (Oxf)* 2010, **73**:85-88.

# 19

# Molecular description of non-autoimmune hyperthyroidism at a neonate caused by a new thyrotropin receptor germline mutation

Heike Biebermann*, Franziska Winkler, Daniela Handke, Annette Grüters, Heiko Krude, Gunnar Kleinau

**Abstract**

**Background:** Constitutively activating germline mutations in the thyrotropin receptor (TSHR) gene result in non-autoimmune hyperthyroidism and can be transmitted as a dominant trait or occur sporadically. These mutations are mostly located in the serpentine part of this G-protein coupled receptor.

**Methods:** Sequencing exon 9 and 10 of the thyrotropin receptor gene in a two months old patient identified a mutation which was functionally characterized after transient transfection into COS-7 cells. Cell surface localization was investigated by an ELISA approach and for signalling properties we measured cAMP by alpha screen technology for Gs/adenylyl cyclase activation and use a reporter gene assay for determination of Gq/11 phospholipase C-β activation.

**Results:** We detected a heterozygous mutation in the first extracellular loop of the TSHR gene leading to an exchange of an isoleucine residue for asparagine at amino acid position 486 (I486N). Cell surface localization was reduced to 51% of wild-type TSHR. Functional characterization of the mutant receptor revealed constitutive activation of the Gs/adenylyl cyclase pathway, in contrast basal activity of the Gq/11 pathway was comparable to the wild-type. The bovine TSH-induced cAMP accumulation was slightly reduced, but IP3 signaling was impaired.

**Conclusion:** We identified a new TSHR germline mutation (I486N) in a neonate with non-autoimmune sporadic hyperthyroidism. The mutation is located at the extracellular loop 1 and exhibits an increase in basal cAMP accumulation, but unexpectedly impairs the capability for TSH induced Gq mediated signaling. The TSHR homology model suggests isoleucine 486 as a potential key-player for induction of signal transduction by an interplay with further activation sensitive extracellular parts.

## Introduction

The thyrotropin receptor (TSHR) is a member of the glycoprotein hormone receptors (GPHRs), a subfamily of the family A G-protein-coupled receptors (GPCRs). In contrast to most other receptors of this family the GPHRs are characterized by a large amino-terminal extracellular part of around 350 amino acids containing high affinity binding sites for hormones and antibodies. The amino-terminal extracellular part can be subdivided into the so-called Leucine-rich repeat domain and the hinge region. The serpentine domain is constituted by seven transmembrane α-helices (TMHs) connected by three intra- (ICLs) and three extracellular (ECLs) loops (reviewed in [1]). The intracellular serpendine domain together with the intracellular C-terminus are involved in G-protein activation.

Hormone binding on the amino-terminal extracellular part induces conformational changes within the 7TMH leading to an active conformation and signaling-state of the receptor [2]. The TSHR couples mainly Gαs to induce activation of adenylyl cyclase, but at higher TSH concentrations also activates the inositol phosphate cascade (IP) via coupling to Gαq [3,4]. So far activation of the Gs/adenylyl cyclase pathway seems to be of highest impact for thyroid growth and function [5]. However, recently it was shown that activation of the Gq/11 pathway is likely an important factor for thyroid growth and thyroid hormone synthesis [6].

* Correspondence: heike.biebermann@charite.de
Institute of Experimental Paediatric Endocrinology, Charité Universitätsmedizin Berlin, Augustenburger Platz 1, 13353 Berlin, Germany
Full list of author information is available at the end of the article

Constitutively activating mutations (CAMs) of the TSHR result in non-autoimmune hyperthyroidism. These mutations are leading to a permanently increased stimulation of the Gs/adenylyl cyclase pathway. The majority of germline CAMs are located in the serpendine domain, but few of such mutations were also found in the ECLs (reviewed in [7]). When occurring in the germline these mutations are found as sporadic carriers or are inherrited as dominant traits in familial cases. Somatic mutations in hyperfunctioning nodules are extremely rare in pediatric patients [8,9]. The phenotypic variability of mutations carriers is ranging from slight signs of hyperthyroidism in later life (mostly in familial occurring mutations) to severe forms of hyperthyroidism in neonates [8].

Here we describe a neonate in whom enhanced tachycardia was the only clinical sign of hyperthyroidism, which is due to the lack of TSH-R stimulating antibodies and was diagnosed as non-autoimmune hyperthyroidism. A new constitutively activating germline TSHR mutation, localized in the ECL1 was identified. Here we describe the patient`s-phenotype, results of molecular characterization and modified structural-functional properties.

## Material and methods

### The patient

The patient was born after an uneventful pregnancy in the 36 week of gestation without signs of prior fetal tachycardia. In utero ultrasound data of the thyroid gland were not available. At the age of one month tachycardia was detected in a routine examination without further clinical signs of hyperthyroidism. At one month of age the weight was 3085 g and length 52 cm length. The thyroid status revealed severely elevated T3 (5.5 µg/L; normal range: 0.8 – 2.0 µg/L) and fT4 (≥ 7.8 ng/dL; normal range: 0.9 – 1.9 ng/d) levels, and supposed TSH below 0.01 mU/L (normal range: 0.27 – 4.2 mU/L). Thyroid autoantibodies were negative. Ultrasound of the thyroid gland showed no increase in volume (1.9 mL; normal range: 0.2 – 2.0 mL).

Due to severe tachycardia with 220/min the child was treated with Propanolol 3.1 mg/kg body weight/d. Antithyroid drug treatment with Thiamazol was initiated with a dose of 0.5 mg/kg body weight per day. In light of severe hyperthyroidism in terms of very high thyroid hormone levels the clinical course beside severe tachycardia was surprisingly asymptomatic including the relatively small volume of the thyroid gland. Actually at the age of two months the patient was treated with 2.5 mg Propanolol four times a day, and with Thiamazol 1 mg/d and D-Fluorette 500 IE/d.

All clinical investigations described were conducted in consultation with the investigated patient and her family and genetic analyses were in accordance with the guidelines proposed in the Declaration of Helsinki.

### Isolation and characterization of genomic DNA encoding the TSHR

Genomic DNA was prepared from peripheral white blood cells from the patient using a commercial kit (Blood amp kit, Qiagen, Hilden, Germany). Exon 9 and 10 of the TSHR gene were PCR-amplified and sequenced using the BigDye Terminator Cycle Sequencing Ready Reaction Kit (Perkin Elmer, Weiterstadt, Germany) and an automatic sequencer (ABI 3710xl, Applied Biosystems, Foster City, CA, USA).

### Cloning of TSHR mutation

The PCR product of the mutation I486N was cloned into the pCR2.1-TOPO vector and then transformed into competent *E.coli* DH5α. DNA was extracted from selected colonies of bacteria using QIAprep Miniprep kit (QIAGEN GmbH, Germany), digested with *Eco*RI (New England Biolabs, MA, USA) and additionally sequenced for the detection of mutation I486N. The mutant was inserted into the eucaryotic expression vector encoding the wild-type (WT) TSHR (N-terminal hemagglutinine (HA)-tagged between amino acid 25 and 26) via Bsu36I and BstEII.

### Cell culture, transfection and functional assays

COS-7 cells were grown in Dulbecco´s modified Eagle medium (DMEM) and HEK-293 cells in Minimum Essential Medium (MEM) Earle´s, both supplemented with 10% fetal bovine serum (FBS), 100 U/ml penicillin, 100 µg/ml streptomycin and 2 mM L-glutamine at 37°C in a 5% $CO_2$ incubator. For functional characterization WT TSHR and mutant receptor were transiently transfected into COS-7 or HEK 293 cells and investigated regarding cell surface expression and TSH-induced accumulation of intracellular cAMP and IP3 accumulation.

For all functional tests $2.5x10^4$ COS-7 cells (for cAMP accumulation) or $5 X 10^4$ HEK 293 cells (for IP accumulation) were seeded in 48-well culture plates. Transient transfection was performed by using metafectene (Biontex, Munich, Germany) according to the manufactures protocol. Cell surface expression was determined by immunological detection of the N-terminal HA-tag as described previously [10]. Intracellular cAMP was determined via alpha-screen technology [11] after stimulation with bovine TSH (bTSH). For investigation of Gq/11 activation, we co-transfected HEK-293 cells with TSHR cDNAs and a reporter construct containing the firefly luciferase gene under the control of NF-AT. Subsequently, the cells were stimulated with bTSH and lysed. Gq/11 activation was reported by luciferase activity expression in the luciferase reporter gene assay according to the manufacturer's instructions (Promega, Madison, USA).

### Design of a molecular TSHR homology model

Using a previously described modeling procedure [12] we designed a new TSHR homology model of the serpentine-domain assembled with the extreme N- and C-terminal parts of the hinge region. As suggested by recently published experimental data [13] a cysteine-bridge between C284 at the N- and C408 at the C- terminus of the hinge region was added. To improve the model and to increase the quality (refined side-chain orientations) we performed in contrast to the previous procedure an extended molecular dynamic simulation of 6ns for the side-chains by fixed backbone atoms. Structure images were produced using the PyMOL Molecular Graphics System, Version 1.3, Schrödinger, LLC.

## Results

### Sequencing of the TSHR gene

Direct sequencing of exon 10 of the TSHR gene in the patient revealed a heterozygous mutation, c.T1458A, that resulted in an exchange of p.**Ile486Asn** in the first extracellular loop. This mutation was not identified in the parents.

### Functional characterization of wild type and mutant TSHR (I486N)

For functional characterization the mutated TSHR (I486N) and wild type TSHR were transiently transfected into either COS-7 cells to detect cell surface localization and cAMP signal transduction or HEK-293 cells to investigate IP3 signaling properties.

### Cell surface localization

The mutant TSHR expression at the cell surface was reduced to 51% ± 7% of WT TSHR (Fig.1 A).

### Signaling properties

We determined a 4-fold increase in ligand independent activation of the Gαs signaling pathway compared with the WT (I486N: 404% ± 67% of WT; Fig.1B). The maximal level of activation of the mutant was slightly reduced compared with WT (I486N: 74% ± 8% of WT; Fig. 1B), whereby the $EC_{50}$ values were similar (EC50 WT: 0.18 ± 0.02 mU/ml; I486N: 0.35 ± 0.17 mU/ml).

In contrast, determination of basal and TSH- induced activation of the Gαq/11 signaling pathway revealed a 13-fold impairment of signaling capability of the I486N mutation (I486N: 8% ± 2% of WT). The basal activity was like wild type (Fig.1C).

### The TSHR homology model suggests an interplay between isoleucine 486 at the extracellular loop 1 with fragments of the extracellular hinge region

It can be assumed that the extreme N- and C-terminus of the extracellular hinge region are localized and tightly embedded between the ECLs (figure 2). Three facts do support this three-dimensional package:

1. The C-terminus of the hinge region directly attaches the extracellular part to the transmembrane helix 1 (TMH1).
2. The experimentally evidenced cysteine bridge (C284-C408) connects the C- with the N-terminus of the hinge region.
3. It has been shown [14,15] that the TSHR without the AtEP can not become activated by mutations at the extracellular loops. At the ECLs as well as on the N- and C-terminus of the hinge region activating mutations were found, which supports there potential interplay as counterparts at the interface between the extracellular and transmembrane region during TSHR activation.

## Discussion

### Occurrence of activating mutations in the first extracellular loop of the Thyrotropin receptor

Constitutively activating mutations in the TSHR are a frequent molecular cause of non-autoimmune hyperthyroidism (reviewed in [16-19]). We here describe a new germline TSHR mutation I486N located in the ECL1. In the affected neonate hyperthyroidism was diagnosed due to tachycardia without further signs of hyperthyroidism and without goiter. Thyroid hormone values were severely elevated revealed non-autoimmune hyperthyroidism.

Three somatic mutations at position 486 were found previously in toxic thyroid adenomas: I486F [20], I486M [20], I486N [21]. Functional characterization for mutations I486F and I486M demonstrated constitutive activation of both Gs and Gq mediated signaling. The mutation I486N we identified in this study as a germline mutation was already found as a somatic mutation [21]. In that study mutation I486N lead to constitutive activation of the Gs pathway, however, activation of Gq activation was not investigated. We here show that I486N did not result in constitutive activation of Gq/11 (figure 1) in contrast to the I486F and I486M mutations. Moreover, the capability for bTSH-induced Gq-mediated signaling was impaired in the I486N mutation.

Interestingly, at the neighbouring position 485 a germline mutation (A485V) was described previously [22]. This mutation also reveals constitutive activation of the Gs mediated pathway, whereas the basal level of IP3 formation remained unchanged. Stimulation of that mutant TSHR with high concentrations of bTSH failed to

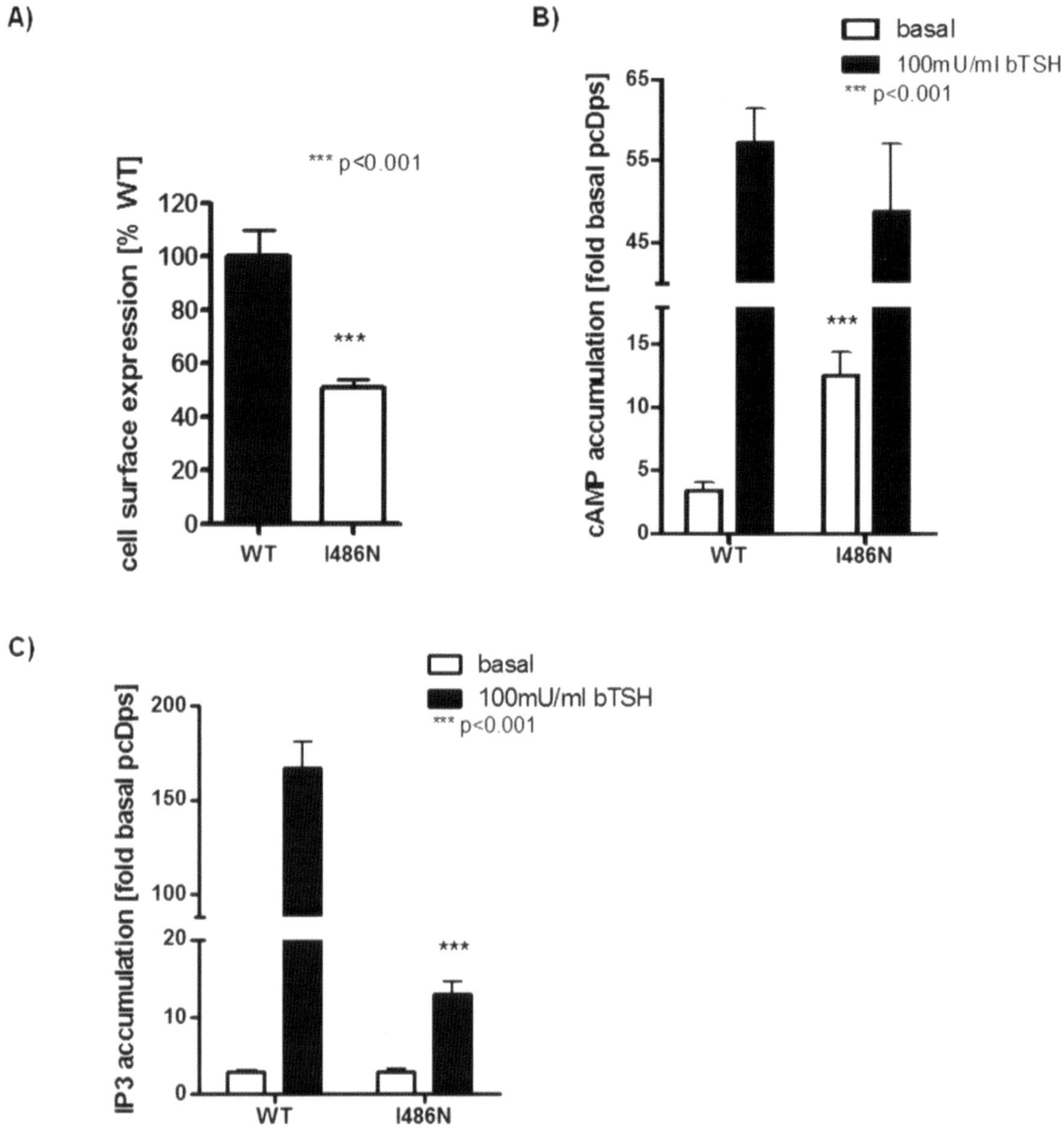


**Figure 1** Functional characterization of WT and mutant TSHR. Cell surface expression (A) and Gs cAMP accumulation (B) were determined in COS-7 cells; Gq/$_{11}$ IP3 accumulation (C) was determined in HEK-293 cells, both expressing WT and mutant (I486N) TSHRs. The cells were transiently transfected with WT TSHR and mutant TSHR-I486N DNA. A: Cell surface expression was measured 72 h after transfection. The cells were fixed, and immunological determination of the N-terminal HA was performed. Results (means ± SD) are expressed as percentage of TSHR-WT (100%). B: Activation of the Gs/adenylyl cyclase pathway was determined 48 h after transfection. Cells were stimulated with bTSH, and intracellular cAMP accumulation was measured. Basal activity is indicated in white bars; activity after stimulation with 100 mU bTSH/ml is indicated in black bars. C: Gq/11 activation was reported 48 h after COS-7 co-transfection with TSHR DNA and a reporter construct containing a response element and the firefly luciferase gene under the control of nuclear factor of activated T-cells (transcription factor). The cells were stimulated with bTSH and lysed, and luciferase activity expression was measured. Basal activity is indicated in white bars, activity after stimulation with 100 mU bTSH/ml in black bars. The figure depicts means ± SD out of duplex or tripletts (n= 2-3). RLU, Relative light units. (*** means p value <0.001). The statistical analysis was made by using a nonparametric One-way-Anova and a tukey-test for column statistic of GraphPad Prism Version 4.03.

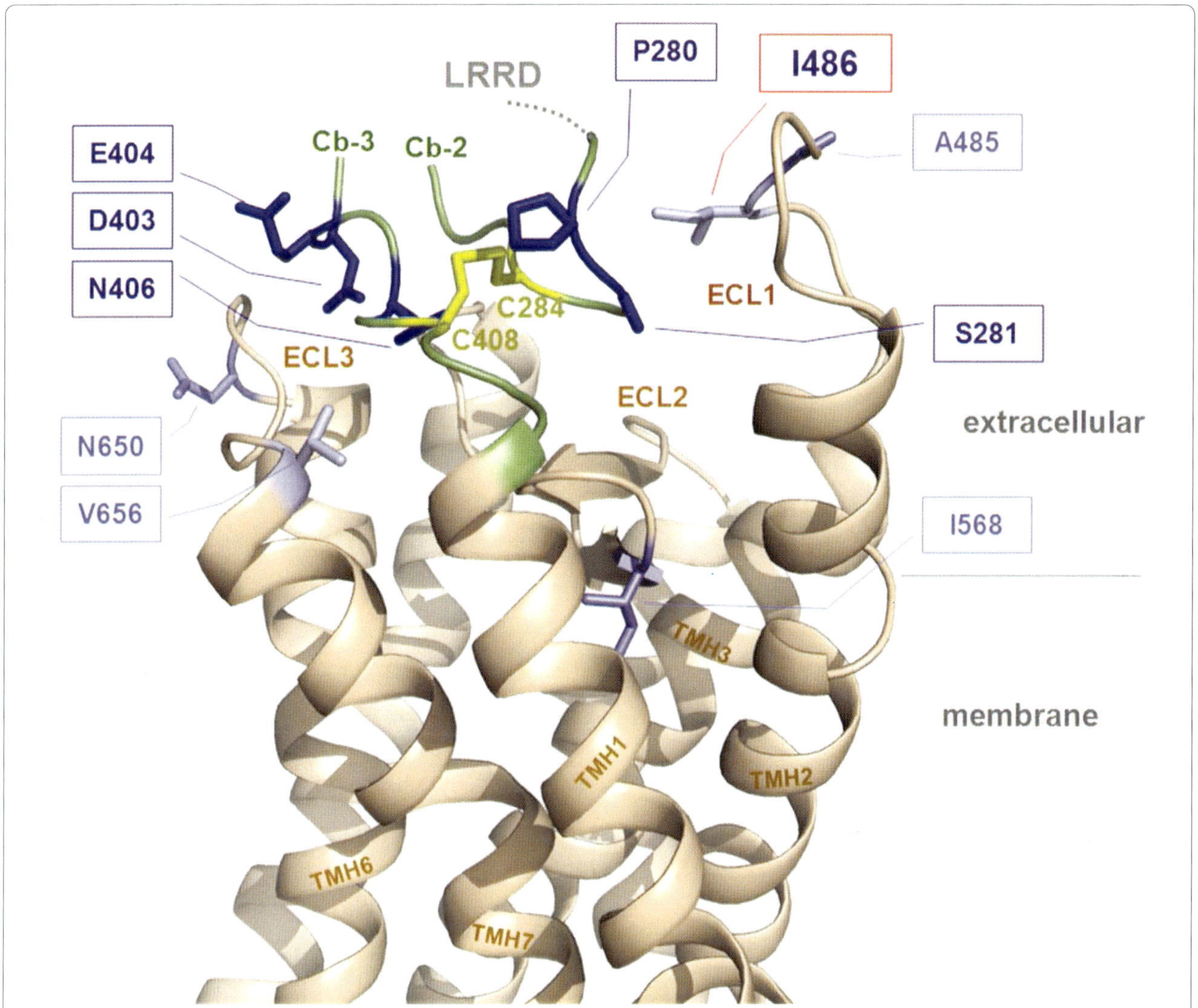


**Figure 2** This TSHR homology model (backbone-ribbon presentation) visualizes the potential arrangement of different structural parts at the interface between the extracellular and transmembrane region. Naturally occurring activating mutations in the extracellular loops (ECLs) were reported several times for the TSHR: ECL1- at positions I486 (red boxed) and A485; ECL2 - at position I568; ECL3 at positions N650 and V656 (wild type amino acids are shown as light blue sticks). Interestingly, the wild type amino acids side-chains are exclusively hydrophobic. The tightly embedded structural-functional counterparts of the loops are the extreme N- and C-terminus (green backbone) of the extracellular hinge region (cysteine-boxes 2 and 3 (Cb-2, Cb-3)) were also activating mutations are known (wild type residues as blue sticks). In conclusion these receptor components are sensitive for activation and they are assembled tightly together at the extracellular site of the receptor. Activation of the TSHR on the extracellular site might be related to a relative spatial shift of these determinants to each other, which mediates signal-transduction to the transmembrane helices.

activate the IP3-Gq pathway. The patient presented with elevated thyroid hormone levels and a suppressed TSH level in the absence of thyroid hormone antibodies, leading to the diagnosis of non-autoimmune hyperthyroidism. No measurable goiter was found in this patient and the phenotype was described as a mild form of hyperthyroidism, although the functional characterization revealed a high constitutive basal activity. This phenotype and functional characterization of the mutated TSHR is similar to our findings regarding the patient-phenotype and molecular characteristics of the TSHR variant I486N. We recently described a patient`s phenotype due to a TSHR mutation with comparable functional characteristics as non-autoimmune and non goitrous hyperthyroidism [23].

#### Implications from naturally occurring mutations for structural-functional aspects of the Thyrotropin receptor and patient phenotypes

To understand the functional and structural role of TSHR-I486N consideration of naturally occurring TSHR mutations in the extracellular loops provides valuable information. Naturally occurring activating mutations in the ECLs are reported several times in the TSHR: ECL1- I486M,F,N [20,21] and A485V [22]; ECL2 - I568T,V [20,24], ECL3 - N650Y [25] and V656F [26]. These activating mutations are indicators that the extracellular loops acting as important determinants for receptor activation. In support to this assumption also few naturally occurring inactivating mutations were published previously: ECL1 - W488R [27], Q489H [28]; ECL3 - L653V [29].

The potential interplaying counterparts of the ECLs (figure 2) are likely the extreme N- and C-terminus of the extracellular hinge region where also activating as well as inactivating mutations were reported (reviewed in [1]). Mutations at I486 likely modify the conformation of loop 1 and by this lead to re-justification of the extracellular receptor parts to each other. This spatial shift induces interruption of side-chain interactions or induces new interactions between amino acids which finally effects the arrangement of connected transmembrane helices (intramolecular signal transduction). The specific importance of the TSHR ECL1 in this scenario was evidenced and specified by site-directed mutagenesis studies [15,30]. In these studies the ECL1 was identified as a key-transducer and amplifier of extracellularly provided signals, which is supported by findings at other GPCRs [31,32].

Of note are the diverse functional characteristics of different I486 mutations tested in cell-systems. Two observations which might be exemplarily also for other pathogenic mutations we would like to highlight:

1. The here described mutation I486N on one hand constitutively activates the Gs pathway, but on the other hand selectively impairs the capacity for bTSH to induced Gq activation. Such selective inactivation for the hormone induced Gq mediated pathway is observed also for the inactivating pathogenic mutation L653V at the ECL3 [29]. Finally, this implicates that on one hand activating, on the other hand inactivating properties for a single side-chain substitution has to be considered. Such dual signal modification is reported recently also for the transmembrane mutant C636W [33]. Unfortunately in most cases of naturally occurring mutants a comprehensive experimental characterization is still missing (see information resource at http://www.ssfa-gphr.de).

2. Furthermore, functional comparison of different mutations at TSHR position 486 reveals substitution-dependent signaling properties. In opposite to mutations I486M and I486F the I486N mutation does not induce constitutive IP accumulation and simultaneously reduces the capacity for Gq activation after TSH binding. This contrast is likely related to the different biophysical properties of the particular substitutions. The methionine and phenylalanine residues are different in bulge and side-chain flexibility, but hydrophobic compared with the wild type isoleucine. In contrast, the hydrophilic asparagine can establish H-bonds or causes repulsion in a hydrophobic micro-environment. In consequence different effects on signaling compared to Met or Phe mutants are to be observed. Strikingly, these findings indicating a position and region were this receptor can be modified selectively for specific signaling properties and this might have impact also on the patient`s thyroid function and thereby the patient`s phenotype.

## Conclusion

Reported activating somatic or germline mutations in the extracellular loops show variable forms of hyperthyroidism-phenotypes. Even the phenotypical variability among carriers of the same germline mutation or even among mutation carriers of one family [22,34] could range from onset of hyperthyroidism as neonate and slight sign of hyperthyroidism as adult [34]. Potential explanations may result from above described differences in the modification of signaling pathways [35], but definitively there is no direct link between the degree of constitutive cAMP activation caused by a certain mutation obtained in an artificial *in vitro* over-expressing system and the severity of hyperthyroidism in patients [26,36]. Therefore it might be that estimation of further molecular aspects of TSHR signal transduction should help to explain the variability in hyperthyroidism-phenotypes.

### Abbreviations

bTSH: bovine TSH; cAMP: cyclic adenosine monophosphate; CAM: Constitutively activating mutations; DMEM: Dulbecco´s modified Eagle medium; ECL: extracellular loop; FBS: fetal bovine serum; fT4: free $T_4$; GPCR: G protein-coupled receptor; GPHR: glycoprotein hormone receptor; HA: hemagglutinin; ICL: intracellular loop; IP: inositol phosphate; IP3: inositol trisphosphate; MEM: Minimum Essential Medium Earle´s; NF-AT: nuclear factor of activated T-cells; TMH: transmembrane helix; TSH: thyroid-stimulating hormone; TSHR: TSH receptor; WT: wild-type.

### Acknowledgement

This work was supported by the Deutsche Forschungsgemeinschaft (KL2334/2-1) and the graduate college 1208 "Hormonal Regulation of Energy Metabolism, Body Weight and Growth", TP1. We also thank Rita Oltjen for her expert technical assistance.

This article has been published as part of *Thyroid Research* Volume 4 Supplement 1, 2011: New aspects of thyroid hormone synthesis and action. The full contents of the supplement are available online at http://www.thyroidresearchjournal.com/supplements/4/S1

### Authors contributions

HB and GK designed and coordinated the study and qualified the patients together with HK and AG. FW and DH did the functional characterization of the TSHR (WT and mutant) and performed statistical analysis. GK designed the TSHR homology model. All authors wrote the manuscript. All authors read and approved the final manuscript.

### Competing interests

The authors confirm that there are no competing interests.

### References


1. Kleinau G, Krause G: Thyrotropin and homologous glycoprotein hormone receptors: structural and functional aspects of extracellular signaling mechanisms. *Endocr Rev* 2009, **30(2)**:133-51.
2. Kleinau G, *et al*: Principles and determinants of G-protein coupling by the rhodopsin-like thyrotropin receptor. *PLoS One* 2010, **5(3)**:e9745.
3. Van Sande J, *et al*: Thyrotropin activates both the cyclic AMP and the PIP2 cascades in CHO cells expressing the human cDNA of TSH receptor. *Mol Cell Endocrinol* 1990, **74(1)**:R1-6.
4. Allgeier A, *et al*: The human thyrotropin receptor activates G-proteins Gs and Gq/11. *J Biol Chem* 1994, **269(19)**:13733-5.
5. Vassart G, Dumont JE: The thyrotropin receptor and the regulation of thyrocyte function and growth. *Endocr Rev* 1992, **13(3)**:596-611.
6. Kero J, *et al*: Thyrocyte-specific Gq/G11 deficiency impairs thyroid function and prevents goiter development. *J Clin Invest* 2007, **117(9)**:2399-407.
7. Biebermann H, Winkler F, Kleinau G: Genetic defects, thyroid growth and malfunctions of the TSHR in pediatric patients. *Front Biosci* 2010, **15**:913-933.
8. Kopp P, *et al*: Brief report: congenital hyperthyroidism caused by a mutation in the thyrotropin-receptor gene. *N Engl J Med* 1995, **332(3)**:150-4.
9. Kraemer S, *et al*: Activating TSH-receptor mutation (Met453Thr) as a cause of adenomatous non-autoimmune hyperthyroidism in a 3-year-old boy. *J Pediatr Endocrinol Metab* 2009, **22(3)**:269-74.
10. Tarnow P, *et al*: A heterozygous mutation in the third transmembrane domain causes a dominant-negative effect on signaling capability of the MC4R. *Obes Facts* 2008, **1(3)**:155-162.
11. Staubert C, *et al*: Evolutionary aspects in evaluating mutations in the melanocortin 4 receptor. *Endocrinology* 2007, **148(10)**:4642-8.
12. Kleinau G, *et al*: Identification of a novel epitope in the thyroid-stimulating hormone receptor ectodomain acting as intramolecular signaling interface. *J Biol Chem* 2004, **279(49)**:51590-600.
13. Bruysters M, Verhoef-Post M, Themmen AP: Asp330 and Tyr331 in the C-terminal cysteine-rich region of the luteinizing hormone receptor are key residues in hormone-induced receptor activation. *J Biol Chem* 2008, **283(38)**:25821-8.
14. Vlaeminck-Guillem V, *et al*: Activation of the cAMP pathway by the TSH receptor involves switching of the ectodomain from a tethered inverse agonist to an agonist. *Mol Endocrinol* 2002, **16(4)**:736-46.
15. Mizutori Y, *et al*: The thyrotropin receptor hinge region is not simply a scaffold for the leucine-rich domain but contributes to ligand binding and signal transduction. *Mol Endocrinol* 2008, **22(5)**:1171-82.
16. Persani L, *et al*: Genetics and phenomics of hypothyroidism due to TSH resistance. *Mol Cell Endocrinol* 2010, **322(1-2)**:72-82.
17. Davies TF, *et al*: Thyrotropin receptor-associated diseases: from adenomata to Graves disease. *J Clin Invest* 2005, **115(8)**:1972-83.
18. Gruters A, Krude H, Biebermann H: Molecular genetic defects in congenital hypothyroidism. *Eur J Endocrinol* 2004, **151(Suppl 3)**:U39-44.
19. Hebrant A, *et al*: Genetic hyperthyroidism: hyperthyroidism due to activating TSHR mutations. *Eur J Endocrinol* 2011, **164(1)**:1-9.
20. Parma J, *et al*: Somatic mutations causing constitutive activity of the thyrotropin receptor are the major cause of hyperfunctioning thyroid adenomas: identification of additional mutations activating both the cyclic adenosine 3',5'-monophosphate and inositol phosphate-Ca2+ cascades. *Mol Endocrinol* 1995, **9(6)**:725-33.
21. Gozu HI, *et al*: Similar prevalence of somatic TSH receptor and Gsalpha mutations in toxic thyroid nodules in geographical regions with different iodine supply in Turkey. *Eur J Endocrinol* 2006, **155(4)**:535-45.
22. Akcurin S, *et al*: A family with a novel TSH receptor activating germline mutation (p.Ala485Val). *Eur J Pediatr* 2008, **167(11)**:1231-7.
23. Winkler F, *et al*: A new phenotype of nongoitrous and nonautoimmune hyperthyroidism caused by a heterozygous thyrotropin receptor mutation in transmembrane helix 6. *J Clin Endocrinol Metab* 2010, **95(8)**:3605-10.
24. Claus M, *et al*: Novel thyrotropin receptor germline mutation (Ile568Val) in a Saxonian family with hereditary nonautoimmune hyperthyroidism. *Thyroid* 2005, **15(9)**:1089-94.
25. Tonacchera M, *et al*: Functional characteristics of three new germline mutations of the thyrotropin receptor gene causing autosomal dominant toxic thyroid hyperplasia. *J Clin Endocrinol Metab* 1996, **81(2)**:547-54.
26. Fuhrer D, *et al*: Somatic mutations in the thyrotropin receptor gene and not in the Gs alpha protein gene in 31 toxic thyroid nodules. *J Clin Endocrinol Metab* 1997, **82(11)**:3885-91.
27. Camilot M, *et al*: Thyrotropin receptor gene mutations and TSH resistance: variable expressivity in the heterozygotes. *Clin Endocrinol (Oxf)* 2005, **63(2)**:146-151.
28. Sura-Trueba S, *et al*: An inactivating mutation within the first extracellular loop of the thyrotropin receptor impedes normal posttranslational maturation of the extracellular domain. *Endocrinology* 2009, **150(2)**:1043-50.
29. Grasberger H, *et al*: A familial thyrotropin (TSH) receptor mutation provides in vivo evidence that the inositol phosphates/Ca2+ cascade mediates TSH action on thyroid hormone synthesis. *J Clin Endocrinol Metab* 2007, **92(7)**:2816-20.
30. Kleinau G, *et al*: Evidence for cooperative signal triggering at the extracellular loops of the TSH receptor. *FASEB J* 2008, **22(8)**:2798-808.
31. Peeters MC, *et al*: GPCR structure and activation: an essential role for the first extracellular loop in activating the adenosine A2B receptor. *FASEB J* 2011, **25**:632-643.
32. Peeters MC, *et al*: Importance of the extracellular loops in G protein-coupled receptors for ligand recognition and receptor activation. *Trends Pharmacol Sci* 2011, **32**:35-42.
33. Winkler F, *et al*: A New Phenotype of Nongoitrous and Nonautoimmune Hyperthyroidism Caused by a Heterozygous Thyrotropin Receptor Mutation in Transmembrane Helix 6. *J Clin Endocrinol Metab* 2010, **95**:3605-3610.
34. Duprez L, *et al*: Germline mutations in the thyrotropin receptor gene cause non-autoimmune autosomal dominant hyperthyroidism. *Nat Genet* 1994, **7(3)**:396-401.
35. Roger PP, *et al*: Signal transduction in the human thyrocyte and its perversion in thyroid tumors. *Mol Cell Endocrinol* 2010, **321(1)**:3-19.
36. Jaeschke H, Mueller S, Eszlinger M, Paschke R: Lack of in vitro constitutive activity for four previously reported TSH receptor mutations identified in patients with nonautoimmune hyperthyroidism and hot thyroid carcinomas. *Clin Endocrinol (Oxf)* 2010, **73**:815-820.

# Riedel's thyroiditis - a case report with genes' expression studies

Katarzyna Wojciechowska-Durczyńska[1], Adam Durczyński[2], Stanisław Sporny[3], Janusz Strzelczyk[2] and Andrzej Lewiński[1*]


## Abstract

**Background:** Genetic background of Riedel's thyroiditis remains unknown. Herein, we describe our results of studies on genes expression levels in Riedel's thyroiditis.

**Case report and genetic findings:** We report the case of 48-year old woman with Riedel's thyroiditis who has presented unusual course of disease with non-specific cervical discomfort, though as with no pain and/or no compression symptoms. After surgery, thyroid specimens were quantitatively evaluated, regarding *PIK3CA, PIK3CD, PIK3CG, Tg, TGFB1, THRB, COL1, CDKN1C, CDH3* and *CACNA2D2* genes expression levels, by real-time PCR in the ABI PRISM® 7500 Sequence Detection System. Out of 10 above genes, in 2 cases the expression was higher than in respective Controls of unchanged thyroid tissue. In the remaining 8 cases, expression in question became comparable or lower as in Controls.

**Discussion:** The association between increased expression levels of *PIK3CA* and *CDH3* genes and Riedel's thyroiditis is not well-defined. However, the increased expression of *PIK3CA* and *CDH3* genes in our case report and in previous studies of other authors on various malignancies may suggest possible molecular relation between Riedel's thyroiditis and certain neoplastic processes, the relation of which requires further genetic evaluation. It is to be stressed that gene expression studies in Riedel's thyroiditis are difficult to perform, mainly due to fibrosis, resulting in scarce thyroid specimens and - in consequence - small amount of genetic material.


**Keywords:** Riedel?'?s thyroiditis, Genes?'? expression, Real-time PCR

## Background

Riedel's thyroiditis is a rare fibrosclerotic infiltrative thyroid disorder of unclear etiology, during which normal thyroid tissues are replaced by fibrous tissue, often expanding outside the thyroid capsule. The diagnosis can be difficult to establish prior to surgical removal of the thyroid and to subsequent histopathological examination of the resected gland [1-3]. Reports on genetic findings in Riedel's thyroiditis are scarce in medical literature. Herein, we describe our results of studies on genes expression levels in Riedel's thyroiditis.

## Case report

We report the case of 48-year old women, diagnosed originally as a goiter with eminently increased consistency on palpation, presented with non-specific cervical discomfort, though with no pain and/or no compression symptoms. Clinically, the thyroid was enlarged, painless, however very firm. Serum thyrotropin (TSH) and free thyroid hormones (FT3 and FT4) concentrations were in normal ranges. Prior to surgery, the result of chest X-ray examination showed no pathological changes and all biochemical laboratory tests were normal. Ultrasound examination of the thyroid gland revealed few normoechoic foci in both lobes. Based on benign cytology of the nodules (normal thyroid follicular cells and colloid - Bethesda II) and the absence of compression symptoms, a subtotal thyroidectomy was performed. During surgery, a stony hard, white thyroid was disclosed. No complications after thyroid surgery were observed. Histopathological findings led to the diagnosis of Riedel's thyroiditis, based on disappearance of thyroid follicles, which were replaced by the fibrous tissue and

* Correspondence: alewin@csk.umed.lodz.pl
[1]Department of Endocrinology and Metabolic Diseases, Polish Mother's Memorial Hospital Research Institute, Medical University of Lodz, Rzgowska St. No. 281/289, 93-338 Lodz, Poland
Full list of author information is available at the end of the article

lymphocytes infiltrations, and features of focal endoarteritis (Figures 1, 2, 3, 4). Postoperatively, the patient was treated with levothyroxine, 100 μg per day. At 4-months follow up, results TSH, FT3, FT4, PTH, calcium-phosphorus homeostasis and autoantibodies against thyroid peroxidase and TSH receptor were in normal ranges; autoantibodies against thyroglobulin (anti-Tg) were elevated. Ultrasound examination of the neck did not showed features of disease recurrence.

## Genetic findings

After surgery, following conventional histopathological examination, thyroid specimen, received from patient with Riedel's thyroiditis, was quantitatively evaluated regarding *PIK3CA, PIK3CD, PIK3CG, Tg, TGFB1, THRB, COL1, CDKN1C, CDH3 and CACNA2D2* genes expression levels by real-time PCR in the ABI PRISM ®7500 Sequence Detection System. Macroscopically unchanged thyroid tissue, surgically removed from the patient with non-toxic nodular goitre (NTG), served as a control for *real-time* PCR experiment.

Total RNA from tissue was extracted by use of an RNeasy Midi Kit (Qiagen, Hilden, Germany) based on modified Chomczyński and Sacchi's according to manufacturers' recommendations. The purity of total RNA was assessed by NanoDrop® ND-100 spectrophotometr and next the RNA was used in the first strand cDNA synthesis with TaqMan® Reverse Transcripton Reagents (Applied Biosystem) according to maufacturers' instruction. Real-time PCR was performed by using *Taq*Man® Universal PCR Master Mix (Applied Biosystem) and *Taq*Man® Gene Expression Assays probe and primer mix (Applied Biosystem) according to the manufacturer' specification. Thermal cycler conditions were as follows: hold for 10 min. at 95°C, follow by two-step PCR for 50 cycles of 95°C for 15 s followed by 60°C for 1 min. Amplification reactions, in triplicate for each sample, were performed and the results were normalized to the *ACTB* gene expression level.

An analysis of relative gene expression data was performed, using the $2^{-\Delta\Delta CT}$ method on an ABI PRISM® 7500 Sequence Detection System Software. The fold change in studied gene expression, normalised to endogenous control, was calculated using: $RQ = 2^{-\Delta\Delta CT}$.

Out of 10 above genes, in 2 cases [*PIK3CA* - responsible for coding alpha catalytic subunit of class I PI3K (phosphoinositide 3-kinase) and *CDH3* - responsible for coding P-cadherin] the expression was higher than in

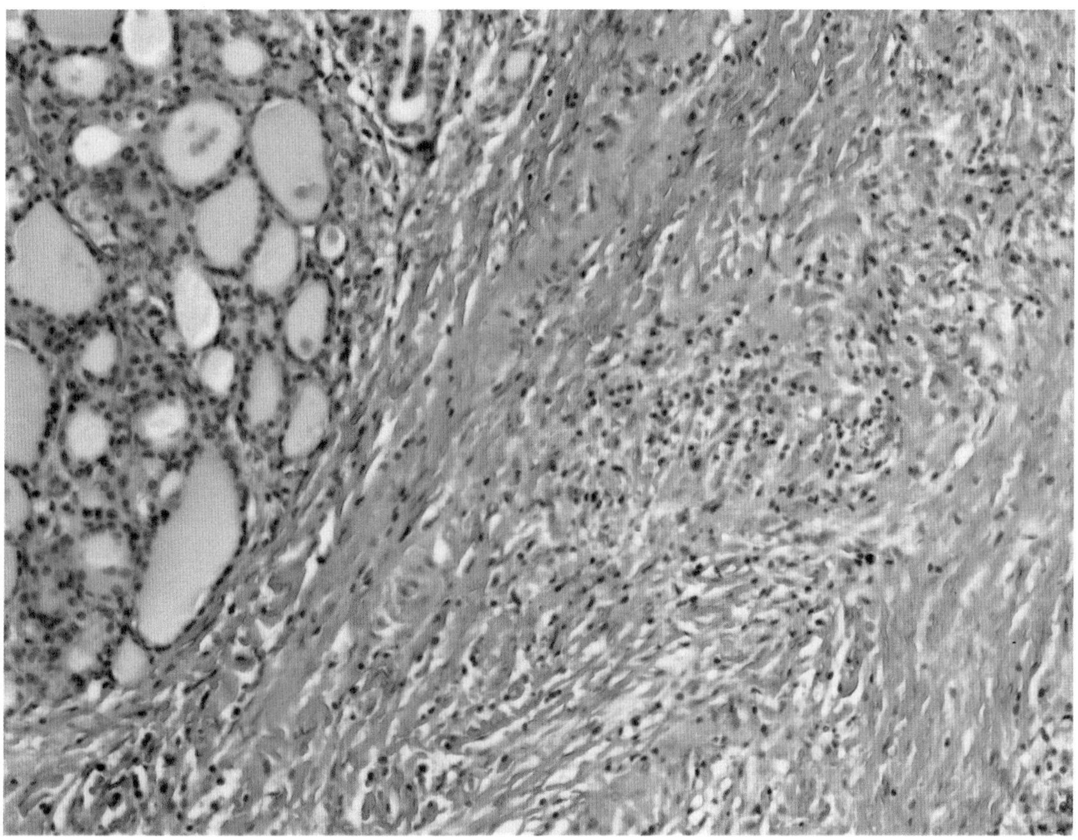

**Figure 1 Thyroid parenchyma peripherally to dense connective tissue hyperplasia.** HE 320 ×.

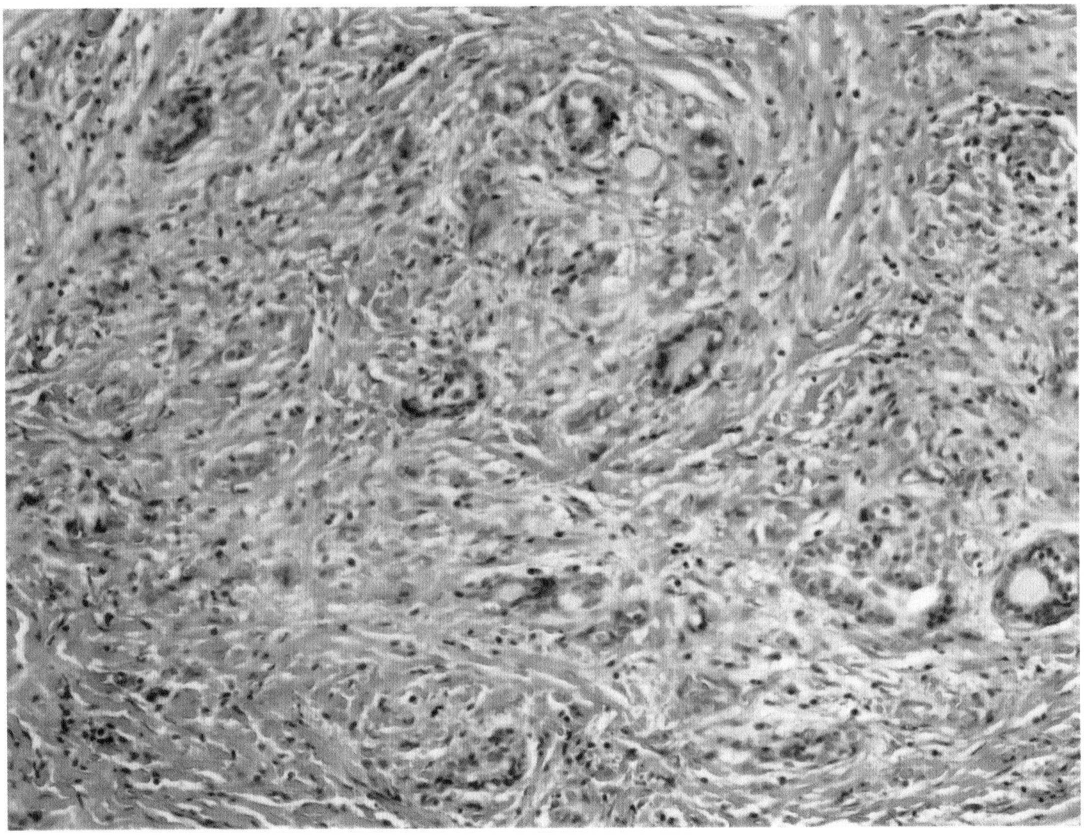

**Figure 2 Thyroid parenchyma remnant among dense connective tissue**. HE 320 ×.

respective Controls of unchanged thyroid tissue. In the remaining 8 cases, expression in question became comparable or lower as in Controls (Figure 5).

## Discussion

Riedel's throiditis is a rare disease that most commonly occurs in females in their fifties and usually demonstrates as a goitre without clinical evidence of thyroid nodules. On palpation, thyroid demonstrates firm or stony consistency ("iron-hard thyroiditis"). Symptoms of regional compression might progressively appear. However, the clinical course of this disease is mostly variable and may include cases with no thyroid-related symptoms, as we have noted in our patient [3]. Before surgery, Riedel's thyroiditis is often difficult to differentiate from aggressive types of thyroid cancers (i.e., undifferentiated thyroid carcinoma), nevertheless, a long-term follow-up shows no disease-specific mortality [4]. Likewise in presented patient, in vast majority of cases, only histopathological, postoperative examination leads to diagnosis of Riedel's thyroiditis, due to no specific symptoms. Cytological evaluation is also of limited use in Riedel's thyroiditis, due to firm thyroid tissue consistency and scanty amount of cellular material thus often non-diagnostic thyroid specimens [5]. According to our opinion, in the case described by us, unusual course of the Riedel's thyroiditis with the absence of compressive symptoms may be related to early-stage of the disease.

A number of hypotheses have been proposed regarding etiology and pathogenesis of Riedel's thyroiditis. The disease may be associated with subacute and chronic thyroiditis, thus some authors proposed the, so called, "intrathyroidal hypothesis". According to that hypothesis, the entity may represent the late stage (i.e., the progression to fibrotic stage) of chronic inflammatory disorder [6-8]. On the contrary, the "pharmacological hypothesis" suggests that some particular medications may trigger Riedel's thyroiditis development [8]. Although not proven, inherited susceptibility and development was hypothesized, as well [8]. Nowadays, the "systemic autoimmune hypothesis" seems to have the most support and it basically views Riedel's thyroiditis as a manifestation of disordered fibroplastic proliferation because of hypersensivity reaction and consequent release of stimulating growth factors [9]. This theory considers a fibroblast not only as a final cell responsible for fibrosis, but also as a main target for well-defined systemic autoimmune attack [8]. In our case, the

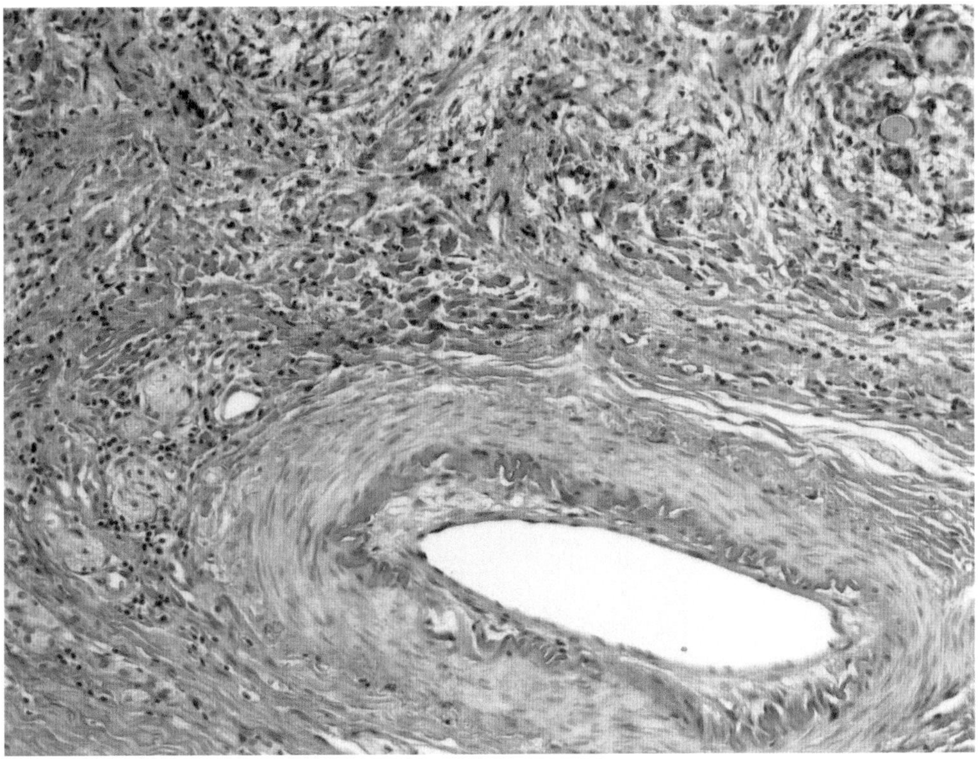

**Figure 3** Arterial vessel among fibrosing thyroid parenchyma. HE 320 ×.

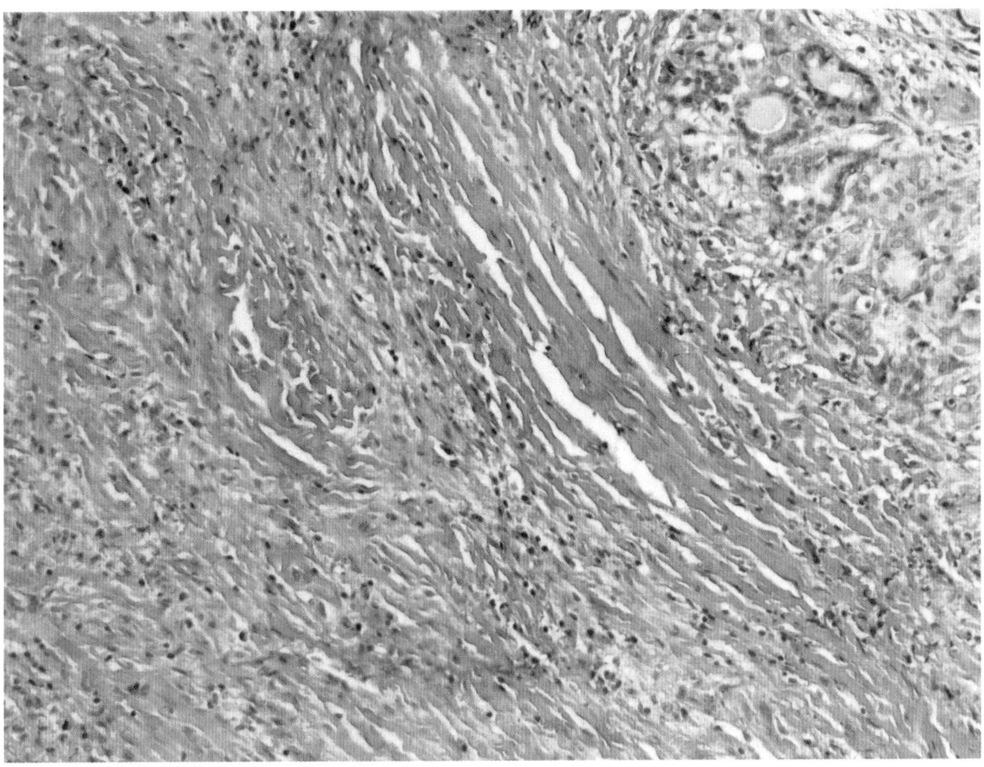

**Figure 4** Thyroid parenchyma peripherally to dense connective tissue hyperplasia. HE 320 ×.

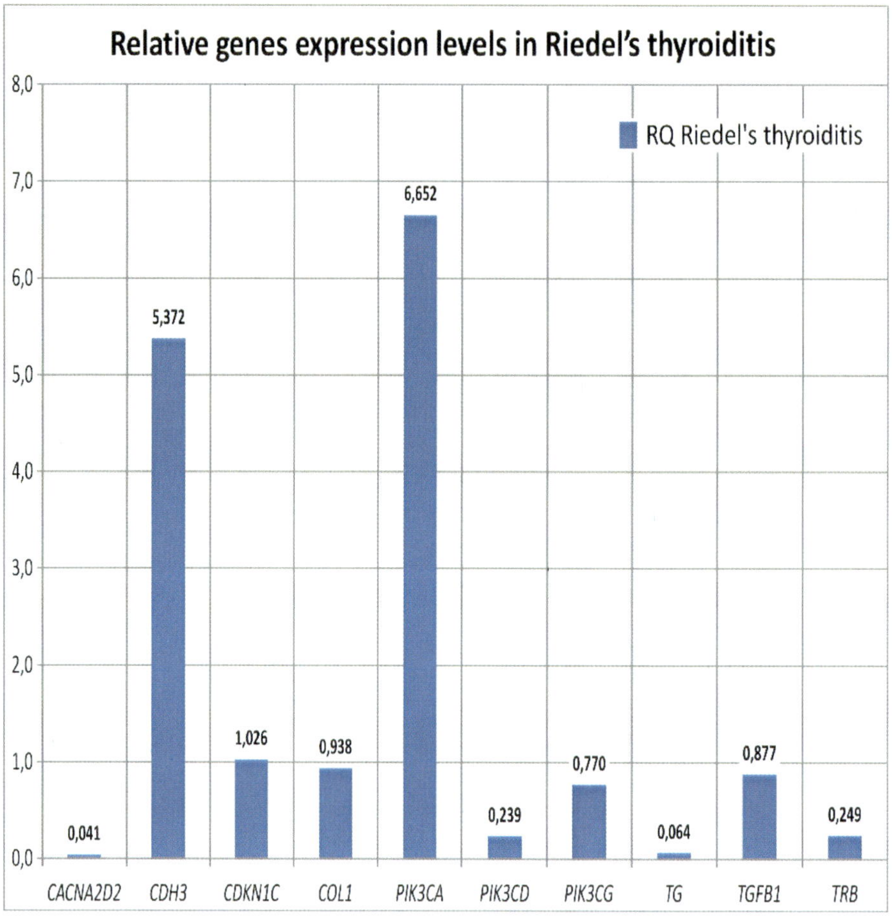


**Figure 5 Real-time PCR relative quantification (RQ) of studied genes levels in Riedel's thyroiditis.** Bars represents quantification values normalized to an endogenous control (β-actin) and relative to a calibrator (control sample, RQ = 1).

"systemic autoimmune hypothesis" of Riedel's thyroiditis is the most plausible, it is supported by laboratory findings of autoimmune thyroid disease (anti-Tg), which have persisted after surgery.

PI3K/Akt (phosphoinositide 3-kinase/serine-threonine protein kinase) pathway participates in cellular signaling in response to various growth factors including FGF (fibroblast growth factor). Activating mutations and amplification of *PIK3CA* gene have been associated with enhancing PIK3CA kinase activity and Akt phosphorylation. Increased PI3K/Akt expression has been observed in both Hashimoto thyroiditis and well-differentiated thyroid cancer [10,11]. Still, little is known about the precise role of *PIK3CA* in fibrosclerotic disorders, however, it has been proved that hepatic Akt expression correlated with advanced liver fibrosis in chronic hepatitis C patient [12].

Our results demonstrate that *CDH3* gene expression may increase in Riedel's thyroiditis, as well. Cadherins, such as *CDH3*, are integral membrane glycoproteins responsible for calcium-dependent cell-cell adhesion. Our contemporary knowledge about the role of P-cadherin in fibrosis and autoimmune processes is scanty and, so far, it has been only demonstrated that aberrant expression of E-cadherin/β-catenin complex is associated with a wide variety of human malignancies and fibrosis [13].

The association between increased expression levels of *PIK3CA* and *CDH3* genes and Riedel's thyroiditis is not well-defined. However, the increased expression of *PIK3CA* and *CDH3* genes in our case report and in previous studies of other authors on various malignancies may suggest possible molecular relation between Riedel's thyroiditis and certain neoplastic processes, the relation which requires further genetic evaluation.

Low expression levels of the remaining studied genes could be associated with destruction of glandular thyroid tissue. The levels of *TGFB1, COL1* and *CDKN1C* genes expression were comparable in Riedel's thyroiditis and in macroscopically unchanged tissue. It is to be emphasized that high expression levels of *TGFB1* and of *COL1A1* genes in chronic thyroiditis and its correlation with thyroid fibrosis has previously been observed [14].

These results call into question the "intrathyroidal hypothesis" of Riedel's disease pathogenesis. One should remind once again that gene expression studies in Riedel's thyroiditis are difficult to perform, mainly due to fibrosis, resulting in scarce thyroid specimens and - in consequence - small amount of genetic material.

## Consent

Written informed consent was obtained from the patient for publication of this report and any accompanying images.

**Author details**

[1]Department of Endocrinology and Metabolic Diseases, Polish Mother's Memorial Hospital Research Institute, Medical University of Lodz, Rzgowska St. No. 281/289, 93-338 Lodz, Poland. [2]Department of General and Transplant Surgery, Medical University of Lodz, Barlicki University Hospital, Lodz, Poland. [3]Department of Dental Pathology, Medical University of Lodz, The Clinical-Didactic Centre, Lodz, Poland.

**Authors' contributions**

KW-D designed and coordinated the study, carried out the molecular genetic studies, writing a manuscript. AD, SS and JS participated in coordination of the study. AL senior supervision, writing a manuscript. All authors have read and approved the final manuscript.

**Competing interests**

The authors declare that they have no competing interests.

**References**

1. Schwaegerle SM, Bauer TW, Esselstyn CB Jr: **Riedel's thyroiditis.** *Am J Clin Pathol* 1988, **6**:715-722, Review.
2. Papi G, Corrado S, Cesinaro AM, Novelli L, Smerieri A, Carapezzi C: **Riedel's thyroiditis: clinical, pathological and imaging features.** *Int J Clin Pract* 2002, **1**:65-67.
3. Fontaine S, Gaches F, Lamant L, Uzan M, Bennet A, Caron P: **An unusual form of Riedel's thyroiditis: a case report and review of the literature.** *Thyroid* 2005, **1**:85-88.
4. Fatourechi MM, Hay ID, McIver B, Sebo TJ, Fatourechi V: **Invasive fibrous thyroiditis (Riedel thyroiditis): the Mayo Clinic experience, 1976-2008.** *Thyroid* 2011, **7**:765-772.
5. Junik R, Juraniec O, Pypkowski J, Krymer A, Marszałek A: **A difficult diagnosis: a case report of combined Riedel's disease and fibrosing Hashimoto's thyroiditis.** *Endokrynol Pol* 2011, **62(4)**:351-356.
6. Zelmanovitz F, Zelmanovitz T, Beck M, Cerski CT, Schmid H, Czepielewski MA: **Riedel's thyroiditis associated with high titers of antimicrosomal and antithyroglobulin antibodies and hypothyroidism.** *J Endocrinol Invest* 1994, **9**:733-737.
7. Papi G, Corrado S, Carapezzi C, De-Gaetani C, Carani C: **Riedel's thyroiditis and fibrous variant of Hashimoto's thyroiditis: a clinicopathological and immunohistochemical study.** *J Endocrinol Invest* 2003, **5**:444-449.
8. Papi G, LiVolsi VA: **Current concepts on Riedel thyroiditis.** *Am J Clin Pathol* 2004, **121**:50-63.
9. Biddinger PW: **Thyroiditis.** In *Diagnostic Pathology and molecular Genetics of the Thyroid.* Edited by: Nikiforov YE. Lippincott Williams 2009:39-59.
10. Larson SD, Jackson LN, Riall TS, Uchida T, Thomas RP, Qiu S, Evers BM: **Increased incidence of well-differentiated thyroid cancer associated with Hashimoto thyroiditis and the role of the PI3k/Akt pathway.** *J Am Coll Surg* 2007, **5**:764-773.
11. Wojciechowska-Durczyńska K, Krawczyk-Rusiecka K, Cyniak-Magierska A, Zygmunt A, Gałecka E, Lewiński A: **Relative quantification of *PIK3C* gene expression level in fine-needle aspiration biopsy thyroid specimens collected from patients with papillary thyroid carcinoma and non-toxic goitre by real-time RT-PCR.** *Thyroid Res* 2010, **3**:5.
12. Huang JF, Chuang YH, Dai CY, Yu ML, Huang CF, Hsiao PJ, Hsieh MY, Huang CI, Yeh ML, Yang JF, Lin ZY, Chen SC, Chuang WL: **Hepatic Akt expression correlates with advanced fibrosis in patients with chronic hepatitis C infection.** *Hepatol Res* 2011, **5**:430-436.
13. Tian X, Liu Z, Niu B, Zhang J, Tan TK, Lee SR, Zhao Y, Harris DC, Zheng G: **E-cadherin/β-catenin complex and the epithelial barrier.** *J Biomed Biotechnol* 2011, **2011**:567305.
14. Cyniak-Magierska A, Januszkiewicz-Caulier J, Brzeziańska E, Lewiński A: **Analysis of correlation between the process of thyroid fibrosis and TGFB1 gene expression level in fine-needle aspiration biopsy (FNAB) thyroid specimens collected from patients with Hashimoto's thyroiditis and non-toxic goitre.** *Exp Clin Endocrinol Diabetes* 2010, **7**:420-426.

# 21

# Extent of surgery in clinically evident but operable MTC – when is central and/or lateral lympadenectomy indicated?

Oliver Gimm[1,2]

*From* 9th Meeting of the European Thyroid Association Cancer Research Network (ETA-CRN)
Lisbon, Portugal.

**Abstract**

Medullary thyroid carcinoma (MTC) metastasizes very early lymphogeneously. It has been shown that the presence of lymph node metastases is associated with a worse outcome. Postoperative biochemical cure, i.e. normalization of posttherapeutical calcitonin levels, has been shown to correlate with a better outcome. The rate of biochemical cure decreases dramatically in the presence of lymph node metastases but can still be achieved in about 30-40% of patients despite the presence of lymph node metastases.

In 2009, the American Thyroid Association (ATA) published guidelines on the management of MTC. Various recommendations in the guidelines are dealing with the extent of lymph node dissection in different clinical settings. This article summarizes and comments on these recommendations.

## Background

Medullary thyroid carcinoma (MTC) metastasizes very early lymphogenously.

The presence of initial lymph node metastases in non-screening patients is generally reported to be higher than 50%, often as high as 75-80% [1,2]. Even bilateral lateral lymph node involvement is quite frequent (>25%) [2] and has been shown to be associated with distant metastases [3]. In these advanced cases, biochemical cure, i.e. normalization of posttherapeutical calcitonin levels, is extremely rare [4].

It has been shown that the presence of lymph node metastases in general is associated with a worse outcome [5]. Interestingly, it has less clearly been shown that lymphadenectomy improves the outcome in patients with MTC [5]. What has been shown is that, depending on patient selection, biochemical cure can be achieved in about 30-40% of patients with regional lymph node metastases [4,6] which, however, is a significantly lower rate than that for patients without lymph node metastases (90-100%) [1,6]. Biochemical cure itself has been shown to correlate with a better outcome [7-9] but late recurrence has been shown.

That the extent of lymph node dissection is part of ongoing discussion has apart from the unknown benefit in a specific patient in part to do with the possible complications that are accompanied with this procedure, mainly hypoparathyroidism and nerve injury [10]. In addition, in the presence of advanced disease, t.ex. distant metastases, the benefit of lymph node dissection is even more questionable.

## ATA guidelines regarding lymphadenectomy

The guidelines published by the American Thyroid Association (ATA) [11] contain various recommendations dealing with the extent of lymphadenectomy.

### Clinically evident or highly suspected MTC

According to the guidelines, patients having MTC or those where MTC is highly likely should undergo total thyroidectomy and prophylactic central compartment (level VI) neck dissection both with and without evidence of cervical lymph node metastases in the absence of advanced local invasion and distant metastases

Correspondence: oliver.gimm@liu.se
[1]Department of Clinical and Experimental Medicine, Faculty of Health Sciences, Linköping University, SE-58185 Linköping, Sweden
Full list of author information is available at the end of the article

(recommendation 61 & 62). The lateral compartment (level II-V) should be included in the case of ultrasound-confirmed lateral lymph node metastases (recommendation 63). Preoperative ultrasound is therefore indicated in all patients prior to surgery (recommendation 19).

Some members of the task force recommended prophylactic inclusion of the lateral compartment recommended in the presence of central compartment lymph node metastases (recommendation 62). This recommendation is based on the finding that the involvement of the ipsilateral cervicolateral compartment correlates with the number of lymph node metastases in the central compartment [12].

#### Advanced disease

In general, a less aggressive approach is advised in the presence of advanced local and/or distant metastases while maintaining locoregional disease control to prevent central neck morbidity (recommendation 64 & 65). In patients with distant metastases, removal of small asymptomatic and nonthreatening lymph node metastases (<1 cm) is of unknown benefit and such lymph nodes may be observed (recommendation 81).

#### Primary incomplete surgery

Following primary incomplete surgery, reoperation including the central lymph node compartment is recommended when neck US is suspicious for persistent local disease in the central or lateral neck compartment (recommendation 71) or when the basal serum calcitonin level is above the normal reference range (recommendation 72).

If not previously performed, node dissection in both the central and lateral compartment should be compartment-oriented. Removal of only grossly metastatic lymph nodes, or other limited procedures, should be avoided in these instances (recommendation 77). This recommendation is based on the fact that removal of only grossly metastatic lymph nodes correlates with a lower calcitonin normalization rate, a higher reoperation rate and a lower survival rate [13].

In view of the ATA guidelines, central lymph node dissection remains controversial if primary surgery only consisted of total thyroidectomy in patients with continuously elevated calcitonin levels in the absence of radiographic findings (recommendation 78). It is explained in the guidelines that controversy also exist due to the increased risk of harm. It is obvious that the surgical experience and expertise plays an important role in this regard. Of note, it must be primarily assumed that continuously elevated calcitonin levels following thyroidectomy mainly are due to lymph node metastases left *in situ*. Calcitonin normalization has in selected patients been observed in up to 35-40% even after reoperation [14,15] and may actually be as low as 6% if one waits for radiographic positive findings [16]. Thus the recommendation to wait for positive imaging as suggested by the ATA guidelines is questionable.

#### Hereditary MTC

In patients with hereditary MTC, early identification of patients, e.g. through family screening, may enable to limit the extent of surgery to the thyroid gland since lymph node metastases may be very unlikely if preoperative calcitonin levels are normal [17,18]. Besides patient's age, primary tumor size and calcitonin levels may be helpful in determining the surgical extent. The ATA guidelines give some recommendations in this regard (recommendations 33, 35, 40-43). Since this review is focusing on clinically evident MTC, these recommendations will not be discussed in detail here.

### Further comments

In general, lymph node dissection should be very restrictive in the presence of advanced local and/or distant disease. This is justified by the very low chance to cure those patients [6] where no benefit might be gained from the lymph node dissection. In these instances, the calcitonin doubling-times may be of help assessing patient's prognosis where doubling-tomes less than 6 months are very unfavourable [19].

#### Clinically evident or highly suspected lymph node metastases

Taken the above into account, dissection is almost always indicated in the presence of cervical lymph nodes metastases. Clinically, the presence of lymph node metastases is most often assumed in the presence of enlarged lymph nodes. Fine-needle aspiration is rarely performed. However, lymph node metastases in MTC are typically rather small in size and, thus, normal lymph node size does not exclude the presence of metastases.

#### Unknown lymph node status

If no enlarged lymph nodes are present, the extent of lymph node dissection is much more difficult to assess. This situation, however, is very common.

Most surgeons would recommend central lymphadenectomy (defined as dissection of level VI) in all patients with sporadic MTC and in all screening patients with elevated calcitonin levels at the time thyroidectomy is performed due to the high likelhood of the presence of positive lymph nodes [20]. The exception are screening patients with normal calcitonin levels that probably have an extremely low risk that lymph node metastases exist [17,18]. These patients may therefore forego lymphadenectomy. As mentioned before, one reason to avoid cervical lymphadenectomy is the observed higher rate of complications [10]. The reason to perform central lymphadenectomy synchronous with thyroidectomy is that metachronous lymphadenectomy confers an even higher risk of complications. This does not apply to the lateral compartments (level II-V) that are not touched if the previous operation consist of thyroidectomy both with and without central lymphadenectomy.

Since the ipsilateral cervicolateral compartment contains almost as often lymph node metastases as the central compartment [21], some surgeons would recommend performing both central and lateral lymphadenactomy synchronous with thyroidectomy. Others have recommended lateral lymph node dissection "on demand", i.e. in the setting of measurable postoperative bCT and/or sCT levels indicating LN metastasis [22]. In the case of contralateral positive lymph nodes, the chance of biochemical cure decreases dramatically [21] and no beneficial outcome has been shown if lymphadenectomy is performed in these patients.

#### Assessing the lymph node status

The question is how the extent of lymph node metastases can be assessed pre- or at the latest intraoperatively in MTC patients.

##### *Imaging techniques*

The accuracy of computed tomography and ultrasonography for evaluating cervical lymph node metastases in patients with papillary thyroid carcinoma is not very high, 74% vs. 68 resp. [23]. Since it is known that lymph mode metastases in MTC are often rather small as compared to papillary thyroid carcinoma, the accuracy is expected to be lower which has indeed been shown [24]. Both, somatostatin receptor scintigraphy and, in particular, FDG-PET have been used with some success in detecting lymph node metastaes preoperatively but the reported series are small [24-28].

In reoperative cases, a variety of imaging techniques (ultrasound, computed tomography, FDG-PET) seems to have a low sensitivity (56%, 42%, and 32%, respectively).

Thus, currently available imaging techniques are of minor value identifying small lymph node metastases. Ultrasound, which is readily available, is the investigation of choice and should always be performed first.

##### *Venous sampling*

In reoperative cases, it has been shown that pentagastrin-stimulated intravenous calcitonin sampling followed by targeted surgery may be beneficial in the diagnostic work-up of MTC after thyroidectomy [29]. However, the number of reported cases is low and the real value is not known yet.

##### *Primary tumor size*

Even small tumors (<1 cm) inherit a risk for lymph node metastases that increases with tumor size [30]. Patients having a primary tumor of less than 5 mm in size have a risk of having lymph node metastases between 13-20% if sporadic and between 6-14% if hereditary. The biochemical cure rates at these early stages are 69-85% and 80-96%, respectively. Concerning tumors smaller than 1 cm in size, lymph node metastases are found in 5-31% and the biochemical cure ranges from 71% to 100% (reviewed in [30]). Thus, even at these early stages, lymph node metastases are not uncommon [31].

Thus, lymph node metastases are not uncommon even in small primary tumors. The tumor size is, hence, of less value in assessing the presence of lymph node metastases in patients with MTC.

##### *Lymph node metastases in the central compartment*

Studies have shown that the involvement of the ipsilateral cervicolateral compartment correlates with the number of lymph node metastases in the central compartment. If more than 3 lymph nodes in the cervicocentral compartment were involved, almost all patients had lateral lymph node metastases in one study [12]. This "marker", however, is of less use in the clinical setting in the absence of macroscopically enlarged lymph nodes since it is not possible to determine the numbers of central lymph node metastases within a decent time period intraoperatively so far. Of note, lateral lymph node metastases were found in about 10% even in the absence of central lymph node metastases. This finding, i.e. the presence of cervicolateral lymph node metastases without cervicocentral compartment involvement, often referred to as skip metastases [32], has even been found in up to 35% by others [33].

##### *Calcitonin levels*

Concerning microMTC (<1 cm), calcitonin levels cannot distinguish between patients with and without lymph node metastases [22]. This is also true for patients with larger primary tumors even though higher basal calcitonin levels correlate better than pentagastrin stimulated calcitonin levels with lymph node involvement [20]. In the latter study, both central and ipsilateral lateral lymph node metastases were present in about 10% of the patients already at a basal level of 20 pg/mL. In patients higher than 200 pg/mL, contralateral lateral lymph node involvement was observed in at least 12% of the patients.

One study showed that intraoperative stimulated calcitonin levels following thyroidectomy and central lymph node dissection correlated well with the presence of lateral lymph node metastases [34]. The intraoperative usefulness of this technique would require quick calcitonin assays. Currently, the analysis takes several hours.

##### *Age*

While age plays an important role assessing timing and extent in patients with hereditary MTC [35], it does not seem to play a role in sporadic MTC.

***Other "markers"***

Beside these more traditional markers, other markers are sought after.

Of interest, one such "marker" has been cervical pain. In one study, the authors reported that roughly 80% of their patients with MTC presented with neck pain (defined as any subjective complaint of anterior neck discomfort, ache, pressure, or sharp, throbbing, or dull sensations in the region of the thyroid gland, with or without palpation) as opposed to only 6% of their patients with papillary thyroid carcinoma [36]. However, even 36% of those without pain had lymph node metastases.

Desmoplastic stromal reaction is one of those intraoperative markers that appear to have more clinical value. In one study analyzing 120 MTCs, it was shown that desmoplastic stromal reaction, which can be assessed intraoperatively, has a low (38%) sensitivity of predicting N0 but a very high (100%) specificity. The authors therefore recommend avoiding lymph node dissection in the absence of desmoplastic stromal reaction [37]. The results where later shown to be reproducible by other pathologists [38] but larger prospective studies are missing yet.

## Conclusions

If advanced disease is absent, central lymph node dissection is almost always indicated at the initial operation in patients with clinically evident MTC. Synchronous inclusion of the ipsilateral lateral compartment is recommended by some but might probably also be done "on demand" if postoperative calcitonin levels remain elevated.

In reoperative cases, the extent of lymph node dissection depends primarily on the extent of previous operation(s). Compartments that have not been operated on in a systematic way, i.e. dissection of all lymph node and the connective tissue *"en bloc"*, should be operated in this manner. Node picking should be reserved to those compartments that have been operated on systematically. I these cases, positive imaging is required. This approach, however, has not been proven to be of any benefit for the patient.

Future research has to concentrate on improving preoperative imaging and on the identification of intraoperative measurable markers that correlate with the presence or absence of lymph node metastases with a high accuracy.

#### Competing interests

The author declares no competing interests.

#### Declarations

This article has been published as part of *Thyroid Research* Volume 6 Supplement 1, 2013: European comments on Medullary Thyroid Cancer Management Guidelines of the American Thyroid Association. The full contents of the supplement are available online at http://www.thyroidresearchjournal.com/supplements/6/S1. Publication of this supplement has been supported by the European Thyroid Association-Cancer Research Network.

#### Author details

[1]Department of Clinical and Experimental Medicine, Faculty of Health Sciences, Linköping University, SE-58185 Linköping, Sweden. [2]Department of Surgery, County Council of Östergötland, SE-58185 Linköping, Sweden.

#### References

1. Weber T, Schilling T, Frank-Raue K, Colombo-Benkmann M, Hinz U, Ziegler R, Klar E: **Impact of modified radical neck dissection on biochemical cure in medullary thyroid carcinomas.** *Surgery* 2001, **130(6)**:1044-1049.
2. Hamy A, Raffaitin P, Floch I, Paineau J, Mirallie E, Visset J: **[The importance of lymph node dissection in medullary thyroid macrocarcinomas].** *Ann Chir* 2003, **128(7)**:447-451.
3. Machens A, Holzhausen HJ, Dralle H: **Contralateral cervical and mediastinal lymph node metastasis in medullary thyroid cancer: systemic disease?** *Surgery* 2006, **139(1)**:28-32.
4. Machens A, Gimm O, Ukkat J, Hinze R, Schneyer U, Dralle H: **Improved prediction of calcitonin normalization in medullary thyroid carcinoma patients by quantitative lymph node analysis.** *Cancer* 2000, **88(8)**:1909-1915.
5. Kandil E, Gilson MM, Alabbas HH, Tufaro AP, Dackiw A, Tufano RP: **Survival implications of cervical lymphadenectomy in patients with medullary thyroid cancer.** *Ann Surg Oncol* 2011, **18(4)**:1028-1034.
6. Gimm O, Ukkat J, Dralle H: **Determinative factors of biochemical cure after primary and reoperative surgery for sporadic medullary thyroid carcinoma.** *World J Surg* 1998, **22(6)**:562-567, discussion 567-568.
7. Dottorini ME, Assi A, Sironi M, Sangalli G, Spreafico G, Colombo L: **Multivariate analysis of patients with medullary thyroid carcinoma. Prognostic significance and impact on treatment of clinical and pathologic variables.** *Cancer* 1996, **77(8)**:1556-1565.
8. Raffaitin P, Hamy A, Mirallie E, Meurette G, Duplessis R, Lemeunier P, Murat A, Le Bodic M, Le Neel JC, Paineau J, *et al*: **[Prognostic factors of survival without clinical recurrences in medullary thyroid carcinoma: apropos of 52 operated cases].** *Ann Endocrinol (Paris)* 1999, **60(6)**:435-442.
9. Rendl G, Manzl M, Hitzl W, Sungler P, Pirich C: **Long-term prognosis of medullary thyroid carcinoma.** *Clin Endocrinol (Oxf)* 2008, **69(3)**:497-505.
10. Cheah WK, Arici C, Ituarte PH, Siperstein AE, Duh QY, Clark OH: **Complications of neck dissection for thyroid cancer.** *World J Surg* 2002, **26(8)**:1013-1016.
11. Kloos RT, Eng C, Evans DB, Francis GL, Gagel RF, Gharib H, Moley JF, Pacini F, Ringel MD, Schlumberger M, *et al*: **Medullary thyroid cancer: management guidelines of the American Thyroid Association.** *Thyroid* 2009, **19(6)**:565-612.
12. Machens A, Hauptmann S, Dralle H: **Prediction of lateral lymph node metastases in medullary thyroid cancer.** *Br J Surg* 2008, **95(5)**:586-591.
13. Dralle H, Damm I, Scheumann GF, Kotzerke J, Kupsch E, Geerlings H, Pichlmayr R: **Compartment-oriented microdissection of regional lymph nodes in medullary thyroid carcinoma.** *Surg Today* 1994, **24(2)**:112-121.
14. Gimm O, Dralle H: **Reoperation in metastasizing medullary thyroid carcinoma: is a tumor stage-oriented approach justified?** *Surgery* 1997, **122(6)**:1124-1130, discussion 1130-1121.
15. Moley JF, Dilley WG, DeBenedetti MK: **Improved results of cervical reoperation for medullary thyroid carcinoma.** *Ann Surg* 1997, **225(6)**:734-740, discussion 740-733.
16. Fleming JB, Lee JE, Bouvet M, Schultz PN, Sherman SI, Sellin RV, Friend KE, Burgess MA, Cote GJ, Gagel RF, *et al*: **Surgical strategy for the treatment of medullary thyroid carcinoma.** *Ann Surg* 1999, **230(5)**:697-707.
17. Dralle H, Gimm O, Simon D, Frank-Raue K, Gortz G, Niederle B, Wahl RA, Koch B, Walgenbach S, Hampel R, *et al*: **Prophylactic thyroidectomy in 75 children and adolescents with hereditary medullary thyroid carcinoma: German and Austrian experience.** *World J Surg* 1998, **22(7)**:744-750, discussion 750-741.
18. Machens A, Lorenz K, Dralle H: **Individualization of lymph node dissection in RET (rearranged during transfection) carriers at risk for medullary thyroid cancer: value of pretherapeutic calcitonin levels.** *Ann Surg* 2009, **250(2)**:305-310.

19. Barbet J, Campion L, Kraeber-Bodere F, Chatal JF: **Prognostic impact of serum calcitonin and carcinoembryonic antigen doubling-times in patients with medullary thyroid carcinoma.** *J Clin Endocrinol Metab* 2005, **90(11)**:6077-6084.
20. Machens A, Dralle H: **Biomarker-based risk stratification for previously untreated medullary thyroid cancer.** *J Clin Endocrinol Metab* 2010, **95(6)**:2655-2663.
21. Machens A, Hinze R, Thomusch O, Dralle H: **Pattern of nodal metastasis for primary and reoperative thyroid cancer.** *World J Surg* 2002, **26(1)**:22-28, Epub 2001 Nov 2022.
22. Scheuba C, Kaserer K, Bieglmayer C, Asari R, Riss P, Drosten R, Niederle B: **Medullary thyroid microcarcinoma recommendations for treatment - a single-center experience.** *Surgery* 2007, **142(6)**:1003-1010, discussion 1010 e1001-1003.
23. Ahn JE, Lee JH, Yi JS, Shong YK, Hong SJ, Lee DH, Choi CG, Kim SJ: **Diagnostic accuracy of CT and ultrasonography for evaluating metastatic cervical lymph nodes in patients with thyroid cancer.** *World J Surg* 2008, **32(7)**:1552-1558.
24. Szakall Jnr. S, Esik O, Bajzik G, Repa I, Dabasi G, Sinkovics I, Agoston P, Tron L: **18F-FDG PET detection of lymph node metastases in medullary thyroid carcinoma.** *J Nucl Med* 2002, **43(1)**:66-71.
25. Czepczynski R, Parisella MG, Kosowicz J, Mikolajczak R, Ziemnicka K, Gryczynska M, Sowinski J, Signore A: **Somatostatin receptor scintigraphy using 99mTc-EDDA/HYNIC-TOC in patients with medullary thyroid carcinoma.** *Eur J Nucl Med Mol Imaging* 2007, **34(10)**:1635-1645.
26. Mucha SA, Kunert-Radek J, Pomorski L: **Positron emission tomography (18FDG-PET) in the detection of medullary thyroid carcinoma.** *Endokrynol Pol* 2006, **57(4)**:452-455.
27. Brandt-Mainz K, Muller SP, Gorges R, Saller B, Bockisch A: **The value of fluorine-18 fluorodeoxyglucose PET in patients with medullary thyroid cancer.** *Eur J Nucl Med* 2000, **27(5)**:490-496.
28. Krausz Y, Rosler A, Guttmann H, Ish-Shalom S, Shibley N, Chisin R, Glaser B: **Somatostatin receptor scintigraphy for early detection of regional and distant metastases of medullary carcinoma of the thyroid.** *Clin Nucl Med* 1999, **24(4)**:256-260.
29. Schott M, Willenberg HS, Sagert C, Nguyen TB, Schinner S, Cohnen M, Cupisti V, Eisenberger CF, Knoefel WT, Scherbaum WA: **Identification of occult metastases of medullary thyroid carcinoma by pentagastrin-stimulated intravenous calcitonin sampling followed by targeted surgery.** *Clin Endocrinol (Oxf)* 2007, **66(3)**:405-409.
30. Machens A, Dralle H: **Biological relevance of medullary thyroid microcarcinoma.** *J Clin Endocrinol Metab* 2012, **97(5)**:1547-1553.
31. Kazaure HS, Roman SA, Sosa JA: **Medullary thyroid microcarcinoma: a population-level analysis of 310 patients.** *Cancer* 2012, **118(3)**:620-627.
32. Machens A, Holzhausen HJ, Dralle H: **Skip metastases in thyroid cancer leaping the central lymph node compartment.** *Arch Surg* 2004, **139(1)**:43-45.
33. Tavares MR, Michaluart P Jr., Montenegro F, Arap S, Sodre M, Takeda F, Brandao L, Toledo S, Ferraz A: **Skip metastases in medullary thyroid carcinoma: a single-center experience.** *Surg Today* 2008, **38(6)**:499-504.
34. Scheuba C, Bieglmayer C, Asari R, Kaczirek K, Izay B, Kaserer K, Niederle B: **The value of intraoperative pentagastrin testing in medullary thyroid cancer.** *Surgery* 2007, **141(2)**:166-171, discussion 171-162.
35. Machens A, Niccoli-Sire P, Hoegel J, Frank-Raue K, van Vroonhoven TJ, Roeher HD, Wahl RA, Lamesch P, Raue F, Conte-Devolx B, *et al*: **Early malignant progression of hereditary medullary thyroid cancer.** *N Engl J Med* 2003, **349(16)**:1517-1525.
36. Guerrero MA, Lindsay S, Suh I, Vriens MR, Khanafshar E, Shen WT, Gosnell J, Kebebew E, Duh QY, Clark OH: **Medullary Thyroid Cancer: It is a pain in the neck?** *J Cancer* 2011, **2**:200-205.
37. Scheuba C, Kaserer K, Kaczirek K, Asari R, Niederle B: **Desmoplastic stromal reaction in medullary thyroid cancer-an intraoperative "marker" for lymph node metastases.** *World J Surg* 2006, **30(5)**:853-859.
38. Koperek O, Scheuba C, Cherenko M, Neuhold N, De Micco C, Schmid KW, Niederle B, Kaserer K: **Desmoplasia in medullary thyroid carcinoma: a reliable indicator of metastatic potential.** *Histopathology* 2008, **52(5)**:623-630.

# 22

# AUF1 and HuR: possible implications of mRNA stability in thyroid function and disorders

Bogusz Trojanowicz, Henning Dralle, Cuong Hoang-Vu*

**Abstract**

RNA-binding proteins may regulate every aspect of RNA metabolism, including pre-mRNA splicing, mRNA trafficking, stability and translation of many genes. The dynamic association of these proteins with RNA defines the lifetime, cellular localization, processing and the rate at which a specific mRNA is translated. One of the pathways involved in regulating of mRNA stability is mediated by adenylate uridylate-rich element (ARE) binding proteins. These proteins are involved in processes of apoptosis, tumorigenesis and development. Out of many ARE-binding proteins, two of them AUF1 and HuR were studied most extensively and reported to regulate the mRNA stability *in vivo*. Our previously published data demonstrate that both proteins are involved in thyroid carcinogenesis. Several other reports postulate that mRNA binding proteins may participate in thyroid hormone actions. However, until now, exacts mechanisms and the possible role of post-transcriptional regulation and especially the role of AUF1 and HuR in those processes remain not fully understood. In this study we shortly review the possible function of both proteins in relation to development and various physiological and pathophysiological processes, including thyroid function and disorders.

## Introduction

Cytoplasmic stability of eukaryotic mRNA is a substantially important check point in the control for gene expression. During differentiation of the cell some mRNAs are expressed stronger and some others are degraded or down regulated. Such a post-transcriptional gene-inactivation (gene silencing) occurs through alterations in translational efficiency and in mRNA stability. Stability of mRNA is mainly controlled by RNA interference processes (e.g. siRNA, microRNA) and RNA binding proteins, which act to selectively degrade or stabilize mRNAs. In mammals, a common feature of many unstable mRNAs is the presence of an Adenylate-Uridylate-rich element (ARE) within the 3'-untranslated region (3'-UTR) [1-3]. This ARE in the 3'-untranslated region is a part of the regulation system, which is responsible for the mRNA degradation or stabilisation and is linked to an interaction with ARE binding proteins. Out of many ARE-binding proteins studied, two of them AUF1 and HuR were investigated most extensively and demonstrated to affect the mRNA stability *in vivo*. AUF1 (A+U rich RNA-binding factor 1, heterogeneous nuclear ribonucleoprotein D) is expressed as a family of four proteins designated by their molecular masses as p37, p40, p42 and p45 arising from a single transcript. HuR (human antigen R) is a ubiquitously expressed member of the embryonic lethal abnormal vision (ELAV) family [4]. Although there are some examples demonstrating stabilizing function of AUF1, it is generally related to degradation of target mRNAs while HuR is known to promote stabilization of several transcripts by enhancing their stability, altering their translation, or performing both functions [5-7]. Both proteins are mainly expressed in nucleus but their function is related with cytoplasmic localisation. Predominantly nuclear AUF1 and HuR shuttle between the nucleus and cytoplasm via nucleocytoplasmic shuttling sequences called DNS and HNS, respectively. In case of AUF1, its nuclear import is mediated by transportin-1 [8,9]. The mechanisms of AUF1 and HuR are believed to be mediated by binding-competition to target mRNAs. It is postulated that AUF1 and HuR could functionally act with target mRNAs both within the nucleus and in the cytoplasm [10]. It suggests that precise mechanism of antagonising and/or cooperative actions of AUF1 and HuR is not entirely understood.

* Correspondence: hoang-vu@medizin.uni-halle.de
Universitätsklinik und Poliklinik für Allgemein-, Viszeral- und Gefäßchirurgie, Martin-Luther Universität, Halle
Full list of author information is available at the end of the article

Both proteins do not posses any enzymatic activity, but were identified with ARE-mRNA-protein-ligand complexes. Previous reports identified the ubiquitin-conjugating enzyme E2I and three RNA binding proteins: NESP-1, NSAP-1 and IMP-2, as AUF1 interacting proteins. Importantly, NSEP-1 revealed an endoribonuclease activity, providing possible explanation for AUF1-mediated poly(A) shortening [11]. With regard to HuR, affinity chromatography and co-immunoprecipitation experiments identified four protein ligands SETa, SETb, pp32 and acidic protein rich in leucine (APRIL) [12]. First three had been previously characterised as inhibitors of protein phosphatase 2A (PP2A) regulating its ability to convert between holoenzyme forms upon stimulation [13,14]. PP2A is known serine/threonine phosphatase participating in diverse cellular processes such as proliferation, cell cycle, DNA replication, development and morphogenesis [15]. Recently, HuR and AUF1 were identified as components of the RNA-induced silencing complex (RISC). In this study HuR employed AUF1 as cofactor to promote p16 mRNA decay [16].

ARE-elements are found in many mRNAs encoding proteins related to normal and neoplastic cell growth and must be considered as a crucial target element in mammalian cells. The human genome project revealed that many mRNAs encoding proto-oncogenes (i.e. c-myc, c-jun, c-fos), growth factors such (i.e. EGF, VEGF), cytokines (i.e. TNFα) and cell cycle regulators (i.e. cyclin A, B1, D1, p21, p27) contain ARE-motifs [17,18]. Analysis of thyroid related genes revealed that many of them contain these motifs and may be regulated at the post-transcriptional level. These include mRNAs related with thyroid function (pendrin, NIS, MCT8, peroxiredoxins, TPO, dual oxidase 1), regulation of thyroid function (TSHR), response to thyroid hormones (selenoprotein P, THR alpha and beta, THR associated protein 6, D1), thyroid development (Nkx2-1, PAX8, HHEX, EYA1, Hox-A3, Hox-A5, PAX9) and thyroid pathology (thyroid adenoma associated protein, papillary thyroid carcinoma encoded protein, thyroid cancer protein) (Table 1). However whether these mRNAs may serve as potential targets for AUF1 and HuR is still unclear. It is worth to note that both proteins may also interact with some mRNAs by employing non-canonical ARE-sites [19,20].

## Developmental expression of AUF1 and HuR

Both proteins are synchronous, but differential expressed during murine development. It had been demonstrated that there is no major translation control of AUF1 and HuR production, but their expression varies noticeably within tissues and at differential developmental stages. The tissue distribution of both proteins demonstrated that yolk-sack and fetal liver possessed very weak levels of AUF1 and HuR, contrary to strong expression in tail, limb bud, brain and heart between E13.5 and E16.5. Adult spleen, thymus, testis and intestine were very abundant in AUF1 and HuR, contrary to brain, liver, heart, kidneys, muscle, lungs and stomach, demonstrating low or no expression of both proteins. AUF1 and HuR revealed a coincident spatio-temporal tissue distribution from 10-somite stage to late embryogenesis [21,22].

The data coming from human tissues revealed that AUF1 and HuR are also strictly involved in liver de-differentiation, development and progression of hepatocellular carcinoma. Those processes are tightly regulated by MAT1A (methionine adenosyltransferase 1A)- and MAT2A (methionine adenosyltransferase 2A. Both enzymes control the levels of S-adenosylmethionine (SAM), the key regulator of hepatocytes proliferation and differentiation. MAT1A is expressed in adult liver, whereas MAT2A is detected extrahepatic and is related with liver proliferation. The analysis of those expression patterns revealed that AUF1 and HuR are crucial post-transcriptional regulators of MAT1A and MAT2A mRNA stability. The authors demonstrated that AUF1 and HuR levels were upregulated in a time-dependent manner during liver de-dedifferentiation and the function of HuR is regulated by its methylation status. The interaction of HuR with MAT2A mRNA in the presence of SAM led unexpectedly to MAT2A mRNA decay, whereas its absence promoted HuR-mediated accumulation of MAT2A mRNA. It is worth to note that addition of SAM reduced the AUF1 interaction with this mRNA. The analysis of rat liver development revealed that there is a switch in the expression from MAT2A to MAT1A during embryogenesis. Proliferating liver express increased levels of SAM-methylated HuR which leads to decreased MAT2A mRNA expression and elevated levels of MAT1A mRNA. Furthermore, increased levels of AUF1 and HuR, and decreased levels of methylated-HuR were detected in hepatocellular carcinoma tissues. Normal liver tissues express very low levels of AUF1 and HuR, and high levels of methylated-HuR [23].

*In vivo* data on AUF1 and HuR knock-out mice models demonstrated that both proteins may play an important role in the development. Investigations of AUF1 -/- mice revealed symptoms which share similarity with human atopic dermatitis such as pruritus, chronic dermatitis, cutaneous atopy, xerosis, elevated serum IgE levels and staphylococcal skin infection [24]. Cunningham et al. observed the presence of thyroid disorders in patients suffering from dermatitis herpetiformis. However the association between the clinical or serological thyroid abnormalities and skin disease could not be explained [25]. Recently different skin findings and accompanying dermatoses could be detected in patients with thyroid diseases. The presence of each dermatosis,

**Table 1 ARE-containing mRNAs related to thyroid function, development and disorders. According to AREsite http://rna.tbi.univie.ac.at/cgi-bin/AREsite.cgi.**

| | ARE-motifs | | | | |
|---|---|---|---|---|---|
| mRNA | AUUUA | WTAUUUATW | WWWWAUUUAWWWW | WWAUUUAWW | Others |
| Selenoproten P | 6 | 1 | 1 | 2 | |
| MCT8 | 5 | | | | |
| ID2 | 3 | 1 | 1 | 1 | 1 |
| Pendrin | 6 | 2 | 1 | 2 | 4 |
| THR alpha | 2 | | | 1 | |
| THR beta | 14 | 1 | | 2 | |
| Thyroid adenoma associated protein | 18 | 1 | 2 | 6 | 6 |
| TTF-1 (Nkx2-1) | 6 | 3 | 2 | 4 | 4 |
| TSH-R | 2 | | | | |
| TPO | 3 | | | 2 | |
| THR associated protein 6 | 2 | | | 1 | |
| Papillary thyroid carcinoma encoded protein | 10 | 2 | 1 | 3 | 2 |
| Dual oxidase 1 | 1 | | | | |
| Thyroid cancer protein | 5 | 1 | 1 | 2 | 2 |
| PAX8 | 3 | 1 | | 2 | 3 |
| NIS | 1 | | | | |
| D1 | 3 | | | | |
| Homebox protein HEX (HHEX) | 2 | | | | |
| Eyes absent homolog EYA1 | 5 | | | 2 | 1 |
| Homebox protein Hox-A3 | 7 | 1 | 1 | 1 | 3 |
| Homebox protein Hox-A5 | 1 | 1 | | 1 | |
| PAX9 | 4 | 1 | | 3 | |
| Peroxiredoxin 6 (PRDX6) | 2 | | | | |
| Peroxiredoxin 3 (PRDX3) | 1 | | | | |
| Peroxiredoxin 4 (PRDX4) | 1 | | | | |

chronic urticaria, vitiligo and pruritus were found to be significantly higher in the patient group with thyroid disorders than in the control group. Autoimmune-hyperthyroidism patients demonstrated significantly higher incidence of vitiligo and diffuse alopecia, while vitiligo alone was found to be significantly higher in autoimmune hypothyroidism patients than in the control group [26]. It had been demonstrated that AUF1-deficient mice revealed abnormal stabilisation of TNFα and IL-1β mRNAs. Such an excessive proinflammatory cytokines production resulted in endotoxic shock, loss of renal and liver function and in end effect caused increased mortality [27]. In studies by Sadri et al. AUF1-deficiency led to disturbance in mature splenic B cell populations and impaired humoral immune responses. The authors observed decreased number of splenic lymphocytes, increased presentation of immature marginal zone lymphocytes and reduced number of mature follicular B lymphocytes [28].

More severe abnormalities were observed in HuR -/- animals. It had been demonstrated that HuR was crucial for midgestational embryonic development. HuR expression increased in murine placenta between E12.5 and E13.5. Immunohistochemical analysis revealed its presence in both embryonic and extraembryonic layers; however HuR nucleo-cytoplasmic localisation varied between maternal and fetal sides. It was dominantly nuclear in maternal decidua cells and embryo-derived trophoblasts giant cells and spongiotrophoblasts. Contrary, labyrinth-trophoblasts showed nuclear and strong cytoplasmic staining. The presence of HuR in cytoplasm at this stage was probably related with its function. Furthermore, the HuR -/- led to midgestational death. In the absence of HuR the labyrinth branching morphogenesis and syncytiotrophoblast differentiation were impaired and caused not sufficient vascularization, labyrinthine apoptosis, and in end effect insufficient nutrient transport and embryos death. Most of the embryos died between E17.5 and E19.5. They revealed reduced size of skeleton and limbs and decreased spleen size. Furthermore, the lungs of HuR -/- mice revealed additional dysmorphologies, whereas the stomach and pancreas were properly located. However, whether the absence of HuR could lead to thyroid abnormalities was not investigated. It is worth to note that HuR was able to interact with several transcription factors crucial not only for proper morphogenesis, patterning and specification, but also for thyroid development such as Hox-A5 [29].The absence of Hox-A5 is related to disorganized follicle formation; decreased TPO; Nkx2.1, Titf2, altered Pax8 gene expression, but normal serum T4 level. As demonstrated in Table 1, these mRNAs bear ARE-sequences and are crucial for thyroid development (Table 2). However, whether their mRNA stability is regulated in ARE-dependent manner, especially in participation of AUF1 and HuR, is not clear.

### Thyroid hormone and TSH-mRNA

There is still a growing body of evidence that actions of thyroid hormone (TH), thyroid function and disorders may also be regulated at post-transcriptional level by mRNA binding proteins. Krane at al. demonstrated that TH is able to regulate the stability of thyroid stimulating hormone (TSH) subunit mRNA. They showed that half-life of the TSH beta mRNA from rat pituitary cultures treated with triiodothyronine (T3) was shorter than that observed in corresponding controls. Furthermore, TSH mRNA was destabilized due to the loss of a portion of the poly(A) tail upon TH treatment [30]. Staton at al. postulated that such a mechanism is highly conserved across the species. In addition to previous studies they observed that simple deadenylation of TSH messenger body is insufficient to induce its decay [31]. This suggests the triggering of additional mechanism such as exonuclease digestion and actions of other still not identified mRNA binding proteins. Recently, Goulart-Silva et al. demonstrated a rapid effect of T3 on TSHβ mRNA stability. They showed that surgically hypothyroided rats revealed an increased TSHβ transcript poly(A) tail, its elevated content in ribosomes and enhanced attachment to cytoskeleton. Furthermore, hypothyroid rats subjected to acute T3 treatment demonstrated a reduction of TSHβ mRNA poly(A) tail and its weakened recruitment to ribosomes. Euthyroid rats did not present any changes in TSHβ mRNA stability, but revealed increased binding of TSHβ transcripts to ribosomes [32]. Although exact mechanisms or proteins participating in mRNA degradation are not fully identified, Leedman et al. isolated a cytoplasmic trans-acting factor (80-85 kDa) capable to bind the 3'-UTR of TSHβ transcripts. Furthermore, its binding to TSHβ transcripts was positively regulated by T3 [33]. With regard to AUF1 and HuR, their actions in regulating the TSHβ transcript stability may be elusive at present, but it is worth to note that AUF1 function is associated with polysomes [10].

**Table 2 Thyroid developmental markers containing ARE-sequences and phenotypes studied on double knock-out mice, modified from [85].**

| Double knock-out | Thyroid phenotype |
|---|---|
| Pax8 -/- | Regression of thyroid primordium at E11.5<br>Thyroid precursor cells disappear at E12<br>No follicles, no Tg, no TPO;<br>thyroids exclusively consist of C-cells (Ttif1-positive) |
| Pax9 -/- | Lack of ultimobranchial body formation |
| Ttif1/Nkx2.1 -/- | Thyroid precursor cells disappear at E10.5-11.5;<br>Mice lack C-cells and thyroid follicular cells |
| Hhex -/- | Thyroid anlage present at E9;<br>Absence of thyroid primordium at E10 |
| Eya1 -/- | lack of fusion between ultimobranchial bodies and thyroid lobes; thyroid hypoplasia; severe reduction in number of C-cells and follicular cells; |
| Hoxa3 -/- | Thyroid hypoplasia; persistent ultimobranchial bodies with C-cells |
| Hoxa5 -/- | Disorganized follicle formation; decreased TPO; Nkx2.1, Titf2, Pax8 gene expression altered, but normal serum T4 level |

### Thyroid hormone and other mRNAs

Murphy et al. observed that growth hormone (GH) mRNA from TH-depleted rats is less abundant than euthyroid controls, but its stability is elevated due to the increased length of poly (A) tail. The authors observed that modulation of GH poly (A) is related to nucleus and its length may be regulated due to the interactions with free ribonucleoproteins. The existence of such a nuclear mechanism resulting in cytoplasmic stabilisation of mature GH mRNA raises the question which mRNA binding proteins may mediate these effects [34]. Recent studies by Goulart da Silva et al., revealed that TH acutely increases GH mRNA translation rate and GH secretion in hypothyroid rats. It had been shown that soon after T3 administration, increased GH labelling was observed in the perinuclear region of somatotrophs and that these events coincided with cytoskeleton rearrangements. Indeed, the authors identified GH mRNA in complexes with F-actin, which provided additional protection for GH mRNA transcripts. Furthermore, as the authors postulated, insufficient GH synthesis in hypothyroid specimens resulted not only from reduced GH transcription rate but also decreased GH mRNA half-life [35]. This novel finding directing GH mRNA soon after T3 administration to polysomes is related with TH nongenomic actions. However, whether additional molecular mechanisms are involved in those processes, remains an open question.

With regard to other mRNAs, the effects of TH on cardiovascular development may also be mediated by actions of mRNA-binding proteins. Minamisawa et al. demonstrated that stability of sarcolipin mRNA, an atrium-specific sarcoplasmic reticulum protein, is affected by thyroid hormone actions. Analysis of atria obtained from hyperthyroidism-induced and T3-treated neonatal rat atrial myocytes revealed accelerated decay of sarcolipin mRNA. The hyperthyroid mice revealed cardiac hypertrophy and sinus tachycardia. Contrary, hypothyroidism did not result in any changes of cardiac morphology and sarcolipin mRNA stability [36]. It had been demonstrated that myocardial relaxation and associated cardiac hypertrophy and heart failure may be related with AUF1-mediated decrease of sarco(endo) plasmic reticulum calcium ATPase 2a (SERCA2a) mRNA stability. In those studies AUF1 was identified as a critical factor of these events. Interaction of AUF1 with SERCA2a 3' UTR was identified predominantly in nucleus, suggesting that AUF1-mediated decay of SERCA2a mRNA starts within the nucleus and further continues during shuttling to the cytoplasm [37].

The further role of AUF1 was shown in studies concerning the mRNA stability of Kv4 channels. Expression of cardiac myocyte Kv4 channels is down-regulated in hypertrophy and leads to decrease in the transient outward current. Studies in vitro demonstrated that employment of angiotensin II may recapitulate these effects and is accompanied by up-regulation of AUF1, which in turn binds and destabilises Kv4 mRNA [38].

Studies on cultured rat brown adipocytes revealed that at higher doses T3 inhibited deiodinase II (D2) activity. Similar effects were induced after administration of triiodothyroacetic acid (Triac) , a natural thermogenic compound in brown adipocytes. Low concentrations of Triac increased D2 activity, while its higher doses inhibited D2 activity. The authors postulate that D2-inhibiton by employing high T3 doses may exist as a regulatory pathway in which D2 triggers down-regulation of T3, against its excess. D2 activity is inhibited in hyperthyroidism, and decreases further after chronic cold exposition. This suggests that high T3 concentrations in brown adipocytes switch off the mechanisms of T3-production via D2. Furthermore, the inhibition of D2 activity was found on post-transcriptional level and was related with proteasome actions. It had been demonstrated that addition of ubiquitin led to D2 inactivation whereas protein deubiquitintating enzyme-1 reversed ubiquitin-mediated inactivation and prolonged D2 half-life. Furthermore, D2 was also stabilised by employing of proteasome inhibitor. Deubiquitintating enzyme-1 was found noticeably increased in brown adipocyte tissue upon cold exposure and was associated with increased D2 stability.

Although there is no direct evidence that T3 regulates proteasome activity or increase D2 decay, the authors could demonstrate that T3 at high doses and THR beta participate in regulation of D2 mRNA stability, T3 by shortening D2 half-life and induction of D2-degradation, and THR beta by stabilisation of D2 activity [39-43].

TH is also implicated in regulation of neuroserpin mRNA stability. Neuroserpin is a serine protease inhibitor of the serpin family playing an important role in neural development and adult neural function. Neuroserpin dysfunction is related with different neurodegenerative diseases. It has been shown that its 3'UTR contains ARE motifs and interacts with HuD protein, belonging as HuR to the ELAV family. HuD is able to bind neuroserpin mRNA and its overexpression was associated with increased mRNA stability. Employment of T3 led to decreased half-life of neuroserpin, probably due to the HuD repression. The authors also suggest the involvement of other mRNA binding proteins [44].

In studies with retinoic acid receptors (RAR) it has been demonstrated that administration of TH led to enhanced mRNA levels of RARβ, decreased RXRγ and had no influence on RXRα. In addition to positive transcriptional regulation of RARβ by TH, investigations concerning the regulation of RXRγ, revealed that TH regulate its mRNA stability post-transcriptional [45]. As RXRγ mRNA bears the ARE-motifs, it is a possible partner for ARE-binding proteins.

## Trace elements

Recent studies revealed that also trace elements such as selenium, calcium or iron may regulate the mRNA stability of proteins related to their transport or metabolism [46-49]. Studies *in vitro* revealed potential roles of calcium and phosphate in AUF1-mediated mRNA stability of parathyroid hormone (PTH). PTH mRNA levels are post-transcriptional increased by hypocalcemia and decreased by hypophosphatemia. AUF1 was identified as a critical factor protecting and stabilizing PTH transcripts [50]. With regard to thyroid function, it has been demonstrated that iodide and selenium may affect the stability of thyroid-related mRNAs. Bermano et al. showed that selenium depletion decreased the stability of cytosolic glutathione peroxidase mRNA. Furthermore, the incorporation of Se-cysteine at specific UGA codons in the selenoenzyme mRNAs was dependent on the presence of stem-loop structures in the 3'-UTRs of these mRNAs. It was demonstrated for selenoenzymes type I (D1) and type III deiodinases (D3) revealing that their translation efficiency was dependent on the structure or sequence of the 3'- UTR [51]. The existence of Se-dependent post-transcriptional mechanisms regulating D1 mRNA stability was also reported in study by Riese et al., suggesting regulation in a sex and tissue specific manner [52]. Although involvement of AUF1 and/or HuR in Se-regulated mRNA stability may be elusive at present, its worth to note that 3'- UTR of D1 bears ARE-motifs and may be regulated in ARE-dependent fashion.

Recent studies demonstrated that acute iodide administration decreased the mRNA stability of sodium-iodide symporter (NIS). The authors observed that NIS transcripts and the length of NIS poly (A) tail were significantly reduced during all periods of iodide treatment. The authors postulate that this mechanism involves the interaction of trace elements such as iodide with proteins bound to untranslated regions of mRNAs. This novel mechanism provide a new insight by which iodide may exert its autoregulatory function on thyroid gland [53]. However whether iodide or other trace elements may bind and regulate the activity of exosome and/or proteasome components in ARE-dependent manner remains to be identified.

### Thyroid cancer

Current data from our group revealed that AUF1 and HuR may be involved in thyroid pathology by regulating the stability of several factors related to cell cycle and proliferation. We demonstrated that thyroid cancer tissues expressed AUF1 significantly stronger than benign tissues. Furthermore, AUF1-knock-down in follicular thyroid carcinoma cells FTC-133 led to decreased proliferation rates accompanied by increased expression of cell cycle inhibitors and down-regulation of cell cycle promoters. The analysis of AUF1-depleted clones revealed that in addition to AUF1-down-regulation, all clones demonstrated also decreased HuR levels [54]. However exact mechanisms, thyroid-specific partners for AUF1 and HuR, the influence of AUF1 and HuR on thyroid specific functions and genes, the role of mRNA stability in thyroid carcinogenesis are still not fully understood. Recent studies by Braun et al. identified altered microRNA signatures as potent post-transcriptional markers for undifferentiated thyroid carcinoma that promote its de-/transdifferentiation and invasion [55].

Our previously published data revealed that expression of several tumor suppressor genes (TSG) and tumor promoting factors, may serve as novel biomarkers for thyroid carcinoma. We demonstrated that down-regulation of CD9, CD82 and RKIP may reflect an increased *in vivo* metastatic potential of thyroid cancer cells [56,57]. Inversely, increased expression of S100A4 and ENO1 was correlated with increased proliferation and metastatic potential of thyroid carcinoma [58]. Investigations performed on AUF1-depleted thyroid cancer cell lines revealed a cross-link between AUF1 and CD9, CD82, S100A4 and ENO1. We demonstrated that AUF1 knock-down led to increased expression of two tumor suppressor genes CD9 and CD82. Subsequently, decreased expression of tumor promoting S100A4, GAPDH and ENO1 was observed (Fig. 1).

It had been demonstrated that retinoic acid (RA) treatment induced beneficial effects in therapy of solid cancers [59,60] including thyroid carcinomas [61-63]. Cell culture experiments performed on thyroid carcinoma cell lines revealed that RA treatment affects thyroid-specific functions, cell-cell or cell-matrix interaction, differentiation markers, growth, and tumorigenicity [64]. Administration of RA demonstrated an anti-proliferative effect on the follicular thyroid carcinoma cell lines FTC-133 and FTC-238. Furthermore, pre-treatment of these cell lines with RA resulted in decreased in-vitro proliferation rates and reduced tumor cell growth of xenotransplants [65]. Our published data revealed that RA led to significantly decreased levels of of glyceraldehyde-3-phpsphate dehydrogenase (GAPDH), pyruvate kinase isoenzymes M1/M2 (PKM1/M2), peptidyl-prolyl cis-trans isomerase A (PPIA), transketolase (TKT), annexin A2 (ANXA2), glutathione S-transferase P (GSTP1) and peroxiredoxin 2 (PRDX2) as compared to untreated control. Investigations on thyroid tissues demonstrated that the same proteins were significantly up-regulated in follicular, papillary and undifferentiated thyroid carcinomas [66]. In addition to previously published data we found that RA pre-treatment led to down-regulation of AUF1 and HuR. Also depletion of ENO1 led to decreased levels of AUF1 and HuR (Fig. 2).

### Other types of cancer

Both proteins were reported to be also related with other malignancies, and like in case of thyroid cancer, were expressed synchronous. Given that both proteins bind to common target mRNAs such an expression pattern is partly explainable. In studies on transgenic mice the overexpression of AUF1 led to development of sarcomas with strong expression of cyclin D1 [67]. Other *in vivo* mice models demonstrated that malignant lung tissues expressed AUF1 significantly stronger as compared with normal and benign lung tissues. The same expression pattern was reported for HuR protein [68]. With regard to HuR expression, its increased levels were demonstrated for malignant tissues of tongue, gingival, colon, breast, ovary and stomach as compared to corresponding controls [69,70].

It had been shown that approximately 80% of anaplastic lymphoma kinase (ALK)-positive lymphomas express the fusion protein called nucleophosmin-anaplastic lymphoma kinase (NPM-ALK), which constitutively activates ALK tyrosine kinase and causes abnormal induction of down-stream signaling resulting in malignant transformation. Studies *in vitro* revealed that AUF1 was co-localised with NPM-ALK in the same cytoplasmic loci. Subsequent hyperphosphorylation of AUF1 in NPM-ALK expressing cells was also observed. It is worth to note that AUF1 hyperphosphorylation was associated with elevated stability of several target mRNAs encoding proteins crucial for cell proliferation and cell survival such as c-myc, and cyclin D1, cyclin A2, cyclin B1, and cyclin D3 [71].

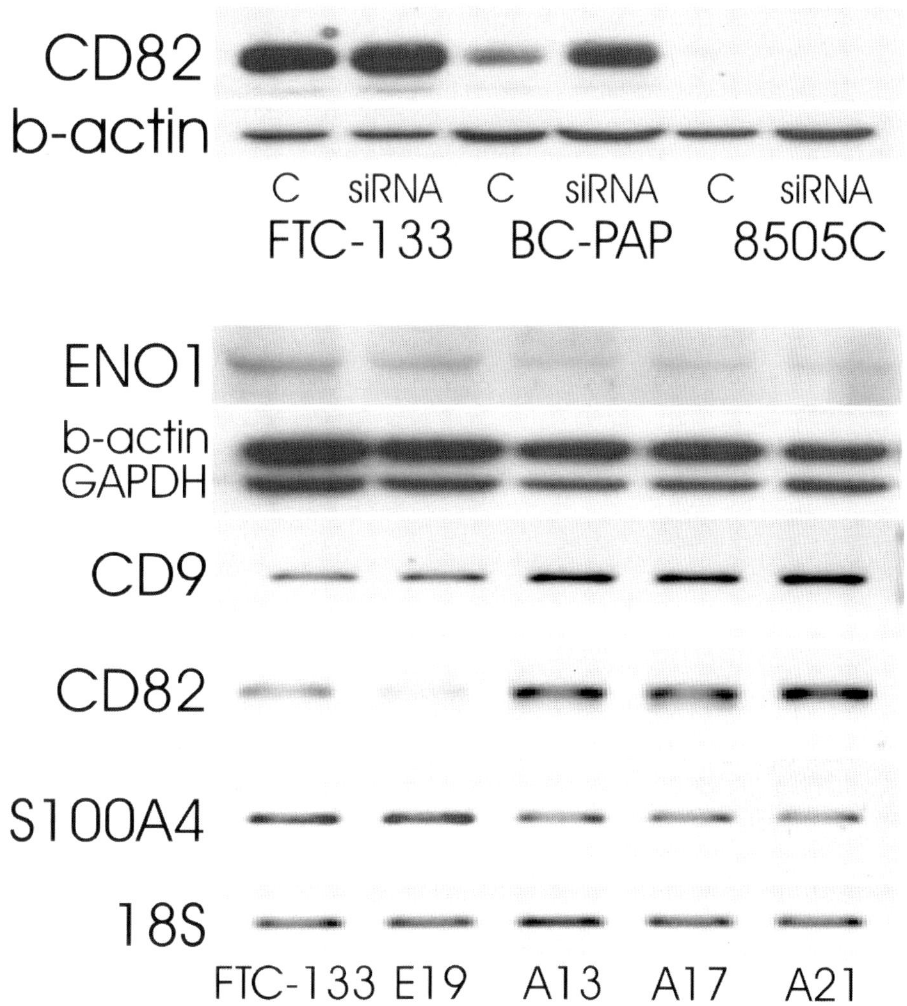


**Figure 1** Upper panel: expression of CD82 in thyroid carcinoma cell lines treated with siRNA targeting AUF1. Lower panel: expression of CD9, CD82, GAPDH, ENO1 and S100A4 in wild type cells FTC-133, FTC-133-EGFP control cells (E19) and FTC-133 transfectants expressing AUF1 targeting shRNAs (A13, A17, A21). Increased levels of tumor suppressors (CD9 and CD82) and subsequent decrease of tumor promoters (ENO1, GAPDH and S100A4) are visible. Note that 8505C control and AUF1-siRNA cells are CD82 negative. 18S and B-actin served as normalizing markers.

Overexpression of AUF1 (especially isoforms p37 and p45) resulted in enhanced translation of internal ribosome entry site (IRES) of Hepatitis C virus (HCV), which is one of the major agents causing a virus-related hepatitis, liver cirrhosis and hepatocellular carcinoma. Depletion of AUF1 significantly hampered infection by HCV [72]. Similar mechanisms were also reported by depletion of insulin-like growth factor 2 mRNA binding protein IGF2BP1 [73].

Increased expression of AUF1, heterogeneous nuclear ribonucleoprotein K (HNRNPK), MutS homolog 2 (MSH2) and grainyhead-like 2 (GRHL2), and subsequently elevated activity of human telomerase reverse transcriptase (hTERT) were detected in human oral squamous cell carcinoma cells (OSCC) when compared to normal cells, which do not exhibit hTERT activity. RNAi mediated knock-down of AUF1, MSH2 and GRHL2 resulted in decreased proliferation rates and hTERT promoter activity. Depletion of HNRNPK inhibited only proliferation of the cells without affecting the hTERT promoter activity [74].

Prostaglandin A2 (PGA2) is an experimental anti-cancer agent associated with decreased levels of cyclin D1 and decreased proliferation of cancer cells. It has been demonstrated that employment of PGA2 induced AUF1 expression and resulted in degradation of cyclin D1 mRNA in non small cell lung cancer (H1299) and breast carcinoma (MCF-7) cells. The other breast carcinoma cell line tested MDA-MB-453, bearing a large deletion in cyclin's D1 3'UTR, responded with unaltered cyclin

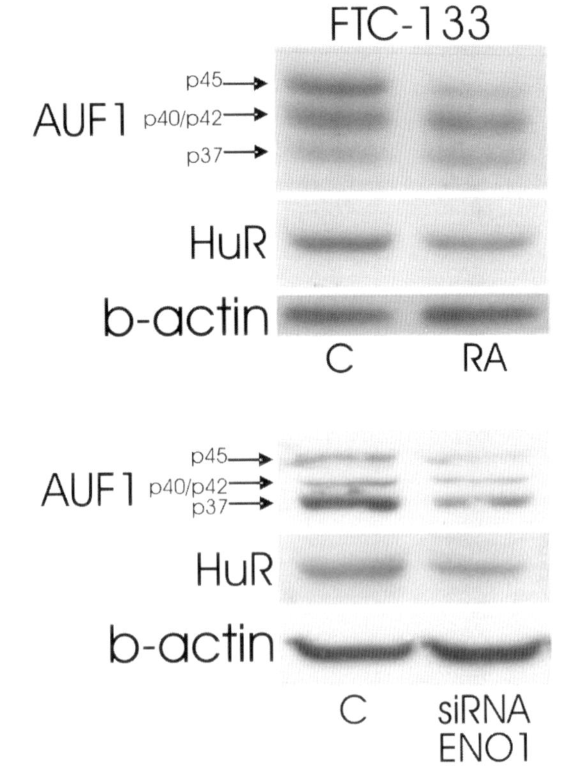


**Figure 2** Expression of AUF1 and HuR after RA pre-treatment and ENO1-siRNA employment. Upper panel: FTC-133 cells pre-treated with RA revealed decreased levels of AUF1 and HuR. Lower panel: ENO1 knock-down led to decreased levels of AUF1 and HuR. B-actin served as normalizing marker.

D1 mRNA upon PGA2 treatment [75]. In melanoma cells increased elevated levels of interleukin 10 (IL-10) resulted in decreased cytosolic AUF1 levels as compared with normal melanocytes [76].

## Non-cancerous actions and disorders

The role and actions of AUF1 and HuR were also reported in other non-cancerous disorders. AUF1 proteins were identified as novel autoantigens in systemic lupus erythematosus (SLE) and other associated autoimmune rheumatic disorders. Autoantibodies to AUF1 were detected in 33% of SLE patients, 20% of patients with rheumatioid arthritis, 17% of patients with mixed connective tissue disorders and below 10% of patients with other related rheumatic diseases. Healthy controls were negative for AUF1 autoantibodies [77]. The presence and the role of HuR autoantibodies are discussed in non-neuronal tissues [78].

The role of post-transcriptional gene regulation was also studied in the cells upon low oxygen levels. It has been demonstrated that in hypoxia conditions, HuR upregulates the expression of two major hypoxia-inducible proteins, VEGF and HIF-1$\alpha$. Furthermore, HuR also regulates the levels and/or translation of other ARE-containing mRNAs which encode hypoxia-inducible proteins such as GLUT1, TGF-$\beta$, c-myc and p53 [79]. With regard to p53, HuR is able to bind Mdm2 mRNA, a critical negative regulator of p53. The authors suggest that by regulation of p53 levels HuR promotes the survival of hematopoietic progenitor cells [80]. Until now the possible role of AUF1 in those processes remains undiscovered.

Both proteins were also identified as critical mediators of replicative senescence. It had been shown that reduction of AUF1 level occurred with replicative senescence and contributed to stabilization and elevated expression of ARE-bearing p16 mRNA in senescence-phenotype cells [81]. Interestingly, exposure of the cells to hydrogen peroxide, which is related with TH production, led to reduced levels of AUF1. Furthermore, the cells overexpressing AUF1 were resistant to hydrogen peroxide-induced senescence. However whether AUF1 protective function against oxidative stress may be linked to thyroid function and disorders remains to be elucidated [82]. HuR was found to interact with the 3'UTR of the HuR mRNA and elevated HuR translation by promoting the nuclear export of HuR mRNA. The authors propose that such a regulatory mechanism may be responsible for the loss of HuR during replicative senescence [83].

Nagaoka et al. showed that AUF1 may be implicated in mammary gland differentiation. It had been demonstrated that stimulation with lactogenic hormone decreased cytoplasmic, but increased nuclear AUF1 levels. Furthermore, depletion of AUF1 correlated with elevated expression of b-casein and decreased levels of c-myc mRNAs. Such a cytoplasmic-nuclear translocation of AUF1 allowed the cells initiation of differentiation followed by induction of milk production and inhibition of proliferation [84].

## Conclusions

The possibility of functional interactions between AUF1 and HuR, and thyroid related mRNAs presented in this study is still speculative, but open new ways to investigate the unrevealed mechanisms, far beyond the known function of both proteins.

**List of abbreviations used**

3'-UTR: 3'-untranslated region; ALK: anaplastic lymphoma kinase; ANXA2: annexin A2; ARE: Adenylate-Uridylate-rich element; AUF1: Adenylate-Uridylate rich RNA-binding Factor 1; D1, D2, D3: deiodinases I, II, III; ELAV: embryonic lethal abnormal vision; EYA1: eyes absent homolog; GAPDH): glyceraldehyde-3-phpsphate dehydrogenase; GRHL2: grainyhead-like 2; GSTP1: glutathione S-transferase P; HCV: Hepatitis C virus; HHEX: homebox protein HEX; HNRNPK: heterogeneous nuclear ribonucleoprotein K; Hox-A3: homebox protein Hox-A3; Hox-A5: homebox protein Hox-A5; hTERT: human telomerase reverse transcriptase; HuR: human antigen R; IGF2BP1: insulin-like growth factor 2 mRNA binding protein; IRES: internal ribosome entry site; MAT1A: methionine adenosyltransferase 1A; MAT1A: methionine adenosyltransferase

1A; MAT2A: methionine adenosyltransferase 2A; MAT2A: methionine adenosyltransferase 2A; MCT8: monocarboxylate transporter 8; MSH2: MutS homolog 2; NIS: sodium-iodide symporter; NPM: nucleophosmin; PGA2: Prostaglandin A2; PKM1/M2: pyruvate kinase isoenzymes M1/M2; PPIA: peptidyl-prolyl cis-trans isomerase A; PRDX2: peroxiredoxin 2; PTH: parathyroid hormone; RA: retinoic acid; RAR: retinoic acid receptors; SAM: S-adenosylmethionine; SERCA2a: sarco(endo)plasmic reticulum calcium ATPase 2a; SLE: systemic lupus erythematosus; T3: triiodothyronine; TH: thyroid hormone; THR: thyroid hormone receptor; TKT: transketolase; TPO: thyroid peroxidise; TSG: tumor suppressor genes; TSH: thyroid stimulating hormone; TSHR: thyroid stimulating hormone receptor.

**Acknowledgements**

We would like to thank Ms. Kathrin Hammje for excellent technical assistance in creation of this manuscript. This study was partly supported by Deutsche Forschungsgemeinschaft (DFG) and Deutsche Krebshilfe. The authors declare that there is no conflict of interest that would prejudice the impartiality of this scientific work.

This article has been published as part of *Thyroid Research* Volume 4 Supplement 1, 2011: New aspects of thyroid hormone synthesis and action. The full contents of the supplement are available online at http://www.thyroidresearchjournal.com/supplements/4/S1

**Competing interests**

The authors declare that they have no competing interests.

**References**

1. Brewer G: **An A+U-rich element RNA-binding factor regulates c-myc mRNA stability in vitro.** *Mol Cell Biol* 1991, **11**:2460-2466.
2. DeMaria CT, Brewer G: **AUF1 binding affinity to A+U-rich elements correlaates with rapid mRNA degradation.** *J Biol Chem* 1996, **271**:12179-12184.
3. Good PJ: **A conserved family of elav-like genes in vetebrates.** *Proc Natl Acad Sci U S A* 1995, **92**:4557-4561.
4. Ma WJ, Cheng S, Campell C, Wrignt A, Furneaux H: **Cloning and characterization of HuR, a ubiquitously expressed Elav-like protein.** *J Biol Chem* 1996, **271**:8144-8151.
5. Loflin P, Chen CYA, Shyu AN: **Unraveling a cytoplasmic rolr for hnRNPD in the in vivo mRNA destabilization directed by the AU-rich element.** *Genes Dev* 1999, **13**:1884-1897.
6. Zhang W, Wagner BJ, Ehrenmann K, Schaefer AW, DeMaria CT, Crater D, DeHaven K, Long L, Brewer G: **Purification, characterization and cDNA cloning of an AU-rich element RNA-binding protein, AUF1.** *Mol Cell Biol* 1993, **13**:7652-7665.
7. Wang W, Caldwell MC, Lin S, Furneaux H, Gorospe M: **HuR regulated Cyclin A and cyclin B1 mRNA stability during cell proliferation.** *EMBO J* 2000, **19(10)**:2340-2350.
8. Suzuki M, Iijima M, Nishimura A, Tomozoe Y, Kamei D, Yamada M: **Two separate regions essential for nuclear import of the hnRNP D nucleocytoplasmic shuttling sequence.** *FEBS J* 2005, **272**:3975-3987.
9. Fan XC, Steitz JA: **HNS, a nuclear-cytoplasmic shuttling sequence in HuR.** *Proc Natl Acad Sci U S A* 1998, **95**:15293-15298.
10. David PS, Tanveer R, Port JD: **FRET-detectable interactions between the ARE binding proteins, HuR and p37AUF1.** *RNA* 2007, **13**:1453-1468.
11. Moraes KC, Quaresma AJ, Maehnss K, Kobarg J: **Identification and characterization of proteins that selectively interact with isoforms of the mRNA binding protein AUF1 (hnRNP D).** *Biol Chem* 2003, **384**:25-37.
12. Dignam JD, Lebovitz RM, Roeder RG: **Accurate transcription initiation by RNA polymerase II in a soluble extract from isolated mammalian nuclei.** *Nucleic Acids Res* 1983, **11**:1475-1489.
13. Li M, Makkinje A, Damuni Z: **Molecular identification of I1PP2A, a novel potent heat-stable inhibitor protein of protein phosphatase 2A.** *Biochemistry* 1996, **35**:6998-7002.
14. Zhu T, Matsuzawa S, Mizuno Y, Kamibayashi C, Mumby MC, Andjelkovic N, Hemmings BA, Onoé K, Kikuchi K: **The interconversion of protein phosphatase 2A between PP2A1 and PP2A0 during retinoic acid-induced granulocytic differentiation and a modification on the catalytic subunit in S phase of HL-60 cells.** *Arch Biochem Biophys* 1997, **339**:210-217.
15. Millward TA, Zolnierowicz S, Hemmings BA: **Regulation of protein kinase cascades by protein phosphatase 2A.** *Trends Biochem Sci* 1999, **24**:186-191.
16. Chang N, Yi J, Guo G, Liu X, Shang Y, Tong T, Cui Q, Zhan M, Gorospe M, Wang W: **HuR uses AUF1 as a cofactor to promote p16INK4 mRNA decay.** *Mol Cell Biol* 2010, **30**:3875-3886.
17. Bakheed T, Frevel M, Williams BR, Greer W, Khabar KS: **ARED: human AU-rich element containing mRNA database reveals an unexpectedly diverse functional repertoire of encoded proteins.** *Nucleic Acids Res* 2001, **29**:246-254.
18. Gruber AR, Fallmann J, Kratochvill F, Kovarik P, Hofacker IL: **AREsite: a database for the comprehensive investigation of AU-rich elements.** *Nucleic Acids Res* 2011, **39(Database issue)**:D66-9.
19. López de Silanes I, Zhan M, Lal A, Yang X, Gorospe M: **Identification of a target RNA motif for RNA-binding protein HuR.** *Proc Natl Acad Sci U S A* 2004, **101**:2987-2992.
20. Mazan-Mamczarz K, Kuwano Y, Zhan M, White EJ, Martindale JL, Lal A, Gorospe M: **Identification of a signature motif in target mRNAs of RNA-binding protein AUF1.** *Nucleic Acids Res* 2009, **37**:204-214.
21. Gouble A, Morello D: **Synchronous and regulated expression of two AU-binding proteins, AUF1 and HuR, throughout murine development.** *Oncogene* 2000, **19**:5377-5384.
22. Hambardzumyan D, Sergent-Tanguy S, Thinard R, Bonnamain V, Masip M, Fabre A, Boudin H, Neveu I, Naveilhan P: **AUF1 and Hu proteins in the developing rat brain: implication in the proliferation and differentiation of neural progenitors.** *J Neurosci Res* 2009, **87**:1296-1309.
23. Vázquez-Chantada M, Fernández-Ramos D, Embade N, Martínez-Lopez N, Varela-Rey M, Woodhoo A, Luka Z, Wagner C, Anglim PP, Finnell RH, Caballería J, Laird-Offringa IA, Gorospe M, Lu SC, Mato JM, Martínez-Chantar ML: **HuR/methyl-HuR and AUF1 regulate the MAT expressed during liver proliferation, differentiation, and carcinogenesis.** *Gastroenterology* 2010, **138**:1943-1953.
24. Sadri N, Schneider RJ: **Auf1/Hnrnpd-deficient mice develop pruritic inflammatory skin disease. Auf1/Hnrnpd-deficient mice develop pruritic inflammatory skin disease.** *J Invest Dermatol* 2009, **129**:657-670.
25. Cunningham MJ, Zone JJ: **Thyroid abnormalities in dermatitis herpetiformis. Prevalence of clinical thyroid disease and thyroid autoantibodies.** *Ann Intern Med* 1985, **102**:194-196.
26. Artantas S, Gül U, Kiliç A, Güler S: **Skin findings in thyroid diseases.** *Eur J Intern Med* 2009, **20**:158-161.
27. Lu JY, Sadri N, Schneider RJ: **Endotoxic shock in AUF1 knockout mice mediated by failure to degrade proinflammatory cytokine mRNAs.** *Genes Dev* 2006, **20**:3174-3184.
28. Sadri N, Lu JY, Badura ML, Schneider RJ: **AUF1 is involved in splenic follicular B cell maintenance.** *BMC Immunol* 2010, **11**:1.
29. Katsanou V, Milatos S, Yiakouvaki A, Sgantzis N, Kotsoni A, Alexiou M, Harokopos V, Aidinis V, Hemberger M, Kontoyiannis DL: **The RNA-binding protein Elavl1/HuR is essential for placental branching morphogenesis and embryonic development.** *Mol Cell Biol* 2009, **29**:2762-2776.
30. Krane IM, Spindel ER, Chin WW: **Thyroid hormone decreases the stability and the poly(A) tract length of rat thyrotropin beta-subunit messenger RNA.** *Mol Endocrinol* 1991, **5**:469-475.
31. Staton JM, Leedman PJ: **Posttranscriptional regulation of thyrotropin beta-subunit messenger ribonucleic acid by thyroid hormone in murine thyrotrope tumor cells: a conserved mechanism across species.** *Endocrinology* 1998, **139**:1093-1100.
32. Goulart-Silva F, de Souza PB, Nunes MT: **T3 rapidly modulates TSHβ mRNA stability and translational rate in the pituitary of hypothyroid rats.** *Mol Cell Endocrinol* 2011, **332**:277-282.
33. Leedman PJ, Stein AR, Chin WW: **Regulated specific protein binding to a conserved region of the 3'-untranslated region of thyrotropin beta-subunit mRNA.** *Mol Endocrinol* 1995, **9**:375-387.
34. Murphy D, Pardy K, Seah V, Carter D: **Posttranscriptional regulation of rat growth hormone gene expression: increased message stability and nuclear polyadenylation accompany thyroid hormone depletion.** *Mol Cell Biol* 1992, **12**:2624-2632.
35. Silva FG, Giannocco G, Luchessi AD, Curi R, Nunes MT: **T3 acutely increases GH mRNA translation rate and GH secretion in hypothyroid rats.** *Mol Cell Endocrinol* 2010, **317**:1-7.
36. Minamisawa S, Uemura N, Sato Y, Yokoyama U, Yamaguchi T, Inoue K, Nakagome M, Bai Y, Hori H, Shimizu M, Mochizuki S, Ishikawa Y: **Post-**

transcriptional downregulation of sarcolipin mRNA by triiodothyronine in the atrial myocardium. *FEBS Lett* 2006, **580**:2247-2252.

37. Blum JL, Samarel AM, Mestril R: **Phosphorylation and binding of AUF1 to the 3'-untranslated region of cardiomyocyte SERCA2a mRNA.** *Am J Physiol Heart Circ Physiol* 2005, **289**:H2543-2550.
38. Zhou C, Vignere CZ, Levitan ES: **AUF1 is upregulated by angiotensin II to destabilize cardiac Kv4.3 channel mRNA.** *J Mol Cell Cardiol* 2008, **45**:832-838.
39. Steinsapir J, Harney J, Larsen PR: **Type 2 iodothyronine deiodinase in rat pituitary tumor cells is inactivated in proteasomes.** *J Clin Invest* 1998, **102**:1895-1899.
40. Gereben B, Goncalves C, Harney JW, Larsen PR, Bianco AC: **Selective proteolysis of human type 2 deiodinase: a novel ubiquitin-proteasomal mediated mechanism for regulation of hormone activation.** *Mol Endocrinol* 2000, **14**:1697-1708.
41. Curcio-Morelli C, Zavacki AM, Christofollete M, Gereben B, de Freitas BC, Harney JW, Li Z, Wu G, Bianco AC: **Deubiquitination of type 2 iodothyronine deiodinase by von Hippel-Lindau protein-interacting deubiquitinating enzymes regulates thyroid hormone activation.** *J Clin Invest* 2003, **112**:189-196.
42. Sagar GD, Gereben B, Callebaut I, Mornon JP, Zeöld A, da Silva WS, Luongo C, Dentice M, Tente SM, Freitas BC, Harney JW, Zavacki AM, Bianco AC: **Ubiquitination-induced conformational change within the deiodinase dimer is a switch regulating enzyme activity.** *Mol Cell Biol* 2007, **27**:4774-4783.
43. Martinez de Mena R, Scanlan TS, Obregon MJ: **The T3 receptor beta1 isoform regulates UCP1 and D2 deiodinase in rat brown adipocytes.** *Endocrinology* 2010, **151**:5074-5083.
44. Navarro-Yubero C, Cuadrado A, Sonderegger P, Muñoz A: **Neuroserpin is post-transcriptionally regulated by thyroid hormone.** *Brain Res Mol Brain Res* 2004, **123**:56-65.
45. Mano H, Mori R, Ozawa T, Takeyama K, Yoshizawa Y, Kojima R, Arao Y, Masushige S, Kato S: **Positive and negative regulation of retinoid X receptor gene expression by thyroid hormone in the rat. Transcriptional and post-transcriptional controls by thyroid hormone.** *J Biol Chem* 1994, **269**:1591-1594.
46. Schmutzler C, Mentrup B, Schomburg L, Hoang-Vu C, Herzog V, Köhrle J: **Selenoproteins of the thyroid gland: expression, localization and possible function of glutathione peroxidase 3.** *Biol Chem* 2007, **388**:1053-1059.
47. Naveh-Many T, Bell O, Silver J, Kilav R: **Cis and trans acting factors in the regulation of parathyroid hormone (PTH) mRNA stability by calcium and phosphate.** *FEBS Lett* 2002, **529**:60-64.
48. Owen D, Kühn LC: **Noncoding 3' sequences of the transferrin receptor gene are required for mRNA regulation by iron.** *EMBO J* 1987, **6**:1287-1293.
49. Mittag J, Behrends T, Hoefig CS, Vennström B, Schomburg L: **Thyroid hormones regulate selenoprotein expression and selenium status in mice.** *PLoS One* 2010, **5**:e12931.
50. Sela-Brown A, Silver J, Brewer G, Naveh-Many T: **Identification of AUF1 as a parathyroid hormone mRNA 3'-untranslated region-binding protein that determines parathyroid hormone mRNA stability.** *J Biol Chem* 2000, **275**:7424-7429.
51. Bermano G, Arthur JR, Hesketh JE: **Selective control of cytosolic glutathione peroxidase and phospholipid hydroperoxide glutathione peroxidase mRNA stability by selenium supply.** *FEBS Lett* 1996, **387**:157-160.
52. Riese C, Michaelis M, Mentrup B, Götz F, Köhrle J, Schweizer U, Schomburg L: **Selenium-dependent pre- and posttranscriptional mechanisms are responsible for sexual dimorphic expression of selenoproteins in murine tissues.** *Endocrinology* 2006, **147**:5883-5892.
53. Serrano-Nascimento C, Calil-Silveira J, Nunes MT: **Posttranscriptional regulation of sodium-iodide symporter mRNA expression in the rat thyroid gland by acute iodide administration.** *Am J Physiol Cell Physiol* 2010, **298**:C893-C899.
54. Trojanowicz B, Brodauf L, Sekulla C, Lorenz K, Finke R, Dralle H, Hoang-Vu C: **The role of AUF1 in thyroid carcinoma progression.** *Endocr Relat Cancer* 2009, **16**:857-871.
55. Braun J, Hoang-Vu C, Dralle H, Hüttelmaier S: **Downregulation of microRNAs directs the EMT and invasive potential of anaplastic thyroid carcinomas.** *Oncogene* 2010, **29**:4237-4244.
56. Trojanowicz B, Fu T, Gimm O, Sekulla C, Finke R, Dralle H, Hoang-Vu C: **Relationship between RKIP protein expression and clinical staging in thyroid carcinoma.** *Open Endocrinology Journal* 2008, **2**:16-20.
57. Trojanowicz B, Winkler A, Hammje K, Chen Z, Sekulla C, Glanz D, Schmutzler C, Mentrup B, Hombach-Klonisch S, Klonisch T, Finke R, Köhrle J, Dralle H, Hoang-Vu C: **Retinoic acid mediated down-regulation of ENO1/MBP-1 gene products caused decreased invasiveness of the follicular thyroid carcinoma cell lines.** *J Mol Endocrinol* 2009, **42**:249-260.
58. Chen Z, Mustafa T, Trojanowicz B, Brauckhoff M, Gimm O, Schmutzler C, Köhrle J, Holzhausen HJ, Kehlen A, Klonisch T, Finke R, Dralle H, Hoang-Vu C: **CD82, and CD63 in thyroid cancer.** *Int J Mol Med* 2004, **14**:517-527.
59. Lengfelder E, Saussele S, Weisser A, Buchner T, Hehlmann R: **Treatment concepts of acute promyelocytic leukemia.** *Crit Rev Oncol Hematol* 2005, **56**:261-274.
60. Hansen LA, Sigman CC, Andreola F, Ross SA, Kelloff GJ, De Luca LM: **Retinoids in chemoprevention and differentiation therapy.** *Carcinogenesis* 2000, **21**:1271-1279.
61. Simon D, Körber C, Krausch M, Segering J, Groth P, Görges R, Grünwald F, Müller-Gärtner HW, Schmutzler C, Köhrle J, Röher HD, Reiners C: **Clinical impact of retinoids in redifferentiation therapy of advanced thyroid cancer: final results of a pilot study.** *Eur J Nucl Med Mol Imaging* 2002, **29**:775-782.
62. Handkiewicz-Junak D, Roskosz J, Hasse-Lazar K, Szpak-Ulczok S, Puch Z, Kukulska A, Olczyk T, Piela A, Paliczka-Cieslik E, Jarzab B: **13-cis-retinoic acid re-differentiation therapy and recombinant human thyrotropin-aided radioiodine treatment of non-Functional metastatic thyroid cancer: a single-center, 53-patient phase 2 study.** *Thyroid Res* 2009, **2**:8.
63. Fernández CA, Puig-Domingo M, Lomeña F, Estorch M, Camacho Martí V, Bittini AL, Marazuela M, Santamaría J, Castro J, Martínez de Icaya P, Moraga I, Martín T, Megía A, Porta M, Mauricio D, Halperin I: **Effectiveness of retinoic acid treatment for redifferentiation of thyroid cancer in relation to recovery of radioiodine uptake.** *J Endocrinol Invest* 2009, **32**:228-233.
64. Schmutzler C, Kohrle J: **Retinoic acid redifferentiation therapy for thyroid cancer.** *Thyroid* 2000, **10**:393-406.
65. Schmutzler C, Hoang-Vu C, Rüger B, Kohrle J: **Human thyroid carcinoma cell lines show different retinoic acid receptor repertoires and retinoid responses.** *Eur J Endocrinol* 2004, **150**:547-556.
66. Trojanowicz B, Sekulla C, Lorenz K, Köhrle J, Finke R, Dralle H, Hoang-Vu C: **Proteomic approach reveals novel targets for retinoic acid-mediated therapy of thyroid carcinoma.** *Mol Cell Endocrinol* 2010, **325**:110-117.
67. Gouble A, Grazide S, Meggetto F, Mercier P, Delsol G, Morello D: **A new player in oncogenesis: AUF1/hnRNPD overexpression leads to tumorigenesis in transgenic mice.** *Cancer Res* 2002, **62**:1489-1495.
68. Blaxall BC, Dwyer-Nield LD, Bauer AK, Bohlmeyer TJ, Malkinson AM, Port JD: **Differential expres-sion and localization of the mRNA binding proteins, AU-rich element mRNA binding protein (AUF1) and Hu antigen R (HuR), in neoplastic lung tissue.** *Mol Carcinog* 2000, **28**:76-83.
69. Yuan Z, Sanders AJ, Ye L, Jiang WG: **HuR, a key post-transcriptional regulator, and its implication in progression of breast cancer.** *Histol Histopathol* 2010, **25**:1331-1340.
70. Kakuguchi W, Kitamura T, Kuroshima T, Ishikawa M, Kitagawa Y, Totsuka Y, Shindoh M, Higashino F: **HuR knockdown changes the oncogenic potential of oral cancer cells.** *Mol Cancer Res* 2010, **8**:520-528.
71. Fawal M, Armstrong F, Ollier S, Dupont H, Touriol C, Monsarrat B, Delsol G, Payrastre B, Morello D: **A "liaison dangereuse" between AUF1/hnRNPD and the oncogenic tyrosine kinase NPM-ALK.** *Blood* 2006, **108**:2780-2788.
72. Paek KY, Kim CS, Park SM, Kim JH, Jang SK: **RNA-binding protein hnRNP D modulates internal ribosome entry site-dependent translation of hepatitis C virus RNA.** *J Virol* 2008, **82**:12082-12093.
73. Weinlich S, Hüttelmaier S, Schierhorn A, Behrens SE, Ostareck-Lederer A, Ostareck DH: **IGF2BP1 enhances HCV IRES-mediated translation initiation via the 3'UTR.** *RNA* 2009, **15**:1528-1542.
74. Kang X, Chen W, Kim RH, Kang MK, Park NH: **Regulation of the hTERT promoter activity by MSH2, the hnRNPs K and D, and GRHL2 in human oral squamous cell carcinoma cells.** *Oncogene* 2009, **28**:565-574.
75. Lin S, Wang W, Wilson GM, Yang X, Brewer G, Holbrook NJ, Gorospe M: **Down-regulation of cyclin D1 expression by prostaglandin A(2) is mediated by enhanced cyclin D1 mRNA turnover.** *Mol Cell Biol* 2000, **20**:7903-7913.
76. Brewer G, Saccani S, Sarkar S, Lewis A, Pestka S: **Increased interleukin-10 mRNA stability in melanoma cells is associated with decreased levels of**

A + U-rich element binding factor AUF1. *J Interferon Cytokine Res* 2003, **23**:553-564.
77. Skriner K, Hueber W, Süleymanoglu E, Höfler E, Krenn V, Smolen J, Steiner G: AUF1, the regulator of tumor necrosis factor alpha messenger RNA decay, is targeted by autoantibodies of patients with systemic rheumatic diseases. *Arthritis Rheum* 2008, **58**:511-520.
78. Nabors LB, Furneaux HM, King PH: HuR, a novel target of anti-Hu antibodies, is expressed in non-neural tissues. *J Neuroimmunol* 1998, **92**:152-159.
79. Masuda K, Abdelmohsen K, Gorospe M: RNA-binding proteins implicated in the hypoxic response. *J Cell Mol Med* 2009, **13**:2759-2769.
80. Ghosh M, Aguila HL, Michaud J, Ai Y, Wu MT, Hemmes A, Ristimaki A, Guo C, Furneaux H, Hla T: Essential role of the RNA-binding protein HuR in progenitor cell survival in mice. *J Clin Invest* 2009, **119**:3530-3543.
81. Wang W, Martindale JL, Yang X, Chrest FJ, Gorospe M: Increased stability of the p16 mRNA with replicative senescence. *EMBO Rep* 2005, **6**:158-164.
82. Guo GE, Ma LW, Jiang B, Yi J, Tong TJ, Wang WG: Hydrogen peroxide induces p16(INK4a) through an AUF1-dependent manner. *J Cell Biochem* 2010, **109**:1000-1005.
83. Yi J, Chang N, Liu X, Guo G, Xue L, Tong T, Gorospe M, Wang W: Reduced nuclear export of HuR mRNA by HuR is linked to the loss of HuR in replicative senescence. *Nucleic Acids Res* 2010, **38**:1547-1558.
84. Nagaoka K, Tanaka T, Imakawa K, Sakai S: Involvement of RNA binding proteins AUF1 in mammary gland differentiation. *Exp Cell Res* 2007, **313**:2937-2945.
85. Klonisch T, Hoang-Vu C, Hombach-Klonisch S: Thyroid stem cells and cancer. *Thyroid* 2009, **19**:1303-1315.

# Treatment of advanced medullary thyroid cancer

Johannes Smit

*From* 9th Meeting of the European Thyroid Association Cancer Research Network (ETA-CRN)
Lisbon, Portugal.

**Abstract**

Therapy decisions in advanced medullary thyroid carcinoma should be guided by a critical appraisal of the natural disease course (slowly progressive vs. aggressive) and benefits and side effects of therapy. Therapy goals should be distinguished between curative and palliative. Local treatments are mainly palliative and may add to quality of life. The advent of novel systemic therapies opens promising perspectives but its place in the therapeutic arsenal must be further determined.

## Introduction

Distant metastases in medullary thyroid carcinoma (MTC) are frequently present at initial presentation in sporadic MTC patients [1,2]. Organs most often affected include the lungs, bones and liver, and infrequently the brain. Distant metastases are frequently associated with persistent locoregional disease [3]. Patients with distant metastases at diagnosis have a poor prognosis, with only 40% surviving 10 years [2].

## Treatment goals

Treatment goals in advanced MTC are ultimately related to promoting the quality of life. It is important to explicitly discuss with the patient the expectations and goals with respect to quality of life in the individual context and to agree on a personalized treatment plan. In general, it is important to document the sites of metastases and the tumor volume as well as tumor progression to get an estimate of total tumor burden and prognosis. In addition, it is necessary to document signs and symptoms and estimate imminent problems. In patients with recurrent disease, an acceptable quality of life can usually be maintained for months or even years. Treatment decisions must therefore balance the usually slow progression rate and the reasonable life expectancy against the efficacy and side effects of therapies.

An important step is to decide whether any therapy will be curative or palliative, as the risk-benefit ratio of curative therapies is essentially different from palliative therapies. Curative therapies will *by definition* be aimed at improved survival and disease-free survival. The main objective of palliative therapies is to improve quality of life by relief of symptoms. When recurrent local disease is present or distant metastases are limited to a single organ curative surgical resection may be considered. Unfortunately, in advanced MTC, curative options are limited as both local recurrent disease and metastases are seldomly amenable to curative surgery. Active treatment is most often indicated in patients with lesions in critical locations such as brain metastases, threatening spinal cord compression, airway obstruction, bleeding, impending or active fracture or hormonal secretion.

## Documenting disease and disease progression

The discovery of metastases is often preceded by detectable or increasing serum levels of calcitonin or CEA. It must however be stressed that elevated levels of tumor markers are not a reason in itself to start therapies. Elevated tumor markers, and especially a low doubling time of serum calcitonin and CEA are rather considered risk factors for the presence and development of metastases and a poor prognosis [4,5]. Indeed, disease progression should always be confirmed by imaging before considering treatment. Patients who have elevated stable tumor markers without demonstrable tumor may have a good prognosis and quality of life [6-8]. Those patients are being followed with serum tumor marker measurements and regular imaging, the interval depending on the serum marker level and doubling time [1,4,5].

Correspondence: J.Smit@aig.umcn.nl
Department of General Internal Medicine, Radboud University Nijmegen Medical Centre P.O. Box 9101, 6500 HB Nijmegen, The Netherlands

Imaging should identify all clinically relevant sites of disease, both for the identification of tumors that require local interventions and the selection of potential target lesions to assess response to systemic therapy. Imaging procedures in metastatic MTC include conventional contrast-enhanced spiral CT scan or MRI of the brain, neck, chest and liver and bone scintigraphy [3]. Diagnostic accuracy of Fluorodeoxyglucose (FDG)- PET scan is questionable [3,9]. F-DOPA-PET scintigraphy is promising and may provide additional information on tumor localization in patients with elevated tumor markers without evidence of disease on conventional imaging. However, the impact on clinical decision making needs to be confirmed [10].

In patients with measurable lesions, it should be evaluated if curative therapy is possible. When no curative options are present, disease progression must be documented. Usually, criteria for the initiation of systemic treatment are defined according to RECIST in combination with considerable tumor burden and/or symptoms.

## Local disease

Recurrent disease in the neck and mediastinum is frequently amenable to surgery, with either curative or palliative intent. Repeat surgery may normalize calcitonin levels in one third of patients and progression free survival may be fairly good, although no controlled studies have been performed. Surgical resection of locoregional recurrent MTC in patients without distant metastases should include compartmental dissection of disease in the neck compartments. In the presence of incurable advanced local or distant disease, less extensive neck surgery may be appropriate to avoid complications [11-13].

The role of external beam radiation therapy (EBRT) in recurrent local MTC is not clear. In patients with local disease in whom no curative surgery is possible, EBRT may improve locoregional disease control, although an improvement in overall survival has not been established [14].

## Distant metastases

Distant metastases limited to a single organ may be considered for curative surgical resection or another local treatment modality. Slow growing or stable metastases without clinical symptoms may be followed, the interval of imaging depending on the size of the tumor and the progression rate.

## Local treatment modalities for distant metastases

### Brain metastases

Clinically overt brain metastases from MTC are reported in 1–5% of MTC patients with local or metastatic disease [3]. Brain metastases are suspected in MTC patients with neurologic symptoms especially when distant metastases are present. Brain imaging should be performed in asymptomatic MTC patients before initiation of systemic therapy [15-17]. When small brain lesions are discovered, it may be decided to follow-up without treatment. In clinical studies in differentiated thyroid carcinoma and other tumors, it has been suggested that surgical resection in patients with solitary or a limited number of brain metastases may be associated with improved survival and quality of life [15-17]. Other treatment options include stereotactic radiosurgery or whole brain EBRT for clinically overt brain metastases.

### Bone metastases

Bone metastases occur in 45% of MTC patients with local or metastatic disease [3]. Small, asymptomatic bone metastases can be followed without treatment. Isolated bone metastases may be surgically resected. In some studies in differentiated thyroid carcinoma, it has been suggested that surgery is worthwhile when 5 or less bone metastases are present [18]. It is not known if these results can be expanded to MTC. EBRT in symptomatic bone lesions may lead to considerable reduction in pain in 80% of patients, which may last for months [14]. Experience from other tumors learns that symptomatic bone metastases can be successfully treated with percutaneous methods including cementoplasty, thermal ablation (radiofrequency or cryotherapy) and arterial embolization followed by surgery, or a combination of these methods, for pain reduction and bone consolidation [19,20]. Intravenous bisphosphonates are prescribed frequently for painful bony metastases in other malignancies, but this has not been investigated in MTC [21].

### Lung metastases

Lung metastases occur in 33% of MTC patients with local or metastatic disease [6]. In solitary lesions, surgical resection, either by open procedure or video assisted thoracoscopy can be considered. Alternatively, asymptomatic, stable or slowly progressive lesions can be followed. Lung or mediastinal lesions causing local compression of an airway or bleeding may be considered for surgery or EBRT, and lesions with central airway invasion may be amenable to the photodynamic therapy or airway stenting (when the tumor is >15 mm from the vocal cord) to improve quality of life [22]. Radiofrequency ablation may be indicated in patients with few ( <5,) predominantly peripheral lung metastases of < 40 mm in size.

### Liver metastases

Liver metastases occur in 45% of MTC patients with local or metastatic disease [6] . In large, progressive liver metastases or metastases associated with symptoms, local treatment is required. Treatment options include resection or percutaneous radiofrequency ablation. RFA may lead to prolonged symptom reduction in 90–95% of patients, including reduction of diarrhoea. Radiofrequency ablation is less effective in lesions > 50 mm [23,24].

## Systemic treatment

Conventional chemotherapy in patients with advanced MTC has limited efficacy, and considerable toxicity and is therefore not recommended [1].

In recent years, several kinase inhibitors have been evaluated in phase I and II clinical trials, including axitinib, cabozantinib (XL-184), lenvatinib (E7080), motesanib, pazopanib, sorafenib, sunitinib and vandetanib [25,26]. In phase II trials, several of these agents have demonstrated partial response rates in the range of 20–50% with a larger number of patients demonstrating prolonged stable disease. Two of these agents, vandetanib and cabozantinib have completed phase III clinical trials.

Vandetanib (300 mg/day) [27] prolonged median progression free survival from 19 months in the placebo arm to a predicted median of 31 months in the vandetanib arm; the improvement of pain and diarrhoea allowed a number of patients in the vandetanib arm to resume a normal social life. However, 12% of patients receiving vandetanib discontinued treatment due to toxicity and 35% required dose reduction because of an adverse event. Vandetanib was approved by the FDA in April 2011 and by the EMEA in February 2012. Cabozantinib (175 mg/day) prolonged PFS prolongation from 4 to 11 months and was approved by the FDA in November 2012 [28]. However, short-term toxicity of these therapies is significant, with dose reduction or treatment withdrawal in a significant proportion of patients; longterm toxicity needs to be investigated. There is currently no evidence for a higher treatment efficacy at an earlier than later stage when the tumor has progressed. This should lead to initiating these treatments only in patients with significant tumor burden and documented tumor progression.

## Other therapies

Therapies with immunization [29] and radiolabelled molecules have been performed in MTC sometimes with promising results. Treatment with 131-I-MIBG is generally regarded as ineffective for MTC [30].

## Treatment of hormonally active metastases

MTC is an endocrine active tumor and secretion of hormones other than calcitonin is frequently observed. Diarrhoea [31] is frequently present when tumor volume is high. Diarrhoea can be treated with anti-motility drugs including somatostatin analogues. When these therapies are not sufficient, local therapies to reduce tumor volume can be considered. Sometimes, CRH or ACTH production leads to Cushing syndrome, which may be a reason for local tumor reduction, cortisol synthesis inhibitors or bilateral adrenalectomy [32].

### List of abbreviations used

MTC: medullary thyroid carcinoma; CEA: carcinoembryonic antigen; EBRT: external beam radiation therapy.

### Competing interests

No conflict of interest.

### Declarations

This article has been published as part of *Thyroid Research* Volume 6 Supplement 1, 2013: European comments on Medullary Thyroid Cancer Management Guidelines of the American Thyroid Association. The full contents of the supplement are available online at http://www.thyroidresearchjournal.com/supplements/6/S1. Publication of this supplement has been supported by the European Thyroid Association-Cancer Research Network.

### References

1. Kloos RT, Eng C, Evans DB, Francis GL, Gagel RT, Gharib H, Moley JF, Pacini F, Ringel MD, Schlumberger M, Wells SA Jr: **Medullary thyroid cancer: management guidelines of the American Thyroid Association.** *Thyroid* 2009, **19**:565-612.
2. Roman S, Lin R, Sosa JA: **Prognosis of medullary thyroid carcinoma: demographic, clinical, and pathologic predictors of survival in 1252 cases.** *Cancer* 2006, **107(9)**:2134-42.
3. Giraudet AL, Vanel D, Leboulleux S, Aupérin A, Dromain C, Chami L, Ny Tovo N, Lumbroso J, Lassau N, Bonniaud G, Hartl D, Travagli JP, Baudin E, Schlumberger M: **Imaging medullary thyroid carcinoma with persistent elevated calcitonin levels.** *J Clin Endocrinol Metab* 2007, **92**:4185-4190.
4. Giraudet AL, Al Ghulzan A, Aupérin A, Leboulleux S, Chehboun A, Troalen F, Dromain C, Lumbroso J, Baudin E, Schlumberger M: **Progression of medullary thyroid carcinoma: assessment with calcitonin and carcinoembryonic antigen doubling times.** *Eur J Endocrinol* 2008, **158**:239-246.
5. Barbet J, Campion L, Kraeber-Bodere F, Chatal JF: **Prognostic impact of serum calcitonin and carcinoembryonic antigen doubling-times in patients with medullary thyroid carcinoma.** *J Clin Endocrinol Metab* 2005, **90**:6077-6084.
6. van Heerden JA, Grant CS, Gharib H, Hay ID, Ilstrup DM: **Long-term course of patients with persistent hypercalcitoninemia after apparent curative primary surgery for medullary thyroid carcinoma.** *Ann Surg* 1990, **212**:395-400, discussion 400-401.
7. Pellegriti G, Leboulleux S, Baudin E, Bellon N, Scollo C, Travagli JP, Schlumberger M: **Long-term outcome of medullary thyroid carcinoma in patients with normal postoperative medical imaging.** *Br J Cancer* 2003, **88**:1537-1542.
8. Fialkowski E, Debenedetti M, Moley J: **Longterm outcome of reoperations for medullary thyroid carcinoma.** *World J Surg* 2008, **32**:754-765.
9. Ong SC, Schoder H, Patel SG, Tabangay-Lim IM, Doddamane I, Gonen M, Shaha AR, Tuttle RM, Shah JP, Larson SM: **Diagnostic accuracy of 18F-FDG PET in restaging patients with medullary thyroid carcinoma and elevated calcitonin levels.** *J Nucl Med* 2007, **48**:501-507.
10. Koopmans KP, de Groot JW, Plukker JT, de Vries EG, Kema IP, Sluiter WJ, Jager PL, Links TP: **18F-dihydroxyphenylalanine PET in patients with biochemical evidence of medullary thyroid cancer: relation to tumor differentiation.** *J Nucl Med* 2008, **49**:524-531.
11. Kebebew E, Kikuchi S, Duh QY, Clark OH: **Long-term results of reoperation and localizing studies in patients with persistent or recurrent medullary thyroid cancer.** *Arch Surg* 2000, **135**:895-901.
12. Dralle H: **Lymph node dissection and medullary thyroid carcinoma.** *Br J Surg* 2002, **89**:1073-1075.
13. Fialkowski E, Debenedetti M, Moley J: **Long-term outcome of reoperations for medullary thyroid carcinoma.** *World J Surg* 2008, **32**:754-765.

14. Brierley J, Tsang R, Simpson WJ, Gospodarowicz M, Sutcliffe S, Panzarella T: **Medullary thyroid cancer: analyses of survival and prognostic factors and the role of radiation therapy in local control.** *Thyroid* 1996, **6**:305-310.
15. McWilliams RR, Giannini C, Hay ID, Atkinson JL, Stafford SL, Buckner JC: **Management of brain metastases from thyroid carcinoma: a study of 16 pathologically confirmed cases over 25 years.** *Cancer* 2003, **98**:356-362.
16. Chiu AC, Delpassand ES, Sherman SI: **Prognosis and treatment of brain metastases in thyroid carcinoma.** *J Clin Endocrinol Metab* 1997, **82**:3637-3642.
17. Salvati M, Frati A, Rocchi G, Masciangelo R, Antonaci A, Gagliardi FM, Delfini R: **Single brain metastasis from thyroid cancer: report of twelve cases and review of the literature.** *J Neurooncol* 2001, **51**:33-40.
18. Bernier MO, Leenhardt L, Hoang C, Aurengo A, Mary JY, Menegaux F, Enkaoua E, Turpin G, Chiras J, Saillant G: **Survival and therapeutic modalities in patients with bone metastases of differentiated thyroid carcinomas.** *J Clin Endocrinol Metab* 2001, **86**:1568-1573.
19. Eustatia-Rutten CFA, Romijn JA, Guijt MJ, Vielvoye GJ, van den Berg R, Corssmit EPM, Pereira AM, Smit JW: **Outcome of palliative embolization of bone metastases in differentiated thyroid carcinoma.** *J Clin Endocrinol Metab* 2003, **88**:3184-3189.
20. Mont'Alverne F, Vallee JN, Cormier E, Guillevin R, Barragan H, Jean B, Rose M, Chiras J: **Percutaneous vertebroplasty for metastatic involvement of the axis.** *AJNR Am J Neuroradiol* 2005, **26**:1641-1645.
21. Vitale G, Fonderico F, Martignetti A, Caraglia M, Ciccarelli A, Nuzzo V, Abbruzzese A, Lupoli G: **Pamidronate improves the quality of life and induces clinical remission of bone metastases in patients with thyroid cancer.** *Br J Cancer* 2001, **84**:1586-1590.
22. Tsutsui H, Kubota M, Yamada M, Suzuki A, Usuda J, Shibuya H, Miyajima K, Sugino K, Ito K, Furukawa K, Kato H: **Airway stenting for the treatment of laryngotracheal stenosis secondary to thyroid cancer.** *Respirology* 2008, **13**:632-638.
23. Wertenbroek MW, Links TP, Prins TR, Plukker JT, van der Jagt EJ, de Jong KP: **Radiofrequency ablation of hepatic metastases from thyroid carcinoma.** *Thyroid* 2008, **18**:1105-1110.
24. Fromigue J, De Baere T, Baudin E, Dromain C, Leboulleux S, Schlumberger M: **Chemoembolization for liver metastases from medullary thyroid carcinoma.** *J Clin Endocrinol Metab* 2006, **91**:2496-2499.
25. Gild ML, Bullock M, Robinson BG, Clifton-Bligh R: **Multikinase inhibitors: a new option for the treatment of thyroid cancer.** *Nat Rev Endocrinol* 2011, **7(10)**:617-24.
26. Kapiteijn E, Schneider TC, Morreau H, Gelderblom H, Nortier JW, Smit JW: **New treatment modalities in advanced thyroid cancer.** *Ann Oncol* 2012, **23(1)**:10-8.
27. Wells SA, Robinson BG, Gagel RF, Dralle H, Fagin JA, Santoro M, Baudin E, Elisei R, Jarzab B, Vasselli JR, Read J, Langmuir P, Ryan AJ, Schlumberger MJ: **Vandetanib in patients with locally advanced or metastatic medullary thyroid cancer: a randomized, double-blind phase III trial (ZETA).** *J Clin Oncol* 2012, **30**:134-141.
28. Schoffski P, Elisei R, Müller S, Brose MS, Shah MH, Licitra LF, Jarzab B, Medvedev V, Kreissl M, Niederle B, Cohen EEW, Wirth LJ, Ali HY, Hessel C, Yaron Y, Ball DW, Nelkin B, Sherman SI, Schlumberger M: **An international, double-blind, randomized, placebo-controlled phase III trial (EXAM) of cabozantinib (XL184) in medullary thyroid carcinoma (MTC) patients (pts) with documented RECIST progression at baseline [abstract].** *J Clin Oncol* 2012, **30(15_suppl 5508)**.
29. Kraeber-Bodere F, Goldenberg DM, Chatal JF, Barbet J: **Pretargeted radioimmunotherapy in the treatment of metastatic medullary thyroid cancer.** *Curr Oncol* 2009, **16**:3-8.
30. Pasieka JL, McEwan AJ, Rorstad O: **The palliative role of 131 I-MIBG and 111 In-octreotide therapy in patients with metastatic progressive neuroendocrine neoplasms.** *Surgery* 2004, **136**:1218-1226.
31. Jensen RT: **Overview of chronic diarrhea caused by functional neuroendocrine neoplasms.** *Semin Gastrointest Dis* 1999, **10**:156-172.
32. Barbosa SL, Rodien P, Leboulleux S, Niccoli-Sire P, Kraimps JL, Caron P, Archambeaud-Mouveroux F, Conte-Devolx B, Rohmer V: **Ectopic adrenocorticotropic hormone syndrome in medullary carcinoma of the thyroid: a retrospective analysis and review of the literature.** *Thyroid* 2005, **15**:618-623.

# 24

# Calcitonin estimation in patients with nodular goiter and its significance for early detection of MTC: european comments to the guidelines of the American Thyroid Association

Rossella Elisei*, Cristina Romei

*From* 9th Meeting of the European Thyroid Association Cancer Research Network (ETA-CRN)
Lisbon, Portugal.

**Abstract**

One of the most discussed and controversial issue in the management of thyroid nodules is the need to perform a routine measurement of serum Calcitonin (Ct) in all cases. The American Thyroid Association guidelines do not recommend in favor or against this procedure since they retain that there are not enough evidences that it can determine an advantage to the health outcomes of these patients. This is not the view of many European experts who met in Lisbon in 2009 at the European Thyroid Association-Cancer Research Network meeting to discuss all the still open controversial issues on the management of medullary thyroid cancer patients.

This paper is focused on the routine measurement of serum Ct in all patients with thyroid nodule(s): the evidences, the rational and the benefits of this procedure are deeply analysed following the discussion that was done in Lisbon. The conclusions reached at that time are reported in detail.

## Introduction

In 2009 the European Thyroid Association endorsed the American Thyroid association guidelines for the management of medullary thyroid cancer (MTC) affected patients [1]. Although the majority of recommendations were absolutely sharable, some of them were matter of discussion because the European experts on MTC had different perspectives. At the European Thyroid Association-Cancer Research Network (ETA-CRN) Meeting held in Lisbon in 2009 an European Panel of Experts (EPE) discussed all these issues and the present paper reports in particular the EPE comments and perspectives related to the routine measurement of serum calcitonin (Ct) in patients with thyroid nodules.

* Correspondence: rossella.elisei@med.unipi.it
Department of Endocrinology and Metabolism, University of Pisa, Lungarno Pacinotti 43 - 56126 Pisa, Italy

## ATA recommendation 52: European comments

The ATA recommendation 52 of the guidelines for the management of MTC patients defers the recommended approach to thyroid nodules, including FNA and serum Ct testing, to the ATA guideline that addresses thyroid nodules [2]. On this regard, the recommendation 4 of the ATA guidelines for the management of thyroid nodules clearly states that the panel of American experts cannot recommend either for or against the measurement of serum Ct (recommendation rating: I). This level of rating indicates that the evidence is insufficient to recommend for or against because evidence is lacking that the intervention (i.e. serum Ct measurement in all thyroid nodules) improves important health outcomes or the evidence is of poor quality or conflicting. However, recommendation 52 of the guidelines for MTC patients management states that if a basal or stimulated serum Ct level >100 pg/ml [equal to >100 ng/L] is obtained it should be interpreted as suspicious for MTC and further evaluation and treatment should ensue (recommendation rating: A). It is worth to note that this rate of recommendation is a very strong rate since the recommendation is based on good evidence that the intervention can improve important health outcomes since the evidence includes consistent results from well-designed and well-conducted studies in representative populations. These two recommendations appear rather conflicting and in particular it is unclear how and why serum Ct should be obtained if not performed inside the diagnostic work up of a thyroid nodule.

At variance with the ATA view, the ETA consensus [3] clearly states that the routine procedure of serum Ct measurement should be applied in the work up of all thyroid nodules since it is more sensitive than fine needle aspiration cytology. It is clear that the European and American views are opposite on the regard of this issue. It is worth to note that in 2010, independently from the ETA-CRN meeting in Lisbon discussion, a new document signed by the American Association of Clinical Endocrinologists (AACE), by the Associazione Medici Endocrinologici (AME) and by the European Thyroid Association (ETA) was published which declared that routine serum Ct may be useful, especially before surgery and strongly recommended its measurement in certain high-risk group [4].

## Why is it important to measure serum Ct in nodular goiter for the EPE?

The aim of the discussion in Lisbon was to better clarify the clinical reasons and evidences to sustain the indication to perform the serum Ct routine measurement in thyroid nodules. There is no doubt that many studies demonstrated that routine measurement of serum Ct is the most accurate diagnostic tool for the detection of MTC in patients with thyroid nodules, even more sensitive than cytology [5-11]. However, low-mild elevated values of serum Ct can be either falsely positive for technical reasons [12-14] (Table 1) or for the presence of other rare pathological settings (i.e other neuroendocrine tumors, hyperparathyroidism, renal failure etc) [15] (Table 2).

To distinguish these situations, subjects with elevated basal serum Ct should be submitted to a stimulation test which should clarify the origin of the detected Ct, especially when the basal value is low-mild elevated (i.e. between 10 and 100 pg/ml). The Ct deriving from MTC usually increases 3-4 times above the basal value after stimulation while artifactual Ct values due to technical problems or serum Ct produced by non thyroid cells usually do not increase after stimulation (Figure 1). Until few years ago the Ct stimulation test was performed with the injection of pentagastrin (Pg) (Peptavlon, Nova Laboratories, LTD, Leichester U,K 0.5 mg/kg ev) and this represented a very important limit for American colleagues because Pg was, and still is, unavailable in USA. Recently, it has been clearly demonstrated that a similar and even stronger stimulation can be obtained with a rapid infusion of calcium (2.3 mg/Kg of calcium ion or 25 mg/Kg of calcium gluconate) [16-19]. Thus, with the possibility to use calcium infusion instead of pentagastrin this limit has been overcome but it is still unresolved the problem of the stimulated Ct operative cut-off. There are several studies in which it has been attempted to clarify this issue [20-22]. However, while approaching this issue it is important to take into account that also normal subjects can have a positive response of serum Ct after stimulation but it never increases over 60 pg/ml [ng/L][17], thus a stimulated Ct between 60 and 100 pg/ml is a grey zone that deserves to be monitored. Furthermore, the rate of increase should also be considered and the clinicians should be aware that only a 3-4 time increase of stimulated Ct with respect to basal Ct should be considered as a positive response [23]. On this regard it is useful to say that these considerations are valid for sporadic cases of suspected MTC while when a hereditary case is under investigation any level of increase of either basal or stimulated Ct should be considered as positive [24].

Although the routine measurement of serum Ct in all subjects with thyroid nodules is still controversial [25,26], evidence has been provided that this approach allows an early diagnosis and treatment, thus significantly improving the outcome of this potentially lethal disease [27,28]. This evidence has been criticized by American colleagues who strongly believe that the serum Ct measurement identifies a lot of microMTC clinically irrelevant [29]. Indeed, one of the aims of measuring serum Ct in all nodules is to early identify MTC

**Table 1 Technical problems in serum Ct measurement**

| |
|---|
| 1. Serum not appropriately stored (i.e -20°C) may give *false negative* results |
| 2. Very high values can give *false negative* results (Hook effect) |
| 3. Some drugs, such as omeprazole, can stimulate Ct and produce *false positive* results* |
| 4. Heterophylic antibodies may give *false positive* results* |
| 5. *Normal range* should be calculated in each laboratory |
| 6. *Analytical and functional sensitivity* of the assay should be verified in each laboratory |

*no positive response to stimulation with either calcium or pentagastrin

**Table 2 Hypercalcitoninemia in pathological conditions other than MTC**

| |
|---|
| 1."Small cells" lung carcinoma* |
| 2. Various neuroendocrine tumors* |
| 3. Chronic renal failure * |
| 4. Pernicious anemia* |
| 5. Zollinger's syndrome* |
| 6. Pancreatitis* |
| 7. Lymphocytic thyroiditis** |
| 8. Micropapillary thyroid carcinoma** |

*no positive response to either calcium or pentagastrin stimulation
** positive response to either calcium or pentagastrin usually due to C cell hyperplasia

so it is conceivable that many MTC revealed by serum Ct measurement are small [30], but it is still controversial if it is true that small MTC are always good tumors [31]. Moreover, while an increase of incidence of small papillary thyroid cancer has been clearly demonstrated worldwide [32] it has never been demonstrated an increase of microMTC neither after the introduction of neck ultrasound nor in MTC series of institution adopting the Ct routine screening in thyroid nodules, which was expected if this procedure was able to bring up the hidden clinically inert microMTC.

Another very important reason to perform serum Ct measurement before surgical treatment is that if this is not done, unsuspected MTC can be unexpectedly found after thyroid lobectomy or total thyroidectomy not followed by central neck lymph node dissection that is the surgical treatment to be performed by principle when a presurgical diagnosis of MTC is available. When an incorrect surgical treatment has been already performed because the surgeon was unaware of the MTC diagnosis a personalized follow up strategy should be identified case by case by considering the serum Ct levels [33,34]. This situation is virtually impossible to be encountered in countries where the routine serum Ct measurement of all thyroid nodules is performed since even small foci of MTC not visible at neck ultrasound can be discovered by this strategy [5-8].

Last but not least is the problem of the cost-effectiveness of this screening. European studies previously demonstrated that it is valuable [22,27] but, recently, also a USA study revealed that routine Ct screening in patients with nodular goiter appeared to be cost-effective and in particular its cost-effectiveness resulted comparable to colonoscopy, and mammography screening [35].

## Conclusions

The conclusions of the EPE at the ETA-CRN meeting were that nowadays we have enough evidences to recommend routine serum Ct measurement in all patients with thyroid nodules. Moreover, it should be mandatory in all thyroid nodules patients for whom surgery has been indicated to be sure to perform the appropriate surgical treatment. However, some considerations should be always taken into account such as: a) Basal serum Ct measurement should never be performed in the absence of thyroid nodules detectable by neck ultrasound; b) Low-medium basal Ct needs to be further analysed by "stimulation"; c) Other causes of increased basal Ct should always be excluded; d) Basal Ct > 100 pg/ml must be considered very suspicious of MTC; e) A stimulated Ct < 60 pg/ml is compatible with normal response to

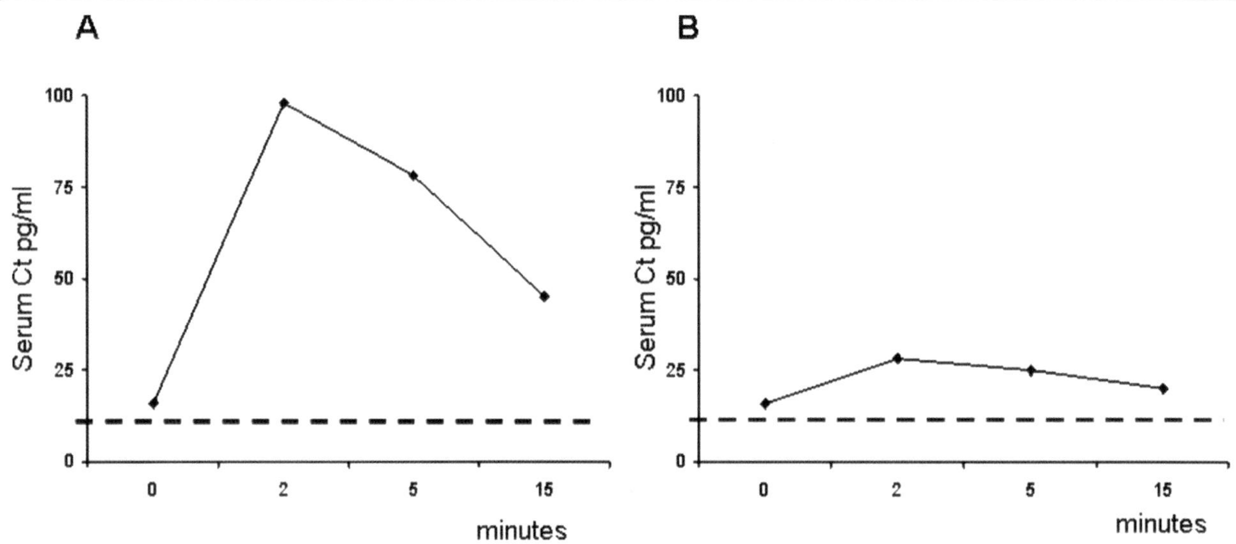


**Figure 1** The pentagastrin stimulation test for serum calcitonin: Panel A) example of a positive stimulation test with an increase from 16 to 98 pg/ml (6 times); panel B) example of a negative stimulation test with an increase from 16 to 28 (1.7 times). The broken line identifies the upper level of our institutional normal range (i.e 10 pg/ml).

stimulation; f) A stimulated Ct > 60 and < 100 pg/ml can be taken under evaluation by repeating the test 6-12 months later; g) The level of increasing of stimulated Ct with respect to the basal value is of great importance since in MTC it is usually greater than 3-4 times the basal value.

### List of abbreviations

Ct: calcitonin; MTC: medullary thyroid carcinoma.

### Competing interests

No competing interests exist for me and my co-authors.

### Declarations

This article has been published as part of *Thyroid Research* Volume 6 Supplement 1, 2013: European comments on Medullary Thyroid Cancer Management Guidelines of the American Thyroid Association. The full contents of the supplement are available online at http://www.thyroidresearchjournal.com/supplements/6/S1. Publication of this supplement has been supported by the European Thyroid Association-Cancer Research Network.

### References


1. American Thyroid Association Guidelines Task Force, Kloos RT, Eng C, Evans DB, Francis GL, Gagel RF, Gharib H, Moley JF, Pacini F, Ringel MD, Schlumberger M, Wells SA Jr: **Medullary thyroid cancer: management guidelines of the American Thyroid Association.** *Thyroid* 2009, **19(6)**:565-612.
2. American Thyroid Association (ATA) Guidelines Taskforce on Thyroid Nodules and Differentiated Tyroid Cancer, Cooper DS, Doherty GM, Haugen BR, Kloos RT, Lee SL, Mandel SJ, Mazzaferri EL, McIver B, Pacini F, Schlumberger M, Sherman SI, Steward DL, Tuttle RM: **Revised American Thyroid Association management guidelines for patients with thyroid nodules and differentiated thyroid cancer.** *Thyroid* 2009, **19(11)**:1167-214.
3. Pacini F, Schlumberger M, Dralle H, Elisei R, Smit JW, European Thyroid Cancer Taskforce: **European consensus for the management of patients with differentiated thyroid carcinoma of the follicular epithelium.** *Eur J Endocrinol* 2006, **154(6)**:787-803.
4. Gharib H, Papini E, Paschke R, Duick DS, Valcavi R, Hegedüs L, Vitti P, AACE/AME/ETA Task Force on Thyroid Nodules: **American Association of Clinical Endocrinologists, Associazione Medici Endocrinologi, and European Thyroid Association medical guidelines for clinical practice for the diagnosis and management of thyroid nodules: executive summary of recommendations.** *J Endocrinol Invest* 2010, **33(5 Suppl)**:51-6.
5. Pacini F, Fontanelli M, Fugazzola L, Elisei R, Romei C, Di Coscio G, Miccoli P, Pinchera A: **Routine measurement of serum calcitonin in nodular thyroid diseases allows the preoperative diagnosis of unsuspected sporadic medullary thyroid carcinoma.** *J Clin Endocrinol Metab* 1994, **78(4)**:826-9.
6. Rieu M, Lame MC, Richard A, Lissak B, Sambort B, Vuong-Ngoc P, Berrod JL, Fombeur JP: **Prevalence of sporadic medullary thyroid carcinoma: the importance of routine measurement of serum calcitonin in the diagnostic evaluation of thyroid nodules.** *Clin Endocrinol (Oxf)* 1995, **42(5)**:453-60.
7. Niccoli P, Wion-Barbot N, Caron P, Henry JF, de Micco C, Saint Andre JP, Bigorgne JC, Modigliani E, Conte-Devolx B: **Interest of routine measurement of serum calcitonin: study in a large series of thyroidectomized patients. The French Medullary Study Group.** *J Clin Endocrinol Metab* 1997, **82(2)**:338-41.
8. Vierhapper H, Raber W, Bieglmayer C, Kaserer K, Weinhäusl A, Niederle B: **Routine measurement of plasma calcitonin in nodular thyroid diseases.** *J Clin Endocrinol Metab* 1997, **82(5)**:1589-93.
9. Kaserer K, Scheuba C, Neuhold N, Weinhäusel A, Vierhapper H, Haas OA, Niederle B: **C-cell hyperplasia and medullary thyroid carcinoma in patients routinely screened for serum calcitonin.** *Am J Surg Pathol* 1998, **22(6)**:722-8.
10. Ozgen AG, Hamulu F, Bayraktar F, Yilmaz C, Tüzün M, Yetkin E, Tunçyürek M, Kabalak T: **Evaluation of routine basal serum calcitonin measurement for early diagnosis of medullary thyroid carcinoma in seven hundred seventy-three patients with nodular goiter.** *Thyroid* 1999, **9(6)**:579-82.
11. Hahm JR, Lee MS, Min YK, Lee MK, Kim KW, Nam SJ, Yang JH, Chung JH: **Routine measurement of serum calcitonin is useful for early detection of medullary thyroid carcinoma in patients with nodular thyroid diseases.** *Thyroid* 2001, **11(1)**:73-80.
12. Bieglmayer C, Scheuba C, Niederle B, Flores J, Vierhapper H: **Screening for medullary thyroid carcinoma: experience with different immunoassays for human calcitonin.** *Wien Klin Wochenschr* 2002, **114(7)**:267-73.
13. Tommasi M, Brocchi A, Cappellini A, Raspanti S, Mannelli M: **False serum calcitonin high levels using a non-competitive two-site IRMA.** *J Endocrinol Invest* 2001, **24(5)**:356-60.
14. Giovanella L, Suriano S: **Spurious hypercalcitoninemia and heterophilic antibodies in patients with thyroid nodules.** *Head Neck* 2011, **33(1)**:95-7.
15. Toledo SP, Lourenço DM Jr, Santos MA, Tavares MR, Toledo RA, Correia-Deur JE: **Hypercalcitoninemia is not pathognomonic of medullary thyroid carcinoma.** *Clinics (Sao Paulo)* 2009, **64(7)**:699-706.
16. Doyle P, Düren C, Nerlich K, Verburg FA, Grelle I, Jahn H, Fassnacht M, Mäder U, Reiners C, Luster M: **Potency and tolerance of calcitonin stimulation with high-dose calcium versus pentagastrin in normal adults.** *J Clin Endocrinol Metab* 2009, **94(8)**:2970-4.
17. Barbot N, Calmettes C, Schuffenecker I, Saint-André JP, Franc B, Rohmer V, Jallet P, Bigorgne JC: **Pentagastrin stimulation test and early diagnosis of medullary thyroid carcinoma using an immunoradiometric assay of calcitonin: comparison with genetic screening in hereditary medullary thyroid carcinoma.** *J Clin Endocrinol Metab* 1994, **78(1)**:114-20.
18. Samaan NA, Castillo S, Schultz PN, Khalil KG, Johnston DA: **Serum calcitonin after pentagastrin stimulation in patients with bronchogenic and breast cancer compared to that in patients with medullary thyroid carcinoma.** *J Clin Endocrinol Metab* 1980, **51(2)**:237-41.
19. Colombo C, Verga U, Mian C, Ferrero S, Perrino M, Vicentini L, Dazzi D, Opocher G, Pelizzo MR, Beck-Peccoz P, Fugazzola L: **Comparison of calcium and pentagastrin tests for the diagnosis and follow-up of medullary thyroid cancer.** *J Clin Endocrinol Metab* 2012, **97(3)**:905-13.
20. Costante G, Meringolo D, Durante C, Bianchi D, Nocera M, Tumino S, Crocetti U, Attard M, Maranghi M, Torlontano M, Filetti S: **Predictive value of serum calcitonin levels for preoperative diagnosis of medullary thyroid carcinoma in a cohort of 5817 consecutive patients with thyroid nodules.** *J Clin Endocrinol Metab* 2007, **92(2)**:450-5.
21. Milone F, Ramundo V, Chiofalo MG, Severino R, Paciolla I, Pezzullo L, Lombardi G, Colao A, Faggiano A: **Predictive value of pentagastrin test for preoperative differential diagnosis between C-cell hyperplasia and medullary thyroid carcinoma in patients with moderately elevated basal calcitonin levels.** *Clin Endocrinol (Oxf)* 2010, **73(1)**:85-8.
22. Verga U, Ferrero S, Vicentini L, Brambilla T, Cirello V, Muzza M, Beck-Peccoz P, Fugazzola L: **Histopathological and molecular studies in patients with goiter and hypercalcitoninemia: reactive or neoplastic C-cell hyperplasia?** *Endocr Relat Cancer* 2007, **14(2)**:393-403.
23. Elisei R: **Routine serum calcitonin measurement in the evaluation of thyroid nodules.** *Best Pract Res Clin Endocrinol Metab* 2008, **22(6)**:941-53.
24. Elisei R, Romei C, Renzini G, Bottici V, Cosci B, Molinaro E, Agate L, Cappagli V, Miccoli P, Berti P, Faviana P, Ugolini C, Basolo F, Vitti P, Pinchera A: **The timing of total thyroidectomy in RET gene mutation carriers could be personalized and safely planned on the basis of serum calcitonin: 18 years experience at one single center.** *J Clin Endocrinol Metab* 2012, **97(2)**:426-35.
25. Hodak SP, Burman KD: **The calcitonin conundrum–is it time for routine measurement of serum calcitonin in patients with thyroid nodules?** *J Clin Endocrinol Metab* 2004, **89(2)**:511-4.
26. Deftos LJ: **Should serum calcitonin be routinely measured in patients with thyroid nodules–will the law answer before endocrinologists do?** *J Clin Endocrinol Metab* 2004, **89(9)**:4768-9, author reply 4769-70.
27. Elisei R, Bottici V, Luchetti F, Di Coscio G, Romei C, Grasso L, Miccoli P, Iacconi P, Basolo F, Pinchera A, Pacini F: **Impact of routine measurement of serum calcitonin on the diagnosis and outcome of medullary thyroid cancer: experience in 10,864 patients with nodular thyroid disorders.** *J Clin Endocrinol Metab* 2004, **89(1)**:163-8.
28. Vierhapper H, Niederle B, Bieglmayer C, Kaserer K, Baumgartner-Parzer S: **Early diagnosis and curative therapy of medullary thyroid carcinoma by routine measurement of serum calcitonin in patients with thyroid disorders.** *Thyroid* 2005, **15(11)**:1267-72.

29. Valle LA, Kloos RT: **The prevalence of occult medullary thyroid carcinoma at autopsy.** *J Clin Endocrinol Metab* 2011, **96(1)**:E109-13.
30. Pacini F: **Screening of thyroid nodules by serum calcitonin measurements: why not?** *Thyroid* 2012, **22(1)**:103.
31. Pillarisetty VG, Katz SC, Ghossein RA, Tuttle RM, Shaha AR: **Micromedullary thyroid cancer: how micro is truly micro?** *Ann Surg Oncol* 2009, **16(10)**:2875-81.
32. Davies L, Welch HG: **Increasing incidence of thyroid cancer in the United States, 1973-2002.** *JAMA* 2006, **295(18)**:2164-7.
33. Ahmed SR, Ball DW: **Clinical review: Incidentally discovered medullary thyroid cancer: diagnostic strategies and treatment.** *J Clin Endocrinol Metab* 2011, **96(5)**:1237-45.
34. Raffel A, Cupisti K, Krausch M, Wolf A, Schulte KM, Röher HD: **Incidentally found medullary thyroid cancer: treatment rationale for small tumors.** *World J Surg* 2004, **28(4)**:397-401.
35. Cheung K, Roman SA, Wang TS, Walker HD, Sosa JA: **Calcitonin Measurement in the Evaluation of Thyroid Nodules in the United States: A Cost-effectiveness and Decision Analysis.** *J Clin Endocrinol Metab* 2008, **93(6)**:2173-80.

# 25

# The optimal range of *RET* mutations to be tested: European comments to the guidelines of the American Thyroid Association

Laura Fugazzola*, Simone De Leo, Michela Perrino

*From* 9th Meeting of the European Thyroid Association Cancer Research Network (ETA-CRN)
Lisbon, Portugal.

**Abstract**

In the 9$^{th}$ ETA-CRN Meeting (September 2009, Lisbon) some recommendations from the American Thyroid Association (ATA) guidelines for the management of medullary thyroid cancer (MTC) were discussed by an European Panel of Experts (EPE). Among the 12 ATA recommendations related to hereditary MTC and to the optimal range of *RET* mutations to be tested (recommendations 1-5 and 9-15), 7 were shared and 5 were not shared by the EPE. In the present paper, the related comments and suggestions will be reported and discussed.

## Introduction

In the 9$^{th}$ ETA-CRN Meeting (September 2009, Lisbon) some recommendations from the American Thyroid Association (ATA) guidelines for the management of medullary thyroid cancer (MTC) [1] were discussed by an European Panel of Experts (EPE). In the present paper, the comments risen on ATA recommendations (ATA-R) related to hereditary MTC and to the optimal range of *RET* mutations to be tested will be reported and discussed (Additional file 1).

## European comments to ATA-R 1-5 and 9-15

### ATA recommendations shared by the EPE

All experts fully agreed with the need to perform RET testing in subjects at risk for autosomal dominant inheritance of MEN 2 (multiple endocrine neoplasia type 2) or FMTC (Familial Medullary Thyroid Cancer) and, in particular, shortly after birth for MEN 2B and before 5 years of age for MEN 2A and FMTC (**ATA-R #3**). Agreement was also found about the need for a pre- and post-RET testing expert genetic counseling (**ATA-R #5**) and it was stated that a list of European laboratories should probably be useful for patients. Nevertheless, though at the Orphanet EuroGentest website (http://www.orpha.net/consor/cgi-bin/index.php) more than 100 European laboratories are listed, this is probably far to be the complete list, also considering that it largely changes over times. No concerns were risen about the need to offer RET mutation analysis to all first-degree relatives of known mutation carriers (**ATA-R #9**). The topic of **ATA-R #12** relates to the indication for the sequencing of the entire coding region of RET in patients with MEN 2 and negative for mutations in exons 8, 10, 11, 13-16. It should be underlined that the remaining 13 exons (1-7, 9, 12, 17-21) have never been found to be mutated [2]. Nevertheless, though this approach was considered poorly cost effective, most experts and the 46% of the participants agreed with the ATA indications, since rare mutations comprise up to 30% of all hereditary cases, based on the literature data [3-5]. An additional recommendation would be to start the analysis of the additional regions of the gene from exon 5, which has been reported to be mutated (G321R) [6]. Strictly related to this topic, the possibility to analyze, in this category of patients, pheocrocytoma (PHAEO)-related genes was also discussed. The background was that 40-45% of apparently sporadic PHAEO or paragangliomas are hereditary and germline mutations are found in VHL (von Hippel-Lindau tumor suppressor, E3 ubiquitin protein ligase), SDHB/C/D (succinate dehydrogenase complex, subunit B, subunit C, subunit D) and RET (ret

* Correspondence: laura.fugazzola@unimi.it
Department of Clinical Sciences & Community Health , University of Milan; Endocrine Unit, Fondazione IRCCS Ca' Granda, Via F. Sforza, 35, 20122 Milan, Italy

proto-oncogene) [7]. Nevertheless, the prevalence of mutated cases is extremely variable among different Countries, and in particular very low for the RET gene. This must be considered when the decision is taken to analyze PHAEO-related genes in RET negative cases.

In the clinical setting of MEN 2B, since virtually all patients harbor mutations in exons 15 and 16 (A883F and M918T, respectively), the panel agreed with ATA indication to analyze both exons and to test the entire *RET* coding region if those 2 exons are negative for mutations **(ATA-R #13 and #14)**. Finally, total agreement was also expressed regarding the **ATA-R #15** which indicates to treat MEN 2B patients harboring codon 804 mutation associated to another mutation similarly to those with the more typical MEN 2B *RET* causing mutations. Indeed, data from the literature report that the phenotype associated to V804M mutation alone is mostly FMTC [8,9], though also MEN 2A cases have been described [9-11]. However, when this mutation is associated to another on the same allele (Y806C, S904C, E805K, V778I) the phenotype resembles that of MEN 2B [12-16].

#### ATA recommendations not shared by the EPE

The **ATA-R #1**, related to the indication to offer the germline *RET* testing to all patients with a personal medical history of primary C cell hyperplasia (CCH), MTC, or MEN2, was extensively discussed. In particular, while no concerns were risen about the need to perform *RET* analysis in a patient with MEN, it was observed that *RET* mutations are extremely rare in patients with CCH (0.03%), as reported by Scheuba et al. in 2009 [17]. Thus, the genetic analysis was not considered cost-effective for CCH cases by about half of the EPE, though the indication to recommend it was shared by other experts and by the majority of the participants. Similarly, there were some pros and cons also regarding apparently sporadic MTC. On one hand, the presentation of sporadic and familial-non MEN2A /2B- forms is almost identical and they cannot be differentiated on a clinical basis. Moreover, it has been reported that 6.5-10% of apparently sporadic cases are indeed hereditary forms [6,18]. On the other hand, it was outlined that the extensive and non-selective use of *RET* testing could lead to a stop in the reimbursement of the genetic screening (at least of the less involved exons) by the National Health Care Systems in patients with MTC, citing a lack of evidence to suggest hereditary disease [19]. The final recommendation was thus to modulate *RET* testing in apparently sporadic MTC according to clinical data and the local General Health System.

The **ATA-R #11** is related to the identification of the optimal range of *RET* mutations to be tested. Most of the experts and about half of the participants suggested to extend the analysis to exon 8, at least in all regions where mutations in that exon have been described, always in non MEN 2A/2B hereditary MTCs (Brazil, Greece, France, Italy) [20-23].

**ATA-R #10** (grade A) suggests to perform the testing of exon 10 in individuals with Hirschprung disease (HSCR), in order to detect families with activating mutations 618 o 620 in whom HSCR and MEN 2A are associated. Nevertheless, it should be highlighted that this association is frequent for MEN 2A (25-40% of families), but it is rare (2%) [24] in a very common disease such as HSCR, which has been related to mutations in at least 10 different genes. *RET* testing was thus considered to be not cost-effective and most experts indicated to downgrade this recommendation, and proposed to test HSCR patients for basal Ct.

Another important topic was related to the lichen planus amyloidosis, in the presence of which ATA guidelines recommend (**#4**, grade C) to perform the *RET* genetic testing for 634 mutation. The EPE and the large majority of participants proposed to upgrade this recommendation based on the data of the literature showing that this early cutaneous manifestation is more frequent than previously suspected, being present in up to 36% of MEN 2A cases [25]. In addition, lichen planus has been associated not only to codon 634, but also to codon 804 mutations [26]. Thus, the presence of lichen planus amyloidosis or pruritis in the central upper back should prompt Ct measurement in adults and genetic testing in children, possibly after 4 mm punch biopsy and staining with thioflavin T in order to identify amyloid deposits.

**ATA-R #2** (grade B) is related to the indication to perform *RET* testing in cases of intestinal ganglioneuromatosis. The background refers to data reporting that in MEN 2B, de novo mutations are extremely more frequent (50-90%) than for the other familial MTCs (2-9%) [27]. For this reason, the early diagnosis of MEN 2B in several cases cannot be based on familial *RET* screening. Moreover, extrathyroidal MEN 2B symptoms develop age dependently, and, though the majority of the "classic" symptoms is not expressed before 4-6 years of age, ganglioneuromatosis is always present and it is one of the earliest signs [28]. In keeping with the general agreement that in MEN 2B the clinical diagnosis of the syndrome is crucial, EPE was concordant in the indication to perform the *RET* screening in cases presenting with one or more signs related to the syndromes, such as ganglioneuromatosis, but also bumpy lips with mucosal neuroma, and corneal nerves thickening (with a prevalence of 69% in MEN 2B and 29% in MEN 2A) [29,30]. Another crucial sign, not reported in the ATA guidelines, is the tearless crying which can be recognized in more than 85% of the MEN 2A/B infants and which seems to be one of the most promising signs [27], though more data are likely needed to include this manifestation as indication for *RET* testing in infants without any other MEN 2 symptoms and with negative family history.

Finally, the EPE discussed the opportunity to include some recommendation about *RET* polymorphism, not reported in the ATA guidelines. Conflicting results have been published in recent years about the possible role of *RET* polymorphisms as genetic modifiers either in sporadic or hereditary MTC. In particular, and only considering familial MTCs, an association between G691S and S904S with an earlier age at onset in MEN2A [31] was observed, in patients with the V804M mutation, the association between L769L and earlier age of onset was reported [32], whereas in patients with G533C mutation, the variant IVS1-126G > T was found to be associated with age at diagnosis and IVS8 +82A > G; 85-86 insC with node metastases at diagnosis [33]. More recently, the RET S836S variant has been found to be associated with early onset and increased risk for metastatic disease [34]. Nevertheless, the data available to date have not been significantly replicated and discordant data have been obtained in different series [35]. Thus, the EPE and most of the participants supported the idea to draw a recommendation highlighting the lack of clinical significance of polymorphic variants.

**List of abbreviations used**

CCH: C cell hyperplasia; FMTC: Familial Medullary Thyroid Cancer; HSCR: Hirschprung disease; MEN 2: multiple endocrine neoplasia type 2; MTC: Medullary Thyroid Cancer; PHAEO: pheocrocytoma

**Competing interests**

No competing interests exist for me and my co-authors.

**Declarations**

This article has been published as part of *Thyroid Research* Volume 6 Supplement 1, 2013: European comments on Medullary Thyroid Cancer Management Guidelines of the American Thyroid Association. The full contents of the supplement are available online at http://www.thyroidresearchjournal.com/supplements/6/S1. Publication of this supplement has been supported by the European Thyroid Association-Cancer Research Network.

**References**


1. American Thyroid Association Guidelines Task Force, Kloos RT, Eng C, Evans DB, Francis GL, Gagel RF, Gharib H, Moley JF, Pacini F, Ringel MD, Schlumberger M, Wells SA Jr: **Medullary thyroid cancer: management guidelines of the American Thyroid Association.** *Thyroid* 2009, **19**:565-612.
2. Stenson PD, Ball EV, Howells K, Phillips AD, Mort M, Cooper DN: **The Human Gene Mutation Database: providing a comprehensive central mutation database for molecular diagnostics and personalized genomics.** *Hum Genomics* 2009, **4**:69-72.
3. Romei C, Mariotti S, Fugazzola L, Taccaliti A, Pacini F, Opocher G, Mian C, Castellano M, degli Uberti E, Ceccherini I, Cremonini N, Seregni E, Orlandi F, Ferolla P, Puxeddu E, Giorgino F, Colao A, Loli P, Bondi F, Cosci B, Bottici V, Cappai A, Pinna G, Persani L, Verga U, Boscaro M, Castagna MG, Cappelli C, Zatelli MC, Faggiano A, Francia G, Brandi ML, Falchetti A, Pinchera A, Elisei R, ItaMEN network: **Multiple endocrine neoplasia type 2 syndromes (MEN 2): results from the ItaMEN network analysis on the prevalence of different genotypes and phenotypes.** *Eur J Endocrinol* 2010, **163**:301-308.
4. Cordella D, Muzza M, Alberti L, Colombo P, Travaglini P, Beck-Peccoz P, Fugazzola L, Persani L: **An in-frame complex germline mutation in the juxtamembrane intracellular domain causing RET activation in familial medullary thyroid carcinoma.** *Endocr Relat Cancer* 2006, **13**:945-953.
5. Lindsey SC, Kunii IS, Germano-Neto F, Sittoni MY, Camacho CP, Valente FO, Yang JH, Signorini PS, Delcelo R, Cerutti JM, Maciel RM, Dias-da-Silva MR: **Extended RET gene analysis in patients with apparently sporadic medullary thyroid cancer: clinical benefits and cost.** *Horm Cancer* 2012, **3**:181-186.
6. Romei C, Cosci B, Renzini G, Bottici V, Molinaro E, Agate L, Passannanti P, Viola D, Biagini A, Basolo F, Ugolini C, Materazzi G, Pinchera A, Vitti P, Elisei R: **RET genetic screening of sporadic medullary thyroid cancer (MTC) allows the preclinical diagnosis of unsuspected gene carriers and the identification of a relevant percentage of hidden familial MTC (FMTC).** *Clin Endocrinol (Oxf)* 2011, **74**:241-247.
7. Opocher G, Schiavi F: **Genetics of pheochromocytomas and paragangliomas.** *Best Pract Res Clin Endocrinol Metab* 2010, **24**:943-956.
8. Feldman GL, Edmonds MW, Ainsworth PJ, Schuffenecker I, Lenoir GM, Saxe AW, Talpos GB, Roberson J, Petrucelli N, Jackson CE: **Variable expressivity of familial medullary thyroid carcinoma (FMTC) due to a RET V804M (GTG->ATG) mutation.** *Surgery* 2000, **128**:93-98.
9. Pinna G, Orgiana G, Riola A, Ghiani M, Lai ML, Carcassi C, Mariotti S: **RET proto-oncogene in Sardinia: V804M is the most frequent mutation and may be associated with FMTC/MEN-2A phenotype.** *Thyroid* 2007, **17**:101-104.
10. Nilsson O, Tisell LE, Jansson S, Ahlman H, Gimm O, Eng C: **Adrenal and extra-adrenal pheochromocytomas in a family with germline RET V804L mutation.** *JAMA* 1999, **281**:1587-1588.
11. Gibelin H, Bezieau S, Misso C, Bouin-Pineau MH, Maréchaud R, Kraimps JL: **Germline RET V804M mutation associated with multiple endocrine neoplasia type 2A.** *Br J Surg* 2004, **91**:1458-1459.
12. Miyauchi A, Futami H, Hai N, Yokozawa T, Kuma K, Aoki N, Kosugi S, Sugano K, Yamaguchi K: **Two germline missense mutations at codons 804 and 806 of the RET proto-oncogene in the same allele in a patient with multiple endocrine neoplasia type 2B without codon 918 mutation.** *Jpn J Cancer Res* 1999, **90**:1-5.
13. Menko FH, van der Luijt RB, de Valk IA, Toorians AW, Sepers JM, van Diest PJ, Lips CJ: **Atypical MEN type 2B associated with two germline RET mutations on the same allele not involving codon 918.** *J Clin Endocrinol Metab* 2002, **87**:393-397.
14. Cranston AN, Carniti C, Oakhill K, Radzio-Andzelm E, Stone EA, McCallion AS, Hodgson S, Clarke S, Mondellini P, Leyland J, Pierotti MA, Whittaker J, Taylor SS, Bongarzone I, Ponder BA: **RET is constitutively activated by novel tandem mutations that alter the active site resulting in multiple endocrine neoplasia type 2B.** *Cancer Res* 2006, **66**:10179-10187.
15. Kasprzak L, Nolet S, Gaboury L, Pavia C, Villabona C, Rivera-Fillat F, Oriola J, Foulkes WD: **Familial medullary thyroid carcinoma and prominent corneal nerves associated with the germline V804M and V778I mutations on the same allele of RET.** *J Med Genet* 2001, **38**:784-787.
16. Mukherjee S, Zakalik D: **RET codon 804 mutations in multiple endocrine neoplasia 2: genotype-phenotype correlations and implications in clinical management.** *Clin Genet* 2011, **79**:1-16.
17. Scheuba C, Kaserer K, Moritz A, Drosten R, Vierhapper H, Bieglmayer C, Haas OA, Niederle B: **Sporadic hypercalcitoninemia: clinical and therapeutic consequences.** *Endocr Relat Cancer* 2009, **16**:243-253.
18. Wiench M, Wygoda Z, Gubala E, Wloch J, Lisowska K, Krassowski J, Scieglinska D, Fiszer-Kierzkowska A, Lange D, Kula D, Zeman M, Roskosz J, Kukulska A, Krawczyk Z, Jarzab B: **Estimation of risk of inherited medullary thyroid carcinoma in apparent sporadic patients.** *J Clin Oncol* 2001, **19**:1374-80.

19. Machens A, Dralle H: **Prophylactic thyroidectomy in RET carriers at risk for hereditary medullary thyroid cancer.** *Thyroid* 2009, **19**:551-554.
20. Da Silva AM, Maciel RM, Da Silva MR, Toledo SR, De Carvalho MB, Cerutti JM: **A novel germ-line point mutation in RET exon 8 (Gly(533)Cys) in a large kindred with familial medullary thyroid carcinoma.** *J Clin Endocrinol Metab* 2003, **88**:5438-5443.
21. Fazioli F, Piccinini G, Appolloni G, Bacchiocchi R, Palmonella G, Recchioni R, Pierpaoli E, Silvetti F, Scarpelli M, Bruglia M, Melillo RM, Santoro M, Boscaro M, Taccaliti A: **A new germline point mutation in Ret exon 8 (cys515ser) in a family with medullary thyroid carcinoma.** *Thyroid* 2008, **18**:775-782.
22. Muzza M, Cordella D, Bombled J, Bressac-de Paillerets B, Guizzardi F, Francis Z, Beck-Peccoz P, Schlumberger M, Persani L, Fugazzola L: **Four novel RET germline variants in exons 8 and 11 display an oncogenic potential in vitro.** *Eur J Endocrinol* 2010, **162**:771-777.
23. Sarika HL, Papathoma A, Garofalaki M, Vasileiou V, Vlassopoulou B, Anastasiou E, Alevizaki M: **High prevalence of exon 8 g533c mutation in apparently sporadic medullary thyroid carcinoma (mtc) in Greece.** *Clin Endocrinol (Oxf)* 2012, 7, doi: 10.1111/j.1365-2265.2012.04462.x. [Epub ahead of print].
24. Amiel J, Sproat-Emison E, Garcia-Barcelo M, Lantieri F, Burzynski G, Borrego S, Pelet A, Arnold S, Miao X, Griseri P, Brooks AS, Antinolo G, de Pontual L, Clement-Ziza M, Munnich A, Kashuk C, West K, Wong KK, Lyonnet S, Chakravarti A, Tam PK, Ceccherini I, Hofstra RM, Fernandez R, Hirschsprung Disease Consortium: **Hirschsprung disease, associated syndromes and genetics: a review.** *J Med Gene* 2008, **45**:1-14.
25. Verga U, Fugazzola L, Cambiaghi S, Pritelli C, Alessi E, Cortelazzi D, Gangi E, Beck-Peccoz P: **Frequent association between MEN 2A and cutaneous lichen amyloidosis.** *Clin Endocrinol (Oxf)* 2003, **59**:156-161.
26. Rothberg AE, Raymond VM, Gruber SB, Sisson J: **Familial medullary thyroid carcinoma associated with cutaneous lichen amyloidosis.** *Thyroid* 2009, **19**:651-655.
27. Brauckhoff M, Gimm O: **Extrathyroidal manifestations of multiple endocrine neoplasia type 2.** *Thyroid* 2009, **19**:555-557.
28. Camacho CP, Hoff AO, Lindsey SC, Signorini PS, Valente FO, Oliveira MN, Kunii IS, Biscolla RP, Cerutti JM, Maciel RM: **Early diagnosis of multiple endocrine neoplasia type 2B: a challenge for physicians.** *Arq Bras Endocrinol Metabol* 2008, **52**:1393-1398.
29. Vasen HF, van der Feltz M, Raue F, Kruseman AN, Koppeschaar HP, Pieters G, Seif FJ, Blum WF, Lips CJ: **The natural course of multiple endocrine neoplasia type IIb. A study of 18 cases.** *Arch Intern Med* 1992, **152**:1250-1252.
30. Kinoshita S, Tanaka F, Ohashi Y, Ikeda M, Takai S: **Incidence of prominent corneal nerves in multiple endocrine neoplasia type 2A.** *Am J Ophthalmol* 1991, **111**:307-311.
31. Robledo M, Gil L, Pollán M, Cebrián A, Ruíz S, Azañedo M, Benitez J, Menárguez J, Rojas JM: **Polymorphisms G691S/S904S of RET as genetic modifiers of MEN 2A.** *Cancer Res* 2003, **63**:1814-1817.
32. Magalhães PK, de Castro M, Elias LL, Soares EG, Maciel LM: **Polymorphisms in the RET proto-oncogene and the phenotypic presentation of familial medullary thyroid carcinoma.** *Thyroid* 2004, **14**:848-852.
33. Tamanaha R, Camacho CP, Pereira AC, da Silva AM, Maciel RM, Cerutti JM: **Evaluation of RET polymorphisms in a six-generation family with G533C RET mutation: specific RET variants may modulate age at onset and clinical presentation.** *Clin Endocrinol (Oxf)* 2009, **71**:56-64.
34. Siqueira DR, Romitti M, da Rocha AP, Ceolin L, Meotti C, Estivalet A, Puñales MK, Maia AL: **The RET polymorphic allele S836S is associated with early metastatic disease in patients with hereditary or sporadic medullary thyroid carcinoma.** *Endocr Relat Cancer* 2010, **17**:953-963.
35. Ceolin L, Siqueira DR, Romitti M, Ferreira CV, Maia AL: **Molecular Basis of Medullary Thyroid Carcinoma: The Role of RET Polymorphisms.** *Int J Mol Sci* 2012, **13**:221-239.

# Molecules important for thyroid hormone synthesis and action - known facts and future perspectives

Klaudia Brix[1†], Dagmar Führer[2†], Heike Biebermann[3*†]

**Abstract**

Thyroid hormones are of crucial importance for the functioning of nearly every organ. Remarkably, disturbances of thyroid hormone synthesis and function are among the most common endocrine disorders affecting approximately one third of the working German population. Over the last ten years our understanding of biosynthesis and functioning of these hormones has increased tremendously. This includes the identification of proteins involved in thyroid hormone biosynthesis like Thox2 and Dehal where mutations in these genes are responsible for certain degrees of hypothyroidism. One of the most important findings was the identification of a specific transporter for triiodothyronine (T3), the monocarboxylate transporter 8 (MCT8) responsible for directed transport of T3 into target cells and for export of thyroid hormones out of thyroid epithelial cells. Genetic disturbances of MCT8 in patients result in a biochemical constellation of high T3 levels in combination with low or normal TSH and thyroxine levels leading to a new syndrome of severe X-linked mental retardation. Importantly mice lacking MCT8 presented only with a mild phenotype, indicating that compensatory mechanisms exist in mice. Moreover, it has become clear that not only genomic actions of T3 exist. T3 is also capable to activate adhesion receptors and it signals via activation of PI3K and MAPK pathways. Most recently, thyroid hormone derivatives were identified, the thyronamines which are decarboxylated thyroid hormones initiating physiological actions like lowering body temperature and heart rate, thereby acting in opposite direction to the classical thyroid hormones. So far it is believed that thyronamines function via the activation of a G-protein coupled receptor, TAAR1. The objective of this review is to summarise the recent findings in thyroid hormone synthesis and action and to discuss their implications for diagnosis of thyroid disease and for treatment of patients.

## Introduction

### Health consequences of disturbed thyroid hormone action

Thyroid hormones are of significant importance for regular functioning of almost all body organs. Thyroxine (T4) is the main hormone released from the thyroid gland and it is transformed into biologically active 3',3,5-triiodothyronine (T3) via 5'-deiodinases of thyroid hormone target cells [1]. For thyroid hormone synthesis, sufficient supply of the thyroid gland with essential micronutrients such as iodine and selenium is crucial.

The most important target tissues of thyroid hormones are the central nervous system, the cardiovascular system and the skeleton. Moreover, due to the increasing incidence of obesity worldwide, thyroid hormone action in adipose tissue has re-gained increasing interest for understanding energy homeostasis [2].

Disturbance of thyroid hormone synthesis and thyroid hormone actions, further referred to as thyroid disorders, are among the most common endocrine afflictions and they require special attention in specific life phases. For instance, undiagnosed hypothyroidism during pregnancy will lead to irreparable central nervous system (CNS) defects in the newborn because the development of the child *in utero* is critically affected by the mother's thyroid status [3]. Therefore and to avoid fatal consequences of a lack of thyroid hormone synthesis after birth, eventually leading to severe mental retardation,

* Correspondence: heike.biebermann@charite.de
† Contributed equally
[3]Institute of Experimental Pediatric Endocrinology, Charité Universitätsmedizin Berlin, Augustenburger Platz 1, 13353 Berlin, Germany
Full list of author information is available at the end of the article

thyroid stimulating hormone (TSH)-screening of newborns [4] was implemented in Germany and in other countries. In action since the late 1970s and with a clear improvement in those areas of the world where TSH-screening was first introduced, a marked decrease in cretinism was observed.

Thyroid hormone (TH) action serves important regulatory functions throughout all phases of life. Disturbed TH action is linked with major health problems especially in critical life phases such as development, disease or ageing. Thus, lack of TH action in the adult brain causes impaired neuro-cognitive function and psychiatric states such as severe depression and dementia [5]. Not only hypothyroidism but also hyperthyroidism affects the CNS and frequently results in agitation, increased irritability and dysregulation of body temperature. There is ample epidemiological evidence that both, hyper- and hypothyroidism confer an increased risk for cardiovascular morbidity (e.g. arrhythmia, heart failure and stroke) and mortality. Moreover, thyroid disorders affect maturation and turnover rates of bone. For example, children with hyperthyroidism show advanced bone age, and post-menopausal women with thyrotoxicosis are at risk for osteoporosis. Furthermore, adiposity is associated with altered levels of measurable thyroid function parameters, whereby it is not known however whether the obesity state influences the set-point for thyroid function parameters or vice versa. Besides the common health issues, life threatening conditions may either arise from severely disturbed thyroid hormone action or are accompanied by altered thyroid hormone action. These include e.g. thyroid storm with a mortality of more than 30%, which at present can only be diagnosed on clinical grounds since measurement of thyroid hormone levels is not useful and may be identical to those in patients with uncomplicated thyrotoxicosis or the non-thyroid illness syndrome in intensive care patients with e.g. sepsis.

Health-economical dimensions of thyroid disorders are shown most plainly by the example of latent hypothyroidism which is evident in about 20% of all individuals at the age of 60-79 years, with higher incidences in women than in men [6]. On top of this, an increase in the number of patients with thyroid disorders is expected in the future. Possible causes are anthropogenic in origin and are represented by a variety of environmental substances, so-called endocrine disruptors such as estrogen-derivates and PBCBs, that affect the endocrine system at large including the thyroid gland and thyroid hormone actions [7].

Furthermore, classical epidemiology on large cohorts (SHIP and KORA) has underlined that manifest and even more so, subclinical thyroid disorders are often associated with other, quite frequently occurring pathophysiological processes [8,9]. These include, but are not limited to left-ventricular hypertrophy, atherosclerosis with increased risk for stroke and coronary heart disease, disorders in lipid metabolism, osteoporosis and neurodegenerative diseases. However, subclinical hyperthyroidism was found not to be associated with e. g. changes in blood pressure in the SHIP cohort study [9] although serum TSH levels in the upper reference range were indicative of endothelial dysfunction [10], highlighting the necessity of further investigations aiming at a better definition of the healthy thyroid state.

## New aspects of thyroid hormone synthesis

A number of molecular causes of thyroid dysgenesis, accounting for approx. 80% of cases suffering from congenital hypothyroidism (CH), have been identified over the last few years and were shown to include mutations in transcription factors important for thyroid development such as *Pax8*, *Nkx2.1*, *FoxE1*, and *HoxA3*[11]. Mutations in these genes often also lead to developmental dysfunction in organs other than the thyroid, thereby affecting the lung and the central nervous system (*Nkx2.1*) [12], or the kidney (*PAX8*) [13]. However, only about 5% of these genetic defects could account for the pathogenesis of thyroid dysgenesis [14]. Therefore, non-classical mechanisms involving epigenetic regulation are to be considered in future as modulators of gene expression during development of the thyroid.

In addition, genetic defects have been detected in all those genes bearing an essential role in the biosynthesis of thyroid hormones (approx. 10 to 15% of CH cases). These include the gene for the prohormone thyroglobulin (Tg) itself [15]; the thyroid stimulating hormone receptor (*TSHR*) [16], and the thyroid peroxidase (*TPO*) [17]; as well as genes relevant for iodide transport, i.e. the sodium-iodide symporter (*NIS*) [18] at the basolateral and *Pendrin*[19] at the apical pole of thyroid epithelial cells. Furthermore, the gene products of *Dehal*[20] and *Thox2*[21] as well as inactivating and activating mutations of the Gs alpha gene [22] have been added to the growing list of candidate proteins with important thyroid-specific functions. Recently, potassium channel subunits *Kcnq1* and *Kcne2* were found to be crucial for TSH-stimulated thyroid hormone biosynthesis. Mice lacking *Kcne2* suffer from impaired iodide uptake into the thyroid gland and exhibit signs of hypothyroidism [23].

A more profound understanding of thyroid hormone biosynthesis has also led to a clearer view on the molecular regulation of the thyroid gland and has increased our knowledge about the differentiated state of thyroid epithelial cells. In this context, novel players have been identified, which are important for the maintenance of thyroid physiology, i.e. molybdenum-dependent enzymes with important functions in the oxidative system of thyrocytes [24] and molecules that play a role in thyroglobulin processing for thyroid hormone liberation and release from the thyroid gland (megalin and cysteine cathepsins) [25-27].

Many of these players have been known for long, but it was only recently that the impact of mutations in thyroid-specific genes for thyroid physiology was set into context for a clearer depiction of the interactions and cross-relations between the many molecules and pathways relevant for thyroid biology. The regulation governing the functions of thyroid-specific proteins and their precise roles in the etiology of thyroid disorders will enable us to understand their mechanisms of action in detail and will advance our knowledge on the molecular biology of the thyroid gland.

## Novel concepts of transmembrane and intracellular thyroid hormone actions

Previous textbook knowledge of thyroid hormone entry into cells included a diffusion-based passive transmembrane passage for thyroid hormones which are lipophilic but charged molecules. However, an eye-opening revelation was the identification of the MCT8 transporter (*SLC16A2*) that selectively enables T3 transport into target cells [28]. This important finding explained at the molecular level the phenotype of severe X-linked mental retardation and disrupted locomotor development of patients with the Allan Herndon Dudley (AHD) syndrome, already described in the 1940s. These patients carry a defect in the MCT8 transporter, which explains why T3 does not reach all of its target cells in sufficient quantities during development. At the same time AHD patients show highly elevated serum T3 levels with unaltered to elevated TSH contradicting the "normal feedback scenario". Thus it needs to be investigated further whether the abnormally high T3 levels in conditions of MCT8 defects that are linked with normal to slightly elevated TSH levels may cause thyrotoxic effects in TH target tissues other than the central nervous system [29]. However this clinical observation prompted thyroidologists to question the classical views on thyroid regulation. Subsequently, other TH transporter candidates have been identified (e.g. Oatp14, Lat1, Lat2, Mct10) in mice and require functional characterization [30-33]. It will be important in future to not only identify the tissue distribution patterns of TH transporters but more so, to clarify their potential contributions to the intracellular compartmentalisation of TH so that a clearer picture is gained on the sub-cellular gradients of TH and how specific compartments within cells, besides the nucleus, are supplied with TH in order to contribute or to withstand non-classical TH actions. Further TH transporters are eagerly awaited to be defined (Figure 1).

Another unexpected finding of recent research projects was the identification of thyroid hormone derivatives, the so-called thyronamines [34]. These are decarboxylated thyroid hormones that exert effects with kinetics different from those of thyroid hormone mediated actions and principally counter-acting them (so called "cool thyroid hormones"). Most obvious effects of thyronamines are observed in decreased heart rates and in negative regulation of body temperature. Thyronamines display their effects via activating a new subfamily of G-protein-coupled receptors (GPCRs), the *trace amine associated receptors* (TAARs) [35-37]. Because of their central roles in signalling resulting in a multitude of regulatory effects on almost all biological processes, GPCRs are interesting targets for pharmacological intervention [38]. Hence, the development of new therapeutic agents for regulation of heart beat frequency and of body temperature is now discussed in light of emergency treatments of stroke or acute myocardial infarction. Moreover, thyronamine-based therapies are expected to enter intensive care medical treatments.

Furthermore several lines of evidence suggest that in addition to the classic nuclear thyroid hormone action, rapid plasma membrane-initiated effects of thyroid hormones exist. Signalling via adhesion receptors ($\alpha v\beta 3$ integrins) and activation of intracellular PI-3 kinase and mitogen activated protein (MAP) kinase pathways have been proposed to account for these effects [39-41]. The precise mechanisms and the physiological implications of non-classical TH actions however remain elusive.

Besides the classic hormones T4 and T3 new data demonstrate that the rare thyroid hormone metabolite 3,5-T2 is effective in the prevention of high fat diet-induced adiposity and prevents hepatic steatosis, however, without exerting the severe side effects on the cardiac system that have been observed with T3-based treatments [42] . The vital importance of thyroid hormones for regulation of thermogenesis and for maintenance of the homeostasis of the mitochondrial energy metabolism has long been established. However, the functional interactions between the activities of uncoupling proteins (UCP) which are triggered by T3 and catecholamines affecting brown adipose tissue (BAT) as well as skeletal muscle of the adult, provide new possibilities for therapeutic intervention in obesity that have only recently become apparent [43].

Thus in the present concept of thyroid hormone action, the cellular thyroid hormone status is defined by thyroid hormone transporters, thyroid hormone membrane receptors, thyroid hormone molecules and TAM mediated actions (Figure 1B). It is highly likely and corroborated by recent experimental results that cell type-specificity, with respect to thyroid hormone signalling,

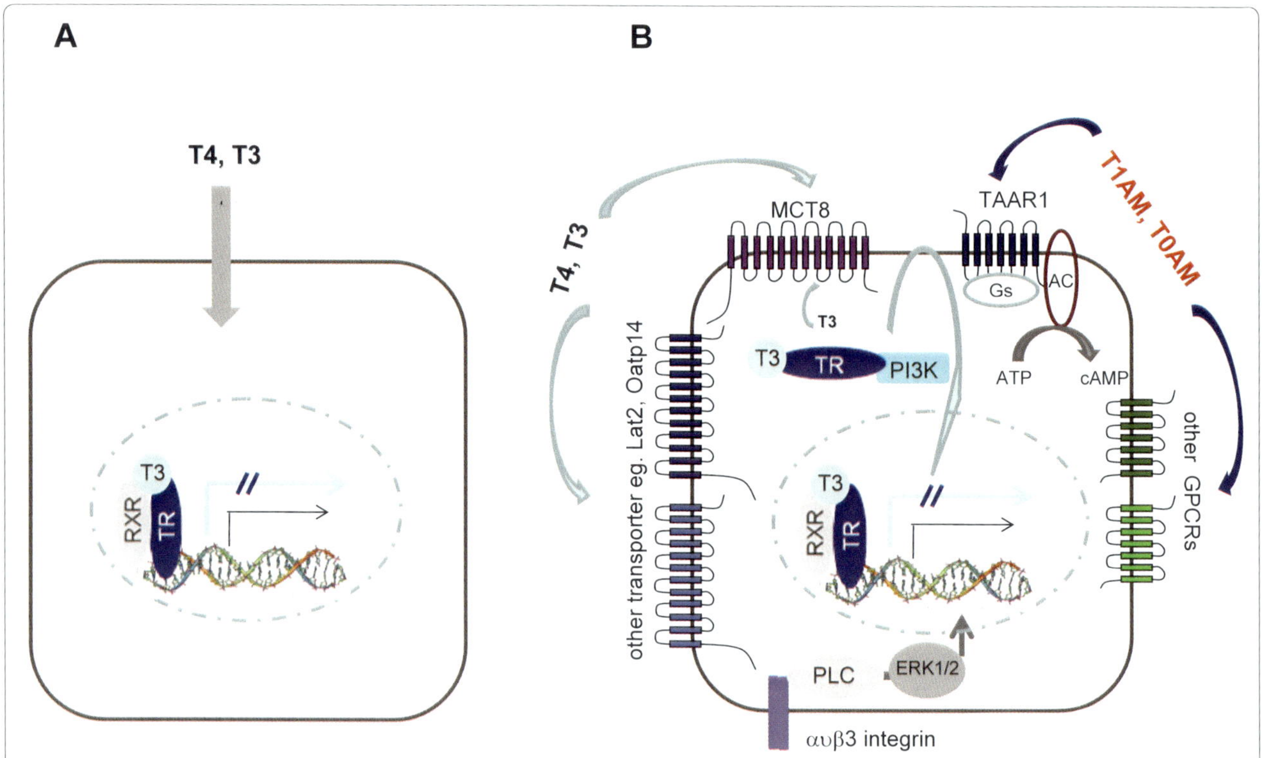


**Figure 1 Old and new concepts of thyroid hormone action. A: Old concept of thyroid hormone action.** In former times it was assumed that thyroid hormones are able to pass the plasma membrane by passive transport. Once in the cytosol T4 is deiodinated to T3 which exerts genomic effects by binding to the thyroid hormone receptor (TR). After hetero-dimerization with other nuclear receptors like retinoic X receptor (RXR), transcriptional regulation is initiated resulting in activation or inactivation of target genes. **B: New concepts of thyroid hormone action.** Thyroid hormones enter a target cell via specific transporters, e.g. T3 uses the monocarboxylate transporter MCT8 while T4 entry is mediated by Lat2 or Oatp14. Moreover, T3 can interact with $\alpha\nu\beta3$ integrins to induce ERK1/2 signalling. Cytosolic T3 exerts genomic effects but can additionally also act by non-genomic means after TR binding and activation of down-stream PI-3 kinase. Likewise, the naturally occurring iodothyronine T2 is believed to stimulate metabolic rates via mitochondrial pathways, thereby bypassing genomic regulation. Besides thyroid hormones, derivatives like the thyronamines T1AM or T0AM, modulate the action of T3, e.g. counter-acting its effects in certain target cells. Thyronamines (TAMs) bind to and activate G-protein coupled receptors (GPCRs) of the trace amine associated receptor (TAAR) family. So far, it is only known that TAAR1 is activated by TAMs and signals via adenylylcyclase (AC) activation with subsequent rise of cAMP levels. However other GPCRs are likely targets for thyroid hormone derivatives.

differs within and in between different organs. Thereby novel avenues are opened for refinement of the concept of organ physiology and the role of thyroid hormone derived signals including their cellular compartmentalization. Such information will complement and add to our current concepts of classical TH actions.

## Perspectives of better understanding of TH action

Epidemiology has shown unequivocally that with age the ratio of subclinical to clinically manifest thyroid disorders increases, thus thyroid disorders are a disease of the ageing population. In light of the demographic changes of our societies, improvements of human health care systems should not be limited to better management of only cardiovascular disorders, cancer, and neurodegenerative diseases. We believe that modern and future-oriented health politics and policy making institutions need to take an endocrine organ into account that has been known for decades, but is still not fully "revealed", the thyroid gland.

The knowledge of known thyroid-specific genes, the discovery of new genes as well as the investigations of thyroid hormone- and thyronamine-mediated actions on their many target tissues will entail therapeutic potentials not only for the prevention and treatment of thyroid disorders but importantly also for major health problems that are, as yet, not well treatable with thyroid hormone molecules.

Further investigations of a seemingly familiar but frequently overlooked endocrine organ, the thyroid gland, bear hopes and promises for better management of future challenges arising from current common environmental stressors of human health such as endocrine disruptors.

### List of abbreviations used

AC: adenylylcyclase; AHD: Allan Herndon Dudley; BAT: brown adipose tissue; CH: congenital hypothyroidism; CNS: central nervous system; GPCRs: G-protein coupled receptors; MAP: mitogen activated protein; NIS: sodium-iodide symporter; RXR: retinoic X receptor; T3: 3',3,5-trioodothyronine; T4: thyroxine; TAAR: trace amine associated receptor; TAMs: thyronamines; Tg: thyroglobulin; TH: thyroid hormone; TPO: thyroid peroxidase; TR: thyroid hormone receptor; TSH: thyroid stimulating hormone; TSHR: thyroid stimulating hormone receptor; UCP: uncoupling proteins;

### Acknowledgements

This work was supported by the Deutsche Forschungsgemeinschaft, graduate college 1208 "Hormonal Regulation of Energy Metabolism, Body Weight and Growth", TP1.

The authors are grateful to Marc Scheibner, Dr. Sofia Tedelind and Dr. Denise Yu for manuscript editing.

This article has been published as part of *Thyroid Research* Volume 4 Supplement 1, 2011: New aspects of thyroid hormone synthesis and action. The full contents of the supplement are available online at http://www.thyroidresearchjournal.com/supplements/4/S1

### Author details

[1]School of Engineering and Science, Jacobs University Bremen, Research II, Campus Ring 6, 28759 Bremen, Germany. [2]Universitätsklinikum Leipzig Medizinische Klinik III, 04103 Leipzig, Germany; as of June 2011: Klinik für Endokrinologie, Zentrum für Innere Medizin, Bereich Forschung und Lehre im Zentrallabor, 45147 Essen, Germany. [3]Institute of Experimental Pediatric Endocrinology, Charité Universitätsmedizin Berlin, Augustenburger Platz 1, 13353 Berlin, Germany.

### Authors' contribution

KBr, DF and HB contributed equally, read and approved the manuscript.

### Competing interests

The authors declare that they have no competing interests.

### References

1. Kohrle J: **The deiodinase family: selenoenzymes regulating thyroid hormone availability and action.** *Cell Mol Life Sci* 2000, **57**:1853-1863.
2. Obregon MJ: **Thyroid hormone and adipocyte differentiation.** *Thyroid* 2008, **18**:185-195.
3. Gartner R: **Thyroid diseases in pregnancy.** *Curr Opin Obstet Gynecol* 2009, **21**:501-507.
4. Gruters A, l'Allemand D, Beyer P, Eibs G, Helge H, Korth-Schutz S, Oberdisse U, Schwartz-Bickenbach D, Weber B: **Screening of newborn infants for hypothyroidism in Berlin (West) 1978-1982.** *Monatsschr Kinderheilkd* 1983, **131**:100-105.
5. Bauer M, Goetz T, Glenn T, Whybrow PC: **The thyroid-brain interaction in thyroid disorders and mood disorders.** *J Neuroendocrinol* 2008, **20**:1101-1114.
6. Biondi B, Cooper DS: **The clinical significance of subclinical thyroid dysfunction.** *Endocr Rev* 2008, **29**:76-131.
7. Boas M, Main KM, Feldt-Rasmussen U: **Environmental chemicals and thyroid function: an update.** *Curr Opin Endocrinol Diabetes Obes* 2009, **16**:385-391.
8. Ittermann T, Haring R, Sauer S, Wallaschofski H, Dorr M, Nauck M, Volzke H: **Decreased serum TSH levels are not associated with mortality in the adult northeast German population.** *Eur J Endocrinol* 2010, **162**:579-585.
9. Volzke H, Ittermann T, Schmidt CO, Dorr M, John U, Wallaschofski H, Stricker BH, Felix SB, Rettig R: **Subclinical hyperthyroidism and blood pressure in a population-based prospective cohort study.** *Eur J Endocrinol* 2009, **161**:615-621.
10. Volzke H, Robinson DM, Spielhagen T, Nauck M, Obst A, Ewert R, Wolff B, Wallaschofski H, Felix SB, Dorr M: **Are serum thyrotropin levels within the reference range associated with endothelial function?** *Eur Heart J* 2009, **30**:217-224.
11. Gruters A, Krude H, Biebermann H: **Molecular genetic defects in congenital hypothyroidism.** *Eur J Endocrinol* 2004, **151(Suppl 3)**:U39-44.
12. Krude H, Schutz B, Biebermann H, von Moers A, Schnabel D, Neitzel H, Tonnies H, Weise D, Lafferty A, Schwarz S, *et al*: **Choreoathetosis, hypothyroidism, and pulmonary alterations due to human NKX2-1 haploinsufficiency.** *J Clin Invest* 2002, **109**:475-480.
13. Al Taji E, Biebermann H, Limanova Z, Hnikova O, Zikmund J, Dame C, Gruters A, Lebl J, Krude H: **Screening for mutations in transcription factors in a Czech cohort of 170 patients with congenital and early-onset hypothyroidism: identification of a novel PAX8 mutation in dominantly inherited early-onset non-autoimmune hypothyroidism.** *Eur J Endocrinol* 2007, **156**:521-529.
14. Kuehnen P, Grueters A, Krude H: **Two puzzling cases of thyroid dysgenesis.** *Horm Res* 2009, **71(Suppl 1)**:93-97.
15. Ieiri T, Cochaux P, Targovnik HM, Suzuki M, Shimoda S, Perret J, Vassart G: **A 3' splice site mutation in the thyroglobulin gene responsible for congenital goiter with hypothyroidism.** *J Clin Invest* 1991, **88**:1901-1905.
16. Biebermann H, Schoneberg T, Krude H, Schultz G, Gudermann T, Gruters A: **Mutations of the human thyrotropin receptor gene causing thyroid hypoplasia and persistent congenital hypothyroidism.** *J Clin Endocrinol Metab* 1997, **82**:3471-3480.
17. Abramowicz MJ, Targovnik HM, Varela V, Cochaux P, Krawiec L, Pisarev MA, Propato FV, Juvenal G, Chester HA, Vassart G: **Identification of a mutation in the coding sequence of the human thyroid peroxidase gene causing congenital goiter.** *J Clin Invest* 1992, **90**:1200-1204.
18. Fujiwara H: **Congenital hypothyroidism caused by a mutation in the Na+/I-symporter.** *Nat Genet* 1997, **16(2)**:124-125.
19. Everett LA, Glaser B, Beck JC, Idol JR, Buchs A, Heyman M, Adawi F, Hazani E, Nassir E, Baxevanis AD, *et al*: **Pendred syndrome is caused by mutations in a putative sulphate transporter gene (PDS).** *Nat Genet* 1997, **17**:411-422.
20. Moreno JC, Klootwijk W, van Toor H, Pinto G, D'Alessandro M, Leger A, Goudie D, Polak M, Gruters A, Visser TJ: **Mutations in the iodotyrosine deiodinase gene and hypothyroidism.** *N Engl J Med* 2008, **358**:1811-1818.
21. Moreno JC, Bikker H, Kempers MJ, van Trotsenburg AS, Baas F, de Vijlder JJ, Vulsma T, Ris-Stalpers C: **Inactivating mutations in the gene for thyroid oxidase 2 (THOX2) and congenital hypothyroidism.** *N Engl J Med* 2002, **347**:95-102.
22. Spada A, Mantovani G, Lania A: **Inactivating and activating mutations of the Gs alpha gene.** *Ann Endocrinol (Paris)* 2005, **66**:258-263.
23. Roepke TK, King EC, Reyna-Neyra A, Paroder M, Purtell K, Koba W, Fine E, Lerner DJ, Carrasco N, Abbott GW: **Kcne2 deletion uncovers its crucial role in thyroid hormone biosynthesis.** *Nat Med* 2009, **15**:1186-1194.
24. Havemeyer A, Bittner F, Wollers S, Mendel R, Kunze T, Clement B: **Identification of the missing component in the mitochondrial benzamidoxime prodrug-converting system as a novel molybdenum enzyme.** *J Biol Chem* 2006, **281**:34796-34802.
25. Friedrichs B, Tepel C, Reinheckel T, Deussing J, von Figura K, Herzog V, Peters C, Saftig P, Brix K: **Thyroid functions of mouse cathepsins B, K, and L.** *J Clin Invest* 2003, **111**:1733-1745.
26. Jordans S, Jenko-Kokalj S, Kuhl NM, Tedelind S, Sendt W, Bromme D, Turk D, Brix K: **Monitoring compartment-specific substrate cleavage by cathepsins B, K, L, and S at physiological pH and redox conditions.** *BMC Biochem* 2009, **10**:23.
27. Marino M, Zheng G, Chiovato L, Pinchera A, Brown D, Andrews D, McCluskey RT: **Role of megalin (gp330) in transcytosis of thyroglobulin by thyroid cells. A novel function in the control of thyroid hormone release.** *J Biol Chem* 2000, **275**:7125-7137.
28. Friesema EC, Ganguly S, Abdalla A, Manning Fox JE, Halestrap AP, Visser TJ: **Identification of monocarboxylate transporter 8 as a specific thyroid hormone transporter.** *J Biol Chem* 2003, **278**:40128-40135.
29. Friesema EC, Grueters A, Biebermann H, Krude H, von Moers A, Reeser M, Barrett TG, Mancilla EE, Svensson J, Kester MH, *et al*: **Association between mutations in a thyroid hormone transporter and severe X-linked psychomotor retardation.** *Lancet* 2004, **364**:1435-1437.
30. Sugiyama D, Kusuhara H, Taniguchi H, Ishikawa S, Nozaki Y, Aburatani H, Sugiyama Y: **Functional characterization of rat brain-specific organic anion transporter (Oatp14) at the blood-brain barrier: high affinity transporter for thyroxine.** *J Biol Chem* 2003, **278**:43489-43495.
31. Friesema EC, Docter R, Moerings EP, Verrey F, Krenning EP, Hennemann G, Visser TJ: **Thyroid hormone transport by the heterodimeric human system L amino acid transporter.** *Endocrinology* 2001, **142**:4339-4348.

32. Ritchie JW, Taylor PM: **Role of the System L permease LAT1 in amino acid and iodothyronine transport in placenta.** *Biochem J* 2001, **356**:719-725.
33. Friesema EC, Jansen J, Jachtenberg JW, Visser WE, Kester MH, Visser TJ: **Effective cellular uptake and efflux of thyroid hormone by human monocarboxylate transporter 10.** *Mol Endocrinol* 2008, **22**:1357-1369.
34. Scanlan TS, Suchland KL, Hart ME, Chiellini G, Huang Y, Kruzich PJ, Frascarelli S, Crossley DA, Bunzow JR, Ronca-Testoni S, *et al*: **3-Iodothyronamine is an endogenous and rapid-acting derivative of thyroid hormone.** *Nat Med* 2004, **10**:638-642.
35. Borowsky B, Adham N, Jones KA, Raddatz R, Artymyshyn R, Ogozalek KL, Durkin MM, Lakhlani PP, Bonini JA, Pathirana S, *et al*: **Trace amines: identification of a family of mammalian G protein-coupled receptors.** *Proc Natl Acad Sci U S A* 2001, **98**:8966-8971.
36. Staubert C, Boselt I, Bohnekamp J, Rompler H, Enard W, Schoneberg T: **Structural and functional evolution of the trace amine-associated receptors TAAR3, TAAR4 and TAAR5 in primates.** *PLoS One* 2010, **5**: e11133.
37. Piehl S, Hoefig CS, Scanlan TS, Kohrle J: **Thyronamines–Past, Present, and Future.** *Endocr Rev* 2011, **32**:64-80.
38. Panetta R, Greenwood MT: **Physiological relevance of GPCR oligomerization and its impact on drug discovery.** *Drug Discov Today* 2008, **13**:1059-1066.
39. Bergh JJ, Lin HY, Lansing L, Mohamed SN, Davis FB, Mousa S, Davis PJ: **Integrin alphaVbeta3 contains a cell surface receptor site for thyroid hormone that is linked to activation of mitogen-activated protein kinase and induction of angiogenesis.** *Endocrinology* 2005, **146**:2864-2871.
40. Furuya F, Lu C, Guigon CJ, Cheng SY: **Nongenomic activation of phosphatidylinositol 3-kinase signaling by thyroid hormone receptors.** *Steroids* 2009, **74**:628-634.
41. Scarlett A, Parsons MP, Hanson PL, Sidhu KK, Milligan TP, Burrin JM: **Thyroid hormone stimulation of extracellular signal-regulated kinase and cell proliferation in human osteoblast-like cells is initiated at integrin alphaVbeta3.** *J Endocrinol* 2008, **196**:509-517.
42. Lanni A, Moreno M, Lombardi A, de Lange P, Silvestri E, Ragni M, Farina P, Baccari GC, Fallahi P, Antonelli A, Goglia F: **3,5-diiodo-L-thyronine powerfully reduces adiposity in rats by increasing the burning of fats.** *FASEB J* 2005, **19**:1552-1554.
43. Ribeiro MO, Bianco SD, Kaneshige M, Schultz JJ, Cheng SY, Bianco AC, Brent GA: **Expression of uncoupling protein 1 in mouse brown adipose tissue is thyroid hormone receptor-beta isoform specific and required for adaptive thermogenesis.** *Endocrinology* 2010, **151**:432-440.

# 27

# Insights into molecular properties of the human monocarboxylate transporter 8 by combining functional with structural information

Gunnar Kleinau[1*], Ulrich Schweizer[2], Anita Kinne[3], Josef Köhrle[2], Annette Grüters[1], Heiko Krude[1], Heike Biebermann[1]

**Abstract**

**Background:** The monocarboxylate transporter 8 (MCT8) is a member of the major facilitator superfamily (MFS) and transports specificly iodothyronines. MCT8 mutations are the underlying cause of a syndrome of severe X-linked psychomotor retardation known as the Allan-Herndon-Dudley syndrome. This syndrome is characterized by abnormally high T3, low/normal T4 serum levels and slightly elevated serum TSH. To date, more than 25 pathogenic mutations in *hMCT8* are known and they are valuable indicators of important regions for structural and functional MCT8 properties.

**Methods:** We designed a structural human MCT8 model and studied reported pathogenic missense mutations with focus on the estimation of those amino acid positions which are probably sensitive for substrate transport. Furthermore, assuming similarities between determinants of T3 binding observed in the published crystal structure of the thyroid hormone receptor beta occupied by its ligand T3 and the structural MCT8 model, we explore potential T3 binding sites in the MCT8 substrate channel cavity.

**Results:** We found that all known pathogenic missense mutations are located exclusively in the transmembrane helices and to a high degree at conserved residues among the MCT family. Furthermore, mutations either of or to prolines/glycines are located mainly at helices 9-12 and are expected to cause steric clashes or structural misfolding. In contrast, several other mutations are close to the potential substrate channel and affected amino acids are likely involved in the switching mechanism between different transporter conformations. Finally, three potential substrate binding sites are predicted for MCT8.

**Conclusions:** Naturally occurring mutations of MCT8 provide molecular insights into protein regions important for protein folding, substrate binding and the switching mechanism during substrate transport. Future studies guided by this information should help to clarify structure-function relationships at MCT8 which may bear broader relevance for other members of the MCT family. This includes decoding of the complete set of transport-sensitive residue positions and description of structural re-arrangements during transport.

## Introduction

The Allan-Herndon-Dudley syndrome is an X-linked mental retardation first described in 1944 [1]. Neonates are lacking head-moving control and they are characterized by feeding problems. Severe psychomotor retardation becomes more obvious with increasing age and some patients never attain speech or the ability to walk. An abnormal thyroid hormone constellation was found as a characteristic signature for this syndrome and guided the identification of mutations in MCT8 in affected patients [2,3]. This constellation is a combination of high T3 levels with low/normal T4 and slightly increased TSH in human serum. To date, more than 25 pathogenic mutations have been identified including missense, nonsense, deletions, insertions, and splice site mutations [4].

* Correspondence: gunnar.kleinau@charite.de
[1]Institut für Experimentelle Pädiatrische Endokrinologie, Charité-Universitätsmedizin Berlin, Germany
Full list of author information is available at the end of the article

MCT8 is a member of the major facilitator superfamily (MFS) of membrane transporters and is structurally characterized by twelve transmembrane helices connected by intra- and extracellular loops. The N- and C-termini are both located intracellularly [5]. MCT8 was described as a specific iodothyronine transporter [6] and known substrates for human MCT8 are thyroxine (3,3',5,5'-tetraiodo-L-thyronine, T4), T3 (3,3',5-triiodo-L-thyronine), rT3 (3,3`,5'-triiodo-L-thyronine), and 3,3'-T2 (3,3'-diiodo-L-thyronine) [6,7].

It is assumed that substrate binding by MFS transporters triggers the transition between an "outside-open" and "inside-open" conformation, the so-called "rocker-switch" model [8,9]. This structural movement must be linked with specific intramolecular events like rearrangement of amino acid interactions and also with substrate trans-localization. Despite the need of more supporting and detailed information for this structural-functional "rocker-switch" model, specific substrate-protein interactions need to be considered as to be causally related to different protein conformations. Of note, this model should be also applicable for the reverse way of substrate transport (i.e. efflux cycle) from the cytosolic to the extracellular site. So far, details and principles of the process are only partially known.

Naturally occurring missense mutations point to functionally and structurally important residues within the MCT8 protein. Mutations may affect protein folding and stability or directly modify the mechanism of iodothyronine transport [10]. We here explored the spatial localization, molecular environment and the potential function of their wild-type amino acids at a three-dimensional "inside-open" MCT8 model, the only structural conformation where templates for homology models are available. We will also discuss the results of previous studies to evaluate the MCT8 homology model and to extent generally our knowledge regarding molecular mechanisms at MCTs.

## Material and methods

### Homology modelling of MCT8

The crystal structure of the Glycerol-3-phosphate transporter (GlpT) in an "inside-open" conformation was used as a structural template for the human MCT8 (hMCT8) homology model (PDB code 1PW4 [8]). Despite low sequence identity between this template and other members of MFS like MCT8, models based on this structural template are supported by experimental data concerning GLUT1 [11], MCT1 [12,13], and OATP1C1 [14]. The potential dimensions of MCT8 transmembrane helices (TMHs) were defined based on helices in the template crystal structure. For consistency we confirmed these dimensions with other available MFS crystal structures (PDB codes 1PV6 and 1PV7 [15]). For further structural information of MCTs see also the internet platform "Membrane transporter systems" at http://www.membranetransport.org.

Gaps of missing residues in loop regions of the template structure were closed either manually or by the 'Loop Search' tool implemented in Sybyl 7.35 (Tripos Inc., St. Louis, MO, USA). Side chains and loops of the homology model were subjected to conjugate gradient minimization (until converging at a termination gradient of 0.05 kcal/(mol*Å)). The side chain orientations were refined during dynamic simulation (8 ns) by fixing all backbone H-bonds of TMHs. This step of model generation is extended compared to the recently published MCT8 model [7] (5 ns) to get more precise potential MCT8 side chain orientations. Finally, the model was minimized without any constraints.

We have mapped naturally occurring single side chain substitutions (figure 1) on our MCT8 model (figures 2 and 3). Pathogenic deletions or insertions (reviewed in [4]) are not considered here, since they lead to incomplete proteins or they modify the particular helix-conformation and arrangements relative to each other. Therefore, such mutations are revoking a consistent structural prediction.

Structure images were produced using the PyMOL Molecular Graphics System, Version 1.3, Schrödinger, LLC.

### Amino acid sequence alignment of human MCTs and the unification of residue numbering

Amino acid sequences of human MCT family members were aligned to analyze shared and divergent features in amino acid composition (figure 4). Details of the alignment procedure are recently described by Kinne and Kleinau et al. [7]. The alignment was used to highlight positions of pathogenic *MCT8* mutations. This alignment enables comparison and analyses of residue conservation among human MCTs (figure 1).

We suggested previously a unifying numbering system for MCTs similar to family A GPCRs [7]. This position identifier scheme uses a highly conserved residue in each TMH as a common reference for all members of the MCT family. The first number is related to the particular helix, the second number after the dot determines the specific position in relation to the conserved residue. For example, the highly conserved tryptophan in TMH1 is defined as 1.50 and the highly conserved proline from TMH2 is defined as 2.50 (figure 4).

## Results and discussion

### The structural MCT8 model: molecular insights and predictivity

Structural models represent potential conformations of the target macro-molecule. Because of the well known

| Substitution | References | Structural localization | Position | Conservation of wild-type MCT8 residues among nine hMCT members hMCT8/all others |
|---|---|---|---|---|
| H192R | review [4] | TMH1 | 1.67 | 1/9 |
| S194F | [21, 22] | TMH1 | 1.69 | 4/9 |
| G221R | [22, 23] | TMH2 | 2.38 | 3/9 |
| A224V | [3, 21] | TMH2 | 2.41 | 3/9 |
| A224T | [24] | TMH2 | 2.41 | 3/9 |
| V235M | [21, 22] | TMH2 | 2.52 | 2/9 |
| R271H | [21, 24] | ECL2/TMH4 | 4.39 | 1/9 |
| G282C | review [4] | TMH4 | 4.50 | **9/9** |
| P321L | [23] | TMH5 | 5.59 | 3/9 |
| G401R | review [4] | ICL3/TMH7 | 7.39 | **6/9** |
| L434W | [21, 22] | ECL4/TMH8 | 8.39 | **6/9** |
| R445C | review [4] | TMH8 | 8.50 | **8/9 (one Lys)** |
| D453V | review [4] | TMH8 | 8.58 | **5/9 (and 3 Asn)** |
| L471P | [3, 21] | TMH9 | 9.49 | 2/9 |
| L512P | [2] | TMH10/ICL5 | 10.63 | **5/9** |
| P537L | [25] | TMH11 | 11.49 | **9/9** |
| G558D | [26] | TMH12 | 12.54 | **7/9** |
| G564R | [27] | TMH12 | 12.60 | **8/9** |
| L568P | [21, 22] | TMH12 | 12.64 | **7/9** |

**Figure 1 Naturally occurring missense substitutions in human MCT8.** In this table naturally occurring pathogenic amino acid substitutions known for MCT8 are summarized. Specific background-colours indicate structural/functional and biophysical specificities: violet – mutations at or to proline/glycines, respectively; red – side chain substitutions in the vicinity of the presumed substrate channel (figures 2 and 3); green – amino acids pointing towards the membrane. We also provide a summary on conservation of respective amino acids within the MCT family based on the alignment in figure 4 (bold are positions where more than half of the MCTs have an identical amino acid). The unified position numbering suggested in a recent study [7] is provided (for description see section Material and Methods).

causal dependency between specific biological functions (like substrate binding or transport mechanisms at MCTs) and particular structural features, structural models are useful to guide experimental approaches or to support the interpretation of experimental data. In our recent study, we identified two functionally important amino acids located at TMH8 and TMH10 [7]. In this study we started with the hypothesis that two specific charged amino acids in the transmembrane region ($R445^{8.50}$ and $D498^{10.49}$) may interact with the amino acid backbone of iodothyronines. To prove this hypothesis, we have mutated both residues to alanine and tested transport of the natural substrate T3, as well as of two substrates lacking either the carboxyl or the

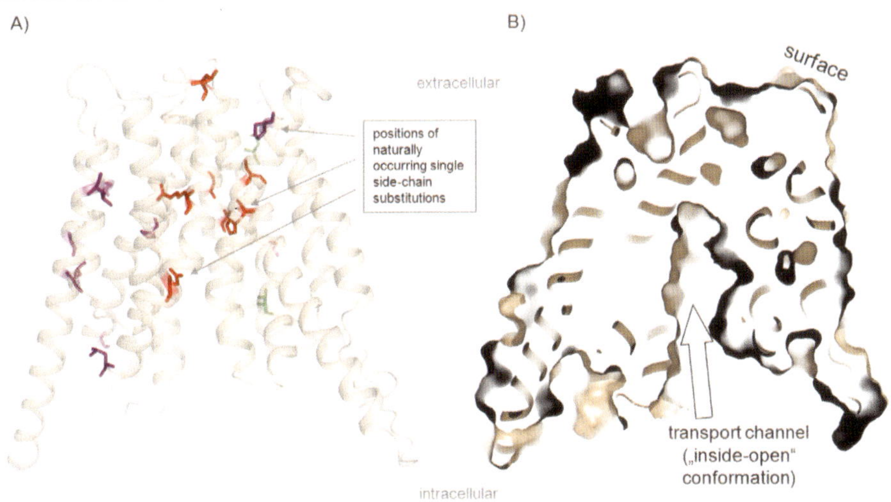


**Figure 2 Homology model of human MCT8 with highlighted naturally occurring side chain substitutions. A)** We highlighted wild-type amino acids of known naturally occurring mutations on the homology model of monocarboxylate transporter 8 in a conformation open to the cytosol (see figure 1). Colours were assigned according to the colour scheme in figure 1. From this three-dimensional mapping it becomes clear that none of these mutations are localized in the extra- or intracellular loops. **B)** The clipped surface-presentation of the MCT8 protein reveals the presumed substrate channel from the intracellular side.

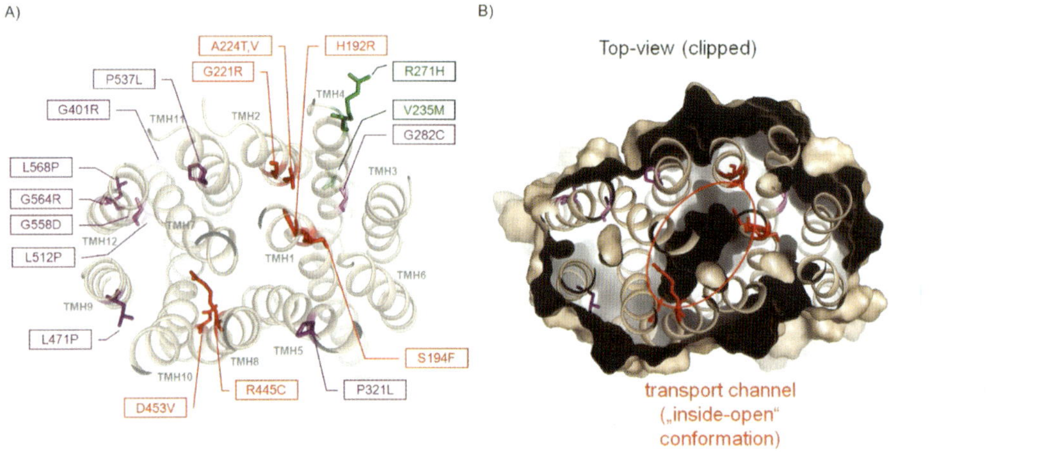


**Figure 3 Homology model of the human MCT8 with mapped details of pathogenic mutations and potential localization of the transport channel switching region. A)** The top-view on the MCT8 homology model with annotated pathogenic side chain substitutions reveals a detailed insight into the distribution of known mutations. The colour code given to the side chains (sticks) is in accordance with described colour scheme in figure 1. **B)** This clipped surface top-view visualizes the spatial relation between the wild-type amino acids of mutant positions and the "inside-open" transport channel conformation. Amino acids that are localized at the transition between the open and closed channel part are coloured red (red circle). These residues might be involved in the switching process between the "inside-open" and "outside-open" conformations.

amino group, 3,3',5-triiodo-thyronamine and 3,3',5-triiodo-thyroacetic acid. Both alanine mutants were inactive towards all three substrates. These findings support our assumption that both amino acids are important for substrate transport. The MCT8 model also predicted a potential salt bridge between both amino acids and an H-bond from R445 to the helix-backbone adjusting the relative orientation between TMH8 and TMH10. In conclusion, these two residues may have a dual function for substrate interaction and for the conformational switch mechanism. Interestingly, positively charged residues corresponding to MCT8 position $445^{8.50}$ can be found in all MCTs. This position and spatial region may bear a fundamental role, since also in other twelve helix-transporters positively charged residues are suggested or evidenced to participate in the transport mechanisms, e.g. for GlpT [8], MCT1 [13], and OATP1C1 [14]. Finally, our findings were supported by the recent report of a naturally occurring mutation at MCT8 position 445 (R445C, reviewed in [4]).

To further evaluate the reliability of our MCT8 model, we retrospectively examined other recently published functional data. An alanine scanning study focussing on all 10 cysteines within hMCT8 [16] was performed to test the contribution to homo-oligomeric MCT8 arrangements. The alanine mutants did not alter MCT8–mediated substrate transport. We have mapped these cysteines on our MCT8 model and found that none of the cysteine side chains participates directly in the substrate channel, except C283 close to the cytosolic entry side (figure 5). Accordingly, the cysteine to alanine substitutions (shorter side chains than of cysteines) did not alter properties of the transport channel and are likely not involved in transport. Finally, seven (C184, C231, C244, C281, C283, C491, C497) out of the ten cysteines are located inside the transmembrane part. Therefore, only the extracellular 3 cysteines (C436, C481, C546) in a non-reducing environment could in principle participate in intermolecular dimer-contacts via disulfide bridges. Of note, they are not in spatial distances to each other (more than 20 Å) to form intramolecular disulfide bridges.

#### Naturally occurring side chain substitutions are indicators for functionally and structurally important MCT regions

We here explored the spatial localization of MCT8 mutations in the three-dimensional "inside-open" MCT8 homology model. First of all, we found by comparison of hMCT amino acid sequences and the MCT8 model that:

1. All single side chain missense mutations are located within TMHs or at helix-loop transitions (figure 2A), but not at extra- or intracellular loops. This finding highlights the transmembrane helices as most important for MCT8 function.
2. Pathogenic MCT8 mutants are localized to a high degree at conserved wild-type amino acids among MCTs (figure 4).

Conserved residues of related proteins (like the MCT family) indicate amino acids of functional and/or structural importance. Wild-type positions of MCT8 mutations at helices 5 to 12 are conserved more than 50%

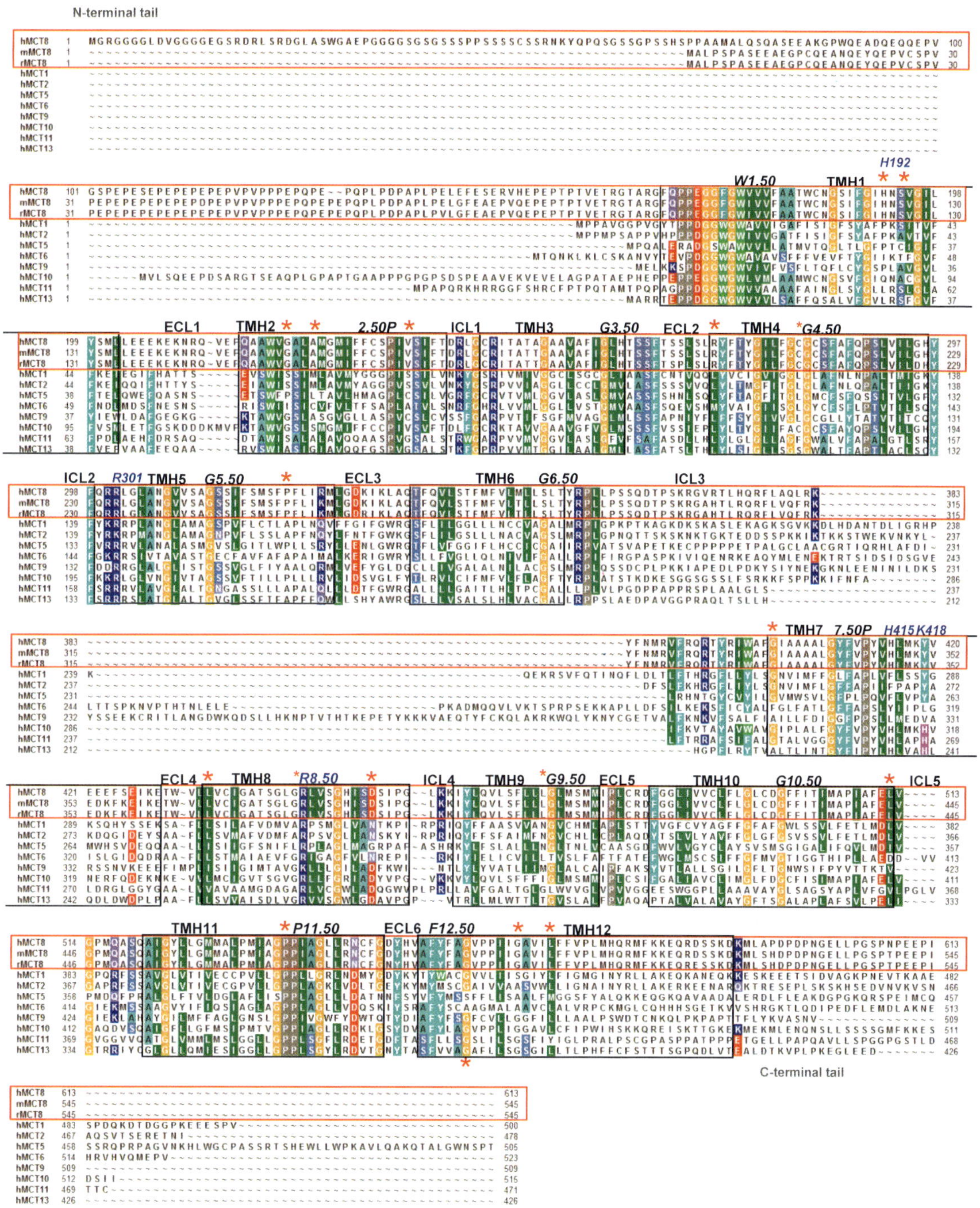


**Figure 4 Alignment of the human MCTs with highlighted positions of pathogenic mutations reported for MCT8.** This alignment compares the human MCT sequences and in addition MCT8 of rat and mice (MCT8 are red boxed). Conserved residues are marked by different colours according to their biophysical properties (blue - positively charged, red - negatively charged, green/orange - hydrophobic, gray - hydrophilic, black – proline, cyan - aromatic). Black boxed are the potential dimensions of the transmembrane helices (TMHs) based on the X-ray structure of the *E.coli* Glycerol-3-phosphate transporter, another member of the major facilitator superfamily which was used as a structural template to build the MCT8 homology model. Red stars above the hMCT8 sequence indicating positions where naturally occurring mutations for the *hMCT8* are reported. Few of them are at positions with a high degree of conservation like R445 (R8.50). In addition, the positively charged residues and histidines hypothesized in this study as to be potentially involved in substrate transport (figure 7) are annotated above the sequences in blue. For each helix the most highly conserved residue is numbered according to a unifying numbering system (see Material and Methods).

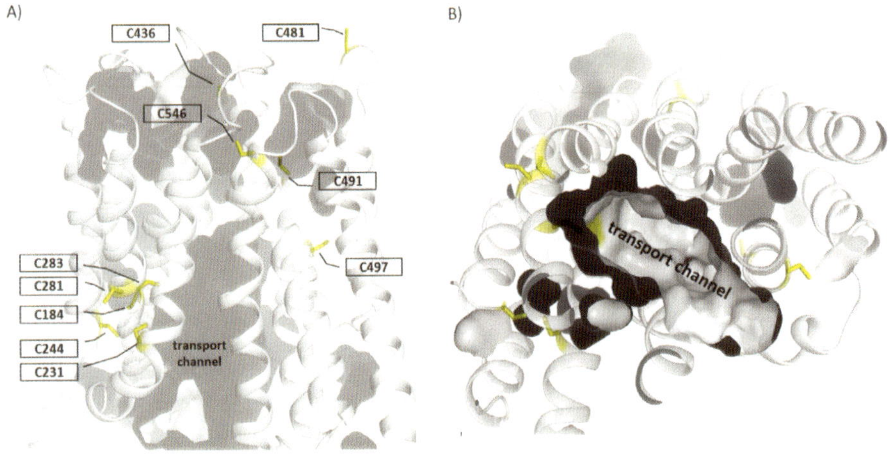


**Figure 5 Distribution of cysteines in the human MCT8 homology model**. To evaluate our MCT8 model on consistency we examined already published functional data. Alanine mutants of all ten cysteines in the hMCT8 did not alter MCT8 functions such as substrate transport [16]. **A)** With the exception of C283 at the cytosolic channel region our "inside-open" MCT8 model suggests that none of the MCT8 cysteine side chains directly participates in the substrate channel. In conclusion the experimental data and the implications from the MCT8 model are in agreement with each other. **B)** The cytosolic view with clipped intracellular loops shows that most of the cysteines are localized at distance from the substrate channel. (Cavities in the model are highlighted by inner surfaces.)

among hMCTs. Three out of nineteen positions are conserved to 100%, four positions are conserved to 90%. In conclusion, it can be speculated that mutations at highly conserved amino acids likely cause pathogenic dysfunction. These positions appear as essential for hMCTs and structural/functional similarities especially at these particular positions are preserved.

Furthermore, we have subdivided pathogenic mutations into two main groups (figure 1): I. mutations either at or to proline/glycine which leads likely to structural changes between helices or directly at helices (prolines in helices supporting kinks); II. side chain substitutions located close to the putative substrate channel which might directly modify substrate transport.

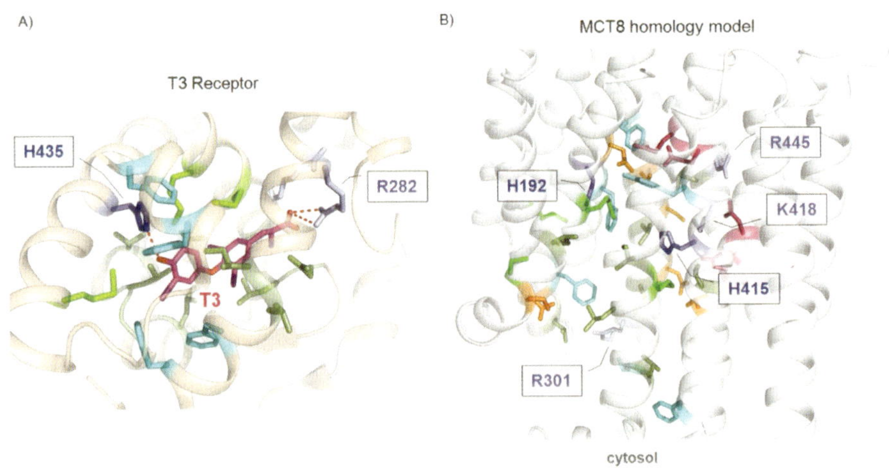


**Figure 6 Details of the T3 receptor beta complex in comparison with determinants of the MCT8 transport channel. A)** The crystal structure of the T3 receptor beta ligand binding domain (PDB code 3GWS [20] backbone-ribbon) reveals detailed insights into the binding mode of this hormone. Surrounded by hydrophobic (green) and aromatic (cyan) amino acids, T3 (magenta) binding is characterized by H-bonds to an arginine and a histidine. According to the assumption of analogy for T3 binding (T3 receptor, A) to different proteins, such specific complementary residues might be generally mandatory for hormone binding/transport. **B)** In the MCT8 homology model two histidines (H192, H415) and three positively charged residues (R445, K418, R301) are predicted to point inside the putative substrate transport channel (sticks with labels). Further amino acids in the transport channel are also highlighted by sticks: orange – hydrophilic residues without charges, magenta – negatively charged residues.

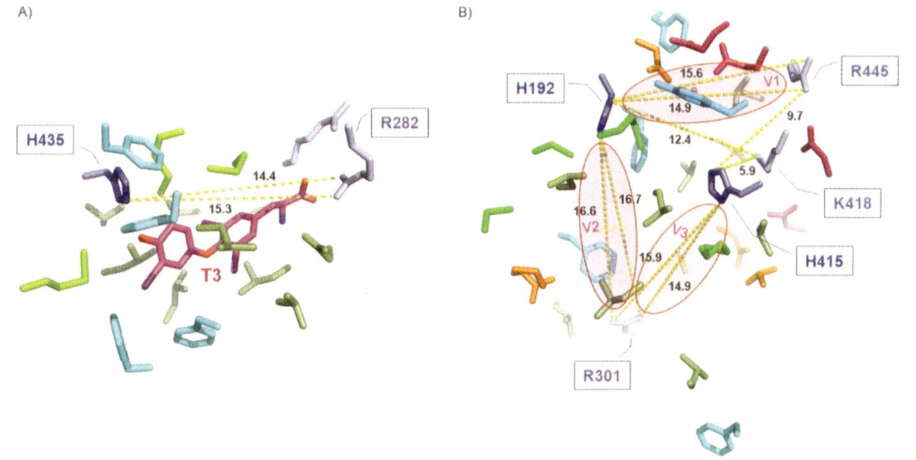


**Figure 7 Applications for potential modes of T3 binding at MCT8 by comparison between the crystallized hormone/receptor complex and the structural MCT8 model. A)** T3 is bound to its receptor in a specific mode characterized by several molecular interactions like H-bonds to a positively charged arginine and a histidine (figure 6A). The amino acid side chains are in a certain distance to each other in a range between 14.4 and 15.3 Å. **B)** Measurement of the distances between the histidines and positively charges residues in the MCT8 model ("inside-open" conformation) reveals three combinations of Arg-His pairings in a similar distance to each other (red translucent regions V1-V3 (V–variant)). Although the distance between R445 (highly conserved among the MCTs) and H192 is around 15 Å, some hydrophilic amino acids are in close spatial distance (V1) which would cause sterical clashes with the T3 substrate. In another transporter conformation this might be different. Of note, R445 and H192 are functionally important as demonstrated by pathogenic mutations (figure 3A). The importance of R445 for transport was also shown by directed mutagenesis.

### Mutations at or to prolines and glycines, respectively, cause structural misfolding

Interestingly, for MCT8 the majority (7 out of 9) of proline/glycine mutations (P/G-X, e.g. P537L) or mutants to proline (X-P, e.g. L512P) are located at helices 9-12 (figure 1, figure 3A). They involve conserved amino acids among the MCTs. Prolines and glycines are known to support kinks and bulges in helices [17-19]. This has strong impact on both the helix (local) and the protein (global) structure. For that reason structural alterations of the helices by mutations at or to proline/glycine, respectively, can be assumed to cause MCT8 misfolding by modification of helix conformation. In consequence deficiencies in cell surface expression of such mutants have been observed [10]. Additionally, for the P/G-X mutants it can be assumed that substitutions of prolines or glycines with enlarged side chains like leucine are predestined to cause sterical clashes in a tight micro-environment of interacting side chains.

### Pathogenic MCT8 mutations indicate important determinants and regions for substrate transport

Wild-type amino acids of those mutants that are close to the transport channel (figures 2A and 3B) might be directly or indirectly involved in substrate transport mechanisms. Interestingly, amino acids H192, S194, G221, A224, and R445 are located at a similar spatial layer which lies at the closed bottom substrate channel viewed from the intracellular side (figures 3B and 5B). These residues are in a specific region that must be modified or "opened" for substrate transport. Therefore, they might be involved in the switching mechanism between an "inside-open" and "outside-open" conformation. Particular residues here may function thereby as gate keepers as already described for R445 [7]. Interactions between neighbouring helices as suggested for R445 may constrain the "bottle neck like" conformation of this region. During the conformational switching such constraints must be re-arranged to enable structural movements of the helices. However, it needs more experimental characterization to clarify the detailed molecular involvement of each of these wild-type amino acids, but we can assume that the pathogenic substitutions do not maintain MCT8 transport function.

### Potential T3 binding sites in the MCT8 substrate transport channel

One may assume that MCT8 substrates bind along the open channel-part in the "inside-open" MCT8 model. In order to identify amino acids which may contribute to substrate binding and transport, we used a comparative strategy. The previously published crystal structure of the T3-bound thyroid hormone receptor (TR) beta ligand binding domain (PDB code 3GWS [20]) reveals detailed insights in T3 binding (figure 6A). Surrounded by hydrophobic aliphatic and aromatic amino acids, T3 is bound by H-bonds to an arginine and a histidine (figure 6A). Side chains of these two residues are in a defined spatial distance to each other of around 14-15 Å (figure 7A). Assuming a certain degree of analogy in T3 binding, such specific residues, their biochemical properties and their arrangement in the binding pocket, might represent a typical pattern for T3 binding. In the MCT8 homology model two histidines ($H192^{1.67}$, $H415^{7.53}$) and three positively charged residues ($R445^{8.50}$, $K418^{8.56}$, $R301^{5.39}$) are predicted to point towards the substrate transport channel (figure 6B). Measurement of the side chain distances between the histidines and positively charged residues ("inside-open" MCT8 conformation, figure 7B) reveals three combinations of Arg-His pairs at a similar distance to each other as in the T3-TR beta complex. These pairs and distances are shown in figure 7B as potential binding regions for T3 in the channel cavity. Of note, although the distance between R445 (highly conserved among the MCTs) and H192 is around 15 Å like in the T3 receptor, few other amino acids are in close spatial proximity likely would lead to sterical clashes with substrate in this conformation. In an "outside-open" conformation this might be different.

Nevertheless, R445 and H192 have already been shown to be functionally important (references in [7]). The present comparative analysis suggests two new potential key-players for substrate transport: $R301^{5.39}$ (highly conserved among the hMCTs 1-13) and $H415^{7.53}$ (conserved in hMCT8, hMCT10, hMCT11, and hMCT13). Both amino acids have not yet been investigated experimentally. R301 at TMH5 is, in contrast to the two other positively charged residues inside the channel, localized more closely to the intracellular side. Noticeably, in all three potential variants of T3 binding modes always one amino acid is linked to the potential "switching sensitive" region at the closed bottle neck of the transport channel.

## Conclusions

Naturally occurring mutations in MCT8 provide molecular insights into protein regions important for protein folding and the switching mechanism during substrate transport. This was shown here by the assignment of mutations especially at TMH9 to TMH12 leading to MCT8 misfolding. Furthermore, by highlighting specific positions of pathogenic mutations in the three-dimensional structure, we have specified a critical region for the transition between the postulated "inside-open" and "outside-open" conformations. These amino acids are located at a bottle neck of the transport channel cavity, surrounded by substrate binding-sensitive amino acids. Our MCT8 model has guided several new insights in the relationship between sequence, structure and function of this transporter. This model is in accordance with experimental data and is predictive to support the identification of functional key-player amino acids. Future studies based on this model are aimed to clarify unknown details of molecular events at MCT8 and likely at other members of the MCT family. This includes: 1. identification of the complete set of transport-sensitive residues, 2. description of structural rearrangements, 3. identification of binding-sensitive residues, 4. details of ligand binding with molecular explanation of substrate specificity. Finally, for comprehensive understanding the relevance of oligomeric MCT8 constellations must be considered.

**Acknowledgement**
This work was supported by the graduate college 1208 "Hormonal Regulation of Energy Metabolism, Body Weight and Growth" (TP1 and TP3), and by the Deutsche Forschungsgemeinschaft (KL2334/2-1).
This article has been published as part of *Thyroid Research* Volume 4 Supplement 1, 2011: New aspects of thyroid hormone synthesis and action. The full contents of the supplement are available online at http://www.thyroidresearchjournal.com/supplements/4/S1

**Author details**
[1]Institut für Experimentelle Pädiatrische Endokrinologie, Charité-Universitätsmedizin Berlin, Germany. [2]Institut für Experimentelle Endokrinologie, Charité-Universitätsmedizin Berlin, Germany. [3]Leibniz-Institut für Molekulare Pharmakologie, Berlin, Germany.

**Authors' contributions**
GK wrote the draft, performed and designed the studies, analyzed the data, prepared the figures; US analyzed the data, wrote the draft; AK analyzed the data; JK performed and designed the studies; AG data evaluation and discussion; HK analyzed the data, project coordination; HB analyzed the data, project coordination. All authors drafted the manuscript and approved the final manuscript.

**Competing interests**
There are no competing interests.

**References**

1. Allan W, H C, Dudley F: **Some examples of the inheritance of mentaldeficiency:apparentlysex-linkedidiocyandmicrocephaly.** *Am J Ment Defic* 1944, **48**:325-334.
2. Dumitrescu AM, Liao XH, Best TB, Brockmann K, Refetoff S: **A novel syndrome combining thyroid and neurological abnormalities is associated with mutations in a monocarboxylate transporter gene.** *Am J Hum Genet* 2004, **74**:168-175.
3. Friesema EC, Grueters A, Biebermann H, Krude H, von Moers A, Reeser M, Barrett TG, Mancilla EE, Svensson J, Kester MH, *et al*: **Association between mutations in a thyroid hormone transporter and severe X-linked psychomotor retardation.** *Lancet* 2004, **364**:1435-1437.
4. Friesema EC, Visser WE, Visser TJ: **Genetics and phenomics of thyroid hormone transport by MCT8.** *Mol Cell Endocrinol* 2010, **322**:107-113.
5. Friesema EC, Jansen J, Milici C, Visser TJ: **Thyroid hormone transporters.** *Vitam Horm* 2005, **70**:137-167.
6. Friesema EC, Ganguly S, Abdalla A, Manning Fox JE, Halestrap AP, Visser TJ: **Identification of monocarboxylate transporter 8 as a specific thyroid hormone transporter.** *J Biol Chem* 2003, **278**:40128-40135.
7. Kinne A, Kleinau G, Hoefig CS, Gruters A, Kohrle J, Krause G, Schweizer U: **Essential molecular determinants for thyroid hormone transport and first structural implications for monocarboxylate transporter 8.** *J Biol Chem* 2010, **285**:28054-28063.
8. Huang Y, Lemieux MJ, Song J, Auer M, Wang DN: **Structure and mechanism of the glycerol-3-phosphate transporter from Escherichia coli.** *Science* 2003, **301**:616-620.

9. Yin Y, He X, Szewczyk P, Nguyen T, Chang G: **Structure of the multidrug transporter EmrD from Escherichia coli.** *Science* 2006, **312**:741-744.
10. Kinne A, Roth S, Biebermann H, Kohrle J, Gruters A, Schweizer U: **Surface translocation and tri-iodothyronine uptake of mutant MCT8 proteins are cell type-dependent.** *J Mol Endocrinol* 2009, **43**:263-271.
11. Salas-Burgos A, Iserovich P, Zuniga F, Vera JC, Fischbarg J: **Predicting the three-dimensional structure of the human facilitative glucose transporter glut1 by a novel evolutionary homology strategy: insights on the molecular mechanism of substrate migration, and binding sites for glucose and inhibitory molecules.** *Biophys J* 2004, **87**:2990-2999.
12. Manoharan C, Wilson MC, Sessions RB, Halestrap AP: **The role of charged residues in the transmembrane helices of monocarboxylate transporter 1 and its ancillary protein basigin in determining plasma membrane expression and catalytic activity.** *Mol Membr Biol* 2006, **23**:486-498.
13. Wilson MC, Meredith D, Bunnun C, Sessions RB, Halestrap AP: **Studies on the DIDS-binding site of monocarboxylate transporter 1 suggest a homology model of the open conformation and a plausible translocation cycle.** *J Biol Chem* 2009, **284**:20011-20021.
14. Westholm DE, Marold JD, Viken KJ, Duerst AH, Anderson GW, Rumbley JN: **Evidence of Evolutionary Conservation of Function between the Thyroxine Transporter Oatp1c1 and Major Facilitator Superfamily Members.** *Endocrinology.* 2010, **151(12)**:5941-5951.
15. Abramson J, Smirnova I, Kasho V, Verner G, Kaback HR, Iwata S: **Structure and mechanism of the lactose permease of Escherichia coli.** *Science* 2003, **301**:610-615.
16. Visser WE, Philp NJ, van Dijk TB, Klootwijk W, Friesema EC, Jansen J, Beesley PW, Ianculescu AG, Visser TJ: **Evidence for a homodimeric structure of human monocarboxylate transporter 8.** *Endocrinology* 2009, **150**:5163-5170.
17. Yohannan S, Yang D, Faham S, Boulting G, Whitelegge J, Bowie JU: **Proline substitutions are not easily accommodated in a membrane protein.** *J Mol Biol* 2004, **341**:1-6.
18. Yohannan S, Faham S, Yang D, Whitelegge JP, Bowie JU: **The evolution of transmembrane helix kinks and the structural diversity of G protein-coupled receptors.** *Proc Natl Acad Sci U S A* 2004, **101**:959-963.
19. Ceruso MA, Weinstein H: **Structural mimicry of proline kinks: tertiary packing interactions support local structural distortions.** *J Mol Biol* 2002, **318**:1237-1249.
20. Nascimento AS, Dias SM, Nunes FM, Aparicio R, Ambrosio AL, Bleicher L, Figueira AC, Santos MA, de Oliveira Neto M, Fischer H, *et al*: **Structural rearrangements in the thyroid hormone receptor hinge domain and their putative role in the receptor function.** *J Mol Biol* 2006, **360**:586-598.
21. Jansen J, Friesema EC, Kester MH, Schwartz CE, Visser TJ: **Genotype-phenotype relationship in patients with mutations in thyroid hormone transporter MCT8.** *Endocrinology* 2008, **149**:2184-2190.
22. Schwartz CE, May MM, Carpenter NJ, Rogers RC, Martin J, Bialer MG, Ward J, Sanabria J, Marsa S, Lewis JA, *et al*: **Allan-Herndon-Dudley syndrome and the monocarboxylate transporter 8 (MCT8) gene.** *Am J Hum Genet* 2005, **77**:41-53.
23. Vaurs-Barriere C, Deville M, Sarret C, Giraud G, Des Portes V, Prats-Vinas JM, De Michele G, Dan B, Brady AF, Boespflug-Tanguy O, Touraine R: **Pelizaeus-Merzbacher-Like disease presentation of MCT8 mutated male subjects.** *Ann Neurol* 2009, **65**:114-118.
24. Raymond L, Whibley A, Price S, Rosser E, Rahman N, Holder S, Stewart F, RTarpey P, Futreal A, Stratton M, Gold I: **Barcelona.** *ESHG2008* 2008.
25. Papadimitriou A, Dumitrescu AM, Papavasiliou A, Fretzayas A, Nicolaidou P, Refetoff S: **A novel monocarboxylate transporter 8 gene mutation as a cause of severe neonatal hypotonia and developmental delay.** *Pediatrics* 2008, **121**:e199-202.
26. Frints SG, Lenzner S, Bauters M, Jensen LR, Van Esch H, des Portes V, Moog U, Macville MV, van Roozendaal K, Schrander-Stumpel CT, *et al*: **MCT8 mutation analysis and identification of the first female with Allan-Herndon-Dudley syndrome due to loss of MCT8 expression.** *Eur J Hum Genet* 2008, **16**:1029-1037.
27. Visser WE, Jansen J, Friesema EC, Kester MH, Mancilla E, Lundgren J, van der Knaap MS, Lunsing RJ, Brouwer OF, Visser TJ: **Novel pathogenic mechanism suggested by ex vivo analysis of MCT8 (SLC16A2) mutations.** *Hum Mutat* 2009, **30**:29-38.

# 28

# Presentation of points of general discussion and voting among the speakers of the European Thyroid Association-Cancer Research Network (ETA-CRN) meeting in Lisbon, 2009, entitled "European comments to ATA medullary thyroid cancer guidelines"

Barbara Jarząb*, Aleksandra Król, Kornelia Hasse-Lazar, Beata Jurecka-Lubieniecka

*From* 9th Meeting of the European Thyroid Association Cancer Research Network (ETA-CRN)
Lisbon, Portugal.

**Abstract**

The main subjects of discussion, held online within the ETA-CRN board invited 16 expert-panelists are shown. The ad hoc emerged ETA-CRN panel of experts (EPE) first congratulated Professor Kloos and the ATA Taskforce for the extensive work on medullary thyroid cancer, and appreciated discussing the ATA guidelines during the ETA-CRN meeting. As it was not possible for all experts to visit the meeting, they enclosed their comments in the online ETA forum. The overall intention was to evaluate certain discrepancies between the ATA guidelines and were biased European clinical practice.

All discussants were aware that the ATA guidelines had followed evidence based medicine rules; however, it was intended to reach an European consensus in this matter. The results of online voting among the EPE are shown. We received answers from nine experts. The particular ATA guidelines devoted to the management of MTC ranged in agreement in 0/9 to 4/9. This did not reflect the general, good assessment of the guidelines, as of votes a set of questions.

The strongest discrepancies were found in assessment of the usefulness of pentagastrin (Peptavlon®) stimulated calcitonin secretion. The majority of the EPE (5/9) chose an option: "the increase of the basal Ct >100 ng/L means the substantial risk of MTC. However, there should also have been a recommendation for the grey zone 10-100 ng/L, where stimulation with pentagastrin is useful. The cut-off to perform stimulation test at ≤ 15-20 ng/L and values >100 ng/L means a significant suspicion of MTC".

Similarly, attention from the EPE was raised towards the surgical procedures in MTC, particularly the extent and indications for lymph node surgical intervention. Four questions were related to the indications to lymphadenectomy and extent of surgery. The equal number (4/8) of EPE agreed with the ATA R61 and half of the ETA-CRN panel of experts disagreed because the indications to lymphadenectomy (Lx) depended in their opinion on the tumors detected by the Ct screening, in which prophylactic Lx might not be necessary.

"Notwithstanding the evidence based guidelines, their final acceptation requires unrestricted discussion and consideration of differences in clinical practice and experience between countries".

* Correspondence: bjarzab@io.gliwice.pl
Department of Nuclear Medicine and Endocrine Oncology, Maria Sklodowska-Curie Memorial Cancer Center and Institute of Oncology, Gliwice Branch, Wybrzeze Armii Krajowej 15, 44-101 Gliwice, Poland

## Introduction

The ATA (American Thyroid Association) MTC Guidelines published 2009 [1] raised a vivid discussion in Europe. This important paper constituted a stimulus for ETA (European Thyroid Association) members to arrange the ETA-CRN (ETA- Cancer Research Network) Meeting in Lisbon to discuss it.

The *ad hoc* emerged ETA-CRN panel of experts (EPE) first congratulated Professor R. Kloos and the ATA Taskforce for the extensive work on medullary thyroid cancer, reflected into the ATA guidelines and appreciated discussing these guidelines during the ETA-CRN meeting. As it was not possible for all experts to visit the meeting, the online ETA forum had been arranged and many ETA members enclosed their comments in the online ETA forum [2].

This paper summarizes the main subjects of discussion, shown in Additional files 1 and 2. The ETA-CRN board invited 16 expert-panelists to answer the questions which were formulated during the online discussion, on the basis of their experience and to comment on them during the ETA-CRN Meeting in Lisbon. All discussants were aware that the ATA guidelines had followed evidence based medicine rules; however, the online discussion was showed, because the guidelines required extensive changes of routine European clinical practice and it was intended to reach a European consensus in this matter. We received answers from nine experts.

As the reader may judge from Additional file 1, which was focused on management of MTC, the ETA-CRN panelists accepted the particular ATA guidelines devoted to the management from 0/9 to 4/9. This did not reflect the general, good assessment of the guidelines, as of votes a set of questions. The overall intention was to evaluate certain discrepancies between the ATA guidelines and were biased European clinical practice.

## Management of MTC

It was understood that the part of ATA Guidelines, described in Additional file 1, Table 1, considered rules of diagnosis and treatment of MTC, which were not different in management of sporadic and hereditary disease.

First, there was a discrepancy in the opinion on the reference range of basal calcitonin (Ct) level. The ATA Guideline R30 recommended that "In the setting of an intact thyroid gland, Ct values should be interpreted in the setting of sex-specific reference ranges, at least in adults (Grade: B) " [1], while the majority (6/9) of ETA-CRN panel of experts preferred to have one Ct reference range (Q1 option A), with normal Ct basal values ≤ 10 ng/l, despite being aware of sex-related differences.

Question 2 was related to ATA Guideline R52 which commented the usefulness of serum calcitonin estimation at the early diagnosis of MTC. This was an issue commented also in this Thyroid Research Supplement by Rosella Elisei and Cristina Romei [3]. The majority of European experts (5/9) agreed on the need for obligatory Ct estimation in nodular goiter and confirmed to perform that test. This was an expected discrepancy because the European consensus [4] on thyroid cancer recommended serum calcitonin measurement.

It seems, the strongest discrepancies were found in assessment of the usefulness of pentagastrin (Peptavlon®) stimulated calcitonin secretion. Thus, the ETA-CRN panel of experts did not agree on question 3, which was referring to Recommendation 52 (R52). "R52 defines a basal or stimulated serum Ct level > 100 ng/L, which should be interpreted as suspicious for MTC needing further evaluation if obtained". This ATA guideline was supported in its full extent (option A) by one of the experts. The majority of the experts (5/9) chose option B: "Indeed, the increase of the basal Ct is >100 ng/L means the substantial risk of MTC. However, we should also have a recommendation for the grey zone 10-100 ng/L, and here the stimulation with pentagastrin is useful. The cut-off to perform stimulation test at ≤ 15-20 ng/L and values >100 ng/L means a significant suspicion of MTC. According to Scheuba et al. [5-9], the risk of MTC was 20% at a stimulated Ct>200 ng/L". It is important to comment that these cut-offs were not valid for hereditary MTC but for sporadic cancer patients. The remaining 3/9 panelists agreed with the above statement but preferred to set the cut-off for stimulated Ct at 50 ng/L (Option C).

Similarly, the attention of the European experts were raised towards the surgical procedures in MTC recommended by ATA [1], particularly the extent and indications for lymph node surgical intervention. As seen from Additional file 1, questions Q4-Q8 were related to the indications to lymphadenectomy and extent of thyroid surgery (ATA Recommendations R61, 62, 66).

Among ETA-CRN panel of experts, the opinions were not unanimous. The equal number (4/8) agreed with the ATA R61 which stated that "Patients with known or highly suspected MTC with no evidence of advanced local invasion by the primary tumor, no evidence cervical lymph node metastases on physical examination and cervical US, and no evidence of distant metastases should undergo total thyroidectomy and prophylactic central compartment (level VI) neck dissection" and half of the ETA-CRN panel of experts disagreed because they stressed that the indications to lymphadenectomy (Lx) depended in their opinion on the tumors detected by the Ct screening, in which prophylactic Lx might not be necessary. Similar discrepancy within EPE was observed at the response to the Question 5, which was related to the ATA R59. Four from eight EPE agreed with the ATA Guideline and 4/8 chose the statement of Machens and

Dralle [10] that liver Ct/ contrast enhanced MRI are necessary only when serum Ct> 1000 – 2000 pg/ml equal to 1000 – 2000 ng/L, because only then, the risk of distant dissemination is substantial.

The question Q6 (Additional file 1) referred to the indications to elective Lx in MTC. The ATA R62 states that if lymph node metastases are not detected by ultrasound, the elective (it means prophylactic) lateral Lx is not necessary. There was an important addition that a minority of the ATA Taskforce had favored prophylactic neck dissection when lymph node metastases were present in the adjacent paratracheal central compartment. There was also a minority (2/9) among the ETA-CRN panel of experts who expressed opinion (Q6 opinion A) "If no enlarged lymph node are detected, elective lateral lymph node dissection is not obligatory in MTC, irrespective of the status of the central neck lymph node". However, the half of EPE (4/8) chose option B: "If no enlarged LN were detected, elective lateral lymph node dissection should be performed when lymph node metastases were present in the adjacent paratracheal central compartment" and the minority (2/8) of ETA-CRN panel of experts chose option C: "Elective lymph node dissection is obligatory in MTC, irrespective of the status of central neck lymph nodes"– one expert stressed it by the sentence "we perform bilateral neck dissection irrespective the lymph node status (skip lesion, micrometastases)". Further, at question Q7, the ATA R66 stated that "in patients with extensive distant metastases a palliative neck operation might still be needed when there was pain, or evidence of tracheal compromise and the need to maintain a safe airway. They added also "Otherwise, in the setting of moderate to high volume extracervical disease, neck disease may be observed and surgery deferred. The ATA Task force opinion was not unanimous and the same was observed among ETA-CRN panel of experts: 2 of 9 of them chose option A, it means they had agreed with the deferral of local surgery in the setting of moderate to high volume extracervical MTC. The majority of ETA-CRN panel of experts (7/9) chose option B – they disagreed with the deferral of local surgery in the setting of moderate to high volume extracervical MTC.

The question Q8 (Additional file 1) referred to the indications to completion thyroidectomy (Tx) ATA R70-72. Two of eight European experts chose the option A: completion "is always indicated after unexpected diagnosis of MTC post less than total Tx, independently from MTC stage and should be completed by appropriate lymph node operation (at least central lymph node dissection, even if postoperative Ct is normal". However, one of the expert surgeons added that completion Tx was always dependent on the basal/ stimulated Ct levels and genetic status and not on morphology. In a different spirit 4/8 experts chose option C: "Indications depend on the size of the primary tumors. The conditions listed in B may be valid only if solitary infracentimetric MTC was found". And option B: "As proposed in ATA R70-71, completion thyroidectomy may be postponed after hemithyroidectomy, if unifocal intrathyroidal sporadic MTC was diagnosed, confined to the thyroid if no C-cell hyperplasia, negative surgical margin, and no suspicion for persistent disease on neck US and the basal serum Ct is below the upper normal of the reference range more than 2 months after surgery" was chosen by 2/8 experts.

The postoperative follow-up was discussed also in terms of usefulness of basal versus stimulated Ct estimation (Additional file 1, Question 9). Two of eight European experts were of the opinion that only basal Ct should be measured as the result of postoperative pentagastrin test does not usually modify the follow-up strategy when basal calcitonin is low. 4/9 chose option B, recommending rather stimulated Ct as more sensitive and 5/9 chose option C (one expert chose simultaneously option B and C). The option C was a compromise between radical options A and B and recommended the pentagastrin test at least at first postoperative evaluation if basal Ct was low to confirm the full success of the operation. It was explained that patients with normal basal, but increased stimulated Ct did not require additional treatment however, they might not be regarded as completely free of disease and required more cautious monitoring. Finally, in the postoperative follow-up, the high sensitivity of Ct testing was related to the difficulties in the localization of the persistent or recurrent disease, especially if Ct level was only moderately increased.

In question Q10 the European experts evaluated the ATA R75, which proposed the cut-off < 150 pg/ml (equal to <150 ng/L), below which the postoperative imaging might be limited to sonography only. Three of nine experts had agreed with the ATA recommendation R75 (Q10, option A). Six of nine ones preferred R76, which stated that post-operative MTC patients with detectable serum Ct levels < 150 ng/L might be considered for additional imaging with Ct or MRI to serve as baseline examinations for future comparison even though these studies were usually negative.

## Hereditary MTC

The other part of online discussion was related to the ATA Guidelines that were devoted to the issues of hereditary MTC, meaning indications to RET genetic diagnostics and treatment of RET mutations carriers.

The EPE consultations were reflected in Additional file 2. The indications for RET testing in patients with primary C cell hyperplasia, contained in the ATA R1, was accepted by 5/9 European experts Additional file 2; Question 20, option A) while the other 4/9 protested, because the risk of finding RET mutations in a C cell hyperplasia patient was assumed to be low.

Also, there has been a discussion on the early symptoms of MEN 2B (Question 21). Three of nine experts accepted the ATA R2, which recommended RET testing in cases of intestinal gangliomatosis (option A), while the majority (6/9) chose option C: "Both bumpy lips with mucosal neuromas and corneal fibres should be also considered. Thickening of corneal fibres is very frequent, with a prevalence of 69% in MEN 2B [11] and 29% in MEN 2A [12]". Tearless crying of small children was not accepted as an indication for RET testing without any other MEN 2 symptoms by 7/9 experts because they needed more evidence (Question 22, option C). However, they found this sign worth mentioning in the European comments to ATA MTC Guidelines.

The ATA R4 recommended RET testing in cases of lichen planus and it was accepted by 5/9 EPE (Question 23, Option A). In fact, further 2/9 experts did not intend to propose a change in ATA R4 recommendation (option C). The R6-R8 Guidelines recommended the ATA risk classes and this new subdivision was accepted by nearly all experts (8/9), but 7 of 9 preferred option B and stressed the necessity to comment it ("To include Ct levels into decision making seems mandatory"). One of the experts argued for a statement to discourage delayed thyroid surgery in RET mutation carriers and this statement was supported by a letter by the Dutch experts [2] (please visit: http://eta-crn.eurothyroid.com for the further reference).

This discussion, encompassed by questions 25-28 has been reflected in a separate article in this Thyroid Research Supplement [13]. The problem of indications to RET testing has been widened by the question of Hirschprung disease (see question 30, Additional file 2). The ATA R10 recommended to consider RET testing in all patients with Hirschprung disease and it was supported by 2 of 9 EPE (Additional file 2, Question 30, option A.). However, the majority of ETA-CRN panel of experts (5/9) chose option B: "Hirschsprung disease (HD) is very common (about 1/5000 births) and at least 10 related genes have been identified. Activating RET mutations have been found in exons 10 and 11 only in in about 2% of cases [14] and this prevalence is too low to recommend the testing as grade A recommendation".

Questions Q31-Q32 were devoted to the problem of extent of DNA testing. The ATA R11 recommended it either a single or multicentered approach and this was supported by 1 of 9 ETA-CRN panel of experts. The majority (5/9) chose option B: "Systematic screening for RET mutations in exon 10, 11, 13, 14, 15, and 16 represents the current gold standard and should be completed by exon 8 analysis in all regions where it was described to be present" while 2/9 meant testing of RET exon 8 as unnecessary in routine DNA diagnosis, as in fact, ATA R11 proposed.

It was also the intention of ETA-CRN panel of experts to widen the discussion by the problem of RET polymorphisms (Additional file 2, Question 33) which was missed by ATA Guidelines. However, the majority of experts 7/9 were of opinion that the data on RET polymorphism are still insufficient to draw any conclusion (option B) and supported the ATA Task force view.

The question of surgical management of RET carriers is reflected in Additional file 2 (Questions Q33, Q35, Q36). The conclusions of the discussion may be summarized in the " both DNA and calcitonin level" concept [10].

## Conclusion

These data serve to illustrate the European consensus on acceptation of ATA MTC Guidelines. The conclusion from the "Result and summary of voting among the audience during presentation and discussion of Medullary Thyroid Carcinoma Clinical Guidelines prepared by American Thyroid Association" [15] should be cited:

"European expert opinion leaders and an audience of specialist in treatment of Medullary Carcinoma welcomes the American Guidelines on the management of MTC, but simultaneously only partially agrees with some of the expert statements. The results of the survey prior to the meeting were biased in that the presenters were selected for presenting the results, but the audience was present upon open invitation through scientific channels. Notwithstanding the evidence based guidelines, their final acceptation requires unrestricted discussion and consideration of differences in clinical practice and experience between countries. These discussion and results subsequently formed the basis for establishing a task force within the ETA, and consequent publication of European guideline mainly for the treatment aspects of metastatic MTC."

#### Competing interests

No competing interests exist for the authors.

#### Declarations

This article has been published as part of *Thyroid Research* Volume 6 Supplement 1, 2013: European comments on Medullary Thyroid Cancer Management Guidelines of the American Thyroid Association. The full contents of the supplement are available online at http://www.thyroidresearchjournal.com/supplements/6/S1. Publication of this supplement has been supported by the European Thyroid Association-Cancer Research Network.

## References


1. American Thyroid Association Guidelines Task Force, Kloos RT, Eng C, Evans DB, Francis GL, Gagel RF, Gharib H, Moley JF, Pacini F, Ringel MD, Schlumberger M, Wells SA Jr: **Medullary thyroid cancer: management guidelines of the American Thyroid Association.** *Thyroid* 2009, **19(6)**:565-612.
2. **ETA-CRN.** [http://eta-crn.eurothyroid.com/meeting_2009.php].
3. Elisei R, Romei C: **Calcitonin estimation in patients with nodular goiter and its significance for early detection of MTC.** *Thyroid Research* 2013, 6(Suppl 1):S2.
4. Pacini F, Schlumberger M, Dralle H, Elisei R, Smit JW, Wiersinga W: **European Thyroid Cancer Taskforce. European consensus for the management of patients with differentiated thyroid carcinoma of the follicular epithelium.** *Eur J Endocrinol* 2006, **154(6)**:787-803.
5. Scheuba C, Kaserer K, Weinhausl A, Pandev R, Kaider A, Passler C, Prager G, Vierhapper H, Haas OA, Niederle B: **Is medullary thyroid cancer predictable? A prospective study of 86 patients with abnormal pentagastrin tests.** *Surgery* 1999, **126**:1089-96.
6. Scheuba C, Kaserer K, Moritz A, Drosten R, Vierhapper H, Bieglmeyer C, Haas OA, Niederle B: **Sporadic hypercalcitoninemia: clinical and therapeutic consequences.** *Endocrine Related Cancer* 2009, **26**:243-253.
7. Scheuba C, Bieglmayer C, Asari R, Kaczirek K, Izay B, Kaserer K, Niederle B: **The value of intraoperative pentagastrin testing in medullary thyroid cancer.** *Surgery* 2007, **141**:166-171.
8. Kaserer K, Scheuba C, Neuhold N, Weinhausel A, Haas O, Vierhapper H, Niederle B: **Sporadic versus familial medullary thyroid microcarcinoma: a histopatological study of 50 consecutive patients.** *Am J Surg Pathol* 2001, **25(10)**:124-1251.
9. Scheuba C, Kaserer K, Bieglmayer C, Asari R, Riss P, Drosten R, Niederle B: **Medullary thyroid microcarcinoma recommendations for treatment - a single-center experience.** *Surgery* 2007, **142**:1003-1010, discussion 1010 e1001–1003.
10. Machens A, Dralle H: **Prophylactic thyroidectomy in RET carriers at risk for hereditary medullary thyroid cancer.** *Thyroid* 2009, **19(6)**:551-554.
11. Vasen HF, van der Feltz M, Raue F, Kruseman AN, Koppeschaar HP, Pieters G, Seif FJ, Blum WF, Lips CJ: **The natural course of multiple endocrine neoplasia type IIb. A study of 18 cases.** *Arch Intern Med* 1992, **152(6)**:1250-2.
12. Kinoshita S, Tanaka F, Ohashi Y, Ikeda M, Takai S: **Incidence of prominent corneal nerves in multiple endocrine neoplasia type 2A.** *Am J Ophthalmol* 1991, **111(3)**:307-11.
13. Jarzab B, Szpak-Ulczok S, Krajewska J, Wloch J: **Timing and criteria for prophylactic thyroidectomy in asymptomatic *RET* carriers – the role of Ct serum level.** *Thyroid Research Suppl* 2013, **6(Suppl 1)**:S9.
14. Amiel J, Sproat-Emison E, Garcia-Barcelo M, Lantieri F, Burzynski G, Borrego S, Pelet A, Arnold S, Miao X, Griseri P, Brooks AS, Antinolo G, de Pontual L, Clement-Ziza M, Munnich A, Kashuk C, West K, Wong KK, Lyonnet S, Chakravarti A, Tam PK, Ceccherini I, Hofstra RM, Fernandez R: **Hirschsprung Disease Consortium: Hirschsprung disease, associated syndromes and genetics: a review.** *J Med Genet* 2008, **45(1)**:1-14.
15. Feldt-Rasmussen U, Soderstrom F: **Result and summary of voting among audience during presentation and discussion of Medullary Thyroid Carcinoma Clinical Guidelines prepared by American Thyroid Association.** *Thyroid Research Suppl* 2013, **6(Suppl 1)**:S12.
16. Brauckhoff M, Machens A, Hess S, Lorenz K, Gimm O, Brauckhoff K, Sekulla C, Dralle H: **Premonitory symptoms preceding metastatic medullary thyroid cancer in MEN 2B: An exploratory analysis.** *Surgery* 2008, **144(6)**:1044-50.
17. Verga U, Fugazzola L, Cambiaghi S, Pritelli C, Alessi E, Cortelazzi D, Gangi E, Beck-Peccoz P: **Frequent association between MEN 2A and cutaneous lichen amyloidosis.** *Clin Endocrinol (Oxf)* 2003, **59(2)**:156-61.
18. Rothberg AE, Raymond VM, Gruber SB, Sisson J: **Familial medullary thyroid carcinoma associated with cutaneous lichen amyloidosis.** *Thyroid* 2009, **19(6)**:651-5.
19. Brandi ML, Gagel RF, Angeli A, Bilezikian JP, Beck-Peccoz P, Bordi C, Conte-Devolx B, Falchetti A, Gheri RG, Libroia A, Lips CJ, Lombardi G, Mannelli M, Pacini F, Ponder BA, Raue F, Skogseid B, Tamburrano G, Thakker RV, Thompson NW, Tomassetti P, Tonelli F, Wells SA Jr, Marx SJ: **Guidelines for diagnosis and therapy of MEN type 1 and type 2.** *J Clin Endocrinol Metab* 2001, **86(12)**:5658-71.

# 29

# Gender-specific regulation of response to thyroid hormone in aging

Satoru Suzuki*, Shin-ichi Nishio, Teiji Takeda and Mitsuhisa Komatsu

**Abstract**

**Background:** Similar to other systems, the endocrine system is affected by aging. Thyroid hormone, the action of which is affected by many factors, has been shown to be associated with longevity. The most useful marker for the assessment of thyroid hormone action is TSH level. Although age and gender are believed to modify the pituitary set point or response to free thyroid hormone concentration, the precise age- and gender-dependent responses to thyroid hormone have yet to be reported.

**Methods:** We analyzed the results of 3564 thyroid function tests obtained from patients who received medication at both out- and inpatient clinics of Shinshu University Hospital. Subjects were from among those with thyroid function test results in the normal or mildly abnormal range. Based on a log-linear relationship between the concentrations of FHs and TSH, we established the putative resistance index to assess the relation between serum FH and TSH levels.

**Results:** Free thyroid hormone and TSH concentration showed an inverse log-linear relation. In males, there was a negative relationship between the free T3 resistance index and age. In females, although there were no relationships between age and FHs, the indices were positively related to age.

**Conclusions:** These findings indicated that there is a gender-specific response to thyroid hormone with aging. Although the TSH level is a useful marker for the assessment of peripheral thyroid hormone action, the values should be interpreted carefully, especially with regard to age- and gender-related differences.

**Keywords:** thyroid hormone, TSH, aging

## Introduction

In common with other systems, the endocrine system is affected by aging. With regard to thyroid hormone, age modifies the pituitary set point or response to comparably reduced free T4 (FT4) concentrations, resulting in lesser serum TSH elevation in older individuals [1]. TSH is suppressed in elderly subjects [2]. The decreased thyroid hormone levels observed in aging are due to lower TSH concentrations [3]. Centenarians exhibit significantly lower TSH levels together with slightly higher reverse T3 levels than aged controls [4]. In contrast to several reports on the association between low TSH level and senescence, heritable longevity has been reported to be associated with high serum TSH and low free T4 levels [5]. Exceptional longevity is associated with raised serum TSH [6,7]. Thus, the relation between the level of TSH and lifespan is controversial.

TSH concentration is higher in women than in men [8]. TSH daily profiling demonstrated that TSH secretion depends on age in women only [9]. These reports suggest that thyroid hormone function, especially TSH level, may be associated with gender differences.

Both T3 and T4 are often loosely referred to as thyroid hormones, although T3 alone has biological thyromimetic activity at the genomic level. The ratio of serum FT3 concentration to FT4 concentration, [FT3]/[FT4] index, is a useful indicator to assess the peripheral metabolism of thyroid hormone, as the index is affected by the magnitude of the conversion of FT4 to FT3 or of the transport of T4 into T3-producing tissues [10].

Serum concentration of thyroid hormone is inversely related to TSH concentration. Although the serum

* Correspondence: suzukis@shinshu-u.ac.jp
Department of Aging Medicine and Geriatrics, Institute on Aging and Adaptation, Shinshu University, Graduate School of Medicine, 3-1-1, Asahi, Matsumoto, 390-8621, Japan

concentration reflects the action of thyroid hormone in cells, clinical manifestations of thyroid hormone action are occasionally not related to the serum hormone concentration. For example, we observe low FT3 concentrations in patients with severe disorders or infection, *i.e.*, *low* T3 syndrome. Moreover, molecular studies have strongly suggested that the nuclear action of thyroid hormone may be affected by numerous factors. MCT8 is a specific transporter of T3 [11]. μ-crystallin is a cytoplasmic thyroid hormone binding protein within cells, which may also affect the action of thyroid hormone [12]. Phosphodiesterase 8B gene variants are associated with serum TSH levels and thyroid function [13]. Molecules that affect the transcriptional machinery also alter the response to thyroid hormone [14]. Taken together, these clinical and molecular findings suggest that factors responsible for the action of thyroid hormone except for thyroid hormone itself are present *in vivo*. The pathophysiological alteration may manifest thyroid hormone resistance, similar to the insulin resistance in diabetic or obese patients.

Free hormones (FHs) are undoubtedly the strongest factors that affect the regulation of TSH expression. There is a log-linear relationship between free thyroxin and TSH over a wide concentration range [15]. Although the resistance factors affect the regulation of TSH secretion, these effects may be diminished in the severe hyper- or hypothyroid state. That is, if the resistance factors exist, these factors may be clearly observed in euthyroid or moderate hyper- and hypothyroid states.

Based on these speculations, we selected data with TSH from 0.04 to 9.99 μIU/ml and FT4 from 0.52 to 2.1 ng/dl. We established the putative resistance index obtained from the serum concentration of thyroid hormone and TSH, and investigated the existence of age- and gender-related factors that affect thyroid hormone resistance. In addition, we discuss the physiological mechanisms of gender-specific and age-oriented thyroid hormone resistance.

## Materials and methods

### Subjects

A total of 1026 male and 2538 female (median age 44 years, range 15 - 92 years) subjects were included in this study. All patients were referred to in- or outpatient clinics of Shinshu University Hospital from January 2004 to January 2005 due to suspected thyroid disease or to receive treatment for various thyroid diseases, including Graves' disease, autoimmune and non-immunogenic thyroiditis, benign diffuse and nodular goiter, and thyroid malignancies. This study was approved by the Ethical Committee of Shinshu University (reference number 818).

### Laboratory methods

Standard laboratory quality evaluation procedures were routinely employed, and regular participation at inter-laboratory tests was also part of the quality management strategy. Inter- and intraassay coefficients of variation were 2.2 and 0.8% for TSH, 4.5 and 1.8% for FT3, 4.6 and 1.3% for FT4, respectively.

### Statistical analysis

For pairs of continuous variables, scatter plots were constructed to visually display the respective relations. If found to be linear with both variables showing a normal distribution, Pearson's correlation was computed to statistically describe the significance, strength, and nature of the relation using SPSS version 18. In the age distribution, statistical significance was determined by *Kruskal-Wallis* followed by the *Games-Howell* multiple comparison test. $P$ values $\geq 0.05$ were considered not significant.

## Results

### Characteristics of the study population

To select the normal and subnormal regulation of thyroid hormone and TSH, we omitted data from subjects with serum TSH concentration ([TSH]) less than 0.04 μIU/ml and greater than 9.99 μIU/ml. We also omitted data from those with serum FT4 concentration ([FT4]) less than 6.7 pM (0.52 ng/dl) and greater than 27.0 pM (2.1 ng/dl). The adopted range was mean ± 2 *S.D.* as shown in Figure 1a. A total of 735 male and 1721 female subjects were included in the analysis. The detailed characteristics of the study population are shown in Table 1.

### Organization of a resistance index

As shown in Figure 1b, the data in this study showed a log-linear relationship between FT4 and TSH (log[TSH] = 1.729 - 0.09[FT4], $P < 0.001$). The linear regression line also showed a good fit to the data points obtained from FT3 and log [TSH] (log[TSH] = 0.429 - 0.034[FT3] $P$ = 0.02). We can express the relation between log[TSH] and the concentration of a free hormone [FH] as follows:

$$\log[\mathrm{TSH}] = \mathrm{b} - \mathrm{a}[\mathrm{FH}]\ (\mathrm{a, b;\ any\ positive\ number})$$

To simplify the equation, we set a = 1:

$$\log[\mathrm{TSH}] = \mathrm{b} - [\mathrm{FH}]$$

We would express a conventional resistance index (Rconv) as follows:

$$\mathrm{Rconv} = [\mathrm{FH}] + \log[\mathrm{TSH}]$$

To be equivalent to the strength of each factor, such as [FH] and log[TSH], we converted each factor to a value ranging from 0 to 1 as follows:

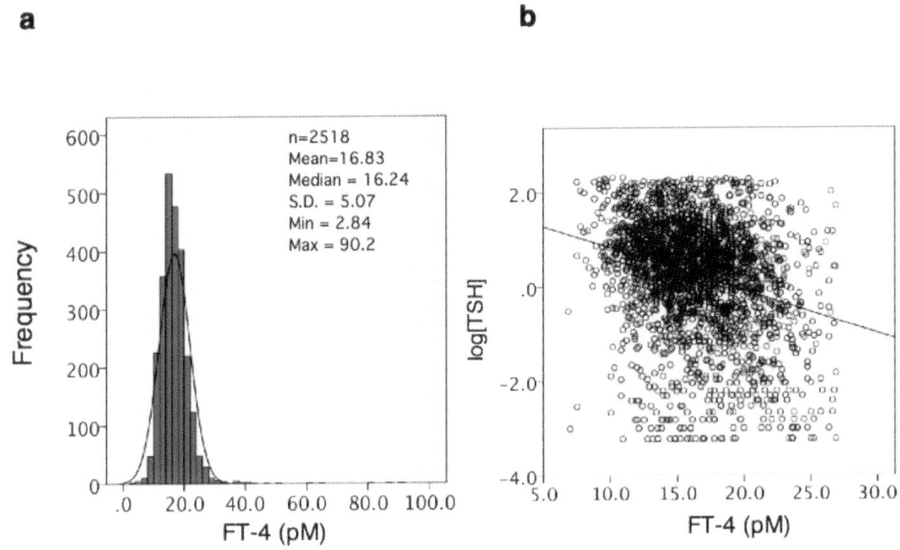


**Figure 1 Frequency distribution of serum free T4 concentration and log-linear relationship of the serum concentration between of free T4 and of TSH in this study**. (a) Frequency distribution of serum free T4 concentration. The gray column represents 2519 samples with TSH ranging from 0.04 to 9.99 selected from the total of 3564 samples. (b) The relationship between [FT4] and log[TSH]. The line represents the linear regression fitted to the data points using SPSS software.

**Table 1 Clinical characteristics of the study population**

| Characteristics | male $n = 735$ | female $n = 1721$ |
|---|---|---|
| Age - years | | |
| Mean ± SD | 46.94 ± 16.24 | 44.05 ± 17.0 |
| Range | 15 - 84 | 15 - 82 |
| Free T3 - pM | | |
| Mean ± SD | 5.91 ± 1.7 | 5.36 ± 1.55 |
| Range | 1.38 - 9.97 | 0.84 - 9.85 |
| Free T4 - pM | | |
| Mean ± SD | 16.85 ± 3.81 | 16.3 ± 3.51 |
| Range | 6.96 - 26.9 | 6.83 - 26.9 |
| TSH - μIU/ml | | |
| Mean ± SD | 2.44 ± 2.14 | 1.99 ± 1.91 |
| Range | 0.04 - 9.99 | 0.04 - 9.95 |
| log [TSH] | | |
| Mean ± SD | 0.464 ± 1.06 | 0.142 ± 1.21 |
| Range | -3.21 - 2.30 | -3.21 - 2.30 |
| ResT3 | | |
| Mean ± SD | 1.22 ± 0.26 | 1.10 ± 0.27 |
| Range | 0.27 - 1.90 | 0.24 - 1.91 |
| ResT4 | | |
| Mean ± SD | 1.16 ± 0.25 | 1.08 ± 0.23 |
| Range | 0.05 - 1.78 | 0.16 - 1.93 |
| [FT3]/[FT4] | | |
| Mean ± SD | 0.37 ± 0.13 | 0.34 ± 0.12 |
| Range | 0.11 - 0.84 | 0.06 - 0.98 |

Res: resistance index

$$R = ([FH] - [FH]_{min}) / ([FH]_{max} - [FH]_{min}) + (\log[TSH] - \log[TSH]_{min}) / (\log[TSH]_{max} - \log[TSH]_{min})$$

In this study,

$[FT3]_{max} = 9.97pM$, $[FT3]_{min} = 0.84pM$, $[FT4]_{max} = 26.93pM$, $[FT4]_{min} = 6.83pM$, $\log[TSH]_{max} = 2.3$ $\log[TSH]_{min} = -3.22$.

Thus, the T3 resistance index (ResT3) and T4 resistance index (ResT4) were defined as follows:

$$ResT3 = ([FT3] - 0.84)/9.13 + (\log[TSH] + 3.22)/5.52$$
$$ResT4 = ([FT4] - 6.83)/20.1 + (\log[TSH] + 3.22)/5.52$$

#### Concentration of free thyroid hormone and resistance indices were decreased with aging in males

We performed linear regression analysis between age and concentrations of free T3, T4, and TSH, values of log [TSH], both resistance indices and the [FT3]/[FT4] index. In males, the concentrations of FHs were negatively related to aging, while the TSH level was not (Figure 2a, b and 2c, Table 2). Both resistance indices decreased significantly with age (Figure 2d and 2e). The [FT3]/[FT4] index decreased significantly (Figure 2f, Table 2).

#### In females, the free thyroid hormone concentration was not altered by aging, but the TSH level increased in an age-dependent manner

We plotted the values of a series of thyroid hormone indices *vs.* age in females. There were no relationships between the concentrations of both FHs and age (Figure 3a and 3b, Table 2). TSH level was significantly

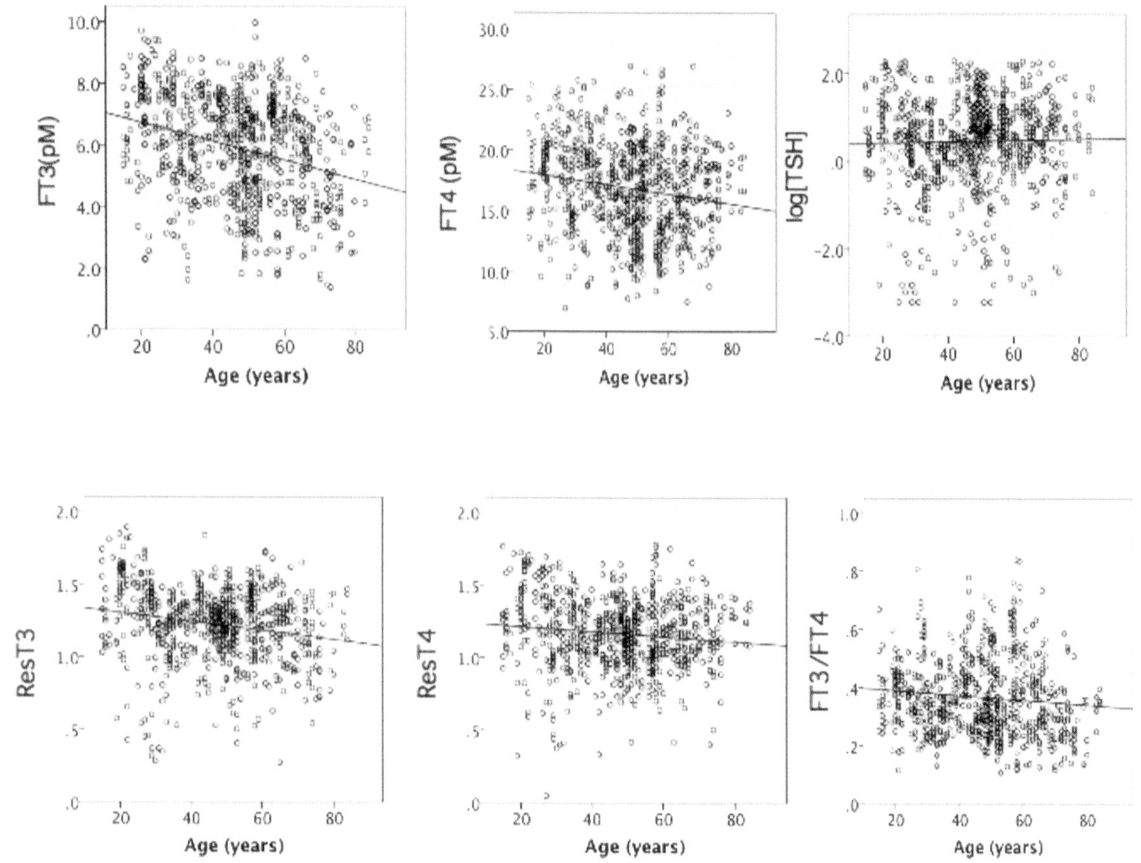


**Figure 2 The relationship between age versus the concentration of FT3 (a), FT4 (b), log[TSH] (c), ResT3 (d), ResT4 (e) and [FT3]/[FT4] index(f) in male subjects.** The line represents the linear regression fitted to the data points calculated by SPSS software.

increased (Figure 3c). Both resistance indices increased with age (Figure 3d and 3e). The [FT3]/[FT4] index did not change significantly with age (Figure 3f).

### Gender-specific differences in resistance indices in the age distribution

According to our mathematical model, the age-dependent distribution revealed a specific pattern in both male and female subjects. As shown in Figure 4a, the mean values of the T3 index decreased in the age group from 15 - 24 to 25 - 34, and then increased slightly in the 25 - 64 age groups in males. The value decreased again over the 55 - 64 age group in males. The mean values of the T3 index increased gradually between the 35 - 44 and 55 - 64 age groups in females. Although there was no statistical significance, the values were decreased in females over 65.

On the other hand, the mean values of the T4 index were reduced in males between 15 - 24 and 25 - 34 (Figure 4b). The values were constant over the 25 - 34 age group. In females, the mean values of the T4 index initially decreased between 15 - 24 and 25 - 34. The values increased gradually over the 25 - 34 age group except in the 65 - 74 and 75 - 84 age groups. The mean values of the [FT3]/[FT4] index decreased in males in the 65 - 74 and 75 - 84 age groups, while the value remained constant in females (Figure 4c). The statistical differences were shown in Table 3.

**Table 2 Spearman's rank correlation coefficient between age and various thyroid hormone indices**

| *vs.* Age | male $n = 735$ | female $n = 1721$ |
|---|---|---|
| Free T3 | -0.292 (0.001>)** | -0.033 (0.174) |
| Free T4 | -0.170 (0.001>)** | 0.014 (0.573) |
| TSH | -0.042 (0.255) | 0.138 (0.001>)** |
| log[TSH] | 0.022(0.548) | 0.099 (0.001>)** |
| ResT3 | -0.194 (0.001>)** | 0.061 (0.012)* |
| ResT4 | -0.111 (0.003)** | 0.106 (0.001>)** |
| FreeT3/FreeT4 | -0.102 (0.006)** | -0.025 (0.298) |

Res: resistance index Parentheses show *P*-values. $^{*}P < 0.05$, $^{**}P < 0.01$.

## Discussion

In this study, we selected the cases with normal or subnormal thyroid function. Despite the narrow range of the study population, an inverse log-linear relation

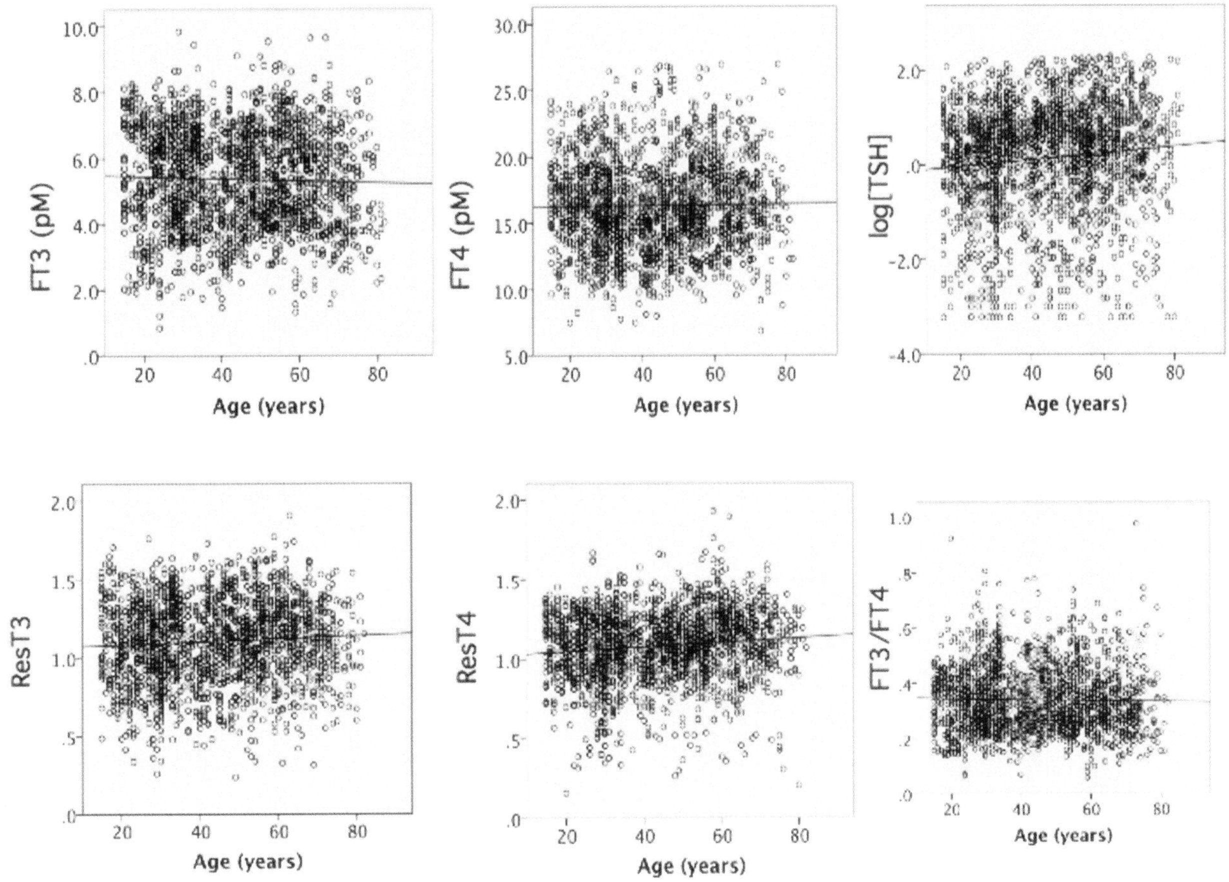


**Figure 3 Relationships between age and the concentration of FT3 (a), FT4 (b), log[TSH] (c), ResT3 (d), ResT4 (e), and [FT3]/[FT4] index (f) in female subjects**. The line represents the linear regression fitted to the data points calculated using SPSS software.

between FH and TSH was observed as described previously [16]. Benhadi *et al.* denoted the straight line as the set point of the hypothalamus-pituitary-thyroid axis [17]. The set point was probably affected by many factors, including genetic and environmental factors.

In this study, when we include the samples whose TSH concentration is less than 0.04 μIU/ml, the value of 2 *S.D* is larger than the mean value in free T4 concentration. Thus we omitted the samples whose TSH concentration is less than 0.04 μIU/ml. There is no mathematical reason why we omitted the samples whose TSH concentration is over 9.99 μIU/ml. We should note that subclinical hypothyroidism is associated with an increased risk of cardiovascular disease events and mortality in those with higher TSH levels, particularly in those with TSH concentration of 10 μIU/ml or greater [18].

In male subjects, negative relationships were observed between aging and serum thyroid hormone concentration. TSH level was not altered by aging. Both resistance indices were suppressed by aging. These data indicated that the age-dependent lower FH concentrations do not induce a compensatory increase in TSH expression in males. There are two possible explanations for these results. One is that age-dependent suppression of TSH secretion is latently present, as described previously [1]. As a result, the lower serum hormone-induced TSH expression may not overcome the suppressed TSH secretion. The other possibility is that lower serum hormone may be sufficient to suppress TSH secretion because the resistance indices are suppressed. It is possible that males show age-dependent sensitization of thyroid hormone action.

Aging did not affect the serum concentrations of free thyroid hormones in female. The TSH levels increased in an aging-dependent manner. Both resistance indices increased significantly with age. These data indicated that age-dependent thyroid hormone resistance in females in contrast to the sensitization in males. The ratio of [FT3] to [FT4] was reduced by aging in males but not in females, suggesting that the deiodination and/or transport of T4 were decreased in males.

The precise age distribution suggests that there are three phases in the lifespan in terms of thyroid hormone

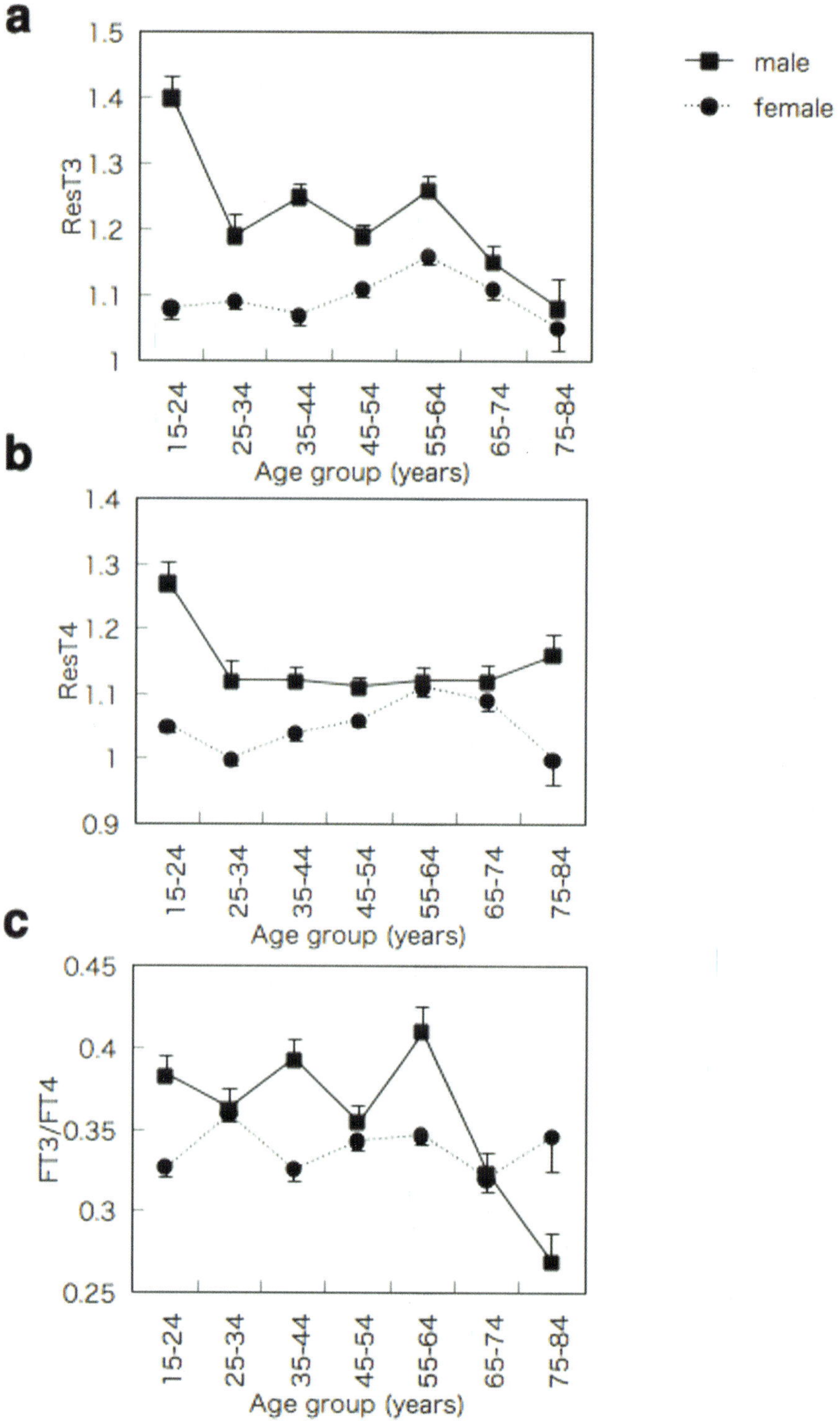


**Figure 4 Age distributions of ResT3 (a), ResT4 (b), and [FT3]/[FT4] index (c) in males and females**. The data represents the means ± *S.E.* of each age group. Bold and broken lines represent the values for males and females, respectively. Statistical significances show in Table 3.

resistance. The first phase is the age between 15-24. The values of both indices were suppressed in male, suggesting that some unknown factors may affect the response to thyroid hormone in adolescent male. It is possible that testosterone plays roles in regulation of response to thyroid hormone, since free dihydrotestosterone concentration peaks at the age group 20-25 [19]. The second phase is the age between 25-64 years old. The mean

**Table 3 Statistical differences between each age group in male (upper area) and in female (lower area).**

| Age group | 15-24 | 25-34 | 35-44 | 45-54 | 55-64 | 65-74 | 75-84 |
|---|---|---|---|---|---|---|---|
| 15-24 ResT3 | | 0.001 > ** | 0.003** | 0.001 > ** | 0.007** | 0.001 > ** | 0.001 > ** |
| 15-24 ResT4 | | 0.011* | 0.001** | 0.001 > ** | 0.002** | 0.003** | 0.189 |
| 15-24 FT3/FT4 | | 0.866 | 0.998 | 0.441 | 0.839 | 0.007** | 0.001 > |
| 25-34 ResT3 | 0.999 | | 0.639 | 1.0 | 0.508 | 0.920 | 0.358 |
| 25-34 ResT4 | 0.399 | | 1.0 | 1.0 | 1.0 | 1.0 | 0.969 |
| 25-34 FT3/FT4 | 0.024* | | 0.557 | 0.999 | 0.218 | 0.251 | 0.001 |
| 35-44 ResT3 | 1.0 | 0.992 | | 0.131 | 1.0 | 0.028* | 0.017** |
| 35-44 ResT4 | 1.0 | 0.668 | | 1.0 | 1.0 | 1.0 | 0.914 |
| 35-44 FT3/FT4 | 1.0 | 0.031* | | 0.154 | 0.981 | 0.001** | 0.001 > ** |
| 45-54 ResT3 | 0.778 | 0.922 | 0.649 | | 0.072 | 0.857 | 0.282 |
| 45-54 ResT4 | 0.980 | 0.030* | 0.875 | | 1.0 | 1.0 | 0.764 |
| 45-54 FT3/FT4 | 0.787 | 0.416 | 0.796 | | 0.046* | 0.383 | 0.001 > ** |
| 55-64 ResT3 | 0.011* | 0.013* | 0.006** | 0.331 | | 0.016* | 0.012* |
| 55-64 ResT4 | 0.011* | 0.001 > ** | 0.004** | 0.074 | | 1.0 | 0.913 |
| 55-64 FT3/FT4 | 0.622 | 0.780 | 0.635 | 1.0 | | 0.001 > ** | 0.001 > ** |
| 65-74 ResT3 | 0.827 | 0.947 | 0.717 | 1.0 | 0.432 | | 0.825 |
| 65-74 ResT4 | 0.175 | 0.001 > ** | 0.083 | 0.541 | 0.985 | | 0.939 |
| 65-74 FT3/FT4 | 0.997 | 0.006** | 0.998 | 0.433 | 0.301 | | 0.165 |
| 75-84 ResT3 | 0.995 | 0.959 | 0.998 | 0.715 | 0.102 | 0.738 | |
| 75-84 ResT4 | 0.957 | 1.0 | 0.985 | 0.834 | 0.189 | 0.379 | |
| 75-84 FT3/FT4 | 0.992 | 0.995 | 0.991 | 1.0 | 1.0 | 0.958 | |

$^{*}P < 0.05$, $^{**}P < 0.01$.

values of both T3 and T4 indices were not altered in males aged between 25 - 34 and 55 - 64. There was, however, a tendency for the resistance indices to increase in the same 25 - 64 age groups, the pre-menopausal phase in females. Many studies have suggested that estrogen may overlap the thyroid hormone action [20]. These data taken together indicate that age-dependent depletion of estrogen may contribute to the progression of resistance to thyroid hormone action in females.

The third phase is over 64 years old. The mean values of the T3 resistance index were suppressed in males over 64 years old, while that of the T4 index was not significantly altered in both genders. The [FT3]/[FT4] index was also decreased in males over 64, but not in females, suggesting that the lack of a reduction in the T4 index in males is probably due to the impaired conversion of FT4 to FT3. In females, both resistance indices were not increased although the reasons remain unclear.

There are two limitations in this study. One is that the subject is heterogeneous in terms of treatment. Obviously, some patients may be administered supplemental T4 or anti-thyroid medication and/or radioiodine therapy. These modifications may somehow affect thyroid function, especially the conversion of FT4 to FT3. These biases may affect the results of the [FT3]/[FT4] index. Although we omitted the data from subjects with extremely low TSH, we may not have excluded patients with mild or moderate hypopituitarism. It is, however, difficult to discriminate physiological hypopituitarism from pathological disorders, as described previously [3]. We consider that age-related pituitary-thyroid regulation may not be affected by pathological thyroid diseases, since the accumulation of vulnerability with age is an all around and non-specific process as described [21]. It is assumed that serum thyroid hormone is the most potent factor to regulate TSH level in all age groups. As both FH and TSH concentrations were normal or mildly abnormal range in the groups, TSH preferentially regulates FH secretion vice versa at the time of sampling the serum. Thus, the data selected in this study were likely appropriate for assessment of negative feedback regulation of thyroid hormone in aging.

Another issue is that the reflex indices in this study may not precisely reflect the strength of the resistance to thyroid hormone. Mathematically, there is a report that log [TSH] is negatively proportional to the square of free T4 concentration [22]. Since there is negative linear relationship between log [TSH] and free concentrations, we conveniently added the two factors after modification of the strength in this study.

In conclusion, we demonstrated the age-dependent sensitization and resistance to thyroid hormone in males and females, respectively. Due to the complexity of negative feedback regulation, TSH level alone could not be used to assess the thyroid hormone action *in vivo*. As TSH level is a convenient marker for assessment of thyroid hormone action, it is necessary to exercise care in interpretation of the values, especially on the basis of age- and gender-related insights. The precise physiological significance of gender-specific resistance to thyroid hormone remains to be elucidated.

### Abbreviations

FH: free hormone; FT3: free T3; FT4: free T4; ResT3: T3 resistance index; ResT4:T4 resistance index.

### Acknowledgements

This research was supported by a Grant-in -Aid for Scientific Research (23591349) from Japan Society for the Promotion of Science.

### Authors' contributions

SN collected and summarized the data obtained from individual patients. TT and MK contributed to discussion and edited the manuscript. SS conceived of the experimental design, analyzed data and wrote the manuscript. All authors read and approved the final manuscript.

### Competing interests

The authors declare that they have no competing interests.

### References

1. Over R, Mannan S, Nsouli-Marktabi H, Burman KD, Jonklaas J: **Age and the thyrotropin response to hypothyroxinemia.** *J Clin Endocrinol Metab* 2010, **95**:3675-3683.
2. Mazzoccoli G, Pazienza V, Piepoli A, Muscarella LA, Inglese M, De Cata A, Giuliani F, Tarquini R: **Hypothalamus-hypophysis-thyroid axis function in healthy aging.** *J Biol Regul Homeost Agents* 2010, **24**:433-439.
3. Sell MA, Schott M, Tharandt L, Cissewski K, Scherbaum WA, Willenberg HS: **Functional central hypothyroidism in the elderly.** *Aging Clin Exp Res* 2008, **20**:207-210.
4. Ferrari E, Cravello L, Falvo F, Barili L, Solerte SB, Fioravanti M, Magri F: **Neuroendocrine features in extreme longevity.** *Exp Gerontol* 2008, **43**:88-94.
5. Rozing MP, Houwing-Duistermaat JJ, Slagboom PE, Beekman M, Frolich M, de Craen AJ, Westendorp RG, van Heemst D: **Familial longevity is associated with decreased thyroid function.** *J Clin Endocrinol Metab* 2010, **95**:4979-4984.
6. Alzmon G, Barzilai N, Surks MI, Gabriely I: **Genetic predisposition to elevated serum thyrotropin is associated with exceptional longevity.** *J Clin Endocrinol Metab* 2009, **94**:4768-4775.
7. Atzmon G, Barzilai N, Hollowell JG, Surks MI, Gabriely I: **Extreme longevity is associated with increased serum thyrotropin.** *J Clin Endocrinol Metab* 2009, **94**:1251-12544.
8. Surks MI, Hollowell JG: **Age-specific distribution of serum thyrotropin and antithyroid antibodies in the US population: implications for the prevalence of subclinical hypothyroidism.** *J Clin Endocrinol Metab* 2007, **92**:4575-4582.
9. Roelfsema F, Pereira AM, Veldhuis JD, Adriaanse R, Endert E, Fliers E, Romijn JA: **Thyrotropin secretion profiles are not different in men and women.** *J Clin Endocrinol Metab* 2009, **94**:3964-3967.
10. Hennemann G, Vos RA, de Jong M, Krenning EP, Docter R: **Decreased peripheral 3,5,3'-triiodothyronine (T3) production from thyroxine (T4): a syndrome of impaired thyroid hormone activation due to transport inhibition of T4- into T3-producing tissues.** *J Clin Endocrinol Metab* 1993, **77**:1431-1435.
11. Friesema EC, Visser WE, Visser TJ: **Genetics and phenomics of thyroid hormone transport by MCT8.** *Mol Cell Endocrinol* 2010, **322**:107-113.
12. Suzuki S, Mori J, Hashizume K: **μ-crystallin, a NADPH-dependent T3-binding protein in cytosol.** *Trends Endocrinol Metab* 2007, **18**:286-289.
13. Amaud-Lopez L, Usala G, Ceresini G, Mitchell BD, Pilia MG, Piras MG, Setsu N, Maschio A, Busonero F, Albai G, Dei M, Lai S, Mulas A, Crisponi L, Tanaka T, Bandinelli S, Guralnik JM, Loi A, Balaci L, Sole G, Prinzis A, Mariotti S, Shuldlner AR, Cao A, Schlessinger D, Uda M, Abecasis GR, Nagaraja R, Sanna S, Naitza S: **Phosphodiesterase 8B gene variants are associated with serum TSH levels and thyroid function.** *Am J Hum Genet* 2008, **82**:1270-1280.
14. Perissi V, Jepsen K, Glass CK, Rosenfeld MG: **Deconstructing repression: evolving models of co-repressor action.** *Nat Rev Genet* 2010, **11**:109-123.
15. Hoermann R, Eckl W, Hoermann C, Larisch R: **Complex relationship between free thyroxine and TSH in the regulation of thyroid function.** *Eur J Endocrinol* 2010, **162**:1123-1129.
16. Spencer CA, LoPresti JS, Patel A, Guttler RB, Eigen A, Shen D, Gray D, Nicoloff JT: **Applications of a new chemiluminometric thyrotropin assay to subnormal measurement.** *J Clin Enodocrinol Metab* 1990, **70**:453-460.
17. Benhadi N, Filers E, Visser TJ, Reitsma JB, Wiersinga WM: **Pilot study on the assessment of the setpoint of the hypothalamus-pituitary-thyroid axis in healthy volunteers.** *Eur J Endocrinol* 2010, **162**:323-329.
18. Arking R: **Measuring age-related changes in population.** In *Biology of Aging.*. 2 edition. Edited by: Sinauer AD. Sunderland: Sinauer Associates, Inc; 1998:27-59.
19. Stárka L, Pospisilová H, Hill M: **Free testosterone and free dihydrotestosterone throughout the life span of men.** *J Steroid Biochem Mol Biol* 2009, **116**:118-120.
20. Davis PJ, Lin HY, Mousa SA, Luidens MK, Hercbergs AA, Wehling M, Davis FB: **Overlapping nongenomic actions of thyroid hormone and steroids.** *Steroids* 2011, **76**:829-833.
21. Rodondi N, den Elzen WP, Bauer DC, Cappola AR, Razvi S, Walsh JP, Asvold BO, Lervasi G, Imaizumi M, Collet TH, Bremner A, Maisonneuve P, Sgarbi JA, Khaw KT, Vanderpump MP, Newman AB, Cornuz J, Franklyn JA, Westendrop RG, Vittinghoff E, Gussekloo J: **Subclinical hypothyroidism and the risk of coronary heart disease and mortality.** *JAMA* 2010, **304**:1365-1374.
22. Leow MK: **A mathematical model of pituitary-thyroid interaction to provide an insight into the nature of the thyrotorpin-thyroid hormone relationship.** *J Theor Biol* 2007, **248**:275-287.

# 30

# Primary and secondary thyroid hormone transporters

Anita Kinne, Ralf Schülein, Gerd Krause*

**Abstract**

Thyroid hormones (TH) are essential for the development of the human brain, growth and cellular metabolism. Investigation of TH transporters became one of the emerging fields in thyroid research after the discovery of inactivating mutations in the Monocarboxylate transporter 8 (MCT8), which was found to be highly specific for TH transport. However, additional transmembrane transporters are also very important for TH uptake and efflux in different cell types. They transport TH as secondary substrates and include the aromatic amino acid transporting MCT10, the organic anion transporting polypeptides (e.g. OATP1C1, OATP1A2, OPTP1A4) and the large neutral amino acid transporters (LAT1 and LAT2). These TH transporters characteristically possess 12 transmembrane spanners but due to the strong differing sequences between the three transporter families we assume an identical conformation is not very likely. In contrast to the others, the LAT family members form a heterodimer with the escort protein 4F2hc/CD98. A comparison of sequence proportions, locations and types of functional sensitive features for TH transport discovered by mutations, revealed that transport sensitive charged residues occur as conserved amino acids only within each family of the transporter types but not in all putative TH transporters. Based on the lack of highly conserved sensitive charged residues throughout the three transporter families as a common counterpart for the amino acid moiety of the substrates, we conclude that the molecular transport mechanism is likely organized either a) by different molecular determinants in the divergent transporter types or b) the counterparts for the substrates` amino acid moiety at the transporter are not any charged side chains but other proton acceptors or donators. However, positions of transport sensitive residues coincide at transmembrane helix 8 in the TH transporter MCT8, OATP1C1 and another amino acid transporter, the L-cystine and L-glutamate exchanger xCT, which is highly homologous to LAT1 and LAT2. Here we review the data available and compare similarities and differences between these primary and secondary TH transporters regarding sequences, topology, potential structures, trafficking to the plasma membrane, molecular features and locations of transport sensitive functionalities. Thereby, we focus on TH transporters occurring in the blood-brain barrier.

## Introduction

Investigation of thyroid hormone (TH) transporters has become one of the emerging fields in thyroid research during the last few years. Molecular studies of TH transporters were enforced after the discovery of inactivating mutations in the TH transporter MCT8 (Monocarboxylate transporter 8). These mutations cause the Allan-Herndon-Dudley syndrome (AHDS) [1], which is an X-linked mental retardation. The affected patients show normal TSH (Thyroid-stimulating hormone, thyrotropin) but elevated $T_3$ (3,3',5-triiodo-L-thyronine) and decreased $T_4$ (3,3',5,5`-tetraiodo-L-thyronine) serum levels [2-6].

TH are essential for the development of the human brain, growth and cellular metabolism. A dysfunction in the availability of TH during early embryonic development leads to neurological deficiency [7]. In the brain, TH are important e.g. for the timely migration of neurons, formation of synaptic contacts and myelination [8]. Neurons are the major target cells for $T_3$ during brain development. According to current concepts, the prohormone $T_4$ enters the neighbouring astrocyte and deiodinase 2 converts $T_4$ to the active form $T_3$ which is then transported into neurons by MCT8 [9].

An impaired uptake of $T_3$ in MCT8-expressing central neurons could explain the neurological deficits found in

* Correspondence: gkrause@fmp-berlin.de
Leibniz-Institut für Molekulare Pharmakologie (FMP), Robert-Roessle-Str. 10, 13125 Berlin, Germany
Full list of author information is available at the end of the article

AHDS patients [1,3]. Surprisingly, the corresponding Mct8-deficient mice show the endocrine changes only, but not the neurological phenotype, observed in affected humans. Symptoms of hyperthyroidism in the peripheral tissues in combination with symptoms of hypothyroidism in the central nervous system were shown in mice. The brain uptake of exogenous $T_3$ is also markedly reduced, whereas the uptake of $T_4$ shows 50% transport activity in comparison to the wild type mice [10-12].

On the basis of these data it was assumed that additional TH transporters ("secondary TH transporters") or differences in their expression patterns and substrate specificity can compensate the loss of Mct8 in mice [13]. Finally, it became obvious that secondary TH transporters are also very important for TH uptake and efflux in different cells types. Whereas the primary TH transporter MCT8 is currently known to be highly specific for TH only [14], the secondary TH transporters are also able to transport different kinds of amino acids and comprise the aromatic amino acid transporting MCT10, the organic anion transporting polypeptide transporters (e.g. OATP1C1, OATP1A2, OPTP1A4), and the large neutral amino acid transporters (LAT1 and LAT2).

Another amino acid transporter, the sodium independent exchanger of L-cystine and L-glutamate (xCT), which can even transport negatively charged amino acids, is also considered here, since xCT shows close similarities to LAT transporters regarding molecular features and plasma membrane trafficking mechanism.

Therefore, we here review the data available on similarities and differences between the primary and secondary TH transporters regarding sequence, trafficking to the plasma membrane, molecular features, predicted membrane topologies, potential structures and functionalities. Thereby, our focus here is on TH transporters occurring in the blood-brain barrier (BBB).

## Expression patterns of primary and secondary TH transporters

It was shown in the brain that MCT8 expression in neurons is essential for neuronal uptake of $T_3$[15]. The reduced brain uptake of $T_3$ and $T_4$ in Mct8-deficient mice suggests that MCT8 transports TH across the BBB. *Roberts et al.* could show an expression of MCT8 in cerebral microvessels and demonstrated the expression of MCT8 at the BBB in the human, mouse, and rat brain [13]. These expression profiles support the suggestion that MCT8 does not only play a major role in TH action in the brain in humans and rodents but also in the uptake of TH in the brain across the BBB in humans. MCT8 is also expressed in the thyroid, liver, testis, and in the skeletal muscle (table 1). Another member of the MCT family which transports TH, MCT10, shows overlapping expression patterns with MCT8, except that MCT10 has not been detected in the thyroid, brain and testis (table 1).

OATP1C1 like MCT8 is expressed at the BBB in mouse and rat, but to a much lesser extent at the human BBB [13]. The strong expression of OATP1C1 in the rodent but less so in the human BBB could explain why Mct8-deficient mice do not show the neurological changes found in AHDS patients. The OATP family members OATP1A2 and OATP1A4 are also expressed in the brain and show transport of TH (table 1) [16].

The TH transporters LAT1 and LAT2 are expressed in various tissues, e.g. in luminal and abluminal membranes of brain capillary endothelial cells, placenta, and intestine, whereas LAT1 also shows high expression levels in tumour cells (table 1). Both transporters are expressed at the BBB, whereby LAT1 expression is higher than LAT2 [17] (figure 1). LAT1 and LAT2 form a heterodimer with the escort protein, 4F2hc (4F2 heavy chain, CD98), which is ubiquitously expressed, e.g. in tumours, brain, kidney, intestine, and placenta (table 1) [18,19].

The amino acid transporter xCT is also expressed in the brain (table 1) [20,21] and it has been suggested that xCT is up-regulated in glial cells upon the oxidative stress and plays an essential role to protect neurons against oxidative stress [22].

## Topology and structures of TH transporters

The TH transporters considered here show a common topology by comprising 12 transmembrane helices (TMHs) while the N- and C-terminal tails are located intracellularly, like a vast number of other known transporters of the major facilitator superfamily (MFS) (see transporter database http://www.tcdb.org/superfamily.php). The MFS is an evolutionary diverse superfamily that includes over 10,000 sequenced members which catalyze uniport, symport and antiport transport mechanisms.

MCT8 and MCT10 belong to the MFS subgroup of Monocarboxylate transporter family. Since the monocarboxylate transport for the members MCT1-4 is proton linked, these MCT transporters are not further considered here.

The OATP family members Oatp1a4 and Oatp1a5 were the first cloned TH transporters [23]. Although the OATP family also belongs to the MFS in terms of sequence similarity it is more distant from MCT8 and MCT10.

LAT1 and LAT2 are even more distant to MCT8. They are members of the Amino Acid-Polyamine-Organocation (APC) superfamily and transport sodium-independent large neutral amino acids such as phenylalanine, tyrosine, leucine, arginine and

**Table 1 Tissue distribution of TH transporters from the MCT (MCT8 and MCT10), OATP (OATP1C1, OATP1A2, OATP1A4), and LAT (LAT1 and LAT2) family and of the xCT transporter and the escort protein 4F2hc.**

| Gene | Protein | Localization | References |
|---|---|---|---|
| SLC16A2 | MCT8 | liver, kidney, brain, heart, skeletal muscle, placenta, thyroid, testis | [14,15,33,64-68] |
| SLC16A10 | MCT10 | intestine, kidney, liver, skeletal muscle, heart, placenta, pancreas | [67-69] |
| SLCO1C1 | OATP1C1 | brain, testis, cochlea | [38,39] |
| SLCO1A2 | OATP1A2 | brain, liver, kidney, intestine | [70-72] |
| SLCO1A4 | OATP1A4 | liver, brain, testis, ovaries, retina | [23,70,73] |
| SLC7A5 | LAT1 | multiple (tumours, brain, spleen, placenta, testis, colon, kidney, intestine, stomach, ovary, thymus, not liver) | [74-81] |
| SLC7A8 | LAT2 | kidney, placenta, brain, intestine, testis, ovary, liver, heart, skeletal muscle, lung, stomach | [74,79-83] |
| SLC7A11 | xCT | brain, kidney, activated macrophages, duodenum | [20,84,85] |

| Gene | Escort protein | Localization | Reference |
|---|---|---|---|
| SLC3A2 | 4F2hc (CD98) | multiple (tumours, brain, intestine, kidney, liver, skeletal muscle, ovary, placenta, testis...) | [74] |

tryptophan from extracellular fluids into the cell, when associated with SLC3A2/4F2hc. The glutamate transporting xCT also belongs to the APC family and shows high similarities to the LATs on the molecular level.

There is a lack of detailed experimental structural information for all TH transmembrane transporters. Therefore, the crystal structure of the Glycerol-3-phosphate transporter (GlpT, PDB code 1PW4 [24]), another member of the MSF superfamily, has been used as a

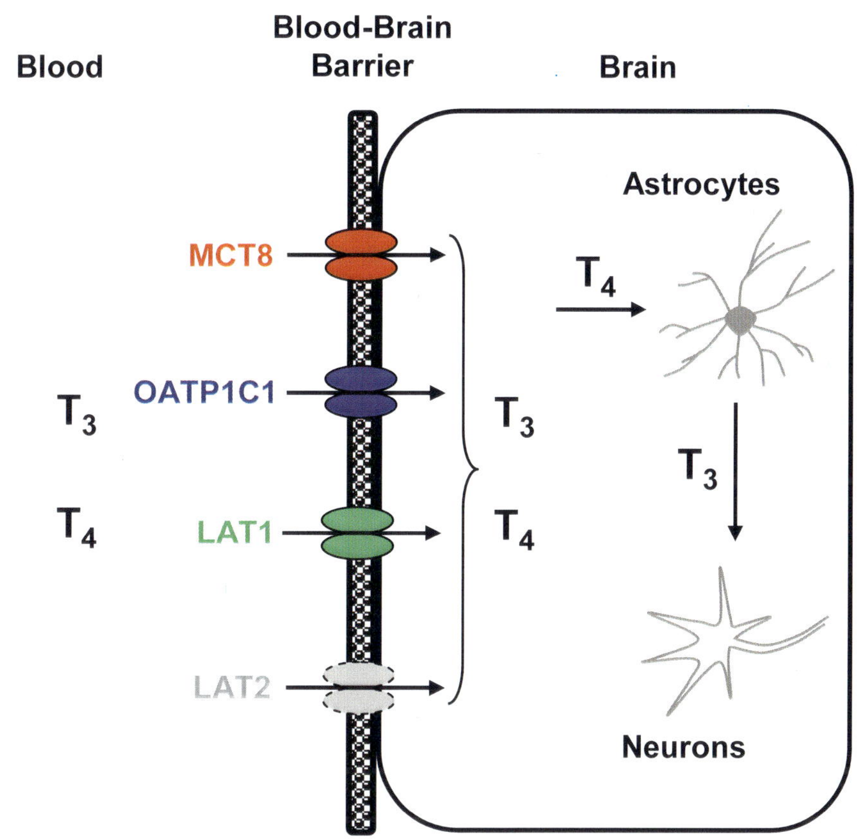


**Figure 1 Illustration of the TH transporters expressed at the blood-brain barrier (BBB).** The TH transporters MCT8, OATP1C1, LAT1, and LAT2 are expressed at the BBB, whereby LAT2 shows lower expression levels than the LAT1. The prohormone $T_4$ enters the astrocyte and is converted to the active form $T_3$ by an outer ring deiodination. According to current concepts, $T_3$ enters the neurons by the TH transporter MCT8.

structural template for homology models for MCT1 [25], MCT8 [26], and OATP1C1 [27]. Although it has been suggested that the substrate translocation at GlpT is associated with conformational changes by an alternating access mechanism with a rocker-switch type of movement of the N- and C-terminal domains [23,25], details for the particular TH transporters are not known yet.

Among the numerous X-ray structures of bacterial transporters the high-resolution three-dimensional structures of another MFS type, the lactose $H^+$ symporter (LacY) [28,29], also shows the closest structural homology to GlpT. The crystal structure of an APC family transporter, the proton-coupled broad-specificity amino acid transporter apo-ApcT [30], shows the 12 TMHs in an inward-facing apo state. It shows a structural similarity to the 12 TMHs within the crystal structure of a bacterial homologue for neurotransmitter transporters, the sodium-dependent leucine transporter (LeuT) from *Aquifex aeolicus*[31]. The ion independent GlpT structure possesses a single binding site for the substrate. The other available structures from MSF and APC families are from proton- or ion-coupled transporters and contain additional binding sites for the symported protons or ions.

## Substrate spectra of TH transporters show a broad range

So far cellular uptake of TH has been shown for the monocarboxylate transporters MCT8 and MCT10, the organic anion transporting polypeptides, e.g. OATP1C1, OATP1A2, and OATP1A4, and the heterodimeric amino acid transporters LAT1 and LAT2 [16].

MCT8 was identified as the first specific transporter of $T_4$ and $T_3$ and was found to transport their inactive TH metabolites such as $rT_3$ (3,3',5`-triiodo-L-thyronine) and 3,3`-$T_2$ (3,3`-diiodo-L-thyronine) [14]. Thereby, the transport of $T_3$ is higher than of $T_4$ or $rT_3$, respectively ($T_3 > T_4 > rT_3 \sim 3,3`\text{-}T_2$) (table 2) [14]. In order to be transported by human MCT8, substrates require at least one iodine atom per aromatic ring preferably at their 3 and 3`position, respectively [26]. Neither thyronamines (except 3-iodothyronamine [32]), decarboxylated metabolites of iodothyronines, nor TH derivatives lacking both chiral center and amino group, are substrates for MCT8 [26,32]. MCT10 was first identified as a T-type transporter for aromatic amino acids [33] and later *Friesema et al.* showed that MCT10 is at least as active for TH transport as MCT8 [34].

The TH transporting OATP family members show a broader substrate spectrum, e.g. in addition to TH they transport bile acids, steroid hormones [35] and drugs [36]. Functional transport analysis of OATP1C1 revealed that $T_4$ and $rT_3$ are high affinity substrates of OATP1C1, whereas the specific uptake of $T_3$ is about 5-fold less than that of $T_4$ and $rT_3$ ($T_4 \sim rT_3 > T_3$) [37-39] (table 2). It has been suggested that OATP1C1 is primarily responsible for $T_4$ uptake from the blood into the brain across the BBB where it is locally converted to the active $T_3$, which is in turn transported into neurons by MCT8 [40].

LAT1 and LAT2 transport large neutral amino acids and amino acid related compounds, whereas LAT2 also transports small amino acids [41,42]. Functional analysis of LAT1 could demonstrate the iodothyronine uptake, which decreased in the order $3,3`\text{-}T_2 > rT_3 \sim T_3 > T_4$. Smaller increments in iodothyronine uptake were noted in transport mediated by LAT2 (table 2) [43].

The amino acid transporter xCT is responsible for the cystine transport through the plasma membrane [44,45]. It mediates an amino acid exchange and prefers cystine and glutamate as its substrates [46].

**Table 2 Uptake of iodothyronines by TH transporters expressed at the blood-brain barrier. The levels of TH transport are indicated as follows: +++ high uptake rate, ++ modest uptake rate, and + low uptake rate; n.d., not determined.**

| Protein | Iodothyronines | | | | Species | References |
|---|---|---|---|---|---|---|
| | 3,3`-$T_2$ | $T_3$ | $rT_3$ | $T_4$ | | |
| MCT8 | +/+ | +++/+++ | +/++ | ++/++ | human/rat | [14,86] |
| OATP1C1 | n.d. | + | +++ | +++ | human, rat, mouse | [37-39] |
| LAT1 | +++ | ++ | ++ | + | human | [43] |
| LAT2 | +++ | ++ | ++ | + | mouse | [43] |

## Similarities and Differences of TH transporters on Molecular Level

### Sequences

A comparison of the different sequence proportions and features among the discussed TH transporters is shown in figure 2. Sequence lengths, proportions and known sensitive features of transport differ between the three TH transporter families (MCT, OATP, and LAT). Due to the very high sequence similarity to the LAT sequences, we also considered the xCT sequences here.

Sequence alignment reveals that the MCT8 and especially the human MCT8 contain a very large N-terminal tail, for which the function is still unknown [47]. Both TH transporting MCT family members, MCT8 and its close homolog MCT10, do not contain extracellular glycosylation sites [34].

Other secondary TH transporters such as those from the OATP family are less similar. They show larger extracellular loops (EL) with numerous conserved cysteines in EL2, EL5 and EL6 (yellow bars in figure 2) that are probably disulfide bridged. Moreover, chances

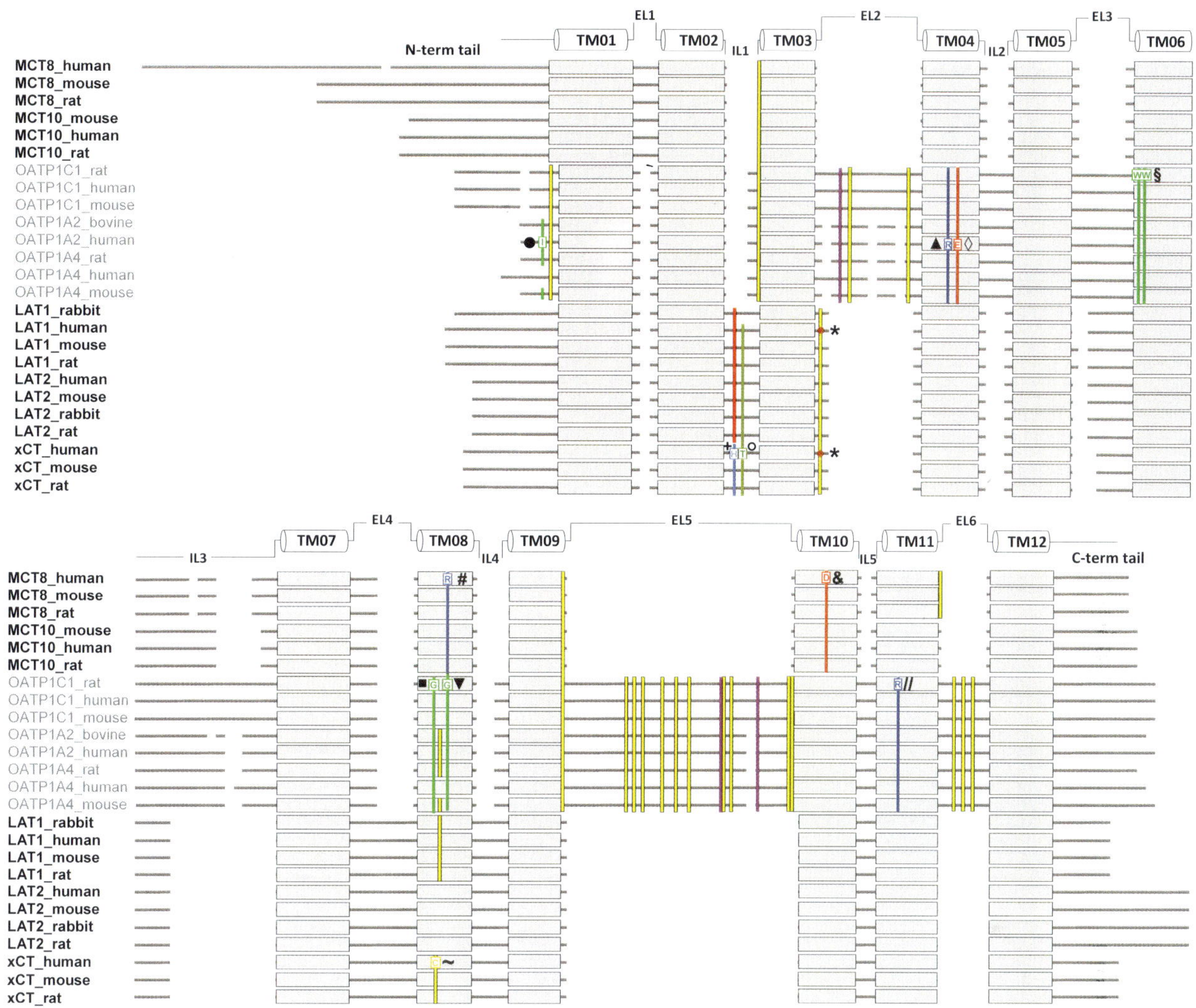


**Figure 2 Comparison of sequence proportions and functional sensitive features of primary and secondary TH transporters.** Sequence scheme of TH transporters expressed at the blood-brain barrier (BBB) is aligned according to the sequences of common 12 transmembrane spanners (pale grey boxes). Sequence lengths, proportions and known sensitive features of transport differ between the three TH transporter families (MCT, OATP, and LAT). The xCT sequences are very homologous to LATs and are therefore added. The human MCT8 possesses a very large N-terminal tail at the intracellular portion. Intra- and extracellularly conserved cysteines are marked in yellow bars. N-glycosylation sites of the OATP family are conserved at large extracellular loops EL2 and EL5 (magenta bars). The proven disulfide bridge formed by the LAT and xCT family to the escort protein 4F2hc are conserved in the EL2 (C165-LAT1_human [49] or C158-xCT_human [50] marked by red dot * at yellow bar). Sensitive positions for TH transport identified by mutations are highlighted: MCT8_human: R445A(# blue bar, TMH8 [26]) and D498A (& red bar, TMH10 [26]), the sensitive arginine and aspartate are conserved at the MCT8 and MCT10 group; Oatp1c1_rat: W277A and W278A (§ green bars, TMH6 [27]), G400A and G410A (■ and ▾green bars, TMH8 [30]), R601A (// blue bar, TMH11 [27]); OATP1A2_human: I13T (◊ N-terminal tail [63]), R168C (▴ blue bar, TMH4 [58]), E172D (◊ red bar, TMH4 [63]). The isoleucine at position 13 (green bar, N-terminal tail) is only conserved at the OATP1A2 group, while the sensitive tryptophan (green bars), arginines (blue bars) and glutamate (red bar) are conserved within the OATP family. At the human xCT may lie close to the substrate binding site H110 (+ blue bar [21]) and T112 (○ green bar [21]) in IL1 and the C327 (~ yellow bar [62]) at TMH8. The accession numbers of these proteins are NM_006517.3 (MCT8_human), NM_009197.2 (MCT8_mouse), NM_147216.1 (MCT8_rat), NM_018593.4 (MCT10_human), NM_001114332.1 (MCT10_mouse), Q91Y77 (MCT10_rat), NM_017435.4 (OATP1C1_human), NM_021471.2 (OATP1C1_mouse), NM_053441.1 (OATP1C1_rat), NM_134431.3 (OATP1A2_human), NM_174654.2 (OATP1A2_bovine), AF205071.1 (OATP1A4_human), NM_030687.1 (OATP1A4_mouse), NM_131906.1 (OATP1A4_rat), BC039692.2 (LAT1_human), BC026131.1 (LAT1_mouse), CH473972.1 (LAT1_rat), NM_001082120.1 (LAT1_rabbit), BC052250.1 (LAT2_human), BC059004.1 (LAT2_mouse), NM_053442.1 (LAT2_rat), NM_001082682.1 (LAT2_rabbit), NM_014331.3 (xCT_human), NM_011990.2 (xCT_mouse), NM_001107673.2 (xCT_rat).

are that several conserved glycosylation sites in EL2 and EL5 are responsible for appropriate traffic of this transporter type towards the cell membrane (magenta bars in figure 2).

The transporters that belong to the APC superfamily, such as LAT1/2 and xCT, are even more evolutionary distant from MCT8. Like the other TH transporters they possess 12 transmembrane α-helical spanners but for suitable membrane expression they need the one helix transmembrane spanner escort protein 4F2hc [48-50]. This transporter type lacks any glycosylation site since the glycosylation sites are only comprised at the large extracellular portion of 4F2hc. Thus, both transporter types (LAT and xCT) are in fact tightly associated by a 13th TMH that is provided by the escort protein 4F2hc. This odd number of transmembrane segments might be one reason why the potential intracellular loop 1 (IL1) between TMH2 and TMH3 is organized as a re-entrant loop in the xCT. In a detailed experimental study elucidating the topology of xCT [21] it was shown that histidin 110 in IL1 (marked + in figure 2) and threonin 112 (marked ° in figure 2) are spatially located in human xCT in such a way that they are accessible from the extracellular side. At the xCT, a part of IL1 is interposed between the transmembrane segments in such a manner that the two residues are accessible from the extracellular side.

The number and properties of residues at IL1 are highly conserved among xCT and LAT1/2. Moreover, at the corresponding amino acid positions, where extracellular accessibility was shown in xCT (H110 and T112), the hydrophilic residues aspartate and serine appear in LAT1 and LAT2 respectively (red and grey bars at IL1 in figure 2). Therefore it is feasible that the IL1 may also functions as a re-entrant loop in LAT1 and LAT2.

#### Escort proteins

Not only differences in the transport of TH within TH transporters are known, but the trafficking mechanisms of these transporter proteins towards the plasma membrane differ also. Trafficking of integral membrane proteins to the plasma membrane is mediated by the secretory pathway. At the beginning, proteins are integrated into the membrane of the endoplasmatic reticulum and are then delivered in the membrane of vesicles through the individual compartments of the Golgi apparatus to the plasma membrane. MCT8, MCT10, LAT1, and LAT2 are non-glycosylated proteins, whereas the OATPs possess potential glycosylation sites [51] (figure 2). Normally, glycosylations are essential for trafficking whereby the trafficking mechanisms for the two TH transporters from the MCT and the LAT families are organized differently. In the case of MCT8 and MCT10 it is speculated that the large N-terminal tail might contain features that facilitate trafficking towards the membrane. Other transporters of the MCT family such as MCT1 and MCT4, which do not transport TH but other substrates e.g. lactate, pyruvate and ketone bodies [52], require an association with the escort protein CD147 for efficient cell surface expression [53] instead. In contrast to the TH transporting MCT family members, the two LAT transporters also need an escort protein for efficient cell surface translocation, the 4F2hc [18,19].

The two escort proteins 4F2hc and CD147 share a common topology. The amino-terminus of 4F2hc is located intracellularly, whereas the very large extracellular carboxy-terminus [48] contains four potential glycosylation sites [54]. Thus, 4F2hc is a multifunctional type II membrane glycoprotein [55]. In the heterodimer complex between LAT1/2 and 4F2hc the 12 helix transport protein is called the light chain and the glycosylated escort protein 4F2hc is called the heavy chain. The heavy chain can form heterodimers with six different non-glycosylated light chains like LAT1, LAT2, y+LAT1, y+LAT2, asc1, and xCT [48].

Both subunits of the heterodimer between the L-type amino acid transporters build a covalent bond via a disulfide bridge through the cysteine residue 109 of the extracellular region of human 4F2hc and the cysteine residue 165 in the second extracellular loop localized between the TMH3 and TMH4 of rat Lat1 (red dot and * in figure 2) [48,49]. This cysteine residue is conserved in all sequences of LAT1, LAT2 and also in all xCT sequences in EL2 (yellow bar in figure 2).

Although these two subunits of the heterodimeric transporters are joined by the highly conserved disulfide bridge, site-directed mutagenesis of these two cysteines on either LAT1 or 4F2hc does not inhibit amino acid transport [56].

Moreover, according to the high sequence homology, it could be shown that the corresponding cysteine in human xCT (cysteine 158, red dot and * in figure 2) [57] also forms a disulfide bridge to 4F2hc.

### Functional data for amino acids potentially involved in substrate interaction and functional transport

Different functional studies of TH transporters could identify amino acid residues potentially involved in substrate interaction. To gain insights into structure-function relationship in TH transport, we designed the first structural model for human MCT8. Thereby, the conserved and charged amino acids R445 at TMH8 (marked # in figure 2) and D498 at TMH10 (marked & in figure 2) have been identified as being involved in substrate interaction. An abrogated $T_3$ transport by the alanine mutants R445A and D498A supported their predicted role in substrate recognition, although both mutants were exposed to the cell surface [26].

The sensitive arginine (blue bar) and aspartate (red bar) are conserved at the MCT8 and MCT10 group in TMH8 and TMH10, respectively (figure 2). The MCT8 model allows to identify transport characteristics of TH and to rationalize potential interactions of amino acids including those mutated in patients with AHDS.

In the high-affinity $T_4$ transporter Oatp1c1 *Westholm et al.* identified amino acid residues to be critical for $T_4$ transport and demonstrated the presence of high and low affinity binding sites [27]. In their study they mapped rat Oatp1c1 substrate interacting sites. W277 and W278 (§ in figure 2) were shown to play a major role in $T_4$ transport with direct binding effects on one binding site.

Oatp1c1 mutations that reach the cell membrane but affect the transport function such as G400A/V and G410A/V at TMH8 (marked ■ and ▾ in figure 2) were proposedly involved in transport kinetics. Their alanine and also valine mutants displayed wild type-like uptake activity but exhibit diminished $T_4$ transport at high substrate concentrations. The authors suggested that a substrate binding site might collapse or is turned to inability to convert between input and output states. Based on mutants of the conserved arginine R601 (marked // in figure 2) at TMH11 of rat Oatp1c1 the authors suggested that this arginine may serve within OATP members as a countercharge for anionic binding to OATP1C1 [27]. Genetic variations by Single nucleotide polymorphisms (SNPs) have been detected to be involved in disturbed substrate transport like methotrexate transport at human OATP1A2 [58] such as R168C at TMH4 [58] (marked ▴ in figure 2). Recently it has been proven that some of these SNPs such as I13T at the intracellular N-terminal tail (marked • in figure 2), and E172D at TMH4 (marked ◊ in figure 2), also effect the $T_3$ and $T_4$ transport [59].

Our sequence comparison scheme showed that the isoleucine (marked • in figure 2) at amino acid position 13 at the N-terminal tail is only conserved at the OATP1A2 group (green bar in figure 2), while the other identified TH sensitive residues such as arginine (blue bars in figure 2) and glutamate (red bar in figure 2) located at TMH4, the two tryptophans (green bars in figure 2) at TMH6, the two glycines (green bars) at TMH8 and the arginine (blue bar) in TMH11 are conserved within the OATP family.

Thereby it is noticeable that the TH transport sensitive position glycine 410 (marked &#9679 in figure 2) of rat Oatp1c1 in TMH8 corresponds to the position of the transport sensitive arginine 445 (marked # in figure 2) in TMH8 at human MCT8.

*Boado et al.* identified amino acids in the L-type amino acid transporter LAT1 from rabbit, which are potentially involved in trafficking mechanisms to the plasma membrane. They showed that the cysteine residue 439 (corresponding to C443 in human LAT1) plays a significant role at TMH11 in either folding or insertion of the transporter protein in the plasma membrane [56]. Mutagenic analysis of the amino acids G219 and W234 in rabbit LAT1, which differ in relation to the human or rat LAT1, demonstrated marked changes in the affinity and capacity of LAT1 [60]. In order to identify domains involved in recognition of the light chains, LAT1, LAT2, and y+LAT2 by 4F2hc were investigated by *Bröer et al.*. They suggested that extracellular domains of the 4F2hc are mainly responsible for recognition of light chains other than LAT1 and that the extracellular domain ensures proper translocation to the plasma membrane [61]. Functional data for xCT demonstrated that H110 located in IL1 which here also represents the re-entrant loop (marked + in figure 2) may lie close to the substrate binding/permeation pathway of xCT [21]. Studies of the cysteine residue 327 at TMH8 of xCT (marked ~ in figure 2) indicated that it is also located close to the substrate binding site of xCT [62]. This transport sensitive cysteine at TMH8 is conserved in xCT and LAT1 transporters but not in LAT2. In addition, it occurs sporadically at the OATP group.

Residues that are sensitive for TH transport have been found for MCT8 on TMH8 and TMH10 and priorily on TMH4, TMH6, TMH8 and TMH11 for Oatp1c1. Until now, no TH transport sensitive residues have been reported for LAT1 and LAT2. For the highly homologous xCT relevant residues for substrate transport have, however, been identified at the re-entrant loop IL1 and on TMH8. When comparing the transport sensitive features by mapping them on a sequence alignment scheme (figure 2), it becomes clear that the identified residues are almost only conserved within one particular TH transporter family. None of the sensitive residues are highly conserved across all three considered families. However, the location of a TH sensitive glycine at TMH8 of the Oatp1c1 and a substrate sensitive cysteine at TMH8 of the xCT corresponds to a similar region, where in TMH8 of the MCT8 a TH transport sensitive arginine was found (figure 2).

## Conclusions

A comparison of TH transporter sequences reveals that with the exception of MCT10 secondary TH transporters belonging to different transporter type families are more divergent to the primary TH transporter MCT8. All different endogenous substrates that are transported by these diverse transporters contain at least one common molecular feature, namely the amino and carboxylate functional group of amino acids. A comparison of locations and types of the identified sensitive TH transporting residues revealed that the known positive or negative charged residues occur as conserved amino acids within each of the transporter types, but not over all TH transporters. Due to the fact that highly diverse amino acid properties (arginine and glycine respectively) have been identified as sensitive for TH transport at a corresponding position of TMH8 for MCT8 and Oatp1c1, we presume that molecular details of the translocation mechanisms are varying between MCT8 and Oatp1c1. From the divergent sequence features among the three secondary TH transporter types and the lack of any highly conserved sensitive positively or negatively charged residues as a common counterpart for the amino acid moiety of the substrates, we conclude that the molecular transport mechanisms are likely organized either a) by different molecular determinants in the divergent transporter types or b) the counterpart for amino acid moiety of the substrates at the transporter are not charged side chains but other proton acceptors or donators. Moreover, even though the TH transporters share the common 12 transmembrane spanners, an identical conformation for all TH transporters is not very likely, particularly at least for the LAT family exhibiting an associated 13th transmembrane helix that is provided by the escort protein. A distinct conformation of the two LATs is also supported by the findings for the homologous xCT suggesting a re-entrant function of the IL1. On the other hand the coincidence of sensitive positions for substrate transport at TMH8 (although by divergent residues) in the different TH transporters MCT8, OATP1C1 and even in xCT could at least be a hint for shared molecular transport events executed at a comparable interior site on TMH8 of the transporters considered here.

Therefore, a detailed knowledge of molecular mechanisms of TH translocation through the membrane transporting proteins by investigation of structure-function relationships between different substrates and their targets is of vital importance to understand the molecular reasons for defects in TH transport. In this respect, future investigations of the molecular mechanisms for different substrate transport in the divergent TH transporters are of great importance to clarify the structural-functional properties of TH transport.

#### Abbreviations

AHDS: Allan-Herndon-Dudley syndrome; APC superfamily: Amino Acid-Polyamine-Organocation superfamily; asc1: asc-type amino acid transporter 1; BBB: blood-brain barrier; LAT: L-type amino acid transporter; MCT: Monocarboxylate transporter; MFS: major facilitator superfamily; OATP: organic anion transporting polypeptide; SNPs: Single nucleotide polymorphisms; TMH: transmembrane helix; $rT_3$: 3,3',5'-triiodo-L-thyronine; 3,3'-$T_2$: 3,3'-diiodo-L-thyronine; $T_3$: 3,3',5-triiodo-L-thyronine; $T_4$: 3,3',5,5'-tetraiodo-L-thyronine; TH: thyroid hormone; TSH: Thyroid-stimulating hormone, thyrotropin; 4F2hc: 4F2 heavy chain, CD98; xCT: cystine/glutamate exchanger; y+LAT1: y(+)L-type amino acid transporter 1.

#### Acknowledgements

This article has been published as part of *Thyroid Research* Volume 4 Supplement 1, 2011: New aspects of thyroid hormone synthesis and action. The full contents of the supplement are available online at http://www.thyroidresearchjournal.com/supplements/4/S1

#### Authors' contributions

AK wrote the draft, analyzed the data, prepared the figures, data evaluation and discussion; RS wrote the draft, data discussion, project coordination; GK wrote the draft, analyzed the data, data evaluation and discussion, project coordination.

#### Competing interests

The authors declare that they have no competing interests.

#### References

1. Friesema EC, Grueters A, Biebermann H, Krude H, von Moers A, Reeser M, Barrett TG, Mancilla EE, Svensson J, Kester MH, *et al*: **Association between mutations in a thyroid hormone transporter and severe X-linked psychomotor retardation.** *Lancet* 2004, **364**:1435-1437.
2. Brockmann K, Dumitrescu AM, Best TT, Hanefeld F, Refetoff S: **X-linked paroxysmal dyskinesia and severe global retardation caused by defective MCT8 gene.** *J Neurol* 2005, **252**:663-666.
3. Dumitrescu AM, Liao XH, Best TB, Brockmann K, Refetoff S: **A novel syndrome combining thyroid and neurological abnormalities is associated with mutations in a monocarboxylate transporter gene.** *Am J Hum Genet* 2004, **74**:168-175.
4. Schwartz CE, May MM, Carpenter NJ, Rogers RC, Martin J, Bialer MG, Ward J, Sanabria J, Marsa S, Lewis JA, *et al*: **Allan-Herndon-Dudley syndrome and the monocarboxylate transporter 8 (MCT8) gene.** *Am J Hum Genet* 2005, **77**:41-53.
5. Herzovich V, Vaiani E, Marino R, Dratler G, Lazzati JM, Tilitzky S, Ramirez P, Iorcansky S, Rivarola MA, Belgorosky A: **Unexpected peripheral markers of thyroid function in a patient with a novel mutation of the MCT8 thyroid hormone transporter gene.** *Horm Res* 2007, **67**:1-6.
6. Maranduba CM, Friesema EC, Kok F, Kester MH, Jansen J, Sertie AL, Passos-Bueno MR, Visser TJ: **Decreased cellular uptake and metabolism in Allan-Herndon-Dudley syndrome (AHDS) due to a novel mutation in the MCT8 thyroid hormone transporter.** *J Med Genet* 2006, **43**:457-460.
7. Zoeller RT, Rovet J: **Timing of thyroid hormone action in the developing brain: Clinical observations and experimental findings.** *Journal of Neuroendocrinology* 2004, **16**:809-818.
8. Zoeller TR, Dowling AL, Herzig CT, Iannacone EA, Gauger KJ, Bansal R: **Thyroid hormone, brain development, and the environment.** *Environ Health Perspect* 2002, **110(Suppl 3)**:355-361.
9. Bernal J: **Iodine and brain development.** *Biofactors* 1999, **10**:271-276.
10. Wirth EK, Roth S, Blechschmidt C, Holter SM, Becker L, Racz I, Zimmer A, Klopstock T, Gailus-Durner V, Fuchs H, *et al*: **Neuronal 3',3,5-triiodothyronine (T3) uptake and behavioral phenotype of mice deficient in Mct8, the neuronal T3 transporter mutated in Allan-Herndon-Dudley syndrome.** *J Neurosci* 2009, **29**:9439-9449.
11. Dumitrescu AM, Liao XH, Weiss RE, Millen K, Refetoff S: **Tissue-specific thyroid hormone deprivation and excess in monocarboxylate transporter (mct) 8-deficient mice.** *Endocrinology* 2006, **147**:4036-4043.
12. Trajkovic M, Visser TJ, Mittag J, Horn S, Lukas J, Darras VM, Raivich G, Bauer K, Heuer H: **Abnormal thyroid hormone metabolism in mice lacking the monocarboxylate transporter 8.** *J Clin Invest* 2007, **117**:627-635.
13. Roberts LM, Woodford K, Zhou M, Black DS, Haggerty JE, Tate EH, Grindstaff KK, Mengesha W, Raman C, Zerangue N: **Expression of the thyroid hormone transporters monocarboxylate transporter-8 (SLC16A2) and organic ion transporter-14 (SLCO1C1) at the blood-brain barrier.** *Endocrinology* 2008, **149**:6251-6261.
14. Friesema EC, Ganguly S, Abdalla A, Manning Fox JE, Halestrap AP, Visser TJ: **Identification of monocarboxylate transporter 8 as a specific thyroid hormone transporter.** *J Biol Chem* 2003, **278**:40128-40135.
15. Heuer H, Maier MK, Iden S, Mittag J, Friesema EC, Visser TJ, Bauer K: **The monocarboxylate transporter 8 linked to human psychomotor**

retardation is highly expressed in thyroid hormone-sensitive neuron populations. *Endocrinology* 2005, **146**:1701-1706.

16. Friesema EC, Jansen J, Visser TJ: **Thyroid hormone transporters.** *Biochem Soc Trans* 2005, **33**:228-232.
17. de Boer AG, van dS I, Gaillard PJ: **The role of drug transporters at the blood-brain barrier.** *Annu Rev Pharmacol Toxicol* 2003, **43**:629-656.
18. Verrey F, Meier C, Rossier G, Kuhn LC: **Glycoprotein-associated amino acid exchangers: broadening the range of transport specificity.** *Pflugers Arch* 2000, **440**:503-512.
19. Nakamura E, Sato M, Yang H, Miyagawa F, Harasaki M, Tomita K, Matsuoka S, Noma A, Iwai K, Minato N: **4F2 (CD98) heavy chain is associated covalently with an amino acid transporter and controls intracellular trafficking and membrane topology of 4F2 heterodimer.** *J Biol Chem* 1999, **274**:3009-3016.
20. Sato H, Tamba M, Ishii T, Bannai S: **Cloning and expression of a plasma membrane cystine/glutamate exchange transporter composed of two distinct proteins.** *J Biol Chem* 1999, **274**:11455-11458.
21. Gasol E, Jimenez-Vidal M, Chillaron J, Zorzano A, Palacin M: **Membrane topology of system xc- light subunit reveals a re-entrant loop with substrate-restricted accessibility.** *J Biol Chem* 2004, **279**:31228-31236.
22. Kim JY, Kanai Y, Chairoungdua A, Cha SH, Matsuo H, Kim DK, Inatomi J, Sawa H, Ida Y, Endou H: **Human cystine/glutamate transporter: cDNA cloning and upregulation by oxidative stress in glioma cells.** *Biochim Biophys Acta* 2001, **1512**:335-344.
23. Abe T, Kakyo M, Sakagami H, Tokui T, Nishio T, Tanemoto M, Nomura H, Hebert SC, Matsuno S, Kondo H, *et al*: **Molecular characterization and tissue distribution of a new organic anion transporter subtype (oatp3) that transports thyroid hormones and taurocholate and comparison with oatp2.** *J Biol Chem* 1998, **273**:22395-22401.
24. Huang Y, Lemieux MJ, Song J, Auer M, Wang DN: **Structure and mechanism of the glycerol-3-phosphate transporter from Escherichia coli.** *Science* 2003, **301**:616-620.
25. Manoharan C, Wilson MC, Sessions RB, Halestrap AP: **The role of charged residues in the transmembrane helices of monocarboxylate transporter 1 and its ancillary protein basigin in determining plasma membrane expression and catalytic activity.** *Mol Membr Biol* 2006, **23**:486-498.
26. Kinne A, Kleinau G, Hoefig CS, Gruters A, Kohrle J, Krause G, Schweizer U: **Essential molecular determinants for thyroid hormone transport and first structural implications for monocarboxylate transporter 8.** *J Biol Chem* 2010, **285**:28054-28063.
27. Westholm DE, Marold JD, Viken KJ, Duerst AH, Anderson GW, Rumbley JN: **Evidence of Evolutionary Conservation of Function between the Thyroxine Transporter Oatp1c1 and Major Facilitator Superfamily Members.** *Endocrinology* 2010, **151(12)**:5941-5951.
28. Abramson J, Smirnova I, Kasho V, Verner G, Kaback HR, Iwata S: **Structure and mechanism of the lactose permease of Escherichia coli.** *Science* 2003, **301**:610-615.
29. Guan L, Mirza O, Verner G, Iwata S, Kaback HR: **Structural determination of wild-type lactose permease.** *Proc Natl Acad Sci U S A* 2007, **104**:15294-15298.
30. Shaffer PL, Goehring A, Shankaranarayanan A, Gouaux E: **Structure and mechanism of a Na+-independent amino acid transporter.** *Science* 2009, **325**:1010-1014.
31. Yamashita A, Singh SK, Kawate T, Jin Y, Gouaux E: **Crystal structure of a bacterial homologue of Na+/Cl–dependent neurotransmitter transporters.** *Nature* 2005, **437**:215-223.
32. Ianculescu AG, Friesema EC, Visser TJ, Giacomini KM, Scanlan TS: **Transport of thyroid hormones is selectively inhibited by 3-iodothyronamine.** *Mol Biosyst* 2010, **6**:1403-1410.
33. Kim DK, Kanai Y, Chairoungdua A, Matsuo H, Cha SH, Endou H: **Expression cloning of a Na+-independent aromatic amino acid transporter with structural similarity to H+/monocarboxylate transporters.** *J Biol Chem* 2001, **276**:17221-17228.
34. Friesema EC, Jansen J, Jachtenberg JW, Visser WE, Kester MH, Visser TJ: **Effective cellular uptake and efflux of thyroid hormone by human monocarboxylate transporter 10.** *Mol Endocrinol* 2008, **22**:1357-1369.
35. Kalliokoski A, Niemi M: **Impact of OATP transporters on pharmacokinetics.** *Br J Pharmacol* 2009, **158**:693-705.
36. König J, Seithel A, Gradhand U, Fromm MF: **Pharmacogenomics of human OATP transporters.** *Naunyn Schmiedebergs Arch Pharmacol* 2006, **372**:432-443.
37. Tohyama K, Kusuhara H, Sugiyama Y: **Involvement of multispecific organic anion transporter, Oatp14 (Slc21a14), in the transport of thyroxine across the blood-brain barrier.** *Endocrinology* 2004, **145**:4384-4391.
38. Sugiyama D, Kusuhara H, Taniguchi H, Ishikawa S, Nozaki Y, Aburatani H, Sugiyama Y: **Functional characterization of rat brain-specific organic anion transporter (Oatp14) at the blood-brain barrier: high affinity transporter for thyroxine.** *J Biol Chem* 2003, **278**:43489-43495.
39. Pizzagalli F, Hagenbuch B, Stieger B, Klenk U, Folkers G, Meier PJ: **Identification of a novel human organic anion transporting polypeptide as a high affinity thyroxine transporter.** *Mol Endocrinol* 2002, **16**:2283-2296.
40. Visser WE, Friesema EC, Jansen J, Visser TJ: **Thyroid hormone transport in and out of cells.** *Trends Endocrinol Metab* 2008, **19**:50-56.
41. Wagner CA, Lang F, Broer S: **Function and structure of heterodimeric amino acid transporters.** *Am J Physiol Cell Physiol* 2001, **281**:C1077-C1093.
42. Segawa H, Fukasawa Y, Miyamoto K, Takeda E, Endou H, Kanai Y: **Identification and functional characterization of a Na+-independent neutral amino acid transporter with broad substrate selectivity.** *J Biol Chem* 1999, **274**:19745-19751.
43. Friesema EC, Docter R, Moerings EP, Verrey F, Krenning EP, Hennemann G, Visser TJ: **Thyroid hormone transport by the heterodimeric human system L amino acid transporter.** *Endocrinology* 2001, **142**:4339-4348.
44. Bannai S, Kitamura E: **Transport interaction of L-cystine and L-glutamate in human diploid fibroblasts in culture.** *J Biol Chem* 1980, **255**:2372-2376.
45. Bannai S, Kitamura E: **Role of proton dissociation in the transport of cystine and glutamate in human diploid fibroblasts in culture.** *J Biol Chem* 1981, **256**:5770-5772.
46. Bannai S: **Exchange of cystine and glutamate across plasma membrane of human fibroblasts.** *J Biol Chem* 1986, **261**:2256-2263.
47. Heuer H, Visser TJ: **Minireview: Pathophysiological importance of thyroid hormone transporters.** *Endocrinology* 2009, **150**:1078-1083.
48. del Amo EM, Urtti A, Yliperttula M: **Pharmacokinetic role of L-type amino acid transporters LAT1 and LAT2.** *Eur J Pharm Sci* 2008, **35**:161-174.
49. Pfeiffer R, Spindler B, Loffing J, Skelly PJ, Shoemaker CB, Verrey F: **Functional heterodimeric amino acid transporters lacking cysteine residues involved in disulfide bond.** *FEBS Lett* 1998, **439**:157-162.
50. Palacin M, Nunes V, Font-Llitjos M, Jimenez-Vidal M, Fort J, Gasol E, Pineda M, Feliubadalo L, Chillaron J, Zorzano A: **The genetics of heteromeric amino acid transporters.** *Physiology (Bethesda)* 2005, **20**:112-124.
51. Konig J, Seithel A, Gradhand U, Fromm MF: **Pharmacogenomics of human OATP transporters.** *Naunyn Schmiedebergs Arch Pharmacol* 2006, **372**:432-443.
52. Halestrap AP, Meredith D: **The SLC16 gene family-from monocarboxylate transporters (MCTs) to aromatic amino acid transporters and beyond.** *Pflugers Arch* 2004, **447**:619-628.
53. Kirk P, Wilson MC, Heddle C, Brown MH, Barclay AN, Halestrap AP: **CD147 is tightly associated with lactate transporters MCT1 and MCT4 and facilitates their cell surface expression.** *EMBO J* 2000, **19**:3896-3904.
54. Hemler ME, Strominger JL: **Characterization of antigen recognized by the monoclonal antibody (4F2): different molecular forms on human T and B lymphoblastoid cell lines.** *J Immunol* 1982, **129**:623-628.
55. Chillaron J, Roca R, Valencia A, Zorzano A, Palacin M: **Heteromeric amino acid transporters: biochemistry, genetics, and physiology.** *Am J Physiol Renal Physiol* 2001, **281**:F995-1018.
56. Boado RJ, Li JY, Chu C, Ogoshi F, Wise P, Pardridge WM: **Site-directed mutagenesis of cysteine residues of large neutral amino acid transporter LAT1.** *Biochim Biophys Acta* 2005, **1715**:104-110.
57. Bassi MT, Gasol E, Manzoni M, Pineda M, Riboni M, Martin R, Zorzano A, Borsani G, Palacin M: **Identification and characterisation of human xCT that co-expresses, with 4F2 heavy chain, the amino acid transport activity system xc-.** *Pflugers Arch* 2001, **442**:286-296.
58. Badagnani I, Castro RA, Taylor TR, Brett CM, Huang CC, Stryke D, Kawamoto M, Johns SJ, Ferrin TE, Carlson EJ, *et al*: **Interaction of methotrexate with organic-anion transporting polypeptide 1A2 and its genetic variants.** *J Pharmacol Exp Ther* 2006, **318**:521-529.
59. van der Deure WM, Peeters RP, Visser TJ: **Molecular aspects of thyroid hormone transporters, including MCT8, MCT10, and OATPs, and the effects of genetic variation in these transporters.** *J Mol Endocrinol* 2010, **44**:1-11.
60. Boado RJ, Li JY, Pardridge WM: **Site-directed mutagenesis of rabbit LAT1 at amino acids 219 and 234.** *J Neurochem* 2003, **84**:1322-1331.

61. Broer A, Friedrich B, Wagner CA, Fillon S, Ganapathy V, Lang F, Broer S: **Association of 4F2hc with light chains LAT1, LAT2 or y+LAT2 requires different domains.** *Biochem J* 2001, **355**:725-731.
62. Jimenez-Vidal M, Gasol E, Zorzano A, Nunes V, Palacin M, Chillaron J: **Thiol modification of cysteine 327 in the eighth transmembrane domain of the light subunit xCT of the heteromeric cystine/glutamate antiporter suggests close proximity to the substrate binding site/permeation pathway.** *J Biol Chem* 2004, **279**:11214-11221.
63. Lee W, Glaeser H, Smith LH, Roberts RL, Moeckel GW, Gervasini G, Leake BF, Kim RB: **Polymorphisms in human organic anion-transporting polypeptide 1A2 (OATP1A2): implications for altered drug disposition and central nervous system drug entry.** *J Biol Chem* 2005, **280**:9610-9617.
64. Bonen A, Heynen M, Hatta H: **Distribution of monocarboxylate transporters MCT1-MCT8 in rat tissues and human skeletal muscle.** *Appl Physiol Nutr Metab* 2006, **31**:31-39.
65. Chan SY, Franklyn JA, Pemberton HN, Bulmer JN, Visser TJ, McCabe CJ, Kilby MD: **Monocarboxylate transporter 8 expression in the human placenta: the effects of severe intrauterine growth restriction.** *J Endocrinol* 2006, **189**:465-471.
66. Di Cosmo C, Liao XH, Dumitrescu AM, Philp NJ, Weiss RE, Refetoff S: **Mice deficient in MCT8 reveal a mechanism regulating thyroid hormone secretion.** *J Clin Invest* 2010, **120**:3377-3388.
67. Halestrap AP, Meredith D: **The SLC16 gene family-from monocarboxylate transporters (MCTs) to aromatic amino acid transporters and beyond.** *Pflugers Arch* 2004, **447**:619-628.
68. Nishimura M, Naito S: **Tissue-specific mRNA expression profiles of human solute carrier transporter superfamilies.** *Drug Metab Pharmacokinet* 2008, **23**:22-44.
69. Gill RK, Saksena S, Alrefai WA, Sarwar Z, Goldstein JL, Carroll RE, Ramaswamy K, Dudeja PK: **Expression and membrane localization of MCT isoforms along the length of the human intestine.** *Am J Physiol Cell Physiol* 2005, **289**:C846-C852.
70. Friesema EC, Docter R, Moerings EP, Stieger B, Hagenbuch B, Meier PJ, Krenning EP, Hennemann G, Visser TJ: **Identification of thyroid hormone transporters.** *Biochem Biophys Res Commun* 1999, **254**:497-501.
71. Glaeser H, Bailey DG, Dresser GK, Gregor JC, Schwarz UI, McGrath JS, Jolicoeur E, Lee W, Leake BF, Tirona RG, *et al*: **Intestinal drug transporter expression and the impact of grapefruit juice in humans.** *Clin Pharmacol Ther* 2007, **81**:362-370.
72. Fujiwara K, Adachi H, Nishio T, Unno M, Tokui T, Okabe M, Onogawa T, Suzuki T, Asano N, Tanemoto M, *et al*: **Identification of thyroid hormone transporters in humans: different molecules are involved in a tissue-specific manner.** *Endocrinology* 2001, **142**:2005-2012.
73. Cheng X, Maher J, Chen C, Klaassen CD: **Tissue distribution and ontogeny of mouse organic anion transporting polypeptides (Oatps).** *Drug Metab Dispos* 2005, **33**:1062-1073.
74. Rossier G, Meier C, Bauch C, Summa V, Sordat B, Verrey F, Kuhn LC: **LAT2, a new basolateral 4F2hc/CD98-associated amino acid transporter of kidney and intestine.** *J Biol Chem* 1999, **274**:34948-34954.
75. Umeki N, Fukasawa Y, Ohtsuki S, Hori S, Watanabe Y, Kohno Y, Terasaki T: **mRNA expression and amino acid transport characteristics of cultured human brain microvascular endothelial cells (hBME).** *Drug Metab Pharmacokinet* 2002, **17**:367-373.
76. Kanai Y, Segawa H, Miyamoto K, Uchino H, Takeda E, Endou H: **Expression cloning and characterization of a transporter for large neutral amino acids activated by the heavy chain of 4F2 antigen (CD98).** *J Biol Chem* 1998, **273**:23629-23632.
77. Yanagida O, Kanai Y, Chairoungdua A, Kim DK, Segawa H, Nii T, Cha SH, Matsuo H, Fukushima J, Fukasawa Y, *et al*: **Human L-type amino acid transporter 1 (LAT1): characterization of function and expression in tumor cell lines.** *Biochim Biophys Acta* 2001, **1514**:291-302.
78. Ohkame H, Masuda H, Ishii Y, Kanai Y: **Expression of L-type amino acid transporter 1 (LAT1) and 4F2 heavy chain (4F2hc) in liver tumor lesions of rat models.** *J Surg Oncol* 2001, **78**:265-271.
79. Pinho MJ, Serrao MP, Gomes P, Hopfer U, Jose PA, Soares-da-Silva P: **Over-expression of renal LAT1 and LAT2 and enhanced L-DOPA uptake in SHR immortalized renal proximal tubular cells.** *Kidney Int* 2004, **66**:216-226.
80. Kobayashi Y: **Localization of the System L Amino Acid Transporters LAT1 and LAT2 in Rat Gastrointestinal Tract.** *Journal of the Kyorin Medical Society* 2007, **38**:75-84.
81. Braun D, Kinne A, Brauer AU, Sapin R, Klein MO, Kohrle J, Wirth EK, Schweizer U: **Developmental and cell type-specific expression of thyroid hormone transporters in the mouse brain and in primary brain cells.** *Glia* 2011, **59**:463-471.
82. Bassi MT, Sperandeo MP, Incerti B, Bulfone A, Pepe A, Surace EM, Gattuso C, De Grandi A, Buoninconti A, Riboni M, *et al*: **SLC7A8, a gene mapping within the lysinuric protein intolerance critical region, encodes a new member of the glycoprotein-associated amino acid transporter family.** *Genomics* 1999, **62**:297-303.
83. Pineda M, Fernandez E, Torrents D, Estevez R, Lopez C, Camps M, Lloberas J, Zorzano A, Palacin M: **Identification of a membrane protein, LAT-2, that Co-expresses with 4F2 heavy chain, an L-type amino acid transport activity with broad specificity for small and large zwitterionic amino acids.** *J Biol Chem* 1999, **274**:19738-19744.
84. Sato H, Tamba M, Kuriyama-Matsumura K, Okuno S, Bannai S: **Molecular cloning and expression of human xCT, the light chain of amino acid transport system xc-.** *Antioxid Redox Signal* 2000, **2**:665-671.
85. Burdo J, Dargusch R, Schubert D: **Distribution of the cystine/glutamate antiporter system xc- in the brain, kidney, and duodenum.** *J Histochem Cytochem* 2006, **54**:549-557.
86. Friesema EC, Kuiper GG, Jansen J, Visser TJ, Kester MH: **Thyroid hormone transport by the human monocarboxylate transporter 8 and its rate-limiting role in intracellular metabolism.** *Mol Endocrinol* 2006, **20**:2761-2772.

# Permissions

All chapters in this book were first published in TR, by BioMed Central; hereby published with permission under the Creative Commons Attribution License or equivalent. Every chapter published in this book has been scrutinized by our experts. Their significance has been extensively debated. The topics covered herein carry significant findings which will fuel the growth of the discipline. They may even be implemented as practical applications or may be referred to as a beginning point for another development.

The contributors of this book come from diverse backgrounds, making this book a truly international effort. This book will bring forth new frontiers with its revolutionizing research information and detailed analysis of the nascent developments around the world.

We would like to thank all the contributing authors for lending their expertise to make the book truly unique. They have played a crucial role in the development of this book. Without their invaluable contributions this book wouldn't have been possible. They have made vital efforts to compile up to date information on the varied aspects of this subject to make this book a valuable addition to the collection of many professionals and students.

This book was conceptualized with the vision of imparting up-to-date information and advanced data in this field. To ensure the same, a matchless editorial board was set up. Every individual on the board went through rigorous rounds of assessment to prove their worth. After which they invested a large part of their time researching and compiling the most relevant data for our readers.

The editorial board has been involved in producing this book since its inception. They have spent rigorous hours researching and exploring the diverse topics which have resulted in the successful publishing of this book. They have passed on their knowledge of decades through this book. To expedite this challenging task, the publisher supported the team at every step. A small team of assistant editors was also appointed to further simplify the editing procedure and attain best results for the readers.

Apart from the editorial board, the designing team has also invested a significant amount of their time in understanding the subject and creating the most relevant covers. They scrutinized every image to scout for the most suitable representation of the subject and create an appropriate cover for the book.

The publishing team has been an ardent support to the editorial, designing and production team. Their endless efforts to recruit the best for this project, has resulted in the accomplishment of this book. They are a veteran in the field of academics and their pool of knowledge is as vast as their experience in printing. Their expertise and guidance has proved useful at every step. Their uncompromising quality standards have made this book an exceptional effort. Their encouragement from time to time has been an inspiration for everyone.

The publisher and the editorial board hope that this book will prove to be a valuable piece of knowledge for researchers, students, practitioners and scholars across the globe.

# List of Contributors

**Rafal Zenon Slapa and Wieslaw Stanislaw Jakubowski**
Department of Diagnostic Imaging, Second Faculty of Medicine with the English Division and the Physiotherapy Division, Medical University of Warsaw, ul. Kondratowicza 8, 03-242 Warsaw, Poland

**Kazimierz Tomasz Szopinski**
Department of Diagnostic Imaging, Second Faculty of Medicine with the English Division and the Physiotherapy Division, Medical University of Warsaw, ul. Kondratowicza 8, 03-242 Warsaw, Poland
Interdisciplinary Centre for Mathematical and Computational Modelling, Warsaw University, Warsaw, Poland

**Jadwiga Slowinska-Srzednicka**
Department of Endocrinology, Centre for Postgraduate Medical Education, Warsaw, Poland

**Artur Bossowski**
Department of Pediatrics, Endocrinology, Diabetology with the Cardiology Division, Medical University Bialystok 15-089. Poland

**Jerzy Harasymczuk**
Department of Pediatric Surgery, Traumatology and Urology. University of Medical Sciences, Poznań 60-967. Poland

**Anna Moniuszko**
Department of Infectious Diseases and Neuroinfections. Medical University. Białystok 15-089. Poland

**Anna Bossowska**
Division of Cardiology. Internal Affair and Administration Ministry Hospital. Białystok 15-089. Poland

**Maciej Hilczer**
Department of Endocrinology and Metabolic Diseases. Medical University. Łódź 93-338. Poland

**Karol Ratomski**
Dep. of Pediatric Laboratory Diagnostic. Medical University. Bialystok 15-089. Poland

**Joanna Smyczyńska, Renata Stawerska and Maciej Hilczer**
Department of Pediatric Endocrinology, Medical University of Lodz, Lodz, Poland
Department of Endocrinology and Metabolic Diseases, Polish Mother's Memorial Hospital - Research Institute in Lodz, Poland

**Andrzej Lewiński**
Department of Endocrinology and Metabolic Diseases, Medical University of Lodz, Lodz, Poland. Department of Endocrinology and Metabolic Diseases, Polish Mother's Memorial Hospital - Research Institute in Lodz, Poland

**Angela M Leung, Stephanie L Lee and Elizabeth N Pearce**
Section of Endocrinology, Diabetes, and Nutrition; Boston University School of Medicine; Boston, MA; USA
Endocrinology; Harvard Vanguard Medical Associates; Boston, MA; USA

**Shalini Dave**
Division of Graduate Medical Sciences; Boston University Medical Center; Boston, MA: USA

**Jeffrey R Garber**
Endocrinology; Harvard Vanguard Medical Associates; Boston, MA; USA
Division of Endocrinology, Diabetes, and Metabolism; Department of Medicine; Beth Israel Deaconess Medical Center; Boston, MA; USA

**Francis X Campion**
Internal Medicine; Harvard Vanguard Medical Associates; Boston, MA; USA

**Kristine Ducena**
Faculty of Medicine, University of Latvia, Raina Bulvaris 19, Riga, LV1586, Latvia

**Arturs Ābols**
Faculty of Medicine, University of Latvia, Raina Bulvaris 19, Riga, LV1586, Latvia
Department of Molecular Biology, Latvian Biomedical Research and Study Centre, Ratsupites 1, Riga, LV1067, Latvia

**Valdis Pīrāgs**
Faculty of Medicine, University of Latvia, Raina Bulvaris 19, Riga, LV1586, Latvia
Surgery Clinics, Pauls Stradins Clinical University Hospital, Pilsonu 13, Riga, LV1002, Latvia

**Diana Andrējeva and Aija Linē**
Department of Molecular Biology, Latvian Biomedical Research and Study Centre, Ratsupites 1, Riga, LV1067, Latvia

**Janis Vilmanis and Zenons Narbuts**
Surgery Clinics, Pauls Stradins Clinical University Hospital, Pilsonu 13, Riga, LV1002, Latvia

**Juris Tārs**
Oncology department, Riga Eastern Clinical University Hospital, Hipokrata 2, Riga, LV1038, Latvia

**Kinga Krawczyk-Rusiecka, Katarzyna Wojciechowska-Durczyńska, Anna Cyniak-Magierska, Zbigniew Adamczewski, Elżbieta Gałecka and Andrzej Lewiński**
Department of Endocrinology and Metabolic Diseases, Medical University of Lodz, Polish Mother's Memorial Hospital - Research Institute, Lodz, Poland

**Theodore T Zava and David T Zava**
ZRT Laboratory, 8605 SW Creekside Place, Beaverton, 97008, USA

**Tadao Yoshida Masaaki Teranishi and Tsutomu Nakashima**
Department of Otorhinolaryngology Nagoya University Graduate School of Medicine, 65 Tsurumai-cho, Showa-ku, Nagoya, Aichi 466-8550, Japan

**Tomoyuki Iwata**
Department of Otorhinolaryngology Nagoya University Graduate School of Medicine, 65 Tsurumai-cho, Showa-ku, Nagoya, Aichi 466-8550, Japan
Inazawa City Hospital, 1-1 Gokusho-cho, Inazawa, Aichi 492-8510, Japan

**Yoshiharu Murata, Yoshitaka Hayashi and Yasuhiko Kanou**
Department of genetics, Research Institute of Environmental Medicine, Nagoya University, Furo-cho, Chikusa-ku, Nagoya, Aichi 464-8601, Japan

**Andrew J Griffith**
National Institute on Deafness and Other Communications Disorders, National Institutes of Health, 5 Research Court, Rockville, MD 20850 USA

**Juliane Braun and Stefan Hüttelmaier**
Institute of Molecular Medicine, Section for Molecular Cell Biology, Martin Luther University of Halle-Wittenberg, ZAMED Heinrich-Damerow-Str.1, 06120 Halle, Germany

**Chaturaka Rodrigo, Champika SSSK Gamakaranage and Dhanesha S Epa**
University Medical Unit, National Hospital of Sri Lanka, Colombo, Sri Lanka

**Ariaranee Gnanathasan and Senaka Rajapakse**
Department of Clinical Medicine, Faculty of Medicine, University of Colombo, Sri Lanka

**Huy A Tran**
Hunter Area Pathology Service and University of Newcastle, Locked Bag Number 1, Hunter Mail Region Centre, Newcastle, New South Wales 2310, Australia

**Tracey L Jones**
Hepatitis C Service, Gastroenterology Department, John Hunter Hospital and University of Newcastle, Locked Bag Number 1, Hunter Mail Region Centre, Newcastle, New South Wales 2310, Australia

**Elizabeth A Ianna**
Hepatitis C Service, Gastroenterology Department, John Hunter Hospital, Locked Bag Number 1, Hunter Mail Region Centre, Newcastle, New South Wales 2310, Australia

**Glenn EM Reeves**
Hunter Area Pathology Service and University of Newcastle, Locked Bag Number 1, Hunter Mail Region Centre, Newcastle, New South Wales 2310, Australia

**Sofia Tedelind, Silvia Jordans, Henrike Resemann and Klaudia Brix**
School of Engineering and Science, Research Center for Molecular Life Science, Jacobs University Bremen, 28759 Bremen, Germany

**Galia Blum**
School of Pharmacy, Faculty of Medicine, The Hebrew University, 91120 Jerusalem, Israel

**Matthew Bogyo**
Departments of Pathology and Microbiology and Immunology, Stanford University School of Medicine, Stanford, California 94305-5324, USA

**Dagmar Führer**
Universitätsklinikum Leipzig Medizinische Klinik III, 04103 Leipzig, Germany; as of June 2011: Klinik für Endokrinologie, Zentrum für Innere Medizin, Bereich Forschung und Lehre im Zentrallabor, 45147 Essen, Germany

**Erika Osada, Naoki Hiroi, Mariko Sue, Natsumi Masai, Ryo Iga, Rika Shigemitsu, Reiko Oka, Masahiko Miyagi, Kaoru Iso, Koji Kuboki and Gen Yoshino**
Division of Diabetes, Metabolism and Endocrinology, Department of Internal Medicine (Omori), Toho University School of Medicine, Tokyo, Japan

**Andrzej Lewiński and Anna Cyniak-Magierska**
Department of Endocrinology and Metabolic Diseases, Medical University of Lodz, Poland

Department of Endocrinology and Metabolic Diseases, Polish Mother's Memorial Hospital - Research Institute, Lodz, Poland

**Joanna Latek**
Department of Endocrinology and Metabolic Diseases, Polish Mother's Memorial Hospital - Research Institute, Lodz, Poland

**Ewa Brzeziańska and Karolina Czarnecka**
Department of Molecular Basis of Medicine, Medical University of Lodz, Poland

**Włodzimierz Koptas**
Department of General and Colorectal Surgery, Medical University of Lodz, Poland

**Alexandra Chrisoulidou, Maria Boudina, Eleni Doumala, Pashalia K Iliadou and Kalliopi Pazaitou-Panayiotou**
Department of Endocrinology and Endocrine Oncology, Theagenio Cancer Hospital, Thessaloniki 54007, Greece

**Athanasios Tzemailas**
Department of Nuclear Medicine, Theagenio Cancer Hospital, Thessaloniki 54007, Greece

**Frideriki Patakiouta**
Department of Pathology, Theagenio Cancer Hospital, Thessaloniki, Greece

**Anna Cyniak-Magierska Katarzyna Wojciechowska-Durczyńska, Kinga Krawczyk-Rusiecka, Arkadiusz Zygmunt and Andrzej Lewiński**
Department of Endocrinology and Metabolic Diseases, Medical University of Lodz, Poland
Polish Mother's Memorial Hospital - Research Institute, Lodz, Poland

**Maximilian Pilhatsch, Michael Marxen, Christine Winter, Michael N Smolka and Michael Bauer**
Department of Psychiatry and Psychotherapy, University Hospital Carl Gustav Carus, Technische Universität Dresden, Dresden, Germany

**Chantal Daumerie and Dominique Maiter**
Department of Endocrinology, Université Catholique de Louvain, Cliniques Universitaires Saint-Luc, Avenue Hippocrate 10, 1200 Brussels, Belgium

**Damien Gruson**
Department of Biochemistry, Université Catholique de Louvain, Cliniques Universitaires Saint-Luc, Avenue Hippocrate 10, 1200 Brussels, Belgium

**Heike Biebermann, Franziska Winkler, Daniela Handke, Annette Grüters, Heiko Krude and Gunnar Kleinau**
Institute of Experimental Paediatric Endocrinology, Charité Universitätsmedizin Berlin, Augustenburger Platz 1, 13353 Berlin, Germany

**Katarzyna Wojciechowska-Durczyńska and Andrzej Lewiński**
Department of Endocrinology and Metabolic Diseases, Polish Mother's Memorial Hospital Research Institute, Medical University of Lodz, Rzgowska St. No. 281/289, 93-338 Lodz, Poland

**Adam Durczyński and Janusz Strzelczyk**
Department of General and Transplant Surgery, Medical University of Lodz, Barlicki University Hospital, Lodz, Poland

**Stanisław Sporny**
Department of Dental Pathology, Medical University of Lodz, The Clinical- Didactic Centre, Lodz, Poland

**Oliver Gimm**
Department of Clinical and Experimental Medicine, Faculty of Health Sciences, Linköping University, SE-58185 Linköping, Sweden
Department of Surgery, County Council of Östergötland, SE-58185 Linköping, Sweden

**Bogusz Trojanowicz, Henning Dralle and Cuong Hoang-Vu**
Universitätsklinik und Poliklinik für Allgemein-, Viszeral- und Gefäßchirurgie, Martin-Luther Universität, Halle

**Johannes Smit**
Department of General Internal Medicine, Radboud University Nijmegen

**Rossella Elisei and Cristina Romei**
Department of Endocrinology and Metabolism, University of Pisa, Lungarno Pacinotti 43 - 56126 Pisa, Italy

**Laura Fugazzola, Simone De Leo and Michela Perrino**
Department of Clinical Sciences and Community Health, University of Milan; Endocrine Unit, Fondazione IRCCS Ca' Granda, Via F. Sforza, 35, 20122 Milan, Italy

**Klaudia Brix**
School of Engineering and Science, Jacobs University Bremen, Research II, Campus Ring 6, 28759 Bremen, Germany

**Dagmar Führer**
Universitätsklinikum Leipzig Medizinische Klinik III, 04103 Leipzig, Germany; as of June 2011: Klinik für Endokrinologie, Zentrum für Innere Medizin, Bereich Forschung und Lehre im Zentrallabor, 45147 Essen, Germany

**Heike Biebermann**
Institute of Experimental Pediatric Endocrinology, Charité Universitätsmedizin Berlin, Augustenburger Platz 1, 13353 Berlin, Germany

**Gunnar Kleinau, Annette Grüters, Heiko Krude and Heike Biebermann**
Institut für Experimentelle Pädiatrische Endokrinologie, Charité- Universitätsmedizin Berlin, Germany

**Ulrich Schweizer and Josef Köhrle**
Institut für Experimentelle Endokrinologie, Charité-Universitätsmedizin Berlin, Germany

**Anita Kinne**
Leibniz-Institut für Molekulare Pharmakologie, Berlin, Germany

**Barbara Jarząb, Aleksandra Król, Kornelia Hasse-Lazar and Beata Jurecka-Lubieniecka**
Department of Nuclear Medicine and Endocrine Oncology, Maria Sklodowska-Curie Memorial Cancer Center and Institute of Oncology, Gliwice Branch, Wybrzeze Armii Krajowej 15, 44-101 Gliwice, Poland

**Satoru Suzuki, Shin-ichi Nishio, Teiji Takeda and Mitsuhisa Komatsu**
Department of Aging Medicine and Geriatrics, Institute on Aging and Adaptation, Shinshu University, Graduate School of Medicine, 3-1-1, Asahi, Matsumoto, 390-8621, Japan

**Anita Kinne, Ralf Schülein and Gerd Krause**
Leibniz-Institut für Molekulare Pharmakologie (FMP), Robert-Roessle-Str. 10, 13125 Berlin, Germany

# Index